CE

of

Medicinal Drugs

SEE WEB LINKS

This is a web-linked dictionary. There is a list of recommended web links in Appendix 5 on page 658. To access the websites, go to the dictionary's web page at www.oup.com/uk/reference/resources/medicinaldrugs, click on **Web links** in the Resources section, then click straight through to the relevant websites.

An A–Z of

Medicinal Drugs

SECOND EDITION

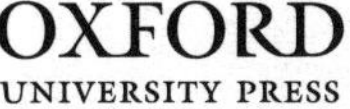

OXFORD
UNIVERSITY PRESS

Great Clarendon Street, Oxford OX2 6DP

Oxford University Press is a department of the University of Oxford.
It furthers the University's objective of excellence in research, scholarship, and education by publishing worldwide in

Oxford New York
Auckland Cape Town Dar es Salaam Hong Kong Karachi
Kuala Lumpur Madrid Melbourne Mexico City Nairobi
New Delhi Shanghai Taipei Toronto

With offices in
Argentina Austria Brazil Chile Czech Republic France Greece
Guatemala Hungary Italy Japan Poland Portugal Singapore
South Korea Switzerland Thailand Turkey Ukraine Vietnam

Oxford is a registered trade mark of Oxford University Press in the UK and in certain other countries

Published in the United States
by Oxford University Press Inc., New York

First edition 2000 (under the title *A Dictionary of Medicines*)
Reissued as *An A–Z of Medicinal Drugs* 2003
Second edition 2010

British Library Cataloguing in Publication Data
Data available

Library of Congress Cataloging in Publication Data
Data available

Typeset by Market House Books Ltd.
Printed in Great Britain by
Clays Ltd, St Ives plc

ISBN 978–0–19–955848–3

10 9 8 7 6 5 4 3 2 1

Contents

Preface

The second edition of *An A–Z of Medicinal Drugs* has been prepared by Market House Books Ltd for Oxford University Press as a companion volume to their highly regarded *Concise Medical Dictionary* (now in its eighth edition). It includes information about both 'prescription only' medicines, which cannot be obtained without a doctor's prescription, and non-prescription medicines, which can be bought from pharmacies and in some cases are available from supermarkets or other stores. For this new edition, all entries have been thoroughly reviewed, discontinued products have been deleted, and over 1000 new preparations have been added. In addition, appendices of online resources and abbreviations have been included. The book is intended primarily as an information source for non-specialists – especially to satisfy the demand from patients and their families for further details of the medicines they are taking. However, like its companion volume, this dictionary should also be of value to nurses, paramedical workers, medical secretaries, and other health-care professionals.

The entries in this book are arranged in a single alphabetical list, making it easier to use than some similar books (which are divided into separate sections).

The alphabetical list consists of three main types of entry:

- medicines, including groups and classes (e.g. **antibiotics**, **ACE inhibitors**), generic names (e.g. **trimethoprim**, **ramipril**), and proprietary names (e.g. **Monomil XL**, **Remicade**);
- conditions that are treated by medicines (e.g. **diabetes mellitus**, **hypertension**), with references to the medicines or classes of medicine used in their treatment;
- terms used in the prescription, supply, and administration of medicines (e.g. **licence**, **modified-release preparation**).

Entries for each medicine include (where relevant) details of some of the possible side effects that could occur in those taking it as well as potential interactions with other medicines, which could be a reason for not taking that medicine with the interacting drug or may require the dosage of the medicine or the interacting drug to be adjusted. There is often also a section on precautions, which may mention some of the conditions (including pregnancy) requiring a medicine to be used 'with caution' or not at all. This means that a person should always tell their doctor, pharmacist, or nurse prescriber if they have any of these conditions before taking that medicine.

Some terms within entries are printed in boldface type; examples are **antiretrovial drugs** in the entry for **antiviral drugs** and **Logynon ED** in the entry **Logynon**. This indicates that such terms are defined in these entries, rather than in their own entries.

An asterisk against a word used in an entry indicates that this term has its own entry in the dictionary, where additional information can be found. Some entries simply refer the reader to another entry in the dictionary (printed in SMALL CAPITAL LETTERS), indicating:

(1) that they are synonyms or abbreviations;

(2) that they are most conveniently explained in one of the dictionary's longer articles; or

(3) that they are proprietary preparations consisting of a single active ingredient.

The generic names of medicines used in Britain have recently been standardized to accord with the Recommended International Non-proprietary Names (rINNs) required by European law. In many cases these new British Approved Names (BANs) are the same as the former BANs. In cases where they differ, the former BAN is given inside angled brackets after the entry word of the medicine; an example is **lidocaine**

<**lignocaine**>. Where the former and new BANs differ considerably, the former name will be an entry in the dictionary referring the reader to the new name, for example:

amethocaine *See* TETRACAINE.

The names of medicines that are registered trade marks have been indicated in the text by the use of an initial capital letter and the inclusion after the relevant headword of the name of the manufacturer, for example:

Lacri-Lube (Allergan)
Lactugal (Intrapharm Laboratories)
Lamictal (GlaxoSmithKline)

While every effort has been made to ensure that the information in the dictionary is accurate, it is never possible to guarantee complete accuracy. We would therefore be grateful if readers would notify us of any errors they find. Readers should under no circumstances use the book to change the dosage of prescribed medicines. A doctor's advice must be followed in relation to the taking of all prescribed medicines.

E.M.
2010

Credits

Consultant Editor

Albert Ferro BSc(Hons), MB, BS, PhD

Contributors

Christopher N. Floyd MA, MBBS
Shalini Solanki BSc(Hons), MBBS
Padman Vamadevan MA, MBBS
Steven Williams BMedSci, MB, ChB(Hons)

Editor

Elizabeth Martin MA

Production editor

Anne Stibbs BA

Keyboarding

Amanda Garner-Hay

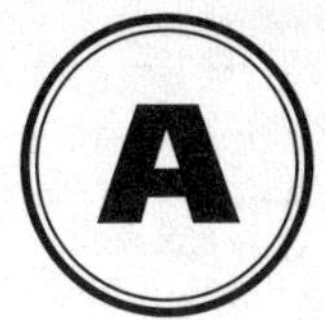

AAA Mouth and Throat Spray (Manx) *See* BENZOCAINE.

abacavir An antiretroviral drug (*see* ANTIVIRAL DRUGS) that prevents retrovirus replication: it is a nucleoside analogue that inhibits the action of reverse transcriptase. Abacavir is used, in combination with other antiretroviral drugs, to treat *HIV infection. It is available as tablets or an oral solution on *prescription only.
Side effects: include allergic reactions (e.g. rash, fever, sore throat, breathlessness, cough; see Precautions below), fatigue, abdominal pain, vomiting, liver damage, headache, dizziness, and blood disorders.
Precautions: abacavir should be used with caution in people with chronic hepatitis B or C or impaired liver or kidney function, and in people at high risk of cardiovascular diseases. It should not be taken by women who are breastfeeding. There is a risk of allergic reactions in some people taking abacavir; treatment should be stopped if symptoms develop.
Interactions with other drugs:
Tipranavir: reduces the plasma concentration of abacavir, and the two drugs are best not taken together.
Proprietary preparations: Ziagen; *Kivexa (combined with lamivudine); *Trizivir (combined with lamivudine and zidovudine).

abatacept A *disease-modifying antirheumatic drug (DMARD) used, in combination with *methotrexate, to treat moderate to severe rheumatoid arthritis that has not responded to other DMARDs. It works by preventing the activation of T lymphocytes (a type of white blood cell), which are involved in the immune response. Abatacept is given under expert supervision by intravenous infusion and is available on *prescription only.
Side effects: include headache, hypertension, dizziness, cough, abdominal pain, nausea, chest infections, and urinary-tract infections.
Precautions: abatacept should not be given to people with severe infections or to women who are pregnant or breastfeeding.
Interactions with other drugs:
Anti-TNF drugs: should not be given with abatacept as they increase the risk of side effects.
Vaccines: should not be given to people receiving abatacept.
Proprietary preparation: Orencia.

abciximab A *monoclonal antibody that has *antiplatelet activity and is used in patients undergoing balloon angioplasty and other forms of heart surgery. It may also be used in the treatment of patients with unstable *angina. Abciximab is used only under specialist supervision, with careful

monitoring of blood clotting; it is available as a solution for intravenous injection or infusion on *prescription only.
Side effects: include excessive bleeding, high blood pressure, nausea, vomiting, blood disorders, and a fast heart rate.
Precautions: abciximab should not be used in people who have had a stroke within the previous two years or recent major surgery, or who have other risk factors for spontaneous bleeding, or by women who are pregnant or breastfeeding. It is also not recommended for patients with certain blood platelet disorders or severe kidney or liver disease.
Proprietary preparation: ReoPro.

Abelcet (Cephalon) *See* AMPHOTERICIN.

Abidec Multivitamin Drops (Chefaro UK) A proprietary combination of *vitamin A, vitamins of the B group (*see* VITAMIN B COMPLEX), *vitamin C, and *vitamin D, used as a multivitamin supplement. It is freely available *over the counter in the form of drops.

Abilify (Bristol-Myers Squibb) *See* ARIPIPRAZOLE.

Abraxane (Abraxis BioScience) *See* PACLITAXEL.

Abstral (ProStrakan) *See* FENTANYL.

acamprosate calcium A drug that is used in the treatment of alcohol dependence, for helping people who have achieved a state of abstinence to refrain from drinking again. It should be started as soon as possible after abstinence has been achieved and is usually taken for a period of one year (this is variable), even if the patient has occasional relapses. Acamprosate is available as tablets on *prescription only.
Side effects: include diarrhoea, nausea, vomiting, abdominal pain, and occasionally rash; there may be fluctuations in libido.
Precautions: acamprosate should not be taken by people with severe liver or kidney impairment or by women who are pregnant or breastfeeding.
Proprietary preparation: Campral EC.

acarbose An *oral hypoglycaemic drug that acts by temporarily inhibiting digestive enzymes in the intestine that break down starch and sucrose into glucose: it therefore delays the absorption of glucose and reduces the high blood-glucose concentrations that occur after a meal. Acarbose is used as an *adjunct to *metformin or *sulphonylureas when these have failed to control blood-glucose concentrations in people with noninsulin-dependent (type II) *diabetes mellitus. It is available as tablets on *prescription only.
Side effects: include flatulence, diarrhoea, and abdominal distension and pain; rarely, liver damage may occur.
Precautions: acarbose should be not be taken by people with impaired liver or severely impaired kidney function, inflammatory bowel disease, or a history of bowel surgery or by women who are pregnant or breastfeeding. It may increase the hypoglycaemic effects of *insulin and sulphonylureas.
Interactions with other drugs:

Neomycin: increases the hypoglycaemic effect of acarbose and the severity of gastrointestinal side effects.

Pancreatin: reduces the effect of acarbose.

Proprietary preparation: Glucobay.

Accolate (AstraZeneca) *See* ZAFIRLUKAST.

Accupro (Pfizer) *See* QUINAPRIL.

Accuretic (Pfizer) A proprietary combination of *quinapril (an ACE inhibitor) and *hydrochlorothiazide (a thiazide diuretic), used in the treatment of *hypertension. It is available as tablets on *prescription only.

Side effects, precautions, and interactions with other drugs: *see* ACE INHIBITORS; THIAZIDE DIURETICS.

See also ANTIHYPERTENSIVE DRUGS; DIURETICS.

Acea (Ferndale) *See* METRONIDAZOLE.

acebutolol A cardioselective *beta blocker used for the treatment and prevention of heart *arrhythmias and the treatment of *angina. It is also used in the treatment of *hypertension. It is available as tablets or capsules on *prescription only.

Side effects, precautions, and interactions with other drugs: *see* BETA BLOCKERS.

Proprietary preparation: Sectral.

See also ANTI-ARRHYTHMIC DRUGS; ANTIHYPERTENSIVE DRUGS.

aceclofenac An *NSAID used for the treatment of pain and inflammation in rheumatoid arthritis, osteoarthritis, and ankylosing spondylitis (a type of arthritis affecting the spine). It is available as tablets on *prescription only.

Side effects, precautions, and interactions with other drugs: *see* NSAIDs.

Proprietary preparation: Preservex.

ACE inhibitors (angiotensin-converting-enzyme inhibitors) A class of drugs that dilate the arteries (*see* VASODILATORS). They act by suppressing the action of an enzyme that converts an inactive chemical, angiotensin, into angiotensin II, a substance in the bloodstream and tissues that normally narrows the arteries. ACE inhibitors are used for treating *hypertension (high blood pressure); the addition of a *thiazide diuretic can enhance the blood-pressure-lowering effects in those who are not well controlled. ACE inhibitors are also used in the treatment of *heart failure as they reduce the workload of the heart. In addition to reducing the blood pressure they also reduce blood volume by improving the blood supply to the kidneys and increasing the excretion of salt in urine. This latter effect reduces excess body fluids and prevents further accumulation of fluid. *See* CAPTOPRIL; CILAZAPRIL; ENALAPRIL MALEATE; FOSINOPRIL; IMIDAPRIL HYDROCHLORIDE; LISINOPRIL; MOEXIPRIL HYDROCHLORIDE; PERINDOPRIL; QUINAPRIL; RAMIPRIL; TRANDOLAPRIL.

Side effects: ACE inhibitors can cause the blood pressure to fall too rapidly, especially when they are first used and when diuretics are also being taken; the first dose is therefore usually taken when the patient is in bed and often

under medical supervision. Other possible side effects include headache, skin rash, dry cough (which is treatable by *sodium cromoglicate) and, less commonly, nausea, muscle cramps, sore throat, and (especially in the elderly and those with kidney disease) impaired kidney function; tests for kidney function should be carried out regularly in the early stages of treatment. There may also be jaundice and other symptoms of liver disease, in which case treatment should be stopped.
Precautions: ACE inhibitors should not be taken by pregnant women or by people with angioedema (a severe allergic reaction that involves swelling of the face, lips, and throat). People taking ACE inhibitors should generally not take *potassium supplements or potassium-sparing diuretics.
Interactions with other drugs:

Anaesthetics: their effects in lowering blood pressure are increased.
Ciclosporin: increases the risk of high concentrations of potassium in the blood.
Diuretics: their effects in lowering blood pressure are increased; potassium-sparing diuretics can increase concentrations of potassium in the blood and cause toxic effects.
Lithium: levels of lithium in the blood may be increased and cause toxic effects.
NSAIDs: increase the risk of kidney damage and reduce the effect of ACE inhibitors.

acemetacin An *NSAID that is a derivative of *indometacin. It is used for the treatment of pain and inflammation in rheumatoid arthritis and other disorders of the joints and muscles and for the relief of pain after an operation. Acemetacin is available as capsules on *prescription only.
Side effects and precautions: *see* INDOMETACIN; NSAIDs.
Interactions with other drugs: *see* NSAIDs.
Proprietary preparation: Emflex.

acenocoumarol <**nicoumalone**> An oral *anticoagulant used for the prevention and treatment of deep-vein *thrombosis and pulmonary embolism and for the prevention of embolism in people with atrial fibrillation (*see* ARRHYTHMIA) and in those who have received an artificial heart valve. It is available as tablets on *prescription only.
Side effects, precautions, and interactions with other drugs: *see* WARFARIN SODIUM.
Proprietary preparation: Sinthrome.

Acepril (Ashbourne Pharmaceuticals) *See* CAPTOPRIL.

acetazolamide A *carbonic anhydrase inhibitor that is used for the treatment of *glaucoma: it reduces pressure inside the eye by reducing the formation of aqueous fluid in the eye. It may be used in the treatment of epilepsy (though rarely) and to prevent mountain sickness (although it does not have a *licence for this use). Acetazolamide produces a moderate loss of fluid as urine but is now little used as a *diuretic. It is available, on

*prescription only, as tablets, *modified-release capsules, or a form for intravenous injection.
Side effects: the main side effect is *potassium loss, which can result in 'pins and needles', weakness, lethargy, and cramps; nausea, vomiting, flushing, headache, and thirst are among the other side effects. Less commonly drowsiness, rashes, and blood disorders have been reported.
Precautions: acetazolamide is not usually recommended for long-term treatment. It should not be taken by people with low blood concentrations of potassium or sodium, severe liver disease, or kidney disease. It should be used with caution in people with lung diseases, such as asthma or emphysema. Anyone taking acetazolamide should report unusual rashes to their doctor.
Interactions with other drugs:

Amiodarone: its adverse effects on the heart are increased due to potassium depletion by acetazolamide.

Antiepileptic drugs: there is an increased risk of potassium loss if carbamazepine is taken with acetazolamide, and acetazolamide increases the plasma concentration of carbamazepine; the risk of osteomalacia may be increased if phenytoin or primidone are taken with acetazolamide.

Digoxin and digitoxin: their adverse effects are increased due to potassium depletion by acetazolamide.

Lithium: its excretion is increased (and therefore its effects may be reduced) by acetazolamide.

Proprietary preparations: Diamox; Diamox SR (modified-release capsules).

acetic acid An organic acid that has weak antimicrobial and antifungal activity. It is used in vaginal gels and douches to treat nonspecific vaginal infections by restoring the normal acidity of the vagina. Acetic acid is an ingredient of solutions and paints for application to the skin or nails and of ear drops to treat infections caused by bacteria, fungi, or protozoa. It is also used as a spermicide, an astringent lotion, and as a treatment for warts and calluses. Weak solutions are used to treat coughs in babies. A solution of 4% acetic acid is also known as **artificial vinegar**. Acetic acid is available without a prescription.
Proprietary preparations: Baby Meltus (cough linctus); Earcalm Spray (ear spray); *Goddard's Muscle Lotion (combined with turpentine oil and dilute ammonia solution); *Otomize (combined with dexamethasone and neomycin sulphate); *Phytex (combined with antifungal drugs).

acetylcholine A substance that conveys messages from nerve cells (i.e. it is a neurotransmitter) in the *parasympathetic nervous system. It acts on very small specialized areas of cells of the target tissues called receptors, of which there are two main types: **muscarinic** receptors, found, for example, in smooth muscle (e.g. of the gut and bladder), heart muscle, and endocrine glands; and **nicotinic** receptors, in (for example) skeletal muscle. Drugs whose action resembles that of acetylcholine are called *cholinergic drugs and include *anticholinesterases (or cholinesterase inhibitors). Drugs that prevent the action of acetylcholine include *antimuscarinic (or anticholinergic) drugs and *muscle relaxants used in general anaesthesia.

acetylcholine chloride A salt of *acetylcholine that is used to keep the pupil of the eye dilated during eye surgery. It is available, on *prescription only, as a solution for bathing the eye.
Proprietary preparation: Miochol-E.

acetylcholinesterase inhibitors A class of drugs that inhibit the action of acetylcholinesterase, an enzyme that breaks down the neurotransmitter *acetylcholine. They therefore increase the amount of acetylcholine that is available for the transmission of nerve impulses. The acetylcholinesterase inhibitors *donepezil hydrochloride, *galantamine, and *rivastigmine exert their effects in the brain. They are used in the treatment of Alzheimer's disease, which is associated with a loss in the activity of acetylcholine-secreting nerve cells in the brain.

acetylcysteine A *mucolytic drug that breaks down the mucus that accumulates as filaments in the eye and causes dry eyes. It is also given intravenously as the antidote to *paracetamol overdosage. Acetylcysteine is available, on *prescription only, as eye drops or a solution for intravenous infusion.
Side effects: intravenous infusion of acetylcysteine may cause rashes or allergic reactions.
Precautions: eye drops should not be used with soft contact lenses; intravenous infusions of acetylcysteine should be used with caution in people with asthma.
Proprietary preparations: Parvolex (injection); *Ilube (combined with hypromellose).

acetylsalicylic acid *See* ASPIRIN.

aciclovir (**acyclovir**) An *antiviral drug that is used specifically to treat herpesvirus infections, including chickenpox, shingles, cold sores, genital herpes, and herpes infections of the eyes or mouth. It works by inhibiting DNA polymerase, the enzyme within human cells that is used by the virus to make viral DNA, which is necessary if the virus is to replicate. Although it may not completely eradicate the virus, aciclovir is more effective if started early after the onset of infection and can be life-saving in patients whose immune systems are compromised. It is also used to prevent infection or recurrence of previous infection in immunocompromised patients. Aciclovir is available, on *prescription only, as dispersible tablets and a suspension for oral use, a solution for intravenous infusion, and as an eye ointment; creams for topical application are available without a prescription, but only from pharmacies.
Side effects: include rashes, nausea and vomiting, headache, dizziness, and fatigue; intravenous infusions may cause local inflammation and (rarely) confusion, hallucinations, and agitation. Local burning, stinging, irritation, or inflammation can occur with topical application; the cream may cause flaking of the skin.

Precautions: people taking aciclovir orally or as an infusion must maintain an adequate intake of fluids. The drug should be used with caution in those with impaired kidney function and in women who are pregnant or breastfeeding. The cream should not be used in the eyes or on mucous membranes (for example in the mouth or vagina) as it may be irritant.

Interactions with other drugs:

Ciclosporin: increases the risk of kidney damage.

Mycophenolate mofetil: the plasma concentrations of both drugs may be increased.

Probenecid: increases the plasma concentration of aciclovir.

Proprietary preparations: Boots Avert (cream); Virovir (tablets); Zovirax; Zovirax Cold Sore Cream.

acid-peptic diseases Conditions associated with the action of gastric (stomach) acid on the lining of the oesophagus (gullet), stomach, or upper sections of the small intestine causing **dyspepsia** (indigestion), marked by pain (**heartburn**) or discomfort. The normal stomach secretes hydrochloric acid as part of the digestive process; however, if the acid enters the lower part of the oesophagus (**gastro-oesophageal reflux**), it can cause pain or actual tissue damage, giving rise to **reflux oesophagitis** (inflammation of the oesophagus). Reflux oesophagitis is more common in people with a **hiatus hernia** (a condition in which a part of the stomach has been pushed upwards through the diaphragm). Pregnant women may suffer reflux and heartburn in the later stages of pregnancy due to the pressure of the fetus on the stomach. **Peptic ulcers**, which most commonly affect the stomach, the lower part of the oesophagus, or the duodenum, may occur when gastric acid is present in abnormally high concentrations but more usually result from other conditions that make the lining of the digestive tract more susceptible to attack by acid. These include the presence of the bacterium *Helicobacter pylori* and the use of *NSAIDs and certain other drugs (e.g. corticosteroids). Ulcers may also be caused or exacerbated by stress, smoking, and alcohol. A rare cause of peptic ulceration is the **Zollinger-Ellison syndrome**, a disorder in which excessive secretion of gastric acid is triggered by the hormone gastrin released by a pancreatic tumour.

Drug treatments for acid-peptic diseases include *antacids, *proton pump inhibitors, and *H_2-receptor antagonists; less commonly *cytoprotectant agents or *antimuscarinic drugs are used. *Helicobacter pylori* is eradicated by a combination of two of the following antibiotics – *clarithromycin, *amoxicillin, *metronidazole – and a proton pump inhibitor.

acipimox A *lipid-lowering drug that is a *nicotinic acid derivative. It lowers both *triglycerides and *cholesterol and is therefore used in the treatment of a variety of *hyperlipidaemias. It acts by inhibiting the breakdown of fats in fatty tissue, thereby typically causing a 20% fall in plasma LDL-cholesterol (*see* LIPOPROTEINS). It is available as capsules on *prescription only.

Side effects: vasodilatation, flushing, itching, and rashes may occur.

Occasional side effects are heartburn, pain in the stomach region, nausea, headache, and diarrhoea.

Precautions: acipimox should not be taken by people with severely impaired kidney function or peptic ulcer or by women who are pregnant or breastfeeding because of a lack of data on its safety.

Proprietary preparation: Olbetam.

acitretin A *retinoid that is used for the treatment of severe extensive *psoriasis that is resistant to other treatments and of severe ichthyosis (abnormal scaling of the skin). It is available as capsules on *prescription only, and treatment must be under hospital supervision.

Side effects: include dryness and thinning of the mucous membranes (for example in the mouth), dryness, redness, and itching of the skin, and dryness of the eyes (which can affect the wearing of contact lenses). Other side effects that may occur include hair loss, muscle or joint aches, nausea, headache, drowsiness, and sweating.

Precautions: acitretin should not be taken by women who are pregnant or breastfeeding, and contraception must be used for one month before and during treatment and for at least two years after stopping treatment (*see* RETINOIDS). It should not be taken by people with impaired liver or kidney function or *hyperlipidaemia and is not recommended for children. Patients should avoid exposure to ultraviolet light (including excessive sunlight). Tests to monitor liver function, blood sugar, and blood fats should be performed before and during treatment. Donation of blood should be avoided during treatment and for at least a year after stopping treatment.

Interactions with other drugs:

Keratolytics: should not be used with acitretin.

Methotrexate: its plasma concentration (and therefore side effects) and the risk of liver damage are increased by acitretin, and the two drugs should not be used together.

Tetracyclines: there is an increased risk of raised pressure in the brain, and these antibiotics should not be used with acitretin.

Vitamin A: the risk of vitamin A poisoning is increased if supplements are taken with acitretin.

Warfarin: its anticoagulant effect may be reduced by acitretin.

Proprietary preparation: Neotigason.

Aclasta (Novartis) *See* ZOLEDRONIC ACID.

Acnamino MR (Dexcel Pharma) *See* MINOCYCLINE.

acne (**acne vulgaris**) A common inflammatory disorder of the sebaceous glands. These grease-producing glands in the skin are under *androgen control, but the cause of acne is unknown. It involves the face, back, and chest and is characterized by the presence of blackheads with papules, pustules, and – in more severe cases – cysts and scars. Mild to moderate acne usually responds to topical therapy with *benzoyl peroxide, *azelaic acid, antibiotics (such as *clindamycin or *erythromycin), or *retinoids; other topical treatments include *nicotinamide. More refractory conditions require treatment with long-term oral antibiotics (such as *oxytetracycline or *tetracycline hydrochloride) or (for treating women only) *Dianette (cyproterone and ethinylestradiol). Severe acne may need treatment with oral *isotretinoin (a retinoid).

Acnecide (Galderma) *See* BENZOYL PEROXIDE.

Acnisal (Alliance) *See* SALICYLIC ACID.

Acnocin (Sandoz) A proprietary combination of *ethinylestradiol (a synthetic oestrogen) and *cyproterone acetate (an anti-androgen), used for the treatment of severe *acne in women that has not responded to prolonged antibiotic therapy. It is also used to treat hirsutism (abnormal growth of facial and body hair in women). Acnocin acts as an *oral contraceptive in women taking it. It is available as tablets on *prescription only.
Side effects: include breast enlargement, fluid retention with a bloated feeling, weight gain, headache, nausea, vomiting, depression, changes in libido, and breakthrough bleeding. The occurrence of a migraine-like headache for the first time, frequent severe headaches, or visual disturbance should be reported immediately to a doctor.
Precautions: Acnocin should not be taken by women who are pregnant or breastfeeding or have a history of thrombosis. For other precautions, *see* ORAL CONTRACEPTIVES.
Interactions with other drugs: *see* ORAL CONTRACEPTIVES.

Acriflex Cream (Thornton & Ross) *See* CHLORHEXIDINE.

acrivastine One of the newer (non-sedating) *antihistamines, used to relieve the symptoms of such allergic conditions as hay fever and urticaria. It is available as capsules on *prescription, and packs containing no more than 10 days' supply can be obtained from pharmacies without a prescription.
Side effects, precautions, and interactions with other drugs: *see* ANTIHISTAMINES.
Proprietary preparations: Benadryl Allergy Relief; *Benadryl Plus Capsules (combined with pseudoephedrine hydrochloride).

Actidose-Aqua Advance (Cambridge Laboratories) *See* ACTIVATED CHARCOAL.

Actifed products (McNeil Ltd) *See* MULTI-ACTION ACTIFED products.

Actilyse (Boehringer Ingelheim) *See* ALTEPLASE.

actinomycin D *See* DACTINOMYCIN.

Actiq (Cephalon) *See* FENTANYL.

activated charcoal An agent that can adsorb (bind) many poisons in the stomach and therefore prevent them from being absorbed. It is used after swallowing poisons or taking an overdose of drugs and should be taken as soon as possible after the poisoning has occurred, although it may still be

effective up to two hours after the poison has been consumed. Activated charcoal is also included in dressings to absorb the odour of infected wounds. Charcoal itself reduces flatulence and abdominal distension and is included as an ingredient in some preparations for the treatment of indigestion. Activated charcoal is available as a powder, effervescent granules, or a suspension and can be obtained without a prescription, but only from pharmacies.
Proprietary preparations: Actidose-Aqua Advance (suspension); Carbomix (powder); Charcodote (suspension); *Carbellon (combined with magnesium hydroxide and peppermint oil).

Actonel Combi (Procter & Gamble) A proprietary preparation of the bisphosphonate *risedronate sodium (tablets) packaged with *calcium carbonate and *colecalciferol (vitamin D_3) (granules in a sachet to be dissolved in water). It is used to prevent spine and hip fractures in postmenopausal women with osteoporosis and is taken once a week. Actonel Combi is available on *prescription only.
Side effects, precautions, and interactions with other drugs: *see* RISEDRONATE SODIUM; CALCIUM; VITAMIN D.

Actonorm Powder (Wallace) A proprietary combination of *atropine sulphate and *peppermint oil (antispasmodics), and *aluminium hydroxide, *calcium carbonate, *magnesium trisilicate, *magnesium carbonate, and *sodium bicarbonate (all antacids), used for the treatment of indigestion (except that caused by ulcers) and flatulence. It is available from pharmacies without a prescription and cannot be prescribed on the NHS.
Side effects and precautions: *see* ATROPINE SULPHATE; MAGNESIUM SALTS; ANTACIDS.
Interactions with other drugs: *see* ATROPINE SULPHATE; ANTACIDS.

Actos (Takeda) *See* PIOGLITAZONE.

Actrapid (Novo Nordisk) *See* INSULIN.

Acular (Allergan) *See* KETOROLAC TROMETAMOL.

Acupan (Meda Pharmaceuticals) *See* NEFOPAM.

acyclovir *See* ACICLOVIR.

Adalat (Bayer) *See* NIFEDIPINE.

adalimumab A *monoclonal antibody that is a *disease-modifying antirheumatic drug (DMARD): it is used to reduce the inflammatory reactions associated with certain autoimmune conditions, including rheumatoid arthritis, psoriatic arthritis, ankylosing spondylitis (a type of arthritis of the spine), Crohn's disease, juvenile arthritis, and psoriasis. It should be used under specialist supervision and is available in liquid form for subcutaneous injection on *prescription only.
Side effects: include airways and other infections, sinusitis, blood disorders,

headache, abdominal pain, nausea and vomiting, altered liver function, rash, and pain in the muscles and joints.
Precautions: adalimumab should not be given to people with moderate or severe heart failure or severe infection or to pregnant or breastfeeding women. It should be used with caution in people with tuberculosis.
Interactions with other drugs:
Anakinra: should not be taken with adalimumab.
Vaccines: should not be given to people who are taking adalimumab.
Proprietary preparation: Humira.

adapalene A drug that resembles the *retinoids and is used for the treatment of mild to moderate acne in which blackheads and pustules predominate. It is available as a cream or gel on *prescription only.
Side effects: adapalene may irritate the skin. If irritation is severe, treatment should be stopped.
Precautions: adapalene should not be used on broken or sunburnt skin, by people with eczema or a personal or family history of skin cancer, or by pregnant women (effective contraception should be used during treatment). It should not be applied near the eyes, lips, nostrils, or mouth, and excessive exposure of treated skin to sunlight should be avoided. Adapalene should not be used with retinoids or *keratolytics.
Proprietary preparation: Differin.

Adartrel (GlaxoSmithKline) *See* ROPINIROLE.

Adcal (ProStraken) *See* CALCIUM CARBONATE.

Adcal-D$_3$ (ProStrakan) A proprietary combination of *calcium carbonate and *colecalciferol (vitamin D$_3$), used as an *adjunct in the treatment of osteoporosis and for the prevention and treatment of vitamin D deficiency, especially in housebound and institutionalized elderly people. It is available as chewable and effervescent tablets without a prescription, but only from pharmacies.
Side effects: include constipation, flatulence, nausea, vomiting, and diarrhoea.
Precautions: Adcal-D$_3$ should be used with caution in people with kidney disease or a history of kidney stones. Adcal-D$_3$ should not be taken by people with hypercalcaemia (high blood calcium levels) due to, for example, cancer.
Interactions with other drugs: Adcal-D$_3$ can reduce the absorption, and therefore efficacy, of thyroxine, bisphosphonates, iron, and quinolone and tetracycline antibiotics.
Antiepileptic drugs: phenytoin and barbiturates decrease the effect of vitamin D in Adcal-D$_3$.
Thiazide diuretics: increase the risk of hypercalcaemia.
Digoxin: its effects on the heart can be accentuated by Adcal-D$_3$.

Adcortyl Intra-articular/Intradermal (E.R. Squibb & Sons) *See* TRIAMCINOLONE ACETONIDE.

a

addiction *See* DEPENDENCE.

adefovir dipivoxil An *antiviral drug that is used for treating chronic hepatitis B infection. It is available as tablets on *prescription only.
Side effects: include vomiting, nausea, abdominal pain, diarrhoea, headache, and allergic reactions.
Precautions: adefovir should not be taken by women who are breastfeeding. Liver and kidney function should be monitored regularly during treatment, which should be stopped if there are signs of deteriorating liver function.
Interactions with other drugs:
Tenofovir disoproxil: should not be taken with adefovir.
Proprietary preparation: Hepsera.

Adenocor (sanofi-aventis) *See* ADENOSINE.

Adenoscan (sanofi-aventis) *See* ADENOSINE.

adenosine A drug that is used for rapid restoration of normal heart rhythm and to help diagnose different types of *arrhythmia. A *prescription only drug in the form of a sterile solution for injection or infusion, it is available only for use in hospitals.
Side effects: include transient flushing, chest pain, breathlessness, a choking sensation, nausea, and light-headedness.
Precautions: adenosine should not be given to people with heart block, severe hypotension (low blood pressure), untreated heart failure, or chronic obstructive pulmonary disease. *See also* ANTI-ARRHYTHMIC DRUGS.
Interactions with other drugs:
Beta Blockers: increase the risk of depression of heart function.
Dipyridamole: enhances the effects of adenosine, therefore a reduction in the dose of adenosine is recommended if it is prescribed with dipyridamole.
Theophylline: inhibits the action of adenosine.
Proprietary preparations: Adenocor; Adenoscan.
See also ANTI-ARRHYTHMIC DRUGS.

Adipine MR, Adipine XL (Chiesi) *See* NIFEDIPINE.

Adizem-XL, Adizem-SR (Napp Pharmaceuticals) *See* DILTIAZEM HYDROCHLORIDE.

adjunct A drug that is used in conjunction with another to provide additional beneficial effects in order to achieve the best treatment of a condition. The adjunct has the role of 'helping' or 'supporting' the main drug used in the treatment. The adjunct may have a mode of action that is different from that of the principal drug. For example, entacapone, a drug that prevents the breakdown of levodopa, is used as an adjunct to levodopa for the treatment of Parkinson's disease.

adrenaline (**epinephrine**) A hormone that is secreted by the centre (medulla) of the adrenal glands into the bloodstream in conditions of stress. It acts on *adrenoceptors to cause constriction of some blood vessels and

dilatation of others, increasing blood flow to the heart and skeletal muscles. The heart rate is increased, while the muscles of the intestine and airways relax. As a drug, adrenaline is available in various forms on *prescription only. It is given by intramuscular injection to relieve the effects of anaphylactic shock (an extreme and potentially fatal allergic reaction; *see* ANAPHYLAXIS) and by intravenous injection to treat cardiac arrest. It is given with *local anaesthetic preparations because it constricts blood vessels and thus confines the local anaesthetic to the area of application. It is also available as eye drops to treat *glaucoma, in which it reduces the production of aqueous fluid in the eye and increases its outflow.
Side effects: when adrenaline is given by injection side effects include dry mouth, palpitation, cold hands and feet, nervousness, tremor, and headache; there may be stomach pain after inhalation. Side effects with eye drops include smarting and redness of the eye and headache.
Interactions with other drugs:

Anaesthetics: irregular heartbeats (*arrhythmias) may occur if adrenaline is given with certain anaesthetics.
Antidepressants: hypertension (raised blood pressure) and arrhythmias may occur if adrenaline is given with tricyclic antidepressants.
Beta blockers: severe hypertension may occur if these drugs are given with adrenaline.
Clonidine: hypertension may occur if this drug is given with adrenaline.
Dopexamine: may increase the effects of adrenaline.
Entacapone: may increase the effects of adrenaline.
Rasagiline: should not be used with adrenaline.

Proprietary preparations: Anapen and Anapen Junior (disposable pens for self-injection); Epipen and Epipen Junior (disposable pens for self-injection); Minijet Adrenaline (injection).

adrenoceptors Specialized areas in the membranes of cells on which noradrenaline, and to a lesser extent adrenaline, act to convey messages from the nerves of the *sympathetic nervous system to their target tissues. There are two main types of adrenoceptors: **alpha receptors** and **beta receptors**. Stimulation of alpha receptors by noradrenaline causes (among other effects) constriction of arteries (*vasoconstriction); stimulation of beta receptors causes an increase in heart rate, widening of airways, relaxation of the muscle of the uterus, and dilatation of arteries (*vasodilatation).

Drugs that act on adrenoreceptors either stimulate them and increase their normal activity or block them and prevent their normal actions. Drugs that mimic the effects of noradrenaline are called *sympathomimetic drugs. There are two classes of drugs that block the effects of noradrenaline they are known as *alpha blockers and *beta blockers (they used to be called sympatholytic drugs). Some drugs (*carvedilol and *labetalol) block both alpha and beta receptors and are used to treat *hypertension.

Adult Meltus Chesty Coughs with Congestion (SSL International) A proprietary combination of *guaifenesin (an expectorant), *pseudoephedrine

(a decongestant), and *menthol, used to relieve the symptoms of coughs and colds. This liquid is available without a prescription, but only from pharmacies. It cannot be prescribed on the NHS.
Side effects and interactions with other drugs: *see* EPHEDRINE HYDROCHLORIDE; GUAIFENESIN.
Precautions: this medicine should not be taken by children under 12 years old. *See also* EPHEDRINE HYDROCHLORIDE.

Advagraf (Astellas Pharma Ltd) *See* TACROLIMUS.

aerosol A suspension of extremely small liquid or solid particles (about 0.001 mm diameter) in a gas. Drugs in aerosol form may be administered by inhalation (*see* INHALER).

Afinitor (Novartis) *See* EVEROLIMUS.

agalsidase Genetically engineered forms of the enzyme α-galactosidase A, **agalsidase alfa** and **agalsidase beta**, used in the treatment of Fabry's disease, an inherited condition due to a lack of this enzyme that has effects on the skin, heart, kidneys, and nervous system. Both drugs are available in forms for intravenous injection on *prescription only.
Side effects: include headache, 'pins and needles', dizziness, sleepiness, a burning sensation, fainting, increased production of tears, tinnitus, vertigo, palpitations, and a fast or slow heart rate.
Precautions: agalsidase alfa and beta carry a risk of allergic reactions. They are not recommended for use in pregnant or breastfeeding women.
Proprietary preparations: Fabrazyme (agalsidase beta); Replagal (agalsidase alfa).

Aggrastat (Merck Sharp & Dohne) *See* TIROFIBAN.

agomelatine A *melatonin agonist and *serotonin antagonist, used for the treatment of major depression (*see* ANTIDEPRESSANT DRUGS). It works by altering circadian (daily) rhythms and increasing levels of dopamine and norepinephrine. Agomelatine is available as tablets on *prescription only.
Side effects: include headache, dizziness, somnolence, insomnia, nausea, diarrhoea, constipation, sweating, back pain, and fatigue.
Precautions: agomelatine should not be taken by people with dementia or impaired liver function or by women who are breastfeeding. It should be used with caution in pregnant women and in people with kidney disease. Liver function should be monitored before and during treatment, which should be stopped if it is severely impaired.
Interactions with other drugs:
Ciprofloxacin: increases the plasma concentration of agomelatine and should not be taken with it.
Fluvoxamine: increases the plasma concentration of agomelatine.
Riamet: should not be taken with agomelatine.
Proprietary preparation: Valdoxan.

agonist A drug that acts at a cell-receptor site to produce an effect that is the same as, or similar to, that of the body's normal chemical messenger. *Cholinergic drugs, which have effects similar to the neurotransmitter acetylcholine, are examples.

AIDS (**acquired immune deficiency syndrome**) *See* HIV.

Airomir (IVAX) *See* SALBUTAMOL.

Aknemin (Almirall) *See* MINOCYCLINE.

Aknemycin Plus (Almirall) A proprietary combination of *erythromycin (an antibiotic) and *tretinoin (a retinoid), used for the treatment of *acne. It is available as a topical solution on *prescription only.
Side effects: include skin irritation and changes in skin colour.
Precautions: Aknemycin Plus should not be used by people with eczema, rosacea, or sunburn or by those with a family history of certain skin cancers. It should not be used during pregnancy or by women who are breastfeeding. Exposure to sunlight or sunlamps should be minimized during treatment. Other skin preparations, especially *keratolytics, should be avoided during treatment.

Alateris (Dee) *See* GLUCOSAMINE.

alclometasone dipropionate A moderately potent *topical steroid used for the treatment of a variety of skin disorders. It is available as a cream or ointment on *prescription only.
Side effects and precautions: *see* TOPICAL STEROIDS.
Proprietary preparation: Modrasone.

Aldactide 25, Aldactide 50 (Pharmacia) *See* CO-FLUMACTONE.

Aldactone (Pharmacia) *See* SPIRONOLACTONE.

Aldara (Meda Pharmaceuticals) *See* IMIQUIMOD.

aldesleukin An *interleukin produced by genetic engineering techniques and used for the treatment of certain patients with cancer of the kidney that has produced secondary tumours. A *prescription only medicine, it is usually given by subcutaneous injection, but only in specialist units.
Side effects: aldesleukin is highly toxic, causing *bone marrow suppression and damage to the liver, kidneys, thyroid gland, brain, and spinal cord.
Interactions with other drugs:
Antihypertensive drugs: aldesleukin increases the blood-pressure-lowering effect of these drugs.
Proprietary preparation: Proleukin.

Aldomet (Merck Sharp & Dohme) *See* METHYLDOPA.

Aldurazyme (Genzyme Therapeutics) *See* LARONIDASE.

alemtuzumab A *monoclonal antibody that specifically destroys B lymphocytes (a type of white blood cell). It is used in the treatment of chronic lymphocytic leukaemia (*see* CANCER) when conventional therapy with

*fludarabine is not appropriate. Alemtuzumab can cause allergic reactions during infusion (*see* RITUXIMAB) and can predispose to infections. Because of this, an analgesic, a corticosteroid, and an antibiotic should be taken before treatment starts. Alemtuzumab is given under expert supervision by slow intravenous infusion and is available on *prescription only.
Side effects and precautions: *see* RITUXIMAB.
Proprietary preparation: MabCampeth.

alendronic acid A *bisphosphonate used for the prevention and treatment of osteoporosis in postmenopausal women: it acts by preventing loss of calcium from bone and therefore increases bone density. It is available as tablets on *prescription only.
Side effects: include ulcers and inflammation of the oesophagus (gullet), abdominal pain and distension, diarrhoea or constipation, flatulence, muscle pain, and headache; rarely, nausea and vomiting, peptic ulcers, or a rash may occur.
Precautions: if there are any signs of irritation of the oesophagus (difficulty in swallowing, new or worsening heartburn), the drug should be discontinued immediately and a doctor contacted. Food and some drugs (see below) bind to alendronic acid in the stomach and intestine and prevent its absorption. Therefore the tablets should be swallowed whole, with a full glass of water, on an empty stomach at least 30 minutes before breakfast. The patient should then remain standing or sitting upright for at least 30 minutes and not lie down until after eating breakfast. The tablets should not be taken at bedtime or before rising. Alendronic acid should not be taken by anyone with disorders of the oesophagus or peptic ulcers. It should be used with caution by those with impaired kidney function and should not be taken by women who are pregnant or breastfeeding.
Interactions with other drugs:

Aminoglycosides: in combination with alendronic acid, they may cause abnormally low concentrations of calcium in the plasma.
Antacids: reduce the absorption of alendronic acid.
Calcium supplements: reduce the absorption of alendronic acid.
Iron supplements: reduce the absorption of alendronic acid.
NSAIDs: alendronic acid may increase the gastrointestinal effects of NSAIDs.

Proprietary preparations: Fosamax; Fosamax Once Weekly; *Fosavance (combined with colecalciferol).

alfacalcidol A derivative of *vitamin D used to prevent and treat the bone disease that may occur in kidney dialysis patients. Alfacalcidol is available as capsules, oral drops, or a solution for intravenous injection on *prescription only.
Side effects, precautions, and interactions with other drugs: *see* VITAMIN D.
Proprietary preparation: One Alpha.

alfentanil A potent *opioid with a very rapid onset of action. It is used for pain relief during short surgical operations and to relieve pain and depress

breathing in patients on ventilators in intensive care. Alfentanil is a *controlled drug; it is available as an intravenous infusion or injection.
Side effects and precautions: *see* MORPHINE.
Interactions with other drugs: *see* OPIOIDS.
Proprietary preparation: Rapifen.

alfuzosin hydrochloride An *alpha blocker used to relieve urinary obstruction in men with an enlarged prostate gland. It is available as tablets or *modified-release tablets on *prescription only.
Side effects: *see* ALPHA BLOCKERS.
Precautions: alfuzosin should not be taken by people with severely impaired liver function. *See also* ALPHA BLOCKERS.
Interactions with other drugs:
Ritonavir: may increase the plasma concentration of alfuzosin and the two drugs should not be used together.
See also ALPHA BLOCKERS.
Proprietary preparations: Besavar XL (modified-release tablets); Xatral; Xatral XL (modified-release tablets).

alginic acid A complex carbohydrate extracted from certain brown seaweeds (kelps). It absorbs water to form a slightly sticky gel. Alginic acid or its compounds, **magnesium alginate** and **sodium alginate**, are included in many *antacid preparations because they form a thick layer on the surface of the stomach contents, providing a mechanical barrier to protect the oesophagus from reflux (*see* ACID-PEPTIC DISEASES).
Proprietary preparations: Gaviscon Infant (sugar-free powder of sodium alginate and magnesium alginate); *Asilone Heartburn (combined with aluminium hydroxide, magnesium trisilicate, and sodium bicarbonate); *Gastrocote (combined with aluminium hydroxide, magnesium trisilicate, and sodium bicarbonate); *Gaviscon Advance (combined with potassium bicarbonate); *Gaviscon Double Action (combined with calcium carbonate and sodium bicarbonate); *Gaviscon Liquid (combined with sodium bicarbonate and calcium carbonate); *Gaviscon Tablets (combined with aluminium hydroxide, magnesium trisilicate, and sodium bicarbonate); *Peptac (combined with sodium bicarbonate and calcium carbonate); *Topal (combined with aluminium hydroxide and magnesium carbonate).

alglucosidase alfa A genetically engineered form of the enzyme alpha-glucosidase used for the treatment of Pompe disease, a rare disorder caused by a deficiency of this enzyme. It is given by intravenous infusion, under expert supervision, and is available on *prescription only.
Side effects: include nausea, vomiting, flushing, an increased heart rate, rapid breathing, swelling of the face, fever, sweating, and rash.
Precautions: severe allergic reactions (*see* ANAPHYLAXIS) may occur during infusion, and an antihistamine, corticosteroid, or antipyretic may be given before treatment starts. Alglucosidase alfa should not be given to women who are pregnant or breastfeeding.
Proprietary preparation: Myozyme.

a

alimemazine tartrate <**trimeprazine tartrate**> One of the original (sedating) *antihistamines, used to relieve the symptoms of such allergic conditions as urticaria and other itching skin conditions. It is available as tablets or a syrup on *prescription only.
Side effects: *see* ANTIHISTAMINES. Alimemazine may also cause *antimuscarinic effects and (more rarely) abnormal heart rhythms, low blood pressure, breathing difficulties, *extrapyramidal reactions, and (in high doses) convulsions.
Precautions: alimemazine should not be taken by people with kidney disease or by women who are pregnant or breastfeeding. *See also* ANTIHISTAMINES.
Interactions with other drugs: *see* ANTIHISTAMINES.
Proprietary preparations: Vallergan; Vallergan Syrup; Vallergan Forte Syrup.

Alimta (Eli Lilly & Co) *See* PEMETREXED.

aliskiren A drug used to treat essential *hypertension. It works by blocking the action of renin, an enzyme that promotes the formation of the hormone angiotensin, which raises blood pressure. Aliskiren is available as tablets on *prescription only.
Side effects: include diarrhoea.
Precautions: aliskiren should not be taken by women who are pregnant or breastfeeding. It should be used with caution in people with kidney disease.
Interactions with other drugs:
Ciclosporin: increases the plasma concentration of aliskiren and should not be taken with it.
Proprietary preparation: Rasilez.

alitretinoin A *retinoid used to treat severe chronic *eczema of the hands that has not responded to topical corticosteroids. It is available as capsules on *prescription only.
Side effects: include headache, raised blood lipids, nausea, vomiting, anaemia, conjunctivitis, dry lips, dry eyes, and flushing.
Precautions: alitretinoin should not be taken by women who are pregnant or breastfeeding and contraception must be used for one month before treatment and for at least one month after stopping treatment (*see* RETINOIDS). It should not be taken by people with liver disease, severe kidney disease, raised blood lipids, an underactive thyroid gland, or raised levels of vitamin A; levels of blood lipids should be monitored during treatment. Alitretinoin should be used with caution by people with depression.
Interactions with other drugs:
Simvastatin: its plasma concentration is reduced by alitretinoin.
Tetracyclines: should not be used with alitretinoin.
Proprietary preparation: Toctino.

alkaloids A group of nitrogen-containing substances that are produced by plants and can have potent effects on body functions. Many alkaloids are medicinally important drugs, including *morphine, *quinine, and *atropine.

Alka-Seltzer (Bayer) *See* ASPIRIN.

Alka-Seltzer XS (Bayer) A proprietary combination of *aspirin and *paracetamol (analgesics) and *caffeine (a stimulant), used for the relief of headache and other symptoms caused by overindulgence in alcohol and food. It is freely available *over the counter as effervescent tablets.
Side effects and precautions: *see* ASPIRIN; PARACETAMOL; CAFFEINE.
Interactions with other drugs: *see* ASPIRIN.

Alkeran (GlaxoSmithKline) *See* MELPHALAN.

alkylating drugs A class of *cytotoxic drugs that prevent cell replication by binding to DNA and preventing the separation of two DNA chains during cell division. They are widely used to treat a variety of cancers. These drugs cause the side effects common to all cytotoxic drugs but are particularly damaging to eggs and sperm and may therefore cause infertility. Their long-term use has also been associated with an increase in the incidence of non-lymphocytic leukaemia. The common alkylating drugs are *cyclophosphamide, *ifosfamide, *chlorambucil, *melphalan, *busulfan, *lomustine, *carmustine, *estramustine, *treosulfan, and *thiotepa.

allantoin An abrasive and *astringent agent that is included in preparations for the treatment of acne, *psoriasis, and other skin disorders and in preparations for the relief of *haemorrhoids and other irritating conditions of the anus or rectum.
Proprietary preparations: Boots Haemorrhoid Suppositories; *Alphosyl HC (combined with coal tar and hydrocortisone).

Allegron (King) *See* NORTRIPTYLINE.

ALLERcalm Allergy Relief Tablets (Actavis) *See* CHLORPHENAMINE.

Alli (GlaxoSmithKline) *See* ORLISTAT.

allopurinol A drug used for the prevention of gout, kidney stones, and high levels of uric acid in the blood in patients receiving chemotherapy; it acts by reducing the formation of uric acid in the body. It is not used to control acute attacks of gout, and may in fact exacerbate symptoms if started during an attack. It may be used in conjunction with *sulfinpyrazone. Allopurinol is available as tablets on *prescription only.
Side effects: rashes may indicate a serious allergic condition and should be reported to a doctor; other side effects include nausea and (rarely) malaise and headache.
Precautions: people taking allopurinol must maintain an adequate fluid intake (at least 2 litres a day) to prevent crystals of uric acid being passed in the urine (which can cause pain and bleeding). Alcohol should be avoided. Allopurinol should be used with caution in people with liver or kidney disease.
Interactions with other drugs:

Anticoagulants: allopurinol may enhance the anticoagulant effects of warfarin and acenocoumarol.

a

Azathioprine: allopurinol increases the risk of azathioprine causing adverse effects; therefore the dosage of azathioprine should be reduced.
Ciclosporin: allopurinol may increase plasma concentrations of ciclosporin and may increase the risk of kidney damage.
Didanosine: allopurinol increases its plasma concentration and therefore adverse effects, and the two drugs should not be used together.
Mercaptopurine: allopurinol prevents the breakdown of mercaptopurine and markedly increases the risk of its adverse effects; therefore the dosage of azathioprine should be reduced.
Proprietary preparations: Caplenal; Cosuric; Rimapurinol; Zyloric.

Almogran (Almirall) *See* ALMOTRIPTAN.

almond oil An oil expressed from almond nuts. It is used as an *emollient in skin creams and is also used to soften earwax.
Proprietary preparations: *Boots Cradle Cap Cream from Birth (combined with lanolin); *Boots Skin Therapy Emollient Cream (combined with lanolin); *Earex Ear Drops (combined with camphor and arachis oil); *Imuderm (combined with liquid paraffin); *Infaderm Therapeutic Body Oil (combined with liquid paraffin).

almotriptan A *5-HT_1 agonist used for the treatment of headache in acute migraine attacks. It is available as tablets on *prescription only.
Side effects: include dizziness, somnolence, nausea, vomiting, fatigue, headache, palpitations, sensations of tingling, and throat tightness.
Precautions: people with severely impaired liver function should not take this medicine, and those with severely impaired kidney function should take no more than one tablet in a 24-hour period. Almotriptan should not be taken by people with a history or symptoms of coronary artery disease, hypertension, previous stroke, or peripheral artery disease.
Interactions with other drugs:
Antimigraine drugs: ergotamine and methysergide should not be taken with almotriptan because of a risk of spasm of the blood vessels.
Proprietary preparation: Almogran.

Alomide (Alcon Laboratories) *See* LODOXAMIDE.

Aloxi (IS Pharmaceuticals) *See* PALONOSETRON.

alpha blockers (α-blockers; in full **alpha-adrenoceptor blockers**) *Vasodilator drugs that act by blocking the effect of noradrenaline on peripheral blood vessels. Noradrenaline normally acts at alpha-*adrenoceptors to constrict blood vessels; therefore opposing these actions causes widening of small arteries (arterioles) and a drop in blood pressure. This arteriolar widening also improves blood flow to areas of poor blood flow and therefore improves oxygen supply. Alpha blockers act on blood vessels and the ring of muscle that controls the opening of the bladder; they are used to treat *hypertension and in the management of bladder problems due to an enlarged prostate. Alpha blockers have beneficial effects on plasma lipids and are suitable for people with diabetes or heart failure.

See ALFUZOSIN HYDROCHLORIDE; DOXAZOSIN; INDORAMIN HYDROCHLORIDE; MOXISYLYTE; PHENOXYBENZAMINE HYDROCHLORIDE; PHENTOLAMINE; PRAZOSIN; TAMSULOSIN HYDROCHLORIDE; TERAZOSIN.

Side effects: sedation, dizziness (especially when standing up suddenly), and hypotension (low blood pressure) are quite common. Less common side effects are drowsiness, weakness and loss of energy, depression, headache, dry mouth, stuffy nose, nausea, urinary frequency and incontinence, and palpitation.

Precautions: the first dose may cause low blood pressure (especially in elderly people) and should be given when the patient is lying down or about to lie down. For this reason people may be started on low dosages and the dosage increased as necessary. Alpha blockers must be taken with caution, after appropriate dosage reduction, by people taking other antihypertensive medication. *See also* ANTIHYPERTENSIVE DRUGS.

Interactions with other drugs: a number of drugs enhance the action of alpha blockers in lowering blood pressure. These include general anaesthetics, beta blockers, calcium antagonists, diuretics, MAOIs, sildenafil, tadalafil, and vardenafil. Moxisylyte can interact with other alpha blockers to cause a severe fall in blood pressure on standing up.

Alphaderm (Alliance) A proprietary combination of *hydrocortisone (a corticosteroid) and *urea (a hydrating agent), used for the treatment of *eczema and dermatitis. It is available as a cream on *prescription only.
Side effects and precautions: *see* TOPICAL STEROIDS.

Alphagan (Allergan) *See* BRIMONIDINE TARTRATE.

Alphanate (Grifols) *See* FACTOR VIII.

AlphaNine (Grifols) *See* FACTOR IX.

alpha stimulants (**alpha agonists**) *See* SYMPATHOMIMETIC DRUGS.

alpha tocopheryl acetate *See* VITAMIN E.

Alphosyl 2-in-1 Shampoo (GlaxoSmithKline) *See* COAL TAR.

Alphosyl HC (GlaxoSmithKline) A proprietary combination of *hydrocortisone (a corticosteroid), *coal tar extract (a keratolytic), and *allantoin (an abrasive and astringent), used for the treatment of *psoriasis. It is available as a cream on *prescription only.
Side effects and precautions: *see* TOPICAL STEROIDS; COAL TAR.

alprazolam A long-acting *benzodiazepine used for the short-term treatment of severe anxiety. It is available as tablets on *prescription only and cannot be prescribed on the NHS.
Side effects and precautions: *see* DIAZEPAM; BENZODIAZEPINES.
Interactions with other drugs:

Antifungal drugs: itraconazole and ketoconazole increase the plasma concentration of alprazolam.
Antiviral drugs: fosamprenavir, indinavir, and ritonavir increase the risk of profound sedation, and the latter two drugs should not be used with alprazolam.
See also BENZODIAZEPINES.
Proprietary preparation: Xanax.

alprostadil A *prostaglandin that produces dilatation of blood vessels. It is used for the treatment of erectile impotence and to aid diagnosis, being administered by injection into the erectile tissue of the penis or by application into the urethra. Treatment is not started until the possibility of any underlying treatable cause of the condition has been excluded. Alprostadil is also available as a solution for infusion to treat newborn babies who are awaiting surgery for congenital heart disease. It acts by preventing the closure of the ductus arteriosus, a blood vessel that enables the circulation to bypass the lungs in the fetus but normally closes after birth to allow the lungs to be included in the circulation. Both forms of alprostadil are only available on *prescription.
Side effects: in men, these may include penile pain, prolonged erection, reactions at the injection site, testicular pain and/or swelling, blood in the urine, nausea, dry mouth, sweating, dizziness, and headache. Men who experience erections lasting four hours or longer should seek immediate medical help; treatment of prolonged erection should not be delayed more than six hours. Side effects in babies include breathlessness (particularly in infants under 2 kg), flushing, a slow heart rate, and low blood pressure; there may be oedema, diarrhoea, fever, and convulsions.
Precautions: alprostadil should not be taken by men with a predisposition to prolonged erection (as seen in sickle-cell anaemia, multiple myeloma, or leukaemia) or anatomical deformity of the penis. It should not be used in conjunction with other drugs for the treatment of erectile dysfunction or when sexual activity is medically inadvisable. Alprostadil should not be given to babies with a history of haemorrhage.
Interactions with other drugs:
Antihypertensive drugs: their effect in lowering blood pressure may be enhanced by alprostadil.
Proprietary preparations: Caverject (intracavernosal injection); MUSE (pellet for direct urethral application); Prostin VR (infusion); Viridal (intracavernosal injection).

Altacite Plus (Peckforton Pharmaceuticals) A proprietary combination of *hydrotalcite (an antacid) and activated *dimeticone (an antifoaming agent), used for the relief of flatulence and heartburn associated with *acid-peptic diseases; this combination is also known as **co-simalcite**. It is available as a suspension and can be obtained without a prescription.
Side effects, precautions, and interactions with other drugs: *see* ANTACIDS.

Altargo (GlaxoSmithKline) *See* RETAPAMULIN.

alteplase A *fibrinolytic drug used to dissolve blood clots in the coronary arteries (which supply the heart) and the carotid arteries (which supply the head) in people who have had a heart attack or a stroke; treatment should be started within 12 hours of the heart attack and within three hours of the stroke. Alteplase is also used to treat pulmonary embolism (*see* THROMBOSIS). It is available in a form for intravenous injection or infusion on *prescription only.
Side effects, precautions, and interactions with other drugs: *see* FIBRINOLYTIC DRUGS.
Proprietary preparation: Actilyse.

Alu-Cap (Meda Pharmaceuticals) *See* ALUMINIUM HYDROXIDE.

aluminium acetate A salt of aluminium that has *astringent properties. It is used to cleanse weeping wounds and patches of eczema and to treat inflammation of the outer ear. Aluminium acetate is available as a lotion or ear drops that can be obtained without a prescription, but only from pharmacies.

aluminium chlorhydroxyallantoinate *See* DERMIDEX.

aluminium chloride A powerful antiperspirant that is used for the treatment of excessive sweating of the armpits, hands, or feet. At lower concentrations, it is included as an ingredient of many proprietary antiperspirant preparations. Aluminium chloride is available as a solution, usually in a roll-on applicator, and can be obtained without a prescription, but only from pharmacies.
Side effects: aluminium chloride may cause skin irritation.
Precautions: aluminium chloride should not be allowed to come in contact with the eyes, mouth, or other mucous membranes and should not be applied to broken or inflamed skin. The armpits should not be shaved or treated with depilatories for 12 hours before or after applying aluminium chloride.
Proprietary preparations: Anhydrol Forte; Driclor.

aluminium hydroxide An *antacid used in the treatment of indigestion (*see* ACID-PEPTIC DISEASES). It is also used as a *phosphate-binding agent to absorb phosphates from the diet. Aluminium hydroxide is available, without a prescription, in the form of tablets or capsules; some preparations that contain aluminium hydroxide as an ingredient can only be obtained from pharmacies. Some preparations cannot be prescribed on the NHS. *See also* CO-MAGALDROX.
Side effects: aluminium hydroxide may cause constipation. *See also* ANTACIDS.
Precautions: aluminium hydroxide should be used with caution in people undergoing kidney dialysis.
Interactions with other drugs: *see* ANTACIDS.
Proprietary preparations: Alu-Cap (capsules); *Asilone Heartburn (combined with alginic acid, magnesium trisilicate, and sodium bicarbonate); *Asilone Suspension (combined with magnesium oxide and simeticone); *Boots Wind Relief Tablets (combined with magnesium hydroxide and simeticone);

*Gastrocote (combined with alginic acid, magnesium trisilicate, and sodium bicarbonate); *Gaviscon Tablets (combined with alginic acid, magnesium trisilicate, and sodium bicarbonate); *Kolanticon Gel (combined with magnesium hydroxide, simeticone, and dicycloverine hydrochloride); Maalox (*see* CO-MAGALDROX); *Maalox Plus (combined with magnesium hydroxide and simeticone); Mucogel (*see* CO-MAGALDROX); *Topal (combined with magnesium carbonate and alginic acid).

aluminium oxide An abrasive agent used for the treatment of acne in the form of a paste containing fine or medium-sized particles in a cleansing base. It is freely available *over the counter.
Precautions: the paste should not be used by people with telangiectasia (in which spidery red spots of distended blood vessels can be seen beneath the skin). It should not come into contact with the eyes.
Proprietary preparation: Brasivol.

Alvedon (AstraZeneca) *See* PARACETAMOL.

alverine citrate An *antispasmodic used in the treatment of irritable bowel syndrome, diverticular disease (which causes abdominal pain and altered bowel habit), and painful periods caused by spasms of the uterus. It is available as capsules and can be obtained without a prescription, but only from pharmacies.
Side effects: include nausea, headache, itching, rash, and dizziness.
Precautions: alverine citrate should not be taken by people with intestinal obstruction due to loss of intestinal movement or during the first three months of pregnancy.
Proprietary preparations: Spasmonal; Spasmonal Forte (a stronger formulation).

Alvesco (Nycomed UK) *See* CICLESONIDE.

amantadine hydrochloride An *antiparkinsonian drug that acts by increasing the activity of *dopamine in the brain. It provides moderate relief of symptoms but *tolerance to its effect may develop. Amantadine is also an *antiviral drug that acts by inhibiting viral replication; it is used particularly in the prevention and treatment of influenza type A_2. It is available, on *prescription only, as capsules or a syrup.
Side effects: include nervousness, inability to concentrate, insomnia, dizziness, and (rarely) convulsions and hallucinations; nausea and loss of appetite may also occur.
Precautions: amantadine should be used with caution in people who have liver or kidney disease, congestive heart disease, or states of confusion or hallucination. It should not be taken by people with epilepsy or a history of peptic ulcers or by women who are pregnant or breastfeeding. Withdrawal of the drug at the end of treatment should be gradual.
Interactions with other drugs:
Antipsychotics: *extrapyramidal reactions can occur.

Memantine: increases the risk of adverse effects on the central nervous system, and these two drugs should not be used together.

Methyldopa: extrapyramidal reactions can occur.

Proprietary preparations: Symmetrel; Lysovir (capsules).

Amaryl (sanofi-aventis) *See* GLIMEPIRIDE.

AmBisome (Gilead Sciences) *See* AMPHOTERICIN.

Ambre Solaire (Laboratoires Garnier) A proprietary *sunscreen preparation consisting of a cream containing avobenzone, 4-methylbenzylidene camphor, terephthalylidene dicamphor sulphonic acid, and *titanium dioxide. It protects against both UVA and UVB (SPF 60) and can be prescribed on the NHS or obtained without a prescription.

ambrisentan A potent *vasodilator used for the treatment of pulmonary arterial hypertension (raised blood pressure in the vessels supplying the lungs). It works by blocking receptors for endothelin, a hormone that stimulates constriction of blood vessels (and hence raises blood pressure). Ambrisentan is available as tablets on *prescription only.

Side effects: include anaemia, palpitations, headache, constipation, dizziness, abdominal pain, swelling of the ankles, insomnia, and flushing.

Precautions: ambrisentan should not be taken by pregnant or breastfeeding women or by people with severe liver disease or anaemia. Blood counts, haemoglobin levels, and liver function should be monitored during treatment.

Proprietary preparation: Volibris.

amethocaine *See* TETRACAINE.

Amias (Takeda) *See* CANDESARTAN CILEXETIL.

amikacin An *aminoglycoside antibiotic used for the treatment of serious infections that are resistant to *gentamicin. It is given as an *intramuscular or *intravenous injection or intravenous *infusion and is available on *prescription only.

Side effects, precautions, and interactions with other drugs: *see* GENTAMICIN.

Amilamont (Rosemont Pharmaceuticals) *See* AMILORIDE HYDROCHLORIDE.

Amil-Co (Norton Healthcare) *See* CO-AMILOZIDE.

amiloride hydrochloride A *potassium-sparing diuretic used in the treatment of *hypertension and *oedema associated with heart failure, liver disease, or kidney disease. It is available, on *prescription only, as tablets or a solution. *See also* CO-AMILOFRUSE; CO-AMILOZIDE.

Side effects, precautions, and interactions with other drugs: *see* POTASSIUM-SPARING DIURETICS.

Proprietary preparations: Amilamont; Frumil (*see* CO-AMILOFRUSE); Moduretic (*see* CO-AMILOZIDE).

See also ANTIHYPERTENSIVE DRUGS; DIURETICS.

aminacrine hydrochloride *See* AMINOACRIDINE HYDROCHLORIDE.

aminoacridine hydrochloride <aminacrine hydrochloride> A disinfectant used in dilute solutions as an *antiseptic. It is included in preparations for treating minor sores and infections of the mouth.
Proprietary preparations: *Iglu Gel (combined with lidocaine); *Medijel (combined with lidocaine hydrochloride).

aminobenzoic acid A vitamin of the B group (*see* VITAMIN B COMPLEX). It is included as an ingredient of some *sunscreen preparations as it absorbs UVB, a range of ultraviolet light of medium wavelength that causes reddening and burning of the skin. Aminobenzoic acid is also included in some vitamin B supplements but there is no evidence of its value.
Side effects: sunscreens containing aminobenzoic acid may cause allergic rashes in the presence of sunlight.
Proprietary preparation: *SpectraBan (combined with padimate-O).

aminoglycosides A group of bactericidal antibiotics (i.e. they kill bacteria, rather than just inhibiting their growth). Because of their toxicity (possible side effects include ear damage, causing impaired hearing and balance, and kidney damage), they are used only when less toxic antibacterials are ineffective or inadvisable. As most of their side effects are dose-related, care must be taken with dosage. Aminoglycosides are excreted by the kidneys, therefore they must be used with caution in people with kidney disease as toxic concentrations of the aminoglycosides can accumulate. Most aminoglycosides are not continued for longer than seven days. Aminoglycosides are not absorbed from the gut unless this is damaged, so they must be administered by injection.

See AMIKACIN; GENTAMICIN; NEOMYCIN SULPHATE; STREPTOMYCIN; TOBRAMYCIN.

aminophylline A *xanthine that is a compound of *theophylline and ethylenediamine and is used for the treatment of *asthma and in some cases of emphysema and chronic bronchitis (*see* BRONCHODILATORS). It is available from pharmacies without a prescription in the form of *modified-release tablets; an injection is available on *prescription only.
Side effects, precautions, and interactions with other drugs: *see* THEOPHYLLINE; XANTHINES.
Proprietary preparations: Minijet Aminophylline (injection); Norphyllin SR (modified-release tablets); Phyllocontin Continus (modified-release tablets).

aminosalicylates A class of drugs used for the treatment of ulcerative colitis (inflammation and ulceration of the large bowel) and to maintain patients in remission from it. They are also used to treat Crohn's disease (inflammation and ulceration of the gastrointestinal tract) that affects the large bowel. The aminosalicylates include *mesalazine (aminosalicylic acid), *balsalazide sodium, *olsalazine sodium, and *sulfasalazine; they are taken by mouth or rectally and are available on *prescription only.
Side effects: include diarrhoea, nausea, headache, allergic reactions

(including rashes), and exacerbation of the symptoms of colitis. Rare side effects include blood disorders (see precautions below).
Precautions: aminosalicylates should not be taken by people who are allergic to *salicylates or by those with severe kidney disease. They should be used with caution in women who are pregnant or breastfeeding. Bleeding, bruising, sore throat, or fever should be reported immediately to a doctor as this can indicate a blood disorder; in this case treatment should be discontinued.

amiodarone A class III *anti-arrhythmic drug, which works by slowing nerve impulses in the heart. It is given to control and prevent ventricular and supraventricular tachycardia and atrial fibrillation (*see* ARRHYTHMIA). This drug can have serious side effects and it should be initiated under hospital or specialist supervision, when it may be given as tablets or by injection. It is available on *prescription only.
Side effects: harmless deposits may form on the cornea of the eyes, which usually cause no symptoms and reverse when the medication is stopped. In the long term amiodarone can have a number of adverse effects on the liver, eyes, lungs, and thyroid gland. About one-third of people taking the drug become more sensitive to the sun, and everyone taking amiodarone should take care in the sun until they have established whether or not they are affected; people who tan easily are no more or less likely to be affected than very fair-skinned people. Sensitivity may be overcome by the use of sunscreens.
Precautions: amiodarone should not be taken by people with thyroid disorders or by women who are pregnant or breastfeeding. It may cause liver disorders, and treatment should be stopped if symptoms of these develop. *See also* ANTI-ARRHYTHMIC DRUGS.
Interactions with other drugs: amiodarone interacts with a number of other drugs to increase the risk of ventricular arrhythmias. These drugs should therefore not be taken with amiodarone (see below).

Antibiotics: amiodarone should not be taken with erythromycin (given by injection), levofloxacin, moxifloxacin, or co-trimoxazole.

Anticoagulants: amiodarone increases the anticoagulant effects of warfarin, acenocoumarol, and phenindione.

Antimalarial drugs: amiodarone should not be taken with mefloquine, chloroquine, quinine, hydroxychloroquine, or Riamet.

Antipsychotic drugs: amiodarone should not be taken with the phenothiazines, amisulpride, benperidol, droperidol, haloperidol, pimozide, sertindole, or zuclopenthixol.

Antiviral drugs: amiodarone should not be taken with fosamprenavir, indinavir, nelfinavir, or ritonavir.

Beta blockers: amiodarone should not be taken with sotalol; the risk of bradycardia (slow heart rate) is increased if amiodarone is taken with other beta blockers.

Calcium antagonists: the risk of bradycardia is increased if amiodarone is taken with diltiazem or verapamil.

Digoxin: amiodarone increases the plasma concentration of digoxin, whose dosage should therefore be reduced.
Disopyramide: should not be taken with amiodarone.
Lithium: should not be taken with amiodarone.
Mizolastine: should not be taken with amiodarone.
Pentamidine isethionate: should not be taken with amiodarone.
Phenytoin: its plasma concentration is increased by amiodarone.
Simvastatin: there is an increased risk of muscle damage if this drug is taken with amiodarone.
Tricyclic antidepressants: should not be taken with amiodarone.

Proprietary preparation: Cordarone X.

amisulpride An atypical *antipsychotic drug that is used in the treatment of schizophrenia; it controls both the positive symptoms (e.g. delusions) and the negative symptoms (e.g. apathy) of the disease. Amisulpride is available as tablets on *prescription only.

Side effects: include weight gain, dizziness, low blood pressure on standing (which can cause fainting in some people), insomnia, anxiety, agitation, sleepiness, constipation, nausea, vomiting, dry mouth, raised concentrations of prolactin in the blood (causing breast pain and enlargement and menstrual problems), and (rarely) slowing of the heart rate.

Precautions: amisulpride should not be taken by women who are pregnant or breastfeeding or by people with phaeochromocytoma (a tumour of the adrenal gland) or tumours that are stimulated by prolactin. It should be used with caution in people with cardiovascular disease, a history of epilepsy, Parkinson's disease, or kidney disease and in the elderly.

Interactions with other drugs: amisulpride interacts with some other drugs to increase the risk of ventricular *arrhythmias. These drugs should therefore not be taken with amisulpride (see below).

Anaesthetics: their effect in lowering blood pressure is increased.
Anti-arrhythmic drugs: amiodarone and disopyramide should not be taken with amisulpride.
Antidepressants: there is an increased risk of *antimuscarinic effects and *arrhythmias if amisulpride is taken with tricyclic antidepressants.
Antiepileptic drugs: amisulpride antagonizes the effects of these drugs in controlling seizures.
Antipsychotic drugs: droperidol and sertindole should not be taken with amisulpride.
Diuretics: the risk of ventricular arrhythmias is increased by the potassium depletion caused by these drugs.
Erythromycin (injection): should not be given with amisulpride.
Methadone: should not be taken with amisulpride.
Pentamidine isethionate: should not be used with amisulpride.
Ritonavir: may increase the effects of amisulpride.
Sedatives: the sedative effects of amisulpride are increased if it is taken with anxiolytic or hypnotic drugs, or any other drug that causes sedation.

Sibutramine: the risk of adverse effects on the central nervous system is increased, and these two drugs should not be used together.

Sotalol: increases the risk of ventricular arrhythmias.

Proprietary preparation: Solian.

amitriptyline hydrochloride A *tricyclic antidepressant drug used for the treatment of pain resulting from nerve damage and bedwetting in children; it is not now recommended for treating depressive illness. It is available, on *prescription only, as tablets or a solution for oral use.

Side effects: include dry mouth, sedation, blurred vision, constipation, nausea, difficulty in urinating, palpitation and fast heart rate, sweating, tremor, rashes and allergic reactions, behavioural disturbances, confusion (especially in the elderly), and interference with sexual function. There may be increased appetite and weight gain, drowsiness, nervousness or insomnia, weakness and fatigue, and changes in blood sugar concentrations.

Precautions and interactions with other drugs: *see* TRICYCLIC ANTIDEPRESSANTS.

Proprietary preparation: *Triptafen (combined with perphenazine).

amlodipine A class II *calcium antagonist used for the prevention of *angina and as a first-line treatment for *hypertension. It has a longer duration of action than *nifedipine or *nicardipine and is therefore usually given once daily. It is available as tablets on *prescription only.

Side effects and interactions with other drugs: *see* CALCIUM ANTAGONISTS.

Precautions: amlodipine should not be used to treat patients with unstable angina and should not be taken by women who are pregnant or breastfeeding.

Proprietary preparations: Amlostin; Istin; *Exforge (combined with valsartan); *Sevikar (combined with olmesartan).

See also ANTIHYPERTENSIVE DRUGS.

Amlostin (Discovery Pharmaceuticals) *See* AMLODIPINE.

ammonia solution A solution that gives off a pungent vapour. Strong or weak ammonia solutions are used in *decongestant and *rubefacient preparations.

Precautions: ammonia can be caustic and irritating, depending on the concentration. It can irritate eyes and mucous membranes and should not be swallowed, as it can burn the lining of the gullet and stomach.

Proprietary preparations: *Blistex Relief Cream (combined with liquefied phenol); *Goddard's Muscle Lotion (combined with dilute acetic acid and turpentine oil); *Mackenzies Smelling Salts (combined with eucalyptus oil).

ammonium acetate *See* EXPECTORANTS.

ammonium carbonate *See* EXPECTORANTS.

ammonium chloride A compound that is included as an *expectorant in some proprietary cough medicines. Ammonium chloride is also used to acidify the urine, which reduces the reabsorption of some drugs from the

a

urine back into the body, and so enhances their excretion; it can therefore be used as an antidote to poisoning by these drugs.
Proprietary preparations: *Benylin Chesty Coughs Original (combined with diphenhydramine and menthol); *Boots Bronchial Cough Mixture (combined with ammonium carbonate and guaifenesin); *Histalix (combined with diphenhydramine and menthol).

amobarbital <**amylobarbitone**> An intermediate-acting *barbiturate. Its sodium salt, **amobarbital sodium**, is used for the short-term treatment of severe insomnia in people who are already taking barbiturates. It is available as capsules and is a *controlled drug.
Side effects, precautions, and interactions with other drugs: *see* BARBITURATES.
Proprietary preparations: Sodium Amytal (capsules); *Tuinal (combined with secobarbital).

Amoram (Eastern Pharmaceuticals) *See* AMOXICILLIN.

amorolfine An *antifungal drug applied topically as the hydrochloride for treating ringworm infections of the nails and skin and pityriasis versicolor (a chronic fungal infection of the skin). It is available as a cream or nail lacquer on *prescription only.
Side effects: amorolfine may rarely cause transient burning or reddening of the skin.
Precautions: amorolfine should be used with caution during pregnancy or breastfeeding. It should not be used in or around the eyes, ears, and mucous membranes.
Proprietary preparations: Curanail Nail Lacquer; Loceryl; Loceryl Lacquer.

amoxicillin <**amoxycillin**> A broad-spectrum *penicillin very similar to *ampicillin but better absorbed when taken by mouth. It is used for the treatment of middle-ear and sinus infections, chest infections (including exacerbations of chronic bronchitis), *Salmonella* infections, urinary-tract infections, and gonorrhoea. It is available, on *prescription only, as capsules, sachets, or an oral suspension and as an injection.
Side effects, precautions, and interactions with other drugs: *see* AMPICILLIN.
Proprietary preparations: Amoram; Amoxil; Galenamox; Augmentin (*see* CO-AMOXICLAV).

Amoxil (GlaxoSmithKline) *See* AMOXICILLIN.

amoxycillin *See* AMOXICILLIN.

amphetamines A group of *sympathomimetic drugs that have a marked *stimulant action on the central nervous system. They alleviate fatigue and produce a feeling of mental alertness and well-being. Amphetamines have limited uses in clinical medicine since they can cause *dependence and psychotic states; the most important member of the group is *dexamfetamine sulphate, which is used in the treatment of narcolepsy in adults and attention deficit hyperactivity disorder in children. Amphetamines should not be used to treat depressive illness, obesity, senility, or tiredness.

amphotericin (**amphotericin B**) An *antifungal drug that is active against a wide range of organisms and can be used to treat most fungal infections; it is especially effective in treating systemic (generalized) infections. When taken orally or applied topically, for treating superficial infections, side effects are rare. For systemic infections amphotericin is given by intravenous infusion, which must be under medical supervision because side effects can be severe. A *prescription only medicine, amphotericin is available as lozenges to be dissolved in the mouth and as solutions or lipid formulations for intravenous infusion.
Side effects: when injected, amphotericin can cause nausea, vomiting, loss of appetite, diarrhoea, stomach pains, fever, headache, muscle and joint pains, anaemia, allergic reactions, kidney damage, and (less frequently) changes in blood pressure, abnormal heart rhythms, blood disorders, liver damage, hearing loss, double vision, and convulsions.
Precautions (with injections): since severe allergic reactions can occur, a test dose of amphotericin should be given before the full dose. Tests for liver and kidney function during treatment are necessary. Amphotericin should be used with caution in people taking corticosteroids or anti-cancer drugs and in women who are pregnant or breastfeeding.
Interactions with other drugs:
Aminoglycoside antibiotics: increase the risk of toxic effects on the kidney.
Ciclosporin: increases the risk of toxic effects on the kidney.
Corticosteroids: increase the risk of low concentrations of potassium in the blood.
Digoxin and digitoxin: the toxic effects of these drugs are increased if amphotericin causes potassium concentrations in the blood to fall.
Diuretics: amphotericin increases the risk of loop and thiazide diuretics causing low potassium concentrations in the blood.
Tacrolimus: increases the risk of toxic effects on the kidney.
Proprietary preparations: Abelcet; AmBisome; Fungilin; Fungizone.

ampicillin A broad-spectrum penicillin that is inactivated by penicillinase (*see* PENICILLINS). It is used for the treatment of middle ear and sinus infections, chest infections (including community-acquired pneumonia and exacerbations of chronic bronchitis), *Salmonella* infections, urinary-tract infections, and gonorrhoea. It is available, on *prescription only, as capsules or a syrup for oral use and as an injection.
Side effects: may include diarrhoea, nausea, and rashes. Rashes, which should be reported to a doctor, are most common in patients suffering from glandular fever, chronic lymphatic leukaemia, and HIV infection and in patients who are also taking *allopurinol.
Precautions: ampicillin should not be taken by anyone with known allergy to penicillins, and it should be used with caution in people with severe kidney disease.

a

Interactions with other drugs:

Methotrexate: concentrations of methotrexate in the blood are increased, which may cause toxic effects.

Oral contraceptives: their contraceptive effect may be reduced. Additional contraceptive precautions should therefore be taken with short courses of ampicillin and for seven days after stopping; if these days run beyond the end of a packet of oral contraceptives, the next packet should be started immediately without a break.

Proprietary preparations: Penbritin; Rimacillin; Flu-Amp (*see* CO-FLUAMPICIL); Magnapen (*see* CO-FLUAMPICIL).

amsacrine A *cytotoxic drug used for the treatment of acute myeloid leukaemia (*see* CANCER). It is similar to *doxorubicin and is available as a solution for intravenous infusion on *prescription only.
Side effects and precautions: *see* DOXORUBICIN.
Proprietary preparation: Amsidine.

Amsidine (Goldshield) *See* AMSACRINE.

amylmetacresol An *antiseptic used as an ingredient of lozenges for the treatment of minor infections of the mouth and throat.
Proprietary preparations: Boots Sore Throat Relief Lozenges; *Strepsils (combined with dichlorobenzyl alcohol).

amylobarbitone *See* AMOBARBITAL.

Anabact (ASTA Medica) *See* METRONIDAZOLE.

anabolic steroids Steroids that promote the growth of tissues, especially muscles. Anabolic steroids are synthetic forms of male sex hormones (*androgens) that have fewer masculinizing effects in women than androgens. They have not proved to be effective for promoting weight gain in severely underweight patients, and their use as body builders by athletes is banned by athletic authorities. *Nandrolone may be used to stimulate production of blood cells by the bone marrow in people with aplastic *anaemia. Prolonged use of anabolic steroids can cause liver damage.
Interactions with other drugs:

Anticoagulants: anabolic steroids increase the anticoagulant effects of warfarin, acenocoumarol, and phenindione.

Anacal (Genus Pharmaceuticals) A proprietary combination of *heparinoid (an anticoagulant) and laureth '9' (a *lauromacrogol), used to relieve the discomfort and pain of *haemorrhoids, anal fissures, proctitis (inflammation of the rectum), or itching of the anal region. It is available as ointment or suppositories and can be obtained without a prescription, but only from pharmacies.

Anadin (Pfizer) A proprietary combination of *aspirin (an analgesic and antipyretic) and *caffeine (a stimulant), used for the treatment of mild to moderate pain (including headache, neuralgia, toothache, and period pains)

and fever and to relieve the symptoms of influenza and colds. It is available as tablets or capsules; **Anadin Maximum Strength** is a stronger formulation in the form of capsules. These preparations are available without a prescription, but larger packs can only be obtained from pharmacies.
Side effects and interactions with other drugs: *see* ASPIRIN.
Precautions: these medicines are not recommended for children, except on medical advice. *See also* ASPIRIN; CAFFEINE.

Anadin Extra, Anadin Extra Soluble (Pfizer) Proprietary combinations of *aspirin and *paracetamol (analgesics and antipyretics) and *caffeine (a stimulant), used for the treatment of mild to moderate pain (including headache, neuralgia, toothache, and period pains) and fever and to relieve the symptoms of influenza and colds. They are available as tablets or soluble tablets without a prescription, but larger packs can only be obtained from pharmacies.
Side effects and interactions with other drugs: *see* ASPIRIN.
Precautions: these medicines should not be given to children, except on medical advice. *See also* ASPIRIN; PARACETAMOL; CAFFEINE.

Anadin Ibuprofen (Pfizer) *See* IBUPROFEN.

Anadin Paracetamol (Pfizer) *See* PARACETAMOL.

Anadin Ultra (Pfizer) *See* IBUPROFEN.

anaemia A condition that arises when the amount of haemoglobin, the oxygen-carrying pigment of the red blood cells, is reduced. Those affected are pale, constantly feel tired, become breathless on exertion, and have poor resistance to infection. There are many causes. **Iron-deficiency anaemia** (*see* IRON) may be due to loss of blood or lack of dietary iron. **Haemolytic anaemias** result from the increased destruction of red blood cells; this occurs, for example, in haemolytic disease of the newborn, in which the red cells of the fetus are destroyed by antibodies in the mother's blood (*see* ANTI-D (RH_0) IMMUNOGLOBULIN). Anaemia can also occur when the production of red cells is impaired. This may be due to a deficiency of the factors necessary for red cell production, such as vitamin B_{12} or intrinsic factor (causing **pernicious anaemia**; *see* VITAMIN B COMPLEX), *folic acid, or *erythropoietin, or by suppression of red cell production in the bone marrow, which occurs in leukaemia (*see* CANCER). Such anaemias are characterized by the presence of abnormal red blood cells; for example megaloblasts are present in the bone marrow in folic acid or vitamin B_{12} deficiency (**megaloblastic anaemias**). In **aplastic anaemia** the numbers of red blood cells are very much reduced due to failure of the bone marrow to produce them.

anaesthetics *See* LOCAL ANAESTHETICS.

Anafranil, Anafranil SR (Novartis) *See* CLOMIPRAMINE HYDROCHLORIDE.

anagrelide A drug used in the treatment of thrombocythaemia, a disorder marked by excess proliferation of platelet-forming cells resulting in

abnormalities in blood clotting. It works by inhibiting the formation of platelets. Anagrelide is available as capsules on *prescription only.
Side effects: include headache, diarrhoea, unusual weakness or fatigue, hair loss, nausea, and dizziness.
Precautions: anagrelide should not be taken by women who are pregnant or breastfeeding. It should be used with caution in people with cardiovascular disease or impaired liver or kidney function.
Interactions with other drugs:
Cilostazol: should not be taken with anagrelide.
Phosphodiesterase inhibitors: enoximone and milrinone should not be taken with anagrelide.
Proprietary preparation: Xagrid.

anakinra A drug that inhibits the action of *interleukin-1 and is used to reduce chronic inflammation in the treatment of rheumatoid arthritis. It is available as a form for injection on *prescription only.
Side effects: include neutropenia (a decrease in the number of neutrophils, a type of white blood cell), headache, and infections.
Precautions: anakinra should not be given to women who are pregnant or breastfeeding. There is a risk of neutropenia; neutrophil counts should be monitored before and during treatment, which should be stopped if signs of neutropenia develop. Anakinra should be used with caution in people with serious infections or impaired kidney function.
Interactions with other drugs:
DMARDs: the use of anakinra with adalimumab, etanercept, and infliximab should be avoided because of the increased risk of side effects.
Vaccines: should not be given to people who are taking anakinra.
Proprietary preparation: Kineret.

analeptic drugs (respiratory stimulants) *See* STIMULANTS.

analgesics Drugs used for controlling pain. **Non-opioid analgesics**, mainly *aspirin and *paracetamol, provide effective relief of such pains as headache, toothache, and mild rheumatic pain. **Opioid analgesics** (sometimes colloquially called narcotic analgesics) include *codeine and more potent drugs (such as *morphine and *pethidine) that are only used under medical supervision (*see* OPIOIDS). The non-steroidal anti-inflammatory drugs (*see* NSAIDs) are a large group of analgesics widely used for treating rheumatic conditions (including rheumatoid arthritis).

analogue A drug that differs structurally in minor ways from its parent compound. These minor differences in molecular structure can result in important changes in action. Examples are *calcipotriol (an analogue of vitamin D) and *betahistine (an analogue of histamine). Useful analogues of existing drugs are either more potent, cause fewer side effects, or are better absorbed after oral administration.

Anapen (Lincoln Medical) *See* ADRENALINE.

anaphylaxis A severe allergic reaction to a particular antigen (foreign protein), which interacts with antibody that is bound to certain cells (mast cells) to bring about the release of *histamine and other chemicals, causing local or widespread symptoms. These range from pain and itchy weals on the face (especially the lips, eyelids, and tongue) accompanied by swelling (**angioedema**) to widespread tissue swelling (which can involve the larynx), constriction of the airways, and a fall in blood pressure leading to circulatory collapse (**anaphylactic shock**). This is a medical emergency requiring prompt treatment (including the injection of *adrenaline).

Substances that can provoke anaphylaxis include insect stings, certain foods (such as peanuts, fish, and eggs), and a variety of drugs (especially if injected), including antibiotics (such as *penicillins), aspirin and other *NSAIDs, vaccines, and blood products.

anastrozole An *aromatase inhibitor used for the treatment of advanced breast *cancer in postmenopausal women. It is usually given to women in whom treatment with *tamoxifen has failed. Anastrozole is available as tablets on *prescription only.
Side effects: include hot flushes, sweating, vaginal dryness and irritation, thinning of the hair, nausea, vomiting, diarrhoea, weakness, insomnia, headache, and rash.
Precautions: anastrozole should not be taken by women who are pregnant or breastfeeding, have moderate to severe liver or kidney disease, or who have not yet reached the menopause.
Proprietary preparation: Arimidex.

Anbesol (SSL International) A proprietary combination of *lidocaine hydrochloride (a local anaesthetic), *cetylpyridinium chloride (an antiseptic), and *chlorocresol (a disinfectant), used for the treatment of mouth pain and minor irritations and infections of the mouth. It is available as a gel, a liquid, or a teething gel formula (in which the lidocaine concentration is lower) and can be obtained without a prescription, but only from pharmacies.

Ancotil (Meda Pharmaceuticals) *See* FLUCYTOSINE.

Andrews Antacid (GlaxoSmithKline) A proprietary combination of *magnesium carbonate and *calcium carbonate, used for the relief of upset stomach, heartburn, indigestion, and trapped wind. It is freely available *over the counter in the form of chewable tablets.
Side effects and precautions: Andrews Antacid is not recommended for children. *See also* MAGNESIUM SALTS.
Interactions with other drugs: *see* ANTACIDS.

Andrews Salts *See* ORIGINAL ANDREWS SALTS.

Androcur (Bayer) *See* CYPROTERONE ACETATE.

androgens The male sex hormones, which stimulate the development of male sex organs and male secondary sexual characteristics (beard, deep voice, body hair). These *steroid hormones are produced primarily in the testes but also, in small amounts, in the ovaries and adrenal cortex. Production is stimulated by a *gonadotrophin secreted by the pituitary gland. The main androgen is *testosterone. Androgens are used mainly as replacement therapy in castrated adult men and to treat men whose testicular function is impaired because of disease of the pituitary gland or testes. When pituitary function is poor androgen therapy can lead to normal sexual development and potency but not fertility (if fertility is desired, treatment is with gonadotrophins). *See also* MESTEROLONE.

Andropatch (GlaxoSmithKline) *See* TESTOSTERONE.

Anexate (Roche Products) *See* FLUMAZENIL.

Angeliq (Bayer) A proprietary combination of *estradiol and drospirenone (a synthetic *progestogen), used as continuous combined *hormone replacement therapy for the treatment of menopausal symptoms and prevention of osteoporosis in women who have not had a hysterectomy and who have not had a period for a year. It is available as tablets on prescription only.
Side effects, precautions, and interactions with other drugs: *see* HORMONE REPLACEMENT THERAPY.

Angettes 75 (Bristol-Myers Squibb) *See* ASPIRIN.

Angeze, Angeze SR (Opus) *See* ISOSORBIDE MONONITRATE.

angina Chest pain that results from lack of oxygen in the heart muscle. It is usually caused by narrowing of the coronary arteries, the vessels that supply blood (and therefore oxygen) to the heart muscle. In **classic** or **exertional angina**, the most common form, pain typically occurs during physical exertion or emotional stress or after a heavy meal; the underlying cause is likely to be *atherosclerosis. **Unstable angina** can occur at rest and results from spasm and constriction of the coronary arteries. Angina is most commonly treated with *nitrates, *beta blockers, or *calcium antagonists.

angioedema *See* ANAPHYLAXIS.

angiogenesis inhibitors *See* VASCULAR ENDOTHELIAL GROWTH FACTOR.

angiotensin II inhibitors (**angiotensin II antagonists**) Drugs that inhibit the action of angiotensin II, a hormone that constricts blood vessels. They have similar effects to *ACE inhibitors and are used in the treatment of *hypertension and heart failure. Unlike ACE inhibitors they do not produce a dry cough. *See* CANDESARTAN CILEXETIL; EPROSARTAN; IRBESARTAN; LOSARTAN POTASSIUM; OLMESARTAN; TELMISARTAN; VALSARTAN.
Side effects: these are usually mild; dizziness occassionally occurs, more rarely rash and oedema (swelling) of the face.
Precautions: angiotensin II inhibitors should be avoided during pregnancy and breastfeeding.
Interactions with other drugs: *see* ACE INHIBITORS.

Angiox (The Medicines Company) *See* BIVALIRUDIN.

Angitak (LPC) *See* ISOSORBIDE DINITRATE.

Angitil SR, Angitil XL (Chiesi) *See* DILTIAZEM HYDROCHLORIDE.

Anhydrol Forte (Dermal Laboratories) *See* ALUMINIUM CHLORIDE.

anidulafungin An *antifungal drug used to treat generalized candidiasis. It is available as a form for intravenous injection on *prescription only.
Side effects: include headache, diarrhoea, vomiting, nausea, rash, itching, flushing, convulsions, and disturbance in kidney function.
Precautions: anidulafungin is not recommended for use in pregnant women and should be used with caution during breastfeeding.
Proprietary preparation: Ecalta.

Anquil (Archimedes Pharma) *See* BENPERIDOL.

Antabuse (Actavis) *See* DISULFIRAM.

antacids Drugs that neutralize stomach acid. Antacids are used to treat any *acid-peptic disease. They produce rapid but brief relief of symptoms by making the stomach less acidic (raising the pH). They are best taken when symptoms are likely to occur, usually after meals or at bedtime, and are often taken four or more times daily. Antacids are alkaline salts of metals. The most commonly used ones are *aluminium hydroxide, magnesium salts (including *magnesium carbonate and *magnesium trisilicate), and carbonates (especially *sodium bicarbonate and *calcium carbonate). Aluminium and magnesium compounds are relatively insoluble in water and therefore long-acting in the stomach. Many antacid preparations contain salts of *alginic acid (e.g. magnesium alginate), which provide protection against reflux oesophagitis. Since bicarbonate salts liberate carbon dioxide, activated *dimeticone, which allows gas bubbles to coalesce and be expelled, is often added to antacid salts. This may cause belching and/or flatulence.
Side effects: magnesium-containing antacids are laxative, whereas aluminium and calcium salts are constipating. The combination of different salts usually results in a preparation with few or no side effects on the bowel. Carbonates cause belching and/or flatulence.
Precautions and interactions with other drugs: antacids can alter the *electrolyte balance and can affect the absorption of some vitamins, minerals, and other drugs. Drugs whose absorption is reported to have been reduced in the presence of antacids, and should therefore not be taken at the same time, include the following: most tetracyclines (which should not be taken within two hours of taking antacids); fosinopril; azithromycin; cefaclor; cefpodoxime; ciprofloxacin; isoniazid; levofloxacin; moxifloxacin; nitrofurantoin; norfloxacin; ofloxacin; rifampicin; gabapentin; phenytoin; itraconazole; ketoconazole; fexofenadine; dipyridamole; chloroquine; hydroxychloroquine; phenothiazines; sulpride; tipranavir; deflazocort; rosuvastatin; bisphosphonates; mycophenolate mofetil; penicillamine. Deferasirox and nilotinib should also not be taken with antacids.

antagonist A drug that opposes the action of another drug or natural body chemical. Examples are the *oestrogen antagonists.

antazoline An *antihistamine used in topical preparations. **Antazoline sulphate** is an ingredient of eye drops for the treatment of allergic conjunctivitis, such as that associated with hay fever. **Antazoline hydrochloride** is used in an ointment for the relief of insect stings and bites. Preparations containing antazoline can be obtained without a prescription, but only from pharmacies.
Side effects: the ointment may cause allergic reactions.
Precautions: the ointment should not be used for longer than three days and should not be used for treating eczema.
Proprietary preparations: Wasp-Eze Ointment; *Otrivine-Antistin (combined with xylometazoline).

Antepsin (Chugai Pharma) *See* SUCRALFATE.

anthelmintics (**antihelminthics**) Drugs used to destroy parasitic worms (such as tapeworms, roundworms, and threadworms) and/or to expel them from the intestine. *See* MEBENDAZOLE; PIPERAZINE.

Anthisan (sanofi-aventis) *See* MEPYRAMINE.

anthracyclines *See* CYTOTOXIC ANTIBIOTICS.

anti-androgens Drugs that antagonize the action of *androgens. They are used for the treatment of severe hypersexuality and sexual deviation in men and can also be used as an *adjunct in the treatment of prostate cancer and excessive body hair and acne in women. *See* BICALUTAMIDE; CYPROTERONE ACETATE; DUTASTERIDE; FINASTERIDE; FLUTAMIDE.

anti-arrhythmic drugs (**anti-arrhythmics**) Drugs used for treating disordered heart rhythms (*see* ARRHYTHMIA). Anti-arrhythmic drugs either slow the flow of electrical impulses to the heart muscle or inhibit the ability of heart muscles to respond to these impulses; they are classified as class I, II, III, or IV anti-arrhythmics, depending on their mode of action. Class I drugs affect the response of the heart muscle to the signal received and may be subdivided into classes Ia (e.g. *disopyramide); Ib (e.g. *lidocaine); and Ic (e.g. *propafenone hydrochloride and *flecainide acetate). Class II anti-arrhythmic drugs are *beta blockers, which reduce the ability of the pacemaker to pass electrical signals to the heart muscle. Class III drugs include *amiodarone. Class IV comprise some, but not all, *calcium antagonists, which interfere with the conduction of nerve impulses in the atria. Other drugs used are *cardiac glycosides (digitalis drugs, such as *digoxin), which affect the way signals are transmitted in the heart, and *adenosine.
Side effects: many of these drugs can depress normal heart function and may produce dizziness on standing (postural hypotension) or breathlessness on exertion. Mild nausea and visual disturbances are quite common. Side effects specific to particular drugs are listed in their entries.
Precautions and interactions with other drugs: the effects of anti-arrhythmic

drugs tend to be additive, therefore specialist care is necessary if two or more are used. Most of the drugs that control arrhythmias can also provoke them in some circumstances. Low *potassium concentrations can enhance this effect; it is important, therefore, that when people are taking diuretics with anti-arrhythmic drugs, a potassium-sparing diuretic is used either alone or in combination with a loop diuretic or a thiazide diuretic. Details of specific interactions are given at entries for individual drugs.

antibacterial drugs *See* ANTIBIOTICS.

antibiotics Originally, natural products secreted by microorganisms (microbes) that inhibit the growth of other microörganisms. The term is now commonly used, however, to denote any drug, natural or synthetic, that has a selective toxic action on bacteria, protozoans, or other single-celled microorganisms. Antibiotics are not active against viruses (*see* ANTIVIRAL DRUGS). The more accurate term is therefore **antimicrobials.** While many are now produced synthetically, they are still based on the natural compounds. Antibiotics used to treat bacterial infections are called **antibacterial** drugs. Antibacterials may kill bacteria, in which case they are described as **bactericidal**, or they may prevent bacterial growth, when they are referred to as **bacteriostatic**. They are usually designed to exploit some aspect of bacterial structure that is not present in mammalian cells and therefore they do not harm human cells. For example, **beta-lactam antibiotics**, including *penicillins and *cephalosporins, attack bacterial cell walls; mammalian cells do not have cell walls. *Aminoglycosides and *tetracyclines attack bacterial ribosomes (the protein-synthesizing machinery of the cell), which are different from mammalian ribosomes. Antibiotics that are active against a wide variety of microorganisms are known as **broad-spectrum antibiotics**; those effective only against particular microbes are called **narrow-spectrum antibiotics.** Widespread use of antibiotics results in bacteria developing resistance to these agents. Antibiotics are therefore, in most Western countries, *prescription only medicines. The normal healthy human body contains several types of bacteria and other microbes, notably in the gut. Use of antibiotics can have a harmful effect on some of these microbes, which results in the overgrowth of others causing **superinfections**, which may present more problems than the original infection. *See* MACROLIDE ANTIBIOTICS; QUINOLONES.

anticholinergic drugs *See* ANTIMUSCARINIC DRUGS.

anticholinesterases Drugs that inhibit the action of cholinesterases, the enzymes that break down *acetylcholine. They therefore prolong the activity of acetylcholine and cause an exaggerated response of the *parasympathetic nervous system, i.e. they are *cholinergic drugs. They have the opposite action to *antimuscarinic drugs. Anticholinesterases are used at the end of surgical operations to reverse the paralysis induced by skeletal *muscle relaxants. They are also used to treat or diagnose myasthenia gravis, an autoimmune condition in which nerve impulses to the muscles are diminished, causing

a

extreme weakness and fatigability of the muscles. By preventing the breakdown of acetylcholine, anticholinesterases enable the transmission of nerve impulses to the muscles to be prolonged. Anticholinesterases have a limited role in relieving urinary retention and paralysis of the bowel, especially after surgery. The commonly used anticholinesterases are *pyridostigmine, *edrophonium, and *neostigmine.

anticoagulants Drugs used to prevent the formation of blood clots, or the extension of an existing blood clot, in the veins. They are widely used for the prevention and treatment of deep-vein *thrombosis in the legs. Anticoagulants are less effective at preventing blood-clot formation in the arteries, but they are used to prevent clots forming in cardiac aneurysms (balloon-like swellings in the walls of the heart) or on artificial heart valves. Anticoagulants may be given before open-heart surgery or kidney dialysis, and patients may be given them after surgery to prevent deep-vein thrombosis.

Oral anticoagulants (mainly *warfarin sodium; *acenocoumarol and *phenindione are now rarely used) act by antagonizing the effects of vitamin K, which is essential for the formation of clotting factors. It may take 72 hours before their full anticoagulant effect occurs. *Dabigatran etexilate is an oral anticoagulant that acts by inhibiting blood clotting. *Heparins, which are given by injection, also directly interfere with the blood-clotting process. They are relatively fast acting. The two types of anticoagulants may be given in combination. Often patients are started on a combination of heparin and warfarin and the heparin is discontinued once the warfarin takes full effect. Other anticoagulants given by injection are the hirudins (*bivalirudin and *lepirudin), *fondaparinux sodium, and *epoprostenol.
Side effects and precautions: the most serious adverse effect of anticoagulants is the risk of excessive bleeding, usually from overdosage. People who are taking anticoagulant therapy therefore need to have the clotting times of their blood measured frequently. Clotting times are usually expressed in terms of the **INR** (International Normalized Ratio). Prolonged clotting times (indicating overdosage) may be shown by easy bruising. For other side effects and precautions, as well as interactions with other drugs, *see* HEPARIN; WARFARIN SODIUM.

anticonvulsant drugs Drugs used to prevent or reduce the severity and frequency of seizures (convulsions). Seizures occur when the electrical activity in the brain that controls the movement of the limbs becomes paroxysmal and chaotic. The most common form of seizures is **epilepsy**. Since not all seizures involve convulsions, and not all types of convulsion are epileptic seizures, the term **antiepileptic** is often preferred to describe medication for treating epilepsy. Most people with epilepsy need to take anticonvulsants on a regular basis until they have been free of seizures for two years. The type of drug used will depend on the type of epilepsy, although a patient's age and response to treatment may also affect the choice of drug.

Tonic-clonic (or major) seizures (formerly called 'grand mal'), in which a period of unconsciousness is followed by convulsions, usually last only a few minutes; prolonged attacks, in which repeated seizures occur with no intervening recovery of consciousness, are called **status epilepticus**. The main drugs used to treat major seizures are *carbamazepine, *sodium valproate, and (more recently) *lamotrigine; *phenobarbital and *primidone may also be used but are more sedating. Drugs used in the treatment of status epilepticus include *lorazepam, *diazepam, *clonazepam, and fosphenytoin (*see* PHENYTOIN). Absence seizures (formerly called 'petit mal'), which usually affect children and consist of a momentary loss of consciousness during which posture and balance are maintained, are treated with *ethosuximide, sodium valproate, and (less commonly) clonazepam. Partial seizures, in which the nature of the seizure depends on the part of the brain that is affected, are most commonly treated with sodium valproate, carbamazepine, *oxcarbazepine, and lamotrigine; phenobarbital and primidone may also be effective. *Phenytoin is effective in treating both tonic-clonic and partial seizures, but dosage requires frequent adjustment and side effects can be severe. *Vigabatrin, *gabapentin, *pregabalin, *lacosamide, *levetiracetam, *zonisamide, *tiagabine, and *topiramate are newer anticonvulsants that may be used as *adjuncts to (or replacements for) older medicines.

antidepressant drugs Drugs that act to relieve the symptoms of moderate to severe depression. Antidepressant drugs usually need to be taken for 2 weeks before their effect is apparent, and full benefit may not be felt for 6–8 weeks. They are generally continued for 4–6 months after the depression has resolved, and if the condition is recurrent, medication may be continued for years. Most antidepressants are dangerous in overdose and should therefore be prescribed in small quantities (prescriptions for one month are common). If stopped suddenly after having been taken for eight weeks or more, withdrawal symptoms (including nausea, vomiting, and weakness) may occur. Depression is thought to be related to abnormal function of the transmitters *noradrenaline and/or *serotonin. After these transmitters have been released in the brain they will stimulate brain cells and then be taken up again by nerve endings, broken down, and hence inactivated. Some antidepressant drugs inhibit the reuptake mechanism, while others prevent breakdown of the transmitters; both actions result in a longer duration of action of these transmitters. The mechanism of action of other antidepressants is less clear.

Antidepressants elevate mood, increase the capacity for physical activity, improve the appetite, and restore activity in everyday life. Some antidepressants are sedative in nature and are especially useful when depression is accompanied by anxiety and insomnia. The main classes of antidepressants are the *tricyclic antidepressants, the *monoamine oxidase inhibitors (MAOIs), the selective serotonin reuptake inhibitors (*SSRIs), and *lithium salts. *See also* AGOMELATINE; DULOXETINE; FLUPENTIXOL; MIRTAZAPINE; REBOXETINE; TRYPTOPHAN; VENLAFAXINE.

antidiabetic drugs *See* INSULIN; ORAL HYPOGLYCAEMIC DRUGS.

antidiarrhoeal drugs Drugs used for the treatment of diarrhoea. *Electrolyte solutions are used to replace fluid and salts that are lost in acute diarrhoea (*see* ORAL REHYDRATION THERAPY). *Bulk-forming laxatives, such as *methylcellulose, are used for treating chronic diarrhoea associated with diverticular disease and irritable bowel syndrome, and to adjust consistency of the faeces in other diseases of the bowel. Adsorbents, such as *kaolin, adsorb irritant substances that cause diarrhoea, but they are not recommended for treating acute diarrhoea. Opioids, such as *codeine phosphate, *loperamide hydrochloride, *co-phenotrope, and *morphine, act by slowing down the movement of the gut and increasing transit time and are used as *adjuncts in the treatment of acute diarrhoea and some chronic diarrhoeas.

anti-D (Rh_0) immunoglobulin An *immunoglobulin that is given to all rhesus-negative pregnant women, especially those who have recently given birth to a baby who is rhesus-positive (or who have miscarried or aborted a rhesus-positive fetus) in order to prevent them from forming antibodies to rhesus-positive fetal cells that may pass into their blood during subsequent pregnancies. The aim is to protect the woman's subsequent children from haemolytic disease of the newborn (*see* ANAEMIA). Anti-D immunoglobulin is available as a solution for injection (usually intramuscular) on *prescription only.
Proprietary preparations: D-GAM; Partobulin SDF; Rhophylac (intramuscular or intravenous injection).

antidiuretic hormone *See* VASOPRESSIN.

antiemetics Drugs that stop or prevent vomiting and, to a lesser extent, nausea. They are used to prevent motion sickness and the nausea associated with Ménière's disease, to prevent or treat the nausea and vomiting caused by *cytotoxic drug therapy for cancer and some other drug treatments, and to treat nausea and vomiting associated with diseases of the stomach, duodenum, liver, and gall bladder or experienced after some types of surgery. Antiemetics should not be taken unless the reason for the vomiting and/or nausea is known. In some circumstances, for example after the ingestion of a poison or contaminated food, vomiting is beneficial and should not be stopped. On the other hand, severe or prolonged vomiting may be a sign of a more serious underlying condition and should be reported to a doctor. Antiemetics should not be given to people with obstruction of the gut, and they are not advised during the first three months of pregnancy unless the vomiting is so severe that a doctor considers them necessary.

Antiemetics include *hyoscine hydrobromide and certain *antihistamines (for motion sickness), *phenothiazines, *droperidol, *domperidone, *metoclopramide, *ondansetron, *granisetron, *palonosetron, *aprepitant, and *fosaprepitant.

antiepileptic drugs *See* ANTICONVULSANT DRUGS.

antifibrinolytic drugs *See* HAEMOSTATIC DRUGS.

a

antifungal drugs Drugs that are used to treat infections caused by fungi (including yeasts). The most common fungal infections are **tinea** (**ringworm**) and **candidiasis** (**thrush**). Tinea is caused by fungi called dermatophytes, which feed on keratin (the principal protein of the skin, hair, and nails). Tinea most commonly affects the skin between the toes (athlete's foot), the scalp, the skin beneath a beard, the groin, and the nail bed (where it can be deep-seated). Thrush is caused by overgrowth of the yeast *Candida albicans*, normally a harmless inhabitant of the gastrointestinal tract and vagina. This can occur when the normal balance of the body's microorganisms is upset, for example in people taking drugs (e.g. antibiotics, oral contraceptives), or when the body's resistance to infection is lowered, for example in people with diabetes and pregnant women. The infection is usually confined to the mouth, vagina, or skin folds (it can infect napkin rash in babies), but in severely immunocompromised people (for example those whose immune systems are impaired by AIDS) candidiasis can spread throughout the body. Such people are also susceptible to other systemic fungal infections (e.g. *Cryptococcus neoformans*).

A variety of drugs is available for treating fungal infections; some of them are also active against bacteria (*see* ANTIBIOTICS). Many of them act on the cell walls of fungi to make them permeable so that the contents of the cell leak out and the fungus dies. The *imidazole antifungal drugs are used mainly to treat candidiasis (especially of the vagina) and various forms of tinea; they are usually applied locally (as pessaries, creams, powders, etc.), although some can also be taken orally for treating persistent infections (*see* CLOTRIMAZOLE; ECONAZOLE NITRATE; KETOCONAZOLE; MICONAZOLE; SULCONAZOLE; TIOCONAZOLE). The triazoles (*see* FLUCONAZOLE; ITRACONAZOLE; POSACONAZOLE; VORICONAZOLE) are usually taken orally. Other antifungal drugs include *griseofulvin and *terbinafine (usually taken orally for treating tinea) and *nystatin. For treating deep-seated or systemic infections, such drugs as *amphotericin, fluconazole, *anidulafungin, *caspofungin, and *micafungin are administered by injection; *flucytosine is used specifically for treating systemic yeast infections. Antifungal drugs applied topically rarely cause side effects, but treatment by mouth or injection may produce severe adverse effects and must be monitored carefully. *See also* AMOROLFINE; TOLNAFTATE; UNDECENOIC ACID.

antihaemophilic factor *See* FACTOR VIII.

antihelminthics *See* ANTHELMINTICS.

antihistamines (**H_1-receptor antagonists**) A class of drugs that antagonize the effect of *histamine, a substance released by the body in large amounts during allergic reactions. Antihistamines act by blocking H_1 receptors in the skin, nose, and airways: these receptors – when stimulated by histamine – produce the symptoms of an allergic response. They relieve the sneezing, running nose, and itching associated with allergic rhinitis, including hay fever (seasonal allergic rhinitis). They are also used to treat urticaria (an itchy rash commonly occurring as an allergic reaction to eating such foods as shellfish and strawberries), other itching skin conditions, and the histamine-induced reaction to insect bites or stings. For allergic reactions antihistamines may be given as nasal sprays or inhaled; they are also taken by mouth to prevent or treat symptoms. Antihistamines may be injected intravenously as an *adjunct to *adrenaline and/or corticosteroids to relieve life-threatening *anaphylaxis – an extreme allergic reaction. Some antihistamines (e.g. *cinnarizine, *cyclizine, and *promethazine) are used as *antiemetics or to treat vertigo or Ménière's disease. The older antihistamines (especially promethazine and *alimemazine and – to a lesser extent – *chlorphenamine and cyclizine) cause drowsiness and some of them are used for their *hypnotic effect, for example in preparations used for treating coughs and colds and in non-prescription sleeping tablets. These antihistamines can impair the ability to drive or operate machinery; alcohol enhances this effect. The newer antihistamines, including *cetirizine, *desloratadine, *fexofenadine, *levocetirizine, *loratadine, and *mizolastine) are less sedating.

See also AZELASTINE HYDROCHLORIDE; CLEMASTINE; CYPROHEPTADINE HYDROCHLORIDE; HYDROXYZINE HYDROCHLORIDE.

Side effects: the older antihistamines cause sedation or drowsiness and (less commonly) headache, antimuscarinic effects (e.g. difficulty in urinating, dry mouth, blurred vision), and stomach upsets. The newer antihistamines are less sedating and are less likely to cause antimuscarinic effects.

Precautions: alcohol enhances the sedating effects of the older antihistamines. Antihistamines should be used with caution by people with epilepsy, an enlarged prostate gland, glaucoma, or liver disease and by women who are pregnant or breastfeeding.

Interactions with other drugs:

Antidepressants: the sedative and antimuscarinic effects of antihistamines are increased if they are taken with monoamine oxidase inhibitors or tricyclic antidepressants.

Anxiolytic and hypnotic drugs: increase the sedative effects of antihistamines.

anti-human thymocyte immunoglobulin An *immunoglobulin, derived from the rabbit, that acts as an antibody against lymphocytes (a type of white blood cell) produced in the thymus. It is used as an *immunosuppressant to prevent rejection of kidney and heart transplants and is available as a form for injection on *prescription only.

Side effects: allergic reactions may occur, which can be minimized by giving an antihistamine and a corticosteroid before treatment. Other side effects include low white blood cell counts, fever, infection, muscle pain, breathlessness, and low blood pressure.

Precautions: this medicine should not be given to patients with infections or to breastfeeding women and should be used with caution in pregnant women. Blood counts should be monitored during treatment.

Proprietary preparation: Thymoglobuline.

antihypertensive drugs (**antihypertensives**) Drugs used in the treatment of *hypertension (high blood pressure), either alone or in combination. They

work in a variety of ways, some of which are not completely understood, and some antihypertensive drugs have more than one action. The main classes of antihypertensive drugs are *ACE inhibitors, *alpha blockers, *angiotensin II inhibitors, *beta blockers, *calcium antagonists, *diuretics, and *vasodilators. Some drugs act centrally (on the brain) to reduce blood pressure (*see* CLONIDINE HYDROCHLORIDE; METHYLDOPA). The overall aim of treatment is to reduce the pressure in the arterial system.
Side effects: see entries for individual classes of drugs.
Precautions: some dosage adjustment may be needed at the start of treatment. It is important to continue taking antihypertensive medication even if the problem appears to be under control. Sudden withdrawal of some of these drugs may cause a potentially dangerous 'rebound' increase in blood pressure; dosage reduction needs to be gradual and under medical supervision.

anti-inflammatory drugs Drugs that act against the body's chemicals that initiate or maintain inflammation. The main class comprises the non-steroidal anti-inflammatory drugs (*see* NSAIDs). Other drugs with anti-inflammatory activity include the glucocorticoids (*see* CORTICOSTEROIDS).

antimetabolites A class of *cytotoxic drugs that act by combining with enzymes in cells to prevent the synthesis of nuclear material (DNA) and cell division. They are used for the treatment of a wide variety of *cancers. The most commonly used antimetabolites are *methotrexate, *cytarabine, *fludarabine, *cladribine, *gemcitabine, *fluorouracil, *raltitrexed, *mercaptopurine, and *tioguanine. *See also* CAPECITABINE; CLOFARABINE; NELARABINE; PEMETREXED; RALTITREXED.

antimicrobial drugs *See* ANTIBIOTICS.

antimuscarinic drugs (**anticholinergic drugs**) A class of drugs that block the activity of *acetylcholine at **muscarinic** receptors (a subdivision of acetylcholine receptors). They tend to relax smooth muscle (including that of the airways and the gut), reduce the secretion of saliva, digestive juices, and sweat, and dilate the pupil of the eye. They are used as *antiparkinsonian drugs, as *antispasmodics in the treatment of gastrointestinal pain, as *bronchodilators, and to treat incontinence; they are also used to dilate the pupil of the eye in ophthalmic examinations, to antagonize the effects of *anticholinesterases, and to increase the heart rate in certain circumstances.
Side effects: characteristic side effects of antimuscarinic drugs include dry mouth, thirst, blurred vision, dry skin, increased heart rate (following an initial slowing of the heart rate), and difficulty in urinating. Side effects occurring more rarely include confusion (especially in elderly people), drowsiness, dizziness, nausea, and vomiting.
Precautions: antimuscarinics should not be taken by people with closed-angle (acute) *glaucoma, myasthenia gravis, intestinal obstruction due to loss of movement in the intestine, pyloric stenosis, and enlargement of the prostate. They should be used with caution in children and the elderly and in

people with reflux oesophagitis, diarrhoea, ulcerative colitis, hypertension (high blood pressure), and conditions causing a fast heart rate.
Interactions with other drugs: taking two or more antimuscarinic drugs together can increase their side effects. Drugs that can increase antimuscarinic effects include amantadine, antihistamines, disopyramide, nefopam, MAOIs, and tricyclic antidepressants.

anti-oestrogens *See* OESTROGEN ANTAGONISTS.

antiparkinsonian drugs Drugs used to treat Parkinson's disease or parkinsonism. These conditions result from a disease process affecting the basal ganglia, the part of the brain responsible for controlling voluntary movement at a subconscious level, and are associated with a deficiency of the neurotransmitter *dopamine. This gives rise to an imbalance between the actions of dopamine and another neurotransmitter, *acetylcholine, and results in disorders of movement, notably tremor, rigidity, and slow movements. A distinction is sometimes made between Parkinson's disease, a degenerative condition associated with ageing, and parkinsonism, parkinsonian symptoms due to other causes; for example, the long-term use of antipsychotic drugs (*see* EXTRAPYRAMIDAL REACTIONS).

A variety of drugs are available for treating the condition. *Levodopa, which is converted to dopamine in the body, is used as replacement therapy. *Selegiline and *rasagiline prevent the breakdown of dopamine in the body; *entacapone and tolcapone prevent the breakdown of levodopa. Dopamine agonists (*see* BROMOCRIPTINE; CABERGOLINE; PERGOLIDE; PRAMIPEXOLE; ROPINIROLE; ROTIGOTINE) increase the action of dopamine by stimulating dopamine receptors in the brain. *Antimuscarinic drugs block the activity of acetylcholine in the brain and thus act to correct the imbalance between dopamine and acetylcholine. They are less effective than levodopa, although they often supplement its action. Patients with mild symptoms may be treated initially with antimuscarinic drugs (alone or with selegiline), levodopa being added at a later stage as symptoms progress. They are also useful in reversing drug-induced extrapyramidal reactions. The common antimuscarinic drugs used in treating parkinsonism are *trihexyphenidyl hydrochloride, *orphenadrine, and *procyclidine. *See also* AMANTADINE HYDROCHLORIDE.

antiplatelet drugs A class of drugs that reduce the ability of platelets (specialized blood cells) to stick together, which occurs normally as part of the blood-clotting process. Antiplatelet drugs are used to prevent the formation of blood clots in arteries, when *anticoagulants are ineffective (*see* THROMBOSIS). The most commonly used antiplatelet drug is *aspirin, which is used (in low daily doses) for the prevention of strokes or heart attacks in people who have had a previous stroke or heart attack. Low-dose aspirin is also given to people at risk of having a heart attack or stroke and after heart bypass surgery or the insertion of stents (tubes) into the coronary arteries to reduce the risk of clots obstructing the grafts or stents, respectively. Other antiplatelet drugs include *clopidogrel, *abciximab, *epoprostenol, *prasugrel, *tirofiban, and *eptifibatide.

antipruritics Agents that relieve itching (pruritus). Examples are *calamine, *crotamiton, *camphor, and *lauromacrogols, applied in creams or lotions. Some *antihistamines, in the form of creams or tablets, are used if the itching is due to an allergy.

antipsychotic drugs (**neuroleptic drugs**) A group of drugs formerly known as **major tranquillizers** (*compare* ANXIOLYTIC DRUGS). Antipsychotic drugs are used in the short term to calm or sedate patients who are severely disturbed, agitated, hostile, or aggressive. They control the acute symptoms of mania (such as extreme overactivity, incoherence, and extravagant behaviour) and relieve acute positive symptoms of schizophrenia (such as disordered thinking, delusions, and hallucinations); long-term treatment is usually required for patients with schizophrenia in order to prevent relapses. Most antipsychotic drugs are less effective in treating the negative symptoms of schizophrenia (e.g. apathy and withdrawal), although some have an alerting effect. Antipsychotic drugs are also used for the short-term treatment of severe anxiety and some also have an *antidepressant effect. Antipsychotic drugs produce their actions by reducing the activity of the neurotransmitter *dopamine in the brain; however, they also affect other body functions controlled by dopamine, which causes a group of troublesome side effects known as *extrapyramidal reactions. These drugs also interfere with the action of other neurotransmitters, including acetylcholine, which produces antimuscarinic effects (*see* ANTIMUSCARINIC DRUGS).

Antipsychotic drugs belong to various different chemical groups, including the *phenothiazines (e.g. *chlorpromazine), **butyrophenones** (e.g. *haloperidol and *benperidol), and **thioxanthenes** (e.g. *flupentixol, *zuclopenthixol); other antipsychotics are *sulpiride and *pimozide. The **atypical antipsychotics** are a group of more recently developed drugs that have less effect on dopamine activity, producing their action by interfering with other neurotransmitters, especially *serotonin (5-hydroxytryptamine). They therefore have less pronounced extrapyramidal reactions than conventional antipsychotic drugs. Atypical antipsychotic drugs are used to treat patients who have not responded to, or cannot tolerate, conventional antipsychotic drugs; they include *amisulpride, *aripiprazole, *olanzapine, *paliperidone, *risperidone, *quetiapine, *clozapine, and *zotepine.
Side effects, precautions, and interactions with other drugs: see entries for individual drugs.

antipyretics Drugs that reduce fever by lowering body temperature. The most commonly used antipyretics are *aspirin and *paracetamol.

antiretroviral drugs *See* ANTIVIRAL DRUGS.

antisecretory drug Any drug that reduces the normal rate of secretion of a body fluid, usually one that reduces acid secretion into the stomach. Such drugs include *antimuscarinic drugs, *H_2-receptor antagonists, and *proton pump inhibitors.

antiseptic A chemical that destroys or inhibits the growth of disease-causing bacteria and other microorganisms and is sufficiently nontoxic to be applied to the skin or mucous membranes to cleanse wounds and prevent infections or to be used internally to treat infections of the intestine and bladder. Examples are *cetrimide, *chlorhexidine, *methenamine hippurate, *triclosan, *cetylpyridinium chloride, and *dequalinium.

antispasmodics Drugs that relax the smooth muscle of the gut. They are used as an *adjunct in the treatment of indigestion not associated with peptic ulcers, of irritable bowel syndrome, and of diverticular disease (which causes abdominal pain and altered bowel habit). The main agents are *antimuscarinic drugs (such as *dicycloverine hydrochloride, *propantheline bromide, *atropine sulphate, and *hyoscine butylbromide), *alverine citrate, *mebeverine hydrochloride, and *peppermint oil.

anti-TNF drugs *See* DISEASE-MODIFYING ANTIRHEUMATIC DRUGS.

antitussives *See* COUGH SUPPRESSANTS.

anti-VEGF drugs *See* VASCULAR ENDOTHELIAL GROWTH FACTOR.

antiviral drugs Drugs used to treat infections caused by viruses. Because viruses can only function within the cells of their hosts, it has been difficult to produce drugs that act specifically against viruses without damaging their host cells. The effectiveness of antiviral drugs is therefore limited: frequently they will contain an outbreak of viral activity but are not capable of totally eradicating the infection, which can recur (as with cold sores). Fortunately, the majority of viral infections resolve spontaneously in most people and do not require specific medication. However, in immunocompromised individuals, whose ability to fight infection is impaired because of drug therapy (e.g. immunosuppressants) or disease (e.g. AIDS), antiviral treatment may be life-saving.

Many antiviral drugs act by interfering with DNA production and thus prevent the virus from replicating (*see* ACICLOVIR; CIDOFOVIR; FAMCICLOVIR; FOSCARNET; GANCICLOVIR; PENCICLOVIR; VALACICLOVIR; VALGANCICLOVIR). Some are **nucleoside** or **nucleotide analogues**: similar to the nucleosides or nucleotides (building blocks) of DNA, they become incorporated into the new DNA being made by the virus, but – since they are not the correct nucleoside or nucleotide – they will stop any further DNA synthesis (*see* ADEFOVIR DIPIVOXIL; ENTECAVIR; IDOXURIDINE; RIBAVIRIN). *Amantadine hydrochloride, *oseltamivir, and *zanamivir act specifically against influenza viruses.

Antiretroviral drugs are antiviral drugs that act specifically against a particular group of viruses, the retroviruses, the best known of which is the human immunodeficiency virus (*HIV), which causes AIDS. Retroviruses contain RNA (rather than DNA) as their genetic material; this is converted to DNA by the virus inside its host cell by means of the enzyme reverse transcriptase. The **nucleoside reverse transcriptase inhibitors** prevent retroviral replication by becoming incorporated into the growing strand of viral DNA (*see* ABACAVIR; DIDANOSINE; EMTRICITABINE; LAMIVUDINE; STAVUDINE; TENOFOVIR DISOPROXIL; ZIDOVUDINE). **Non-nucleoside reverse transcriptase**

inhibitors (*see* EFAVIRENZ; ETRAVIRINE; NEVIRAPINE) bind directly to the enzyme to prevent its action. The **protease inhibitors** act by preventing the action of a protease, a protein-cleaving enzyme that is needed by the virus to produce mature virus particles (*see* ATAZANAVIR; DARUNAVIR; FOSAMPRENAVIR; INDINAVIR; NELFINAVIR; RITONAVIR; SAQUINAVIR; TIPRANAVIR). These drugs are used in combination with other antiretroviral drugs (known as **highly active antiretroviral therapy**) for the treatment of HIV infection. However they also inhibit an enzyme system in the liver that is involved in metabolizing many drugs; there is therefore a potential for drug interactions in people taking protease inhibitors. *Enfuvirtide, *maraviroc, and *raltegravir are used for treating HIV that has not responded to combinations of other antiretroviral drugs.

See also INTERFERONS.

Anturan (Amdipharm) *See* SULFINPYRAZONE.

Anugesic-HC (Pfizer) A proprietary combination of *zinc oxide and *bismuth oxide (astringents), *pramocaine hydrochloride (a local anaesthetic), *hydrocortisone (a corticosteroid), *Peru balsam, and benzyl benzoate (a *surfactant), used to relieve the discomfort of *haemorrhoids, anal itching, and other painful conditions of the anorectal region. It is available as a cream on *prescription only.
Side effects: *see* CORTICOSTEROIDS.
Precautions: Anugesic-HC should not be used when viral or fungal infection is present and should not be used for longer than seven days. It is not recommended for children.

Anugesic-HC Suppositories (Pfizer) A proprietary combination of *zinc oxide, *bismuth subgallate, and *bismuth oxide (astringents), *pramocaine hydrochloride (a local anaesthetic), *hydrocortisone (a corticosteroid), *Peru balsam, and benzyl benzoate (a *surfactant), used to relieve the discomfort of *haemorrhoids, anal itching, and other conditions of the anorectal region. It is available on *prescription only.
Side effects: *see* CORTICOSTEROIDS.
Precautions: these suppositories should not be used when viral or fungal infection is present and should not be used for longer than seven days. They are not recommended for children.

Anusol (McNeil Ltd) A proprietary combination of *zinc oxide and *bismuth oxide (astringents) and *Peru balsam, used to relieve the discomfort of *haemorrhoids, anal itching, and other painful anorectal conditions. It is available as a cream; Anusol ointment and suppositories also contain *bismuth subgallate. All these preparations are freely available *over the counter.

Anusol-HC (McNeil Ltd) A proprietary combination of *zinc oxide, *bismuth subgallate, and *bismuth oxide (astringents), *hydrocortisone (a corticosteroid), *Peru balsam, and benzyl benzoate (a *surfactant), used for the relief of *haemorrhoids and other painful anorectal conditions. It is

available as an ointment or suppositories on *prescription only; **Anusol Plus HC** ointment or suppositories can be obtained from pharmacies without a prescription.
Side effects: *see* CORTICOSTEROIDS.
Precautions: Anusol-HC should not be used when viral or fungal infection is present and should not be used for longer than seven days. It is not recommended for children.

anxiolytic drugs (**sedatives**) Drugs that reduce anxiety; they were formerly known as **minor tranquillizers** (*compare* ANTIPSYCHOTIC DRUGS). Anxiolytics should only be used to relieve anxiety that is severe or disabling. They will also induce sleep when taken at night (*see* HYPNOTIC DRUGS). Physical and psychological *dependence can develop with prolonged use, and these drugs should only be used for short periods and then withdrawn gradually. The lowest effective dosage should be used and discontinued as soon as possible. Anxiolytics may impair judgment and increase reaction time, affecting the ability to drive or operate machinery. They increase the effects of alcohol, and the hangover effects of a night-time dose may impair driving the following day. The most commonly used anxiolytics are the *benzodiazepines and *buspirone.

Apidra (sanofi-aventis) *See* INSULIN.

apomorphine hydrochloride An *antiparkinsonian drug used for the treatment of 'off' episodes in Parkinson's disease, when the condition is poorly controlled by *levodopa. It acts by stimulating *dopamine receptors in the brain. *Domperidone is given before, and during the first weeks of, treatment with apomorphine in order to minimize the nausea that this drug causes (see below). Apomorphine is available as a solution for injection on *prescription only.
Side effects: include nausea and vomiting, drowsiness, confusion, instability of posture with a tendency to fall, impairment of cognitive abilities, and personality changes.
Precautions: apomorphine should not be given to people who are hypersensitive to opioids or who have depressed breathing or liver disease or to women who are breastfeeding. It should be used with caution in people who have a tendency to nausea and vomiting, in those with psychiatric problems, lung, liver, or heart disease, and in the elderly.
Interactions with other drugs:
Antipsychotics: these drugs antagonize the action of apomorphine.
Methyldopa: antagonizes the action of apomorphine.
Proprietary preparation: APO-go.

apraclonidine A *sympathomimetic drug, similar to *brimonidine, that stimulates alpha *adrenoceptors. It is used to reduce the pressure inside the eye in the short-term treatment of chronic (open-angle) *glaucoma and following some types of eye surgery: it is thought to act by reducing the production of aqueous fluid and also by aiding the drainage of fluid from the

eye. Unlike brimonidine, it may dilate the pupil. Its benefits usually diminish after one month. Apraclonidine is available as eye drops on *prescription only.
Side effects: include allergic reactions in the eye, dry mouth, and taste disturbances.
Precautions: apraclonidine should not be used by people with a history of unstable angina or severe heart disease and should be used with caution in those with liver or kidney disease and by women who are pregnant or breastfeeding. It should not be used by those who wear soft contact lenses.
Interactions with other drugs:
MAOIs: should not be used with apraclonidine.
Tricyclic antidepressants: should not be used with apraclonidine.
Proprietary preparation: Iopidine.

aprepitant An *antiemetic drug used as an *adjunct to *dexamethasone and *ondansetron (or a similarly acting drug) for the prevention of nausea and vomiting in patients receiving chemotherapy. It is available as capsules on *prescription only.
Side effects: include headache, dizziness, hiccups, constipation, diarrhoea, indigestion, loss of appetite, and fatigue.
Precautions: aprepitant should not be taken by women who are pregnant or breastfeeding. It reduces the effectiveness of oral contraceptives, therefore other methods of contraception should be used during treatment.
Interactions with other drugs:
Pimozide: should not be taken with aprepitant.
St John's wort: should not be taken with aprepitant.
Proprietary preparation: Emend.

Apresoline (Amdipharm) *See* HYDRALAZINE HYDROCHLORIDE.

Aprinox (Sovereign Medical) *See* BENDROFLUMETHIAZIDE.

Aprovel (Bristol-Myers Squibb; sanofi-aventis) *See* IRBESARTAN.

Aptivus (Boehringer Ingelheim) *See* TIPRANAVIR.

Aquadrate (Alliance) *See* UREA.

aqueous cream A mixture of *liquid paraffin and *white soft paraffin (both emollients), used for the relief of dry skin disorders. It is freely available *over the counter.
Side effects: *see* LIQUID PARAFFIN; WHITE SOFT PARAFFIN.

arachis oil (**peanut oil**) An oil extracted from peanuts. It is an ingredient of emulsions used in nutrition. It is also used in an enema, as a *faecal softener for the treatment of constipation and impacted faeces, as an *emollient in creams, and as an ingredient of ear drops for softening earwax.
Precautions: arachis oil should not be used by people allergic to peanuts.
Proprietary preparations: Fletchers' Arachis Oil Retention Enema; Oilatum Cream (emollient); *Cerumol (combined with paradichlorobenzene and chlorobutanol); *Earex Ear Drops (combined with camphor and almond oil);

*Hydromol Cream (combined with isopropyl myristate, liquid paraffin, sodium lactate, and sodium pyrrolidone); *Polytar (combined with tar, coal tar, and oleyl alcohol).

Aranesp (Amgen) *See* ERYTHROPOIETIN.

Arava (sanofi-aventis) *See* LEFLUNOMIDE.

Arcoxia (Merck Sharp & Dohme) *See* ETORICOXIB.

Aredia (Novartis) *See* DISODIUM PAMIDRONATE.

argipressin *See* VASOPRESSIN.

Aricept, Aricept Evess (Eisai) *See* DONEPEZIL HYDROCHLORIDE.

Arimidex (AstraZeneca) *See* ANASTROZOLE.

aripiprazole An atypical *antipsychotic drug used for the treatment of schizophrenia in adults and in adolescents 15 years and older, as well as for the treatment of moderate to severe manic episodes in patients with bipolar disorder. It is available, on *prescription only, as tablets, dispersible tablets, an oral solution, or an injection.
Side effects: include restlessness, insomnia, anxiety, akathisia (involuntary movements), tremor, dizziness, somnolence, sedation, headache, blurred vision, indigestion, constipation, and fatigue.
Precautions: aripiprazole should be used with caution in people with cardiovascular disease, cerebrovascular disease, or a history of seizures or conditions associated with seizure development. Aripiprazole may cause an increase in blood-glucose levels and therefore people with diabetes should be monitored for worsening of their glucose control. This medicine should not be used in pregnancy unless the expected benefit clearly justifies the potential risk to the fetus. Women are advised not to breastfeed if they are taking aripiprazole.
Interactions with other drugs:
Antihypertensives: aripiprazole has the potential to enhance the effect of certain antihypertensive drugs.
Proprietary preparation: Abilify.

Arixtra (GlaxoSmithKline) *See* FONDAPARINUX SODIUM.

Arlevert (Hampton) A proprietary combination of *cinnarizine and dimenhydrinate (both antihistamines), used for the treatment of nausea, vomiting, and vertigo associated with disorders of the ear (including Ménière's disease). It is available as tablets on *prescription only.
Side effects: drowsiness is the most common side effect. *See also* ANTIHISTAMINES.
Precautions and interactions with other drugs: *see* ANTIHISTAMINES.

Arnica Ointment (Weleda) A proprietary preparation of the traditional herbal remedy arnica, used for the relief of muscular pain, stiffness, sprains, and bruises. It is freely available *over the counter.

Side effects and precautions: *see* RUBEFACIENTS.

Aromasin (Pharmacia) *See* EXEMESTANE.

aromatase inhibitors A class of drugs that inhibit the action of aromatase, an enzyme required for the conversion of *androgens to *oestrogens. Aromatase inhibitors thus decrease the concentrations of oestrogens in the body and are effective against tumours that depend on oestrogen for growth. They are usually used as second-line therapy (after *tamoxifen) for the treatment of breast cancer in postmenopausal women (*see* CANCER). The aromatase inhibitors include *anastrozole, *letrozole, and *exemestane.

Arpicolin (Rosemont Pharmaceuticals) *See* PROCYCLIDINE.

arrhythmia An abnormal heartbeat that may be slower or faster than normal, or just irregular. Normally, electrical impulses originate in the sinoatrial node (natural pacemaker) of the heart and pass along conducting pathways to coordinate the pumping action of the two atria and the two ventricles – the four chambers of the heart. If this coordination breaks down, arrhythmias occur. There are four major types of arrhythmia: **atrial fibrillation**, the most common, when the atria contract irregularly and too rapidly for the ventricles to keep pace; **ventricular tachycardia**, when abnormal electrical activity causes the ventricles to contract too rapidly; **supraventricular tachycardia**, when extra electrical signals arise in the atria, stimulating the ventricles to contract rapidly; and **heart block**, when signals are not conducted from the atria to the ventricles, so that the ventricles beat slowly. Minor disturbances of heart rhythm are common and do not normally require treatment. However, if the pumping action of the heart is seriously altered the circulation of the blood may be compromised and treatment with *anti-arrhythmic drugs is necessary. Arrhythmias may be due to a birth defect (congenital), to coronary heart disease, or to other less common heart disorders. Overactivity of the thyroid gland and some drugs can disturb heart rhythm.

arsenic trioxide A drug used for the treatment of promyelocytic leukaemia (*see* CANCER) that has relapsed or failed to respond to tretinoin and chemotherapy. It is given by intravenous infusion and is available on *prescription only.
Side effects: common side effects include low counts of platelets and neutrophils (a type of white blood cell), raised blood glucose levels, 'pins and needles', breathlessness, joint pain, fever, and arrhythmia (an abnormal heart rhythm).
Precautions: *see* CYTOTOXIC DRUGS. Arsenic trioxide should not be taken by women who are pregnant or breastfeeding and should be used with caution in people with impaired liver or kidney function and in those taking drugs that may cause arrhythmias.
Proprietary preparation: Trisenox.

Artelac (Pharma-Global) *See* HYPROMELLOSE.

artemether *See* RIAMET.

Arthrofen (Ashbourne Pharmaceuticals) *See* IBUPROFEN.

Arthrotec (Pharmacia) A proprietary combination of *diclofenac sodium (an NSAID) and *misoprostol (a prostaglandin analogue), used for the treatment of rheumatoid arthritis and osteoarthritis; the misoprostol is added to prevent the gastric bleeding and ulceration that may result from the use of diclofenac alone. Arthrotec is available, on *prescription only, as tablets of two strengths of diclofenac (**Arthrotec 50** and **Arthrotec 75**).
Side effects and precautions: *see* NSAIDs; MISOPROSTOL.
Interactions with other drugs: *see* NSAIDs.

Arthroxen (CP Pharmaceuticals) *See* NAPROXEN.

Arythmol (Abbott) *See* PROPAFENONE HYDROCHLORIDE.

Asacol (Procter & Gamble) *See* MESALAZINE.

Asasantin Retard (Boehringer Ingelheim) A proprietary combination of *dipyridamole and *aspirin (both antiplatelet drugs), used to prevent the recurrence of strokes in people who have already had a stroke. It is available as *modified-release capsules on *prescription only.
Side effects, precautions, and interactions with other drugs: *see* DIPYRIDAMOLE; ASPIRIN.

ascorbic acid *See* VITAMIN C.

Asilone Heartburn (Thornton & Ross) A proprietary combination of *alginic acid, *aluminium hydroxide, *magnesium trisilicate, and *sodium bicarbonate, used as an antacid for the relief of indigestion, heartburn, gastritis, flatulence, and peptic ulceration (*see* ACID-PEPTIC DISEASES). It is freely available *over the counter in the form of a suspension (**Asilone Heartburn Liquid**) or tablets (**Asilone Heartburn Tablets**); it cannot be prescribed on the NHS.
Side effects, precautions, and interactions with other drugs: *see* ANTACIDS.

Asilone Suspension (Thornton & Ross) A proprietary combination of *aluminium hydroxide and *magnesium oxide (antacids) and activated *dimeticone (an antifoaming agent), used for the treatment of indigestion, heartburn, gastritis, flatulence, and peptic ulceration (*see* ACID-PEPTIC DISEASES). It is freely available *over the counter. This combination is also available as **Asilone Antacid Liquid** and **Asilone Antacid Tablets**, which cannot be prescribed on the NHS.
Side effects and interactions with other drugs: *see* ANTACIDS.
Precautions: Asilone is not recommended for children under 12 years old.

Asmabec Clickhaler (UCB Pharma) *See* BECLOMETASONE DIPROPIONATE.

Asmanex Twisthaler (Schering-Plough) *See* MOMETASONE FUROATE.

Asmasal Clickhaler (UCB Pharma) *See* SALBUTAMOL.

aspirin (**acetylsalicylic acid**) An *analgesic drug that also reduces fever (i.e. it is antipyretic). It is the most common of the group of drugs known as *salicylates and is also classed as a non-steroidal anti-inflammatory drug (*see* NSAIDs), although other drugs of this class are usually preferred to aspirin for treating chronic inflammatory conditions because of its adverse side effects (see below). Aspirin is widely used for treating mild to moderate pain – particularly headache, period pains, and painful (but short-lasting) conditions of muscles and joints – and feverish conditions (such as influenza and colds). Aspirin is also a valuable *antiplatelet drug, used to prevent the formation of blood clots (*thrombosis). Low doses of aspirin (75–100 mg/day) are given to people who have had a heart attack or stroke, after a single high dose, to prevent a recurrence of these conditions; they are also used to prevent thrombosis in people who are at high risk, for example following bypass surgery.

Aspirin is available in a variety of forms – tablets (including *enteric-coated tablets), dispersible tablets, *modified-release capsules, powders, and suppositories – and can be obtained without a prescription, although there are restrictions on the quantities of tablets that can be supplied. Packs containing 16 tablets are freely available *over the counter; packs containing up to 32 (or exceptionally up to 100) tablets can only be obtained from pharmacies. Larger quantities are available on *prescription only. Aspirin is combined with paracetamol, codeine, or other ingredients in a variety of compound analgesic preparations and cold remedies. *See also* CO-CODAPRIN.

Side effects: aspirin can irritate the lining of the stomach, causing indigestion, stomach pain, nausea and vomiting, and (rarely) gastrointestinal bleeding. Rashes, wheezing, or breathing problems may develop in people who are allergic to NSAIDs. *See also* SALICYLATES.

Precautions: aspirin should not be given to children under 12 years old (unless specifically prescribed by a doctor) because it has been associated with Reye's syndrome (a disorder causing liver and brain damage); *paracetamol is the recommended alternative. Aspirin should not be taken by people who are allergic to it or to other NSAIDs or who have an active peptic ulcer, severe liver or kidney disease, or haemophilia, or by women who are breastfeeding. Aspirin should be used with caution in pregnant women and in people with asthma or a history of peptic ulceration.

Interactions with other drugs:

Anticoagulants: the risk of bleeding is increased if aspirin is taken with anticoagulants (especially warfarin).

Antidepressants: the risk of bleeding is increased if aspirin is taken with SSRIs or venlafaxine.

Methotrexate: aspirin increases the side effects of methotrexate.

NSAIDs: aspirin should not be taken with other NSAIDs as this increases the likelihood of stomach irritation and bleeding.

Proprietary preparations: Alka-Seltzer; Angettes 75 (antiplatelet); Bayer Aspirin (standard and antiplatelet); Boots Back Pain Relief; Caprin (standard and antiplatelet); Disprin, Disprin Direct; Flamasacard (modified-release capsules; antiplatelet); Micropirin (antiplatelet); Nu-Seals Aspirin (standard and antiplatelet). For details of these and other preparations of which aspirin is an ingredient, see Appendix 1.

asthma A condition marked by widespread narrowing of the bronchial airways, which changes in severity over short periods of time (either spontaneously or under treatment) and leads to cough, wheezing, and difficulty in breathing. Bronchial asthma may be precipitated by exposure to one or more of a wide range of stimuli, including allergens, drugs (such as aspirin and other NSAIDs), exertion, emotion, infections, and air pollution.

Treatment of asthma is with sympathomimetic drugs that stimulate beta receptors, such as *salbutamol, *salmeterol, or *terbutaline (*see* BRONCHODILATORS), with or without *corticosteroids (such as *beclometasone dipropionate and *budesonide); all these drugs are usually administered via aerosol or dry-powder *inhalers, or – if the condition is more severe – via a *nebulizer. Other drugs that can be used for the prevention of asthmatic attacks include *sodium cromoglicate or *nedocromil, *theophylline, the antimuscarinic drug *ipratropium bromide, and the *leukotriene receptor antagonists. Oral corticosteroids are reserved for those patients who fail to respond adequately to these measures. Severe asthmatic attacks may need large doses of oral corticosteroids (such as *prednisolone).

astringents Drugs that cause cells to shrink by precipitating proteins on their surfaces, making the surface less permeable to liquids, especially water. The cells therefore dry up but do not die. Astringents in various dilutions are used in soothing preparations to treat haemorrhoids (*see* BISMUTH OXIDE; BISMUTH SUBGALLATE; HAMAMELIS), in eye drops to treat watering eyes (*see* ZINC SULPHATE), in lotions to treat weeping skin conditions (*see* ALUMINIUM ACETATE; POTASSIUM PERMANGANATE), and in ear drops to clean the ear canal (aluminium acetate). Other salts of zinc and aluminium are used in antiperspirants (*see* ALUMINIUM CHLORIDE) or skin creams and lotions (*see* ZINC OXIDE; CALAMINE). *See also* ALLANTOIN.

AT 10 (Intrapharm) *See* DIHYDROTACHYSTEROL.

Atarax (Alliance) *See* HYDROXYZINE HYDROCHLORIDE.

atazanavir A protease inhibitor (*see* ANTIVIRAL DRUGS) used, in combination with other antiretroviral drugs, in the treatment of *HIV infection. It is available as capsules on *prescription only.
Side effects: include diarrhoea, nausea, vomiting, abdominal pain, loss of appetite, blood disorders, fatigue, headache, dizziness, breathlessness, and peripheral neuropathy (causing numbness and tingling of the limbs).
Precautions: atazanavir should not be taken by people with porphyria or by women who are breastfeeding. It should be used with caution by pregnant women and by people with diabetes, haemophilia, or liver disease and by those taking drugs that may cause *arrhythmias.
Interactions with other drugs: atazanavir inhibits several enzyme systems in the liver that are involved in metabolizing drugs, resulting in increased

plasma concentrations of these drugs and possibly an increase in their adverse effects. A doctor should therefore be consulted before atazanavir is taken with any other drug.
Proprietary preparation: Reyataz.

Atenix (Ashbourne Pharmaceuticals) *See* ATENOLOL.

atenolol A cardioselective *beta blocker used for the treatment and prevention of cardiac *arrhythmias and *angina and the treatment of *hypertension. It is available on *prescription only as tablets, syrup, or a solution for injection.
Side effects, precautions, and interactions with other drugs: *see* BETA BLOCKERS.
Proprietary preparations: Atenix; Tenormin; *Beta-Adalat (combined with nifedipine); *Tenif (combined with nifedipine); Tenoret 50 (*see* CO-TENIDONE); Tenoretic (*see* CO-TENIDONE).
See also ANTI-ARRHYTHMIC DRUGS; ANTIHYPERTENSIVE DRUGS.

atherosclerosis A disease of the arteries in which their inner walls degenerate with the formation of fatty plaques and scar tissue, which obstructs the flow of blood and predisposes to arterial *thrombosis. It is associated with high concentrations of *cholesterol in the blood (*see* HYPERLIPIDAEMIA), which may require treatment with *lipid-lowering drugs.

Atimos Modulite (Chiesi) *See* FORMOTEROL FUMARATE.

atomoxetine A drug used for the treatment of attention-deficit/hyperactivity disorder (ADHD) in children aged 6 years or more. It acts by inhibiting the reuptake of *noradrenaline and thus prolonging its action. Atomoxetine is available as capsules on *prescription only; its use should be supervised by a specialist.
Side effects: include loss of appetite, dry mouth, nausea, vomiting, abdominal pain, constipation, increased heart rate or palpitations, sleep disturbances, dizziness, headache, and behavioural disturbance.
Precautions: atomoxetine should be used with caution in children with cardiovascular disease and heart disorders, liver disease, glaucoma, or mental health problems. There is a small risk of liver disorders and suicidal thoughts in children taking atomoxetine, and carers should be alert to signs of liver damage (e.g. malaise, darkening of the urine) and behavioural changes (e.g. depression) in these children and seek medical advice.
Interactions with other drugs: the risk of ventricular *arrhythmias is increased if certain drugs are taken with atomoxetine. These drugs include methadone, some anti-arrhythmic and antipsychotic drugs, erythromycin, sotalol, and diuretics. The risk of convulsions is increased if antidepressants are taken with atomoxetine.
Proprietary preparation: Strattera.

atorvastatin A *statin used for treatment of primary and familial

a

hypercholesterolaemia and mixed *hyperlipidaemia that has not responded to dietary measures. It is available as tablets on *prescription only.
Side effects and precautions: *see* STATINS.
Interactions with other drugs:

Antifungal drugs: itraconazole and posaconazole increase the risk of muscle damage and should not be taken with atorvastatin.
See also STATINS.

Proprietary preparation: Lipitor.

atosiban A drug used to prevent premature labour in women who are 24–33 weeks pregnant. It works by blocking the action of *oxytocin, which causes contractions of the uterus. Atosiban is given by intravenous injection and infusion and is available on *prescription only.
Side effects: include headache, dizziness, nausea, vomiting, low blood pressure, and an increased heart rate.
Precautions: atosiban should be used with caution in women with liver or kidney disease.
Proprietary preparation: Tractocile.

atovaquone An *antibiotic with activity against certain types of protozoa. Atovaquone is used for the treatment of mild to moderate pneumonia caused by *Pneumocystis jirovecii* (which is most common in people with AIDS); it is prescribed for people who cannot tolerate *co-trimoxazole, and it should be taken with food. It is available as a suspension on *prescription only. Atovaquone is also used in combination with *proguanil hydrochloride for the treatment of falciparum *malaria.
Side effects: include diarrhoea, nausea, and vomiting (which may hinder its absorption), headache, insomnia, rash, and fever.
Precautions: atovaquone should be used with caution by elderly people, pregnant women, and people with liver or kidney disease. It should not be taken by women who are breastfeeding.
Interactions with other drugs:

Antibiotics: rifabutin, rifampicin, and tetracycline reduce the plasma concentration of atovaquone to the extent that it may not be effective.
Metoclopramide: reduces the plasma concentration (and possibly the effectiveness) of atovaquone.

Proprietary preparations: Wellvone; *Malarone (combined with proguanil).

atracurium besilate *See* MUSCLE RELAXANTS.

atrial fibrillation *See* ARRHYTHMIA.

Atriance (GlaxoSmithKline) *See* NELARABINE.

Atripla (Gilead Sciences) A proprietary combination of *tenofovir disoproxil, *efavirenz, and *emtricitabine (all antiretroviral drugs; *see* ANTIVIRAL DRUGS), used in the treatment of HIV infection and chronic hepatitis B infection. It is available as tablets on *prescription only.

Side effects, precautions, and interactions with other drugs: *see* TENOFOVIR DISOPROXIL; EFAVIRENZ; EMTRICITABINE.

atropine sulphate An *antimuscarinic drug; atropine is one of the components of *belladonna. Atropine sulphate is applied to the eye to dilate the pupil before examination of the interior of the eye, especially in young children. Since its action is long-lasting and it paralyses the ciliary muscles (which control the focusing ability of the eye) as well as the muscle of the iris (which controls the size of the pupil), it is also used for treating inflammation of the ciliary muscles and iris. Atropine is taken by mouth for the relief of gut spasms (*see* ANTISPASMODICS). Injections of atropine are occasionally used during surgery for drying up secretions in the airways and for preventing or reversing the effects of *neostigmine in slowing the heart rate; atropine injections are also given to patients who have a slow heart rate associated with *arrhythmias after a heart attack and to treat cardiac arrest. Atropine is available as eye drops or ointment, tablets, or an injection on *prescription only; compound antispasmodic preparations containing atropine are available from pharmacies without a prescription.
Side effects: for *systemic effects, *see* ANTIMUSCARINIC DRUGS. Eye drops or ointment can cause transient stinging and an increase in pressure in the eye; with prolonged use, local irritation and conjunctivitis can occur.
Precautions: *see* ANTIMUSCARINIC DRUGS. Eye ointment (rather than drops) should be used in children under three months, since they are more likely to develop systemic effects with eye drops.
Interactions with other drugs: *see* ANTIMUSCARINIC DRUGS.
Proprietary preparations: Minims Atropine Sulphate (single-dose eye drops); Minijet Atropine (injection); *Actonorm Powder (combined with antacids and peppermint oil).

Atrovent (Boehringer Ingelheim) *See* IPRATROPIUM BROMIDE.

attapulgite A purified form of magnesium aluminium silicate. It is highly adsorbent and is used in pharmaceutical preparations, especially in preparations to treat diarrhoea (*see* ANTIDIARRHOEAL DRUGS).
Proprietary preparation: *Diocalm Dual Action (combined with morphine).

Augmentin (GlaxoSmithKline) *See* CO-AMOXICLAV.

Aureocort (Goldshield) A proprietary combination of *triamcinolone acetonide (a potent steroid) and *chlortetracycline (an antibiotic), used for the treatment of inflammatory skin conditions when infection is present. It is available as a cream on *prescription only.
Side effects and precautions, and interactions with other drugs: *see* TOPICAL STEROIDS; TETRACYCLINES.

aurothiomalate *See* SODIUM AUROTHIOMALATE.

Avamys (GlaxoSmithKline) *See* FLUTICASONE PROPIONATE.

Avandamet (GlaxoSmithKline) A proprietary combination of *rosiglitazone

and *metformin hydrochloride (both oral hypoglycaemic drug), used in the treatment of type 2 *diabetes mellitus not controlled by metformin alone. It is available as tablets on *prescription only.
Side effects, precautions, and interactions with other drugs: *see* METFORMIN HYDROCHLORIDE; ROSIGLITAZONE.

Avandia (GlaxoSmithKline) *See* ROSIGLITAZONE.

Avastin (Roche Products) *See* BEVACIZUMAB.

Aveeno (Johnson & Johnson) A proprietary preparation consisting of an extract of oatmeal, used as an *emollient for the relief of *eczema and dry skin conditions, including those associated with itching. It is available as an oil, to be added to the bath or applied directly to the skin before bathing, or as a cream to be rubbed into the skin. **Aveeno Oilated**, containing added mineral oil, is a powder to be added to the bath. All preparations are freely available *over the counter.

Avelox (Bayer) *See* MOXIFLOXACIN.

Avloclor (AstraZeneca) *See* CHLOROQUINE.

Avoca (Bray Health & Leisure) *See* SILVER NITRATE.

Avodart (GlaxoSmithKline) *See* DUTASTERIDE.

Avomine (Manx) *See* PROMETHAZINE TEOCLATE.

Avonex (Biogen Idec) *See* INTERFERON BETA.

Axid (Flynn Pharma) *See* NIZATIDINE.

Axsain (Cephalon) *See* CAPSAICIN.

azacitidine An *antimetabolite used for the treatment of disorders in the blood-forming cells of the bone marrow and some types of leukaemia (*see* CANCER). It is given by subcutaneous injection and is available on *prescription only.
Side effects: *see* CYTOTOXIC DRUGS. There may also be diarrhoea or constipation, abdominal pain, indigestion, loss of appetite, headache, and breathlessness.
Precautions: *see* CYTOTOXIC DRUGS. Azacitidine should not be given to people with liver cancer or to breastfeeding women. It should be used with caution in people with impaired liver or kidney function and heart or lung disease.
Proprietary preparation: Vidaza.

azapropazone An *NSAID that is used only for the treatment of rheumatoid arthritis, ankylosing spondylitis (a type of arthritis that affects the spine), and acute gout, but only when these conditions have failed to respond to other NSAIDs. It is available as capsules on *prescription only.
Side effects: azapropazone is more likely than other NSAIDs to cause severe gastrointestinal bleeding and ulceration. Other side effects include rashes, sensitivity to sunlight (people taking azapropazone should avoid exposure to

sunlight or use a sunblock), fluid retention, and (rarely) inflammation of the lungs and blood disorders. *See also* NSAIDs.
Precautions: azapropazone must not be taken by people with a history of peptic ulcers, inflammatory bowel disease, or blood disorders. *See also* NSAIDs.
Interactions with other drugs: *see* NSAIDs. In addition:

Clozapine: there is an increased risk of agranulocytosis (a blood disorder), and clozapine should not be taken with azapropazone.
Methotrexate: should not be taken with azapropazone, as its excretion is reduced by azapropazone, causing amounts of methotrexate to build up and have adverse effects.
Phenytoin: should not be taken with azapropazone as its effects are enhanced by azapropazone.
Tolbutamide: its effects are enhanced by azapropazone and these two drugs should not be taken together.
Warfarin: should not be taken with azapropazone as its anticoagulant effects are greatly enhanced by azapropazone.

Proprietary preparation: Rheumox.

Azarga (Alcon Laboratories) A proprietary combination of *brinzolamide (a carbonic anhydrase inhibitor) and *timolol maleate (a beta blocker), used to reduce the pressure inside the eye in the treatment of chronic (open-angle) *glaucoma and raised blood pressure in the eye when a beta blocker alone has failed to do this. It is available as eye drops on *prescription only.
Side effects, precautions, and interactions with other drugs: *see* BRINZOLAMIDE; BETA BLOCKERS.

azathioprine An *immunosuppressant that is a powerful *cytotoxic drug. It is used to prevent the rejection of transplants (and to minimize the use of *corticosteroids for this purpose) and also to treat a number of autoimmune conditions, usually when corticosteroids have been inadequate, including myasthenia gravis and rheumatoid arthritis. Azathioprine is available as tablets on *prescription only.
Side effects: include nausea and vomiting, loss of appetite, malaise, dizziness, fever, muscular aches and pains, rashes, and hair loss. Azathioprine can suppress production of white blood cells and platelets in the bone marrow, leading to increased susceptibility to infections and unusual bruising or bleeding.
Precautions: azathioprine should only be taken under specialist supervision, and blood counts should be monitored during the treatment period. Any evidence of infection or unusual bruising or bleeding should be reported to a doctor immediately.
Interactions with other drugs:

Allopurinol: increases the toxic effects of azathioprine, whose dosage will therefore need to be reduced.
Co-trimoxazole: increases the risk of blood disorders.
Warfarin: its anticoagulant effect may be reduced by azathioprine.

Proprietary preparations: Immunoprin; Imuran.

a

azelaic acid An antibacterial drug used for the *topical treatment of mild to moderate *acne. It is also used in the treatment of rosacea. Azelaic acid is available as a cream or gel on *prescription only.
Side effects: azelaic acid may irritate the skin and (rarely) make the skin more sensitive to sunlight.
Precautions: azelaic acid should not be applied near the eyes or mouth.
Proprietary preparations: Finacea Gel; Skinoren.

azelastine hydrochloride An *antihistamine used to relieve the symptoms of allergic rhinitis, including hay fever, and allergic conjunctivitis. It is available in a metered-dose pump spray and as eye drops on *prescription only; a nasal spray specifically for the treatment of hay fever is available from pharmacies without a prescription.
Side effects: include local irritation and the spray may cause taste disturbances.
Interactions with other drugs: *see* ANTIHISTAMINES.
Proprietary preparations: Optilast (eye drops); Rhinolast Allergy (nasal spray).

azidothymidine (**AZT**) *See* ZIDOVUDINE.

Azilect (Teva Pharmaceuticals) *See* RASAGILINE.

azithromycin A *macrolide antibiotic used for the treatment of infections of the respiratory tract, ear, skin, and soft tissues and for genital infections. It is similar to *erythromycin, but has a longer duration of action and can be taken only once daily. It is available, on *prescription only, as capsules, tablets, or a suspension.
Side effects, precautions, and interactions with other drugs: *see* ERYTHROMYCIN.
Proprietary preparation: Zithromax.

Azopt (Alcon Laboratories) *See* BRINZOLAMIDE.

AZT **1.** (**azidothymidine**) *See* ZIDOVUDINE. **2.** An abbreviation sometimes used for *azathioprine and *azithromycin.

aztreonam A beta-lactam *antibiotic that is similar to the *penicillins but may be less likely to produce allergic reactions in people sensitive to pencillins. It is used for the treatment of infections of the lower respiratory tract, including lung infections in patients with cystic fibrosis. It is also used to treat bone, skin, and soft-tissue infections, abdominal and urinary-tract infections (including gonorrhoea and cystitis), and meningitis. It is given by *intramuscular or *intravenous injection and is available on *prescription only.
Side effects: may include nausea, vomiting, diarrhoea, abdominal cramps, mouth ulcers, altered taste, jaundice, hepatitis, blood disorders, and rashes.
Precautions: aztreonam should not be taken by women who are pregnant or

breastfeeding or by anyone who is allergic to it, and it should be used with caution in those who have liver or kidney disease.

Interactions with other drugs:

Anticoagulants: the effects of warfarin and acenocoumarol may be increased by aztreonam.

Azzalure (Galderma) *See* BOTULINUM TOXIN TYPE A.

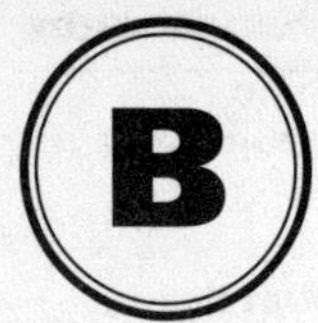

Baby Meltus (SSL International) *See* ACETIC ACID.

bacitracin zinc An *antibiotic used for the treatment of bacterial infections of the skin and eyes. It is available, on *prescription only, in the form of compound preparations with other antibiotics.
Side effects and precautions: see entries for individual compound preparations.
Proprietary preparation: *Polyfax (combined with polymyxin B sulphate)

baclofen A skeletal *muscle relaxant used to relieve muscle spasm, especially when due to trauma or disease of the central nervous system, such as multiple sclerosis, meningitis, or cerebral palsy. Dosages should be increased slowly to avoid side effects. It is available, on *prescription only, as tablets, an oral solution, or injection into the membranes surrounding the spinal cord.
Side effects: sedation, drowsiness, and nausea are the most common. Less common side effects include confusion, dizziness, headache, insomnia, tremor, loss of sensation in the extremities, muscle pain and weakness, and (rarely) hallucinations and convulsions.
Precautions: baclofen should not be taken by people with peptic ulcer and it should be used with caution in those with psychiatric illness, liver or kidney disease, stroke, diabetes, epilepsy, and porphyria and in women who are pregnant or breastfeeding. The drug should be withdrawn gradually at the end of treatment. Alcohol enhances the sedative effect of baclofen, which may affect tasks such as driving.
Interactions with other drugs:
Antihypertensives: baclofen increases their effect in lowering blood pressure.
Anxiolytics and hypnotics: increase the sedative effect of baclofen.
Tricyclic antidepressants: increase the effect of baclofen.
Proprietary preparations: Lioresal; Lyflex (solution).

Bactroban (GlaxoSmithKline) *See* MUPIROCIN.

BAL *See* DIMERCAPROL.

balanced salt solution A sterile solution of *sodium chloride, sodium acetate, *sodium citrate, *calcium chloride, and magnesium chloride, used to wash out the eyes to remove foreign bodies or harmful substances. It is also used for irrigating the eyes during surgery. The solution is available without a prescription, but only from pharmacies.
Proprietary preparation: Iocare.

Balmosa (Avicenna Plc) A proprietary combination of *methyl salicylate, *camphor, *menthol, and *capsicum oleoresin, used for the relief of rheumatic, muscular and mild arthritic pain, lumbago, and sciatica (*see* RUBEFACIENTS). It is freely available *over the counter in the form of a cream.
Side effects and precautions: *see* RUBEFACIENTS; SALICYLATES.

Balneum (Almirall) *See* SOYA OIL.

Balneum Plus Cream (Almirall) A proprietary combination of *urea (an emollient) and *lauromacrogols (antipruritic agents), used for soothing dry skin conditions associated with scaling and itching. It is freely available *over the counter.

Balneum Plus Oil (Almirall) A proprietary combination of *soya oil (an emollient) and *lauromacrogols (antipruritic agents), used for soothing dry skin conditions, including those associated with itching. It is freely available, in the form of a bath oil, *over the counter.

balsalazide sodium An *aminosalicylate that is used for the treatment of mild to moderate ulcerative colitis; it is converted to *mesalazine in the body. Balsalazide is available as capsules on *prescription only.
Side effects: include abdominal pain and vomiting; *see also* AMINOSALICYLATES.
Precautions: *see* AMINOSALICYLATES.
Proprietary preparation: Colazide.

balsam of Peru *See* PERU BALSAM.

Bambec (AstraZeneca) *See* BAMBUTEROL HYDROCHLORIDE.

bambuterol hydrochloride A drug that is converted to *terbutaline in the body; it is used as a *bronchodilator for the treatment of asthma attacks and the relief of wheezing and breathlessness in bronchitis and emphysema. Bambuterol is available as tablets on *prescription only.
Side effects, precautions, and interactions with other drugs: *see* SALBUTAMOL.
Proprietary preparation: Bambec.

Baraclude (Bristol-Myers Squibb) *See* ENTECAVIR.

Baratol (Amdipharm) *See* INDORAMIN HYDROCHLORIDE.

barbiturates A class of drugs that depress activity of the central nervous system; they are classified into three groups according to their duration of action: short-, intermediate-, and long-acting. Barbiturates were formerly widely used as *hypnotic drugs but have largely been superseded by the *benzodiazepines; they are now only prescribed for patients who are already taking them (*see* AMOBARBITAL; BUTOBARBITAL; SECOBARBITAL). They produce *tolerance and *dependence; abrupt withdrawal causes severe effects similar to those seen in alcoholics deprived of alcohol. Toxic effects leading to coma and death are common after overdose, especially when accompanied by alcohol. The long-acting barbiturate *phenobarbital is occasionally used in the treatment of epilepsy, and the short-acting **thiopental sodium** is used to

induce general anaesthesia. Barbiturates are *controlled drugs; they are available as tablets, capsules, or solutions for injection.
Side effects: include 'hangover' effects with drowsiness, dizziness, shaky movements, unsteady gait, depression of breathing, headache, paradoxical excitement, and confusion. Tolerance and dependence may develop.
Precautions: barbiturates should not be used to treat insomnia caused by uncontrolled pain; they should not be taken by women who are pregnant or breastfeeding, by people with a history of drug or alcohol abuse, or by children, young adults, or elderly people. Barbiturates should be used with caution in people who have liver or kidney disease.
Interactions with other drugs:
Anticoagulants: the anticoagulant effects of warfarin and acenocoumarol are reduced by barbiturates.
Antiviral drugs: the plasma concentrations of indinavir, nelfinavir, and saquinavir may be reduced by barbiturates; phenobarbital may reduce the plasma concentrations of other antivirals, including Kaletra.
Calcium antagonists: the effects of diltiazem, felodipine, isradipine, verapamil, and probably nicardipine and nifedipine are reduced by barbiturates.
Ciclosporin: its effects are reduced by barbiturates.
Corticosteroids: their effects are reduced by barbiturates.
Oral contraceptives: their effects are reduced by barbiturates.
Sodium oxybate: its effects are enhanced by barbiturates and it should not be used with these drugs.

barrier preparations Creams, ointments, or sprays used to protect the skin against water-soluble irritants (e.g. detergents, breakdown products of urine). Barrier preparations often contain a silicone (such as *dimeticone). They are used for preventing and treating such conditions as napkin rash and pressure sores and for protecting the skin around a *stoma.

basiliximab A *monoclonal antibody that prevents proliferation of T lymphocytes (a type of white blood cell). It is used to prevent rejection of kidney transplants (*see* IMMUNOSUPPRESSANTS). Basiliximab is given by intravenous injection or infusion under specialist supervision and is available on *prescription only.
Side effects: common side effects include constipation, urinary tract infections, nausea, swelling of the ankles, hypertension, anaemia, headache, weight increase, diarrhoea, and upper airways infections.
Precautions: basiliximab should not be given to women who are pregnant or breastfeeding, and women should use contraception during and for up to 16 weeks after treatment.
Proprietary preparation: Simulect.

Baxan (Bristol-Myers Squibb) *See* CEFADROXIL.

Bayer Aspirin (Bayer) *See* ASPIRIN.

Bazuka Gel (Diomed Developments) A proprietary combination of *salicylic

acid and *lactic acid (both keratolytics), used for the treatment of warts, verrucas, corns, and calluses. **Bazuka Extra Strength Gel** is a stronger formulation. Both medicines can be obtained without a prescription, but only from pharmacies.
Side effects and precautions: *see* SALICYLIC ACID.

BCNU *See* CARMUSTINE.

becaplermin A genetically engineered form of platelet-derived growth factor, a protein that promotes wound healing. It is used to stimulate the healing of chronic ulcers in people with diabetes. Becaplermin is available as a topical gel on *prescription only.
Side effects: include pain, infections, and reddening of the skin in the treated area.
Precautions: becaplermin should not be applied to infected skin or skin tumours.
Proprietary preparation: Regranex.

beclometasone dipropionate <**beclomethasone dipropionate**> A *corticosteroid used mainly for the prevention of *asthma attacks and the treatment of allergic rhinitis (including hay fever). It may be used in conjunction with *bronchodilators and/or *sodium cromoglicate. Beclometasone is also used to treat ulcerative colitis. It is administered by aerosol or powder inhalation (for asthma), by nasal spray (for rhinitis), or as tablets (for ulcerative colitis), and most preparations are available on *prescription only.
Side effects: the most common side effects with an inhaler are hoarseness (due to weakness of the vocal muscles), fungal (*Candida*) infections of the mouth or throat (which can be reduced by rinsing out the mouth after doses), nasal discomfort, or irritation. Disturbances in taste and smell may occur with nasal sprays. The tablets may cause nausea, constipation, headache, and drowsiness. *See also* CORTICOSTEROIDS; TOPICAL STEROIDS.
Precautions: beclometasone should not be taken by people who have untreated nasal infections or who have had nasal surgery or by people who have (or have had) tuberculosis. *See also* CORTICOSTEROIDS.
Interactions with other drugs: *see* CORTICOSTEROIDS.
Proprietary preparations: Asmabec Clickhaler (metered standard-dose and high-dose dry powder for inhalation); Becodisks (discs containing powder blisters, of varying strengths, for use in a breath-activated inhaler); Beconase (nasal spray available from pharmacies without a prescription); Clenil Modulite (inhaler); Clipper (modified release tablets); Nasobec (nasal spray); Pulvinal Beclometasone (inhaler); Qvar (aerosol inhalation); Qvar Autohaler (breath-activated inhaler); Qvar Easi-Breath (breath-activated inhaler); *Fostair (combined with formoterol).

Becodisks (Allen & Hanburys) *See* BECLOMETASONE DIPROPIONATE.

Beconase (Allen & Hanburys) *See* BECLOMETASONE DIPROPIONATE.

b

Bedol (ReSource Medical) *See* ESTRADIOL; HORMONE REPLACEMENT THERAPY.

Bedranol SR (Sandoz) *See* PROPRANOLOL HYDROCHLORIDE.

Beechams All-in-One (GlaxoSmithKline) A proprietary combination of *paracetamol (an analgesic and antipyretic), *guaifenesin (an expectorant), and *phenylephrine (a decongestant), used to relieve the symptoms of colds, chills, and influenza. It is freely available *over the counter in the form of a liquid.
Side effects: *see* GUAIFENESIN; PHENYLEPHRINE.
Precautions: this medicine should not be given to children under six years old except on medical advice. *See also* PARACETAMOL; GUAIFENESIN; PHENYLEPHRINE.
Interactions with other drugs: *see* PHENYLEPHRINE.

Beechams Flu-Plus Caplets (GlaxoSmithKline) A proprietary combination of *paracetamol (an analgesic and antipyretic), *caffeine (a stimulant), and *phenylephrine (a decongestant), used to relieve the symptoms of colds and influenza. including chills, fever, headache, aches and pains, nasal congestion, sinus pain, and sore throat. It is freely available *over the counter in the form of tablets.
Side effects and interactions with other drugs: *see* PHENYLEPHRINE.
Precautions: this medicine should not be given to children, except on medical advice. *See also* PARACETAMOL; PHENYLEPHRINE; CAFFEINE.

Beechams Flu-Plus Hot Lemon, Beechams Flu-Plus Hot Berry Fruits (GlaxoSmithKline) Proprietary combinations of *paracetamol (an analgesic and antipyretic), *phenylephrine (a decongestant), and ascorbic acid (*vitamin C), used to relieve the symptoms of influenza. Both are freely available *over the counter in the form of powders to be dissolved in hot water.
Side effects and interactions with other drugs: *see* PHENYLEPHRINE.
Precautions: these powders should not be given to children, except on medical advice. *See also* PARACETAMOL; PHENYLEPHRINE.

Beechams Powders (GlaxoSmithKline) A proprietary combination of *aspirin (an analgesic and antipyretic) and *caffeine (a stimulant), used to relieve the symptoms of influenza, chills, and colds. It is also be used for the treatment of mild to moderate pain, such as headache, neuralgia, toothache, rheumatic pains, sore throat, and period pains. It is freely available *over the counter.
Side effects and interactions with other drugs: *see* ASPIRIN.
Precautions: Beechams Powders should not be given to children, except on medical advice. *See also* ASPIRIN; CAFFEINE.

Beechams Powders Capsules (GlaxoSmithKline) A proprietary combination of *paracetamol (an analgesic and antipyretic), *caffeine (a stimulant), and *phenylephrine (a decongestant), used to relieve the symptoms of influenza, fevers, chills, and colds, including nasal congestion, sinus pain, and catarrh. It is freely available *over the counter.

Side effects and interactions with other drugs: *see* PHENYLEPHRINE.
Precautions: these capsules should not be given to children, except on medical advice. *See also* PARACETAMOL; CAFFEINE; PHENYLEPHRINE.

Beechams Throat-Plus Sugar Free Lozenges (GlaxoSmithKline) A proprietary combination of the antiseptics *hexylresorcinol and *benzalkonium chloride, used for the relief of sore throats. It is freely available *over the counter.
Precautions: these lozenges are not recommended for children under seven years old.

Beechams Veno's Expectorant (GlaxoSmithKline) *See* GUAIFENESIN.

Beechams Veno's Honey and Lemon (GlaxoSmithKline) A proprietary combination of lemon juice, honey, and liquid glucose used as a *demulcent for the relief of dry irritating coughs. It is freely available *over the counter as a syrup.

belladonna extract A collection of *alkaloids extracted from deadly nightshade (*Atropa belladonna*): they include *atropine sulphate, *hyoscine hydrobromide, and *hyoscine butylbromide, which are *antimuscarinic drugs. Belladonna is used in plasters for the relief of aches, pains, and stiffness.
Side effects and precautions: *see* ANTIMUSCARINIC DRUGS.
Proprietary preparation: Cuxson Gerrard Belladonna Plasters.

bemiparin sodium A *low molecular weight heparin used for the prevention and treatment of deep-vein *thrombosis and for the prevention of blood clots in patients undergoing kidney dialysis. It is available as a solution for subcutaneous injection on *prescription only.
Side effects, precautions, and interactions with other drugs: *see* HEPARIN.
Proprietary preparation: Zibor.

Benadryl Allergy Oral Syrup, Benadryl for Children Allergy Solution, Benadryl One A Day (McNeil Ltd) *See* CETIRIZINE HYDROCHLORIDE.

Benadryl Allergy Relief (McNeil Ltd) *See* ACRIVASTINE.

Benadryl Plus Capsules (McNeil Ltd) A proprietary combination of *acrivastine (a nonsedating antihistamine) and *pseudoephedrine (a decongestant), used for the relief of allergic rhinitis (hay fever). It is available without a prescription, but only from pharmacies.
Side effects: include drowsiness and (more rarely) skin rash and urinary retention.
Precautions: Benadryl Plus should not be taken by people with severe hypertension (high blood pressure) or severe coronary artery disease, overactivity of the thyroid gland, or glaucoma. It should be avoided by people with kidney disease. People should not drive or operate machinery if drowsiness occurs.

b

Interactions with other drugs:
Monoamine oxidase inhibitors: may cause a rise in blood pressure and should therefore be avoided.
Tricyclic antidepressants: may cause a rise in blood pressure and should therefore be avoided.

Benadryl Skin Allergy Relief Cream (McNeil Ltd) A proprietary combination of *diphenhydramine (an antihistamine), *zinc oxide (a soothing astringent compound), and *camphor (a rubefacient), used for the relief of irritation associated with urticaria (hives), shingles, sunburn, insect bites, and nettle stings. It is available without a prescription, but only from pharmacies.
Precautions: the cream should not be applied to broken skin, the mouth lining or other mucous membranes, or to measles or chickenpox rashes.

bendrofluazide *See* BENDROFLUMETHIAZIDE.

bendroflumethiazide <**bendrofluazide**> A *thiazide diuretic used to treat *oedema and *hypertension. It is available as tablets on *prescription only.
Side effects, precautions, and interactions with other drugs: *see* THIAZIDE DIURETICS.
Proprietary preparations: Aprinox; *Neo-Naclex-K (combined with potassium chloride); *Prestim (combined with timolol).
See also ANTIHYPERTENSIVE DRUGS; DIURETICS.

BeneFIX (Pfizer) *See* FACTOR IX.

Benerva (Roche Products) *See* THIAMINE.

benperidol A butyrophenone *antipsychotic drug sometimes used for the treatment of patients with unacceptable deviant sexual behaviour. It is available as tablets on *prescription only.
Side effects: as for *chlorpromazine, but benperidol has more pronounced *extrapyramidal reactions, fewer antimuscarinic effects, and is less sedating.
Precautions: *see* CHLORPROMAZINE HYDROCHLORIDE.
Interactions with other drugs:
Anaesthetics: their effect in lowering blood pressure is enhanced.
Antidepressants: there is an increased risk of antimuscarinic effects and arrhythmias if benperidol is taken with tricyclic antidepressants.
Antiepileptic drugs: their anticonvulsant effects are antagonized by benperidol.
Ritonavir: may increase the effects of benperidol.
Sedatives: the sedative effects of benperidol are increased if it is taken with anxiolytic or hypnotic drugs, or any other drug that causes sedation.
Sibutramine: there is an increased risk of adverse effects on the central nervous system, and benperidol should not be taken with sibutramine.
Proprietary preparation: Anquil.

benserazide hydrochloride A drug that inhibits the enzyme that breaks down *levodopa (an antiparkinsonian drug) to *dopamine in the peripheral tissues. Given in combination with levodopa (*see* CO-BENELDOPA), it increases

the amount of levodopa available to cross into the brain and also helps prevent the side effects of nausea, vomiting, and low blood pressure seen with levodopa therapy.
Proprietary preparations: Madopar and Madopar CR (*see* CO-BENELDOPA).

Benylin Chesty Coughs Non Drowsy (McNeil Ltd) A proprietary combination of *guaifenesin (an expectorant) and *menthol, used for the relief of productive coughs. It is freely available *over the counter in the form of a syrup.
Side effects and precautions: *see* GUAIFENESIN. This medicine is not recommended for children under six years old.

Benylin Chesty Coughs Original (McNeil Ltd) A proprietary combination of *diphenhydramine (a sedative antihistamine), *ammonium chloride (an expectorant), and *menthol, used for the relief of productive coughs and other symptoms of congestion. It is available as a syrup without a prescription, but only from pharmacies. It cannot be prescribed on the NHS.
Side effects and interactions with other drugs: *see* ANTIHISTAMINES.
Precautions: this syrup is not recommended for children under six years old. *See also* ANTIHISTAMINES.

Benylin Children's Chesty Coughs (McNeil Ltd) *See* GUAIFENESIN.

Benylin Children's Coughs and Colds (McNeil Ltd) A proprietary combination of *dextromethorphan (a cough suppressant) and *triprolidine (an antihistamine), used to relieve the symptoms of dry unproductive coughs. It is available as a liquid without a prescription, but only from pharmacies.
Side effects and interactions with other drugs: *see* DEXTROMETHORPHAN; ANTIHISTAMINES.
Precautions: this medicine is not recommended for children under one year old. *See also* ANTIHISTAMINES; OPIOIDS.

Benylin Children's Dry Coughs (McNeil Ltd) *See* PHOLCODINE.

Benylin Children's Night Coughs (McNeil Ltd) A proprietary combination of *diphenhydramine (a sedative antihistamine) and *menthol, used for the relief of coughs in children that interfere with sleep. It is available as a syrup without a prescription, but only from pharmacies.
Side effects and interactions with other drugs: *see* ANTIHISTAMINES.
Precautions: this medicine should not normally be given to children under one year old. *See also* ANTIHISTAMINES.

Benylin Day & Night Tablets (McNeil Ltd) A proprietary combination of *paracetamol (an analgesic and antipyretic) and *pseudoephedrine (a decongestant) in day tablets, and paracetamol and *diphenhydramine (a sedative antihistamine) in night tablets, used to relieve the symptoms of colds and influenza (the night tablets facilitate sleep). The tablets are available without a prescription, but only from pharmacies.
Side effects, precautions, and interactions with other drugs: *see* PARACETAMOL; EPHEDRINE HYDROCHLORIDE; DECONGESTANTS; ANTIHISTAMINES.

Benylin Dry Coughs Non Drowsy (McNeil Ltd) *See* DEXTROMETHORPHAN.

Benylin Dry Coughs Original (McNeil Ltd) A proprietary combination of *dextromethorphan (a cough suppressant), *diphenhydramine (a sedative antihistamine), and *menthol, used for the relief of dry persistent coughs. It is available as a syrup without a prescription, but only from pharmacies. It cannot be prescribed on the NHS.
Side effects and interactions with other drugs: *see* DEXTROMETHORPHAN; OPIOIDS; COUGH SUPPRESSANTS; ANTIHISTAMINES.
Precautions: this medicine is not recommended for children under six years old. *See also* OPIOIDS; ANTIHISTAMINES.

Benylin Four Flu (Benylin 4 Flu) (McNeil Ltd) A proprietary combination of *paracetamol (an analgesic and antipyretic), *pseudoephedrine (a decongestant), and *diphenhydramine (a sedative antihistamine), used to relieve the symptoms of colds and influenza. It is available as tablets or a liquid and can be obtained without a prescription, but only from pharmacies.
Side effects: *see* EPHEDRINE HYDROCHLORIDE; ANTIHISTAMINES.
Precautions: this preparation is not recommended for children under six years old. *See also* PARACETAMOL; EPHEDRINE HYDROCHLORIDE; DECONGESTANTS; ANTIHISTAMINES.
Interactions with other drugs: *see* EPHEDRINE HYDROCHLORIDE; ANTIHISTAMINES.

Benylin Mucus Cough (McNeil Ltd) A proprietary combination of *guaifenesin (an expectorant) and *menthol, used for the relief of productive coughs. It is freely available as a syrup *over the counter.
Side effects: *see* GUAIFENESIN.
Precautions: this medicine should not to be taken by children under the age of 12 years. It should be used with caution by people with severely impaired liver or kidney function. It should not be taken during pregnancy unless the potential benefit of treatment to the mother outweighs the possible risks to the developing fetus.

Benylin Mucus Cough Night (McNeil Ltd) A proprietary combination of *guaifenesin (an expectorant), *diphenhydramine (a sedative antihistamine), and *menthol, used for the night-time relief of coughs and to aid restful sleep. It is available as a syrup without a prescription, but only from pharmacies.
Side effects and interactions with other drugs: *see* ANTIHISTAMINES; GUAIFENESIN.
Precautions: alcohol should be avoided when taking this medicine, which should be used with caution by people with moderate to severe impairment of kidney or liver function or urinary retention. *See* ANTIHISTAMINES.

benzalkonium chloride An *antiseptic that is used in the form of lozenges for treating mouth ulcers, gum disease, and infections of the mouth and throat. It is also an ingredient in creams, paints, and lotions for treating a variety of skin conditions. Benzalkonium is included as a preservative in eye drops. Some preparations containing benzalkonium can be obtained without

a prescription, but some combined preparations can only be bought from pharmacies.
Precautions: eye drops containing benzalkonium should not be used by wearers of soft contact lenses.
Proprietary preparations: Bradosol (lozenges); *Beechams Throat-Plus Sugar Free Lozenges (combined with hexylresorcinol); *Boots Dual Action Athlete's Foot Cream (combined with tolnaftate); *Conotrane (combined with dimeticone); *Dermax Therapeutic Shampoo (combined with sodium lauryl ether sulphate); *Dermol (combined with liquid paraffin, isopropyl myristate, and chlorhexidine hydrochloride); *Drapolene Cream (combined with cetrimide); *Emulsiderm (combined with liquid paraffin and isopropyl myristate); *Oilatum Plus (combined with liquid paraffin and triclosan); *Timodine (combined with nystatin, hydrocortisone, and dimeticone).

benzhexol hydrochloride *See* TRIHEXYPHENIDYL HYDROCHLORIDE.

benzocaine A *local anaesthetic applied to the skin or mucous membranes, particularly around the mouth and throat, for the relief of pain. It is available, alone or combined with other drugs, in the form of sprays, gels, lotions, or lozenges and can be obtained without a prescription, but only from pharmacies.
Precautions: benzocaine should be used with caution by women who are pregnant or breastfeeding.
Proprietary preparations: AAA Mouth and Throat Spray; Burneze Spray; Oragard-B (gel); Boots Anaesthetic & Antibiotic Throat Lozenges (combined with tyrothricin); *Dequacaine (combined with dequalinium chloride); *Merocaine (combined with cetylpyridinium chloride); *Rinstead Adult Gel (combined with chloroxylenol); *Tyrozets (combined with tyrothricin); *Wasp-Eze Spray (combined with mepyramine).

benzodiazepines A group of drugs that are used in the short-term treatment of anxiety and insomnia (*see* ANXIOLYTIC DRUGS; HYPNOTIC DRUGS). They are also used to relax patients before surgery or diagnostic procedures. Benzodiazepines should only be used to relieve anxiety or insomnia that is severe, disabling, or causing unacceptable distress. The lowest effective dosage should be used for the shortest possible time (preferably no more than 2 weeks for insomia, 2–4 weeks for anxiety); the drug should then be withdrawn gradually. Physical and psychological *dependence can develop with prolonged use, and sudden withdrawal can produce 'rebound' insomnia and anxiety. Benzodiazepines have a low incidence of side effects and are relatively safe in overdose when compared with older drugs, such as *barbiturates, although a paradoxical increase in hostility and aggression has been reported by some people taking benzodiazepines (see below); dosage adjustment usually overcomes this problem.

Benzodiazepines vary in their duration of action. Short-acting benzodiazepines, such as *lorazepam and *oxazepam, are effective for 6–10 hours; they have mild residual effects but carry a greater risk of withdrawal reactions. Long-acting drugs include *diazepam, *alprazolam, and

b

*chlordiazepoxide. They have a prolonged action, with persistent sedative effects, but withdrawal reactions are less of a problem. Benzodiazepines are available, on *prescription only, as tablets, capsules, syrups, or injections. Drug abuse with benzodiazepines, especially *temazepam has increased recently. Many benzodiazepines can no longer be prescribed on the NHS, and temazepam is now a *controlled drug.
Side effects and precautions: side effects include drowsiness and light-headedness (which may persist the next day), confusion, shaky movements, and unsteady gait (especially in elderly people), amnesia, and a paradoxical increase in hostility and aggression. This may range from talkativeness and excitement to aggressive and antisocial acts; increased anxiety, hallucinations, and delusions may also occur. Dependence can develop, and it is important that benzodiazepines are stopped gradually to avoid withdrawal reactions; these can include worsening of insomnia and anxiety, sweating, tremor, and weight loss. Drowsiness can impair judgment and dexterity, and the sedative effects of benzodiazepines are increased by alcohol.
Interactions with other drugs: the sedative effects of benzodiazepines are increased by a number of other drugs, including anaesthetics, opioid analgesics, antidepressants, antihistamines, antipsychotics, cimetidine, and most importantly ritonavir, which may in some cases cause profound sedation (see entries for individual drugs).

Sodium oxybate: its effects are enhanced by benzodiazepines, which should therefore not be taken with it.

benzoic acid An antifungal and antibacterial agent that is used mainly as a preservative in medicines and foods. In combination with *salicylic acid, it is used in the form of an ointment for treating fungal infections of the skin, such as ringworm; it is also included in some soothing preparations for *haemorrhoids. Benzoic acid also has *keratolytic properties and is used in combination with *malic acid and salicylic acid for removing dead skin from ulcers, burns, and wounds.
Proprietary preparation: *Hemocane (combined with lidocaine, cinnamic acid, zinc oxide, and bismuth oxide).

benzoin tincture compound (**friars' balsam**) A combination of balsamic acids in the form of a *tincture, used as an aromatic inhalation to relieve nasal congestion or soothe bronchitis. The tincture is added to hot water and the vapour is inhaled. Benzoin tincture compound is available without a prescription, but only from pharmacies.

benzoyl peroxide A mild *keratolytic that also has some antibacterial and antifungal activity and is used mainly for the treatment of *acne. It is available as a gel, solution, or cream and can be obtained without a prescription, but only from pharmacies.
Side effects: benzoyl peroxide may cause transient irritation and peeling of the skin.
Precautions: benzoyl peroxide should not come into contact with the eyes, mouth, or other mucous membranes.

Proprietary preparations: Acnecide (gel); Brevoxyl Cream; Clearasil Max 10 (cream); PanOxyl (gel, cream, or wash); *Duac Once Daily (combined with clindamycin); *Quinoderm (combined with hydroxyquinoline sulphate).

benzthiazide A *thiazide diuretic used for the treatment of *oedema associated with heart failure, liver disease, or kidney disease.
Side effects, precautions, and interactions with other drugs: *see* THIAZIDE DIURETICS. *See also* DIURETICS.

benzydamine hydrochloride An *NSAID used for the relief of painful conditions of the mouth and throat associated with inflammation and ulceration. Benzydamine is available as a mouthwash and a throat and mouth spray; it can be obtained without a prescription, but only from pharmacies.
Side effects: the mouthwash may occasionally cause stinging or numbness. *See also* NSAIDs.
Precautions: the mouthwash is not recommended for children under 12 years old. *See* NSAIDs.
Proprietary preparation: Difflam.

benzyl alcohol An antimicrobial preservative. It is included in many pharmaceutical preparations to keep them free of bacteria. It is also mildly anaesthetic and possesses antipruritic activity (i.e. it relieves itching) and is used as an ingredient in some topical preparations.
Side effects: benzyl alcohol may cause local irritation.

benzyl benzoate A drug used in the treatment of *scabies. It is available as an emulsion to be applied to the body and can be obtained without a prescription, but only from pharmacies.
Side effects: benzyl benzoate can irritate the skin and produces a burning sensation when applied to the genital area or to scratched skin. Rashes may rarely occur.
Precautions: benzyl benzoate should not be used to treat children and should be used with caution by women who are pregnant or breastfeeding (which should be suspended until the emulsion is washed off). It should not come into contact with the eyes, mucous membranes, or broken skin.

benzylpenicillin (**penicillin G**) The first *antibiotic of the *penicillin group to be used therapeutically. It is active against a number of bacteria, including streptococci, gonoccoci, and meningococci, and is used for the treatment of infections of the skin, soft tissues, respiratory tract, ear, nose, or throat, septicaemia, meningitis, and endocarditis (inflammation of the membranes surrounding the heart). It is also effective against anthrax, diphtheria, gas gangrene, leptospirosis, and Lyme disease. Benzylpenicillin is inactivated by penicillinases and therefore can only be used to treat infections caused by bacteria that do not produce penicillinase. It is given by injection or intravenous infusion and is available on *prescription only.
Side effects: allergic reactions may occur, including nettle rash, fever, joint pain, oedema (swelling) of the face, and *anaphylaxis.
Precautions: benzylpenicillin should not be taken by people allergic to

penicillins because of the risk of anaphylaxis (*see* PENICILLINS). It should be used with caution in those with impaired kidney function.
Interactions with other drugs:
  Methotrexate: concentrations of methotrexate in the blood are increased, which may cause adverse effects.
Proprietary preparation: Crystapen.

beractant A synthetic pulmonary *surfactant that is used to treat breathing difficulties in premature babies who are receiving mechanical ventilation (*see* VENTILATOR). Beractant is available, on *prescription only, as a suspension that is administered through a tube placed in the trachea (windpipe).
Side effects: beractant may very occasionally cause bleeding in the lungs.
Precautions: constant monitoring of heart rate and blood gases is necessary during treatment as beractant can cause a rapid improvement in the baby's condition and high concentrations of oxygen in the tissues have toxic effects.
Proprietary preparation: Survanta.

Berinert (CSL Behring) *See* C1-ESTERASE INHIBITOR.

Beriplex (CSL Behring) *See* PROTHROMBIN COMPLEX.

Beromun (Boehringer Ingelheim) *See* TASONERMIN.

Besavar XL (Winthrop Pharmaceuticals) *See* ALFUZOSIN HYDROCHLORIDE.

Beta-Adalat (Bayer) A proprietary combination of *atenolol (a *beta blocker) and *nifedipine (a *calcium antagonist), used for the treatment of *angina or *hypertension, usually when either of these drugs singly has been inadequate. It is available as tablets on *prescription only.
Side-effects, precautions, and interactions with other drugs: *see* BETA BLOCKERS; CALCIUM ANTAGONISTS.
  See also ANTIHYPERTENSIVE DRUGS.

beta agonists (**beta stimulants**) *See* SYMPATHOMIMETIC DRUGS.

beta blockers (**β-blockers**; in full **beta-adrenoceptor blockers**) Drugs that act on the heart, reducing its force and speed of contraction, and on blood vessels, preventing *vasodilatation. They produce their effects by blocking the stimulation of beta-adrenergic receptors by noradrenaline in the *sympathetic nervous system (*see* ADRENOCEPTORS). There are two types of beta receptors: 1 and 2. Beta 1 receptors are located mainly in the heart muscle; beta 2 receptors are found in the airways and blood vessels. Drugs acting only on the beta 1 receptors are described as **cardioselective**; drugs acting on both types of receptor are called **non-cardioselective**. Beta blockers are used to control abnormal heartbeats (*arrhythmias), to treat *angina, and to reduce high blood pressure (*hypertension). (Although they prevent the dilatation of blood vessels, beta blockers are used in the treatment of hypertension as their action on the heart is usually sufficient to correct raised blood pressure.) They are useful for treating people who have both hypertension and arrhythmias. They are also used after a heart attack to prevent a recurrence and may be used to improve heart function in the heart disorders known as cardiomyopathies. Beta blockers reduce symptoms of anxiety (such as palpitations) and are sometimes taken by people to make them feel more calm. They can also be taken to prevent *migraine headaches. In the form of eye drops, beta blockers are used to reduce fluid pressure inside the eyes in people with *glaucoma. Drugs whose name ends in '-alol' or '-olol' are usually beta blockers.

See ACEBUTOLOL; ATENOLOL; BISOPROLOL FUMARATE; BETAXOLOL HYDROCHLORIDE; CARTEOLOL HYDROCHLORIDE; CARVEDILOL; CELIPROLOL HYDROCHLORIDE; ESMOLOL HYDROCHLORIDE; LABETALOL HYDROCHLORIDE; LEVOBUNOLOL HYDROCHLORIDE; METIPRANOLOL; METOPROLOL TARTRATE; NADOLOL; NEBIVOLOL; OXPRENOLOL HYDROCHLORIDE; PINDOLOL; PROPRANOLOL HYDROCHLORIDE; SOTALOL HYDROCHLORIDE; TIMOLOL MALEATE.

Side effects: beta blockers may reduce the capacity for strenuous exercise or cause tiredness; many people experience cold hands and/or feet due to restriction of the blood supply to the limbs. Temporary reversible impotence and odd dreams may occur.

Precautions: beta blockers cause constriction of the air passages, although cardioselective beta blockers are less likely to cause such problems. For this reason, non-cardioselective beta blockers should not be taken by people with obstructive airways disease (such as asthma, chronic bronchitis, or emphysema), and cardioselective drugs should be used with extreme care and only when no alternative treatment is available. Beta blockers reduce the ability of the liver to release sugar when blood sugar is low and may mask some of the signs of *hypoglycaemia; they should therefore be used with caution in people with diabetes. Beta blockers should not be stopped suddenly after prolonged use as this may provoke sudden and severe recurrence of original symptoms and even a heart attack.

Interactions with other drugs:

Anti-arrhythmic drugs: the risk of bradycardia (slow heart rate) and depression of heart function is increased if these drugs are taken with beta blockers.

Antihypertensive drugs: the blood-pressure-lowering effects of alpha blockers, angiotensin II inhibitors, and calcium antagonists are enhanced by beta blockers; there is an increased risk of hypertension with clonidine if beta blockers are stopped suddenly; beta blockers should not be taken with verapamil as this can cause a severe fall in blood pressure and heart failure.

Diuretics: their effect in lowering blood pressure is enhanced by beta blockers.

Moxisylyte: may cause a severe fall in blood pressure on standing up.

Sympathomimetic drugs: severe hypertension can result if adrenaline, noradrenaline, or dobutamine are taken with beta blockers.

For other interactions, see entries for individual beta blockers.

See also ANTI-ARRHYTHMIC DRUGS; ANTIHYPERTENSIVE DRUGS.

Betacap (Dermal Laboratories) *See* BETAMETHASONE.

b

Beta-Cardone (UCB Pharma) *See* SOTALOL HYDROCHLORIDE.

Betadine (Molnlychke Health Care) *See* POVIDONE–IODINE.

Betaferon (Bayer) *See* INTERFERON BETA.

Betagan (Allergan) *See* LEVOBUNOLOL HYDROCHLORIDE.

betahistine An *analogue of *histamine that increases blood flow through the inner ear and is used to reduce the build-up of pressure that is thought to cause the vertigo and tinnitus (ringing in the ears) associated with Ménière's disease. It is available as tablets on *prescription only.
Side effects: include indigestion, headache, and itching or rashes.
Precautions: betahistine should not be taken by people with phaeochromocytoma (a tumour of the adrenal glands) and should be used with caution by people with asthma or peptic ulcers and by women who are pregnant or breastfeeding.
Proprietary preparation: Serc.

betaine A drug used in the treatment of homocystinuria, a hereditary disease caused by an enzyme deficiency and resulting in the presence of the amino acid homocysteine in the urine and high levels in the blood. Betaine is used only under specialist supervision. It is available as an oral powder to be dissolved in water on *prescription only.
Side effects: may include loss of appetite, nausea and vomiting, abdominal discomfort, agitation, depression, disturbed sleep, incontinence, and hair loss.
Precautions: plasma levels of the amino acid methionine should be monitored during treatment, and treatment should be stopped if levels rise and there are signs of fluid accumulating in the brain, which happens very rarely. The drug should be used with caution during pregnancy and breastfeeding.
Proprietary preparation: Cystadane.

beta-lactam antibiotics *See* ANTIBIOTICS.

Betaloc (AstraZeneca) *See* METOPROLOL TARTRATE.

betamethasone A *corticosteroid with potent anti-inflammatory activity, widely used for the treatment of severe asthma, allergic conditions, rheumatoid arthritis, connective-tissue diseases, and other disorders. It is also applied topically to treat infections or inflammation of the eyes and ears, rhinitis and hay fever, and a variety of eczematous inflammations and other skin conditions. Betamethasone and its salts (the dipropionate, the valerate, and the sodium phosphate) are available, on *prescription only, in the form of tablets, an injection, eye, ear, and nose drops, and ointments, plasters, creams, and lotions.
Side effects, precautions, and interactions with other drugs: *see* CORTICOSTEROIDS; TOPICAL STEROIDS.
Proprietary preparations: Betacap (scalp lotion); Betesil (medicated plaster);

Betnelan; Betnesol; Betnovate; Bettamousse (scalp mousse); Diprosone; Vistamethasone (eye or nose drops); *Betnesol-N (combined with neomycin); *Betnovate-C (combined with clioquinol); *Betnovate-N (combined with neomycin); *Diprosalic (combined with salicylic acid); *Dovobet (combined with calcipotriol); *Fucibet (combined with fusidic acid); *Lotriderm (combined with clotrimazole); Xamiol (combined with calcipotriol).

Beta-Prograne (Tillomed Laboratories) *See* PROPRANOLOL HYDROCHLORIDE.

beta stimulants (**beta agonists**) *See* SYMPATHOMIMETIC DRUGS.

betaxolol hydrochloride A cardioselective *beta blocker used for the treatment of chronic (open-angle) *glaucoma. It is available, on *prescription only, as eye drops.
Side effects, precautions, and interactions with other drugs: *see* BETA BLOCKERS.
Proprietary preparation: Betoptic.
See also ANTIHYPERTENSIVE DRUGS.

Betesil (Genus Pharmaceuticals) *See* BETAMETHASONE.

bethanechol chloride A *cholinergic drug that enhances motility of the intestines and contraction of the bladder and has been used as a stimulant laxative and for the treatment of urinary retention (it is now seldom used). Bethanechol is available as tablets on *prescription only.
Side effects: include nausea, vomiting, sweating, blurred vision, and slowing of the heart rate.
Precautions: bethanechol chloride should not be taken by people with peptic ulcer, cardiovascular disorders, respiratory diseases, epilepsy, Parkinson's disease, an overactive thyroid gland, intestinal or urinary obstruction, or when increased muscular activity of the urinary or gastrointestinal tract would be harmful. It should not be taken by women who are pregnant or breastfeeding.
Proprietary preparation: Myotonine.

Betim (Valeant Pharmaceuticals) *See* TIMOLOL MALEATE.

Betnelan (UCB Pharma) *See* BETAMETHASONE.

Betnesol (UCB Pharma) *See* BETAMETHASONE.

Betnesol-N (UCB Pharma) A proprietary combination of *betamethasone (a corticosteroid) and *neomycin sulphate (an antibiotic), used for the treatment of infected allergic conditions of the eyes or ears. It is available, on *prescription only, as eye drops or an ointment.
Side effects: allergic reactions may develop; *see also* TOPICAL STEROIDS; NEOMYCIN SULPHATE.
Precautions: *see* TOPICAL STEROIDS; NEOMYCIN SULPHATE. In addition, soft contact lenses should not be worn during treatment.

Betnovate (GlaxoSmithKline) *See* BETAMETHASONE.

Betnovate-C (Chemidex Pharma) A proprietary combination of *betamethasone (a corticosteroid) and *clioquinol (an antifungal agent), used for the treatment of inflammatory conditions of the skin when candidal and/or bacterial infection is present. It is available as a cream or ointment on *prescription only.
Side effects and precautions: *see* TOPICAL STEROIDS; CLIOQUINOL.

Betnovate-N (Chemidex Pharma) A proprietary combination of *betamethasone (a corticosteroid) and *neomycin sulphate (an antibiotic), used for the treatment of inflammatory conditions of the skin when infection is present. It is available as a cream or ointment on *prescription only.
Side effects, precautions, and interactions with other drugs: *see* TOPICAL STEROIDS; NEOMYCIN SULPHATE.

Betoptic (Alcon Laboratories) *See* BETAXOLOL HYDROCHLORIDE.

Bettamousse (UCB Pharma) *See* BETAMETHASONE.

bevacizumab A *monoclonal antibody that causes abnormal blood vessels supplying a tumour to regress and inhibits the formation of new blood vessels, thereby inhibiting tumour growth. It does this primarily by neutralizing the biological activity of *vascular endothelial growth factor. In combination with suitable chemotherapy, bevacizumab is used for treatment of advanced cancer of the colon or rectum. In combination with *paclitaxel or *docetaxel, it is used for the *first-line treatment of advanced breast cancer. In addition to platinum-based chemotherapy, bevacizumab is used for the first-line treatment of a type of lung cancer. In combination with *interferon alfa-2a, it is used for the first-line treatment of advanced kidney cancer. Bevacizumab is given by intravenous infusion and is available on *prescription only.
Side effects: *see* CYTOTOXIC DRUGS. There may also be hypertension, weakness, diarrhoea, nausea, vomiting, loss of appetite, headache, peripheral neuropathy (causing tingling and numbness of the limbs), and breathlessness.
Precautions: this medicine should not be given to women who are pregnant or breastfeeding and should be used with caution in people with cardiovascular disease or heart failure. *See also* CYTOTOXIC DRUGS.
Proprietary preparation: Avastin.

bexarotene A *retinoid used for the treatment of cutaneous T cell lymphoma (a type of lymphoma (*see* CANCER) that affects the skin). It is available as capsules on *prescription only.
Side effects: include low white blood cell counts, underactivity of the thyroid gland, raised blood lipids, headache, itching, and rash. *See also* CYTOTOXIC DRUGS.
Precautions: bexarotene should not be taken by people with a history of pancreatitis, uncontrolled *hyperlipidaemia, liver disease, or uncontrolled thyroid disease, or by women who are pregnant or breastfeeding. *See also* CYTOTOXIC DRUGS.

Interactions with other drugs:
Clozapine: should not be taken with bexarotene as this combination increases the risk of agranulocytosis (a blood disorder).
Gemfibrozil: increases the plasma concentration of bexarotene and should not be taken with it.
Proprietary preparation: Targretin.

bezafibrate A *fibrate used for the treatment of a wide variety of *hyperlipidaemias that have not responded to dietary modification and other appropriate measures. It is available as tablets and *modified-release tablets on *prescription only.
Side effects and precautions: see FIBRATES.
Interactions with other drugs:
Anticoagulants: the effects of warfarin, phenindione, and acenocoumarol are enhanced.
Antidiabetic agents: the effects of these drugs are enhanced.
See also FIBRATES.
Proprietary preparations: Bezalip; Bezalip-Mono (modified-release tablets twice the strength of Bezalip); Fibrazate XL (modified-release tablets); Zimbacol XL (modified-release tablets).

Bezalip, Bezalip-Mono (Actavis) *See* BEZAFIBRATE.

bicalutamide An *anti-androgen used for the treatment of advanced *cancer of the prostate gland, usually in conjunction with an analogue of *gonadorelin. It is available as tablets on *prescription only.
Side effects: include hot flushes, itching, breast tenderness and enlargement, diarrhoea, nausea, weakness, and (more rarely) jaundice, angina, heart failure, irregularities in heart rhythm, and blood disorders. Other side effects, which are more common in the elderly, include loss of appetite, dry mouth, indigestion, constipation, impotence, breathlessness, and rashes.
Precautions: liver function should be monitored in people with liver disease.
Interactions with other drugs:
Warfarin: its anticoagulant effect may be enhanced.
Proprietary preparation: Casodex.

bicarbonate *See* POTASSIUM BICARBONATE; SODIUM BICARBONATE.

biguanides *See* METFORMIN HYDROCHLORIDE.

bile acids A group of acidic compounds that are normally secreted by the gall bladder and aid the digestion and absorption of fats. The bile acid *ursodeoxycholic acid is used in the treatment of gallstone disease, but is suitable only for those who have small or medium-sized stones. Treatment may take months to complete (typically 3–18 months), and after the stones have dissolved some people may need to take long-term medication in order to prevent recurrence. People taking bile acids should restrict their intake of foods rich in cholesterol and calories.

bile-acid sequestrants A class of *lipid-lowering drugs. They are resins

b

that combine with bile acids and decrease the absorption of fats, thus increasing the amount of fat excreted in the faeces and lowering plasma *cholesterol concentrations. The main drugs in this class are *colestyramine, *colestipol, and *colesevelam hydrochloride. They can reduce plasma LDL-cholesterol by up to 25% (*see* LIPOPROTEINS).
Side effects: bile-acid sequestrants have effects on the gastrointestinal tract, causing discomfort, flatulence, dyspepsia, and constipation, which makes high doses hard to tolerate. The taste and texture of resins is often unacceptable; many people mix them with fruit juice to overcome this problem, but with limited success.
Precautions: the intestinal absorption of fat-soluble vitamins is reduced by resins, so that supplemental vitamins A, D, K, and possibly E may need to be taken by those receiving long-term treatment.
Interactions with other drugs: other drugs should be taken at least 1 hour before or 4–6 hours after resins to reduce possible interference with drug absorption.

Anticoagulants: the anticoagulant effects of warfarin, acenocoumarol, and phenindione may be increased.
Sodium valproate: absorption of this drug may be reduced.
Thiazide diuretics: absorption of these drugs is reduced; resins and thiazides should be taken at least two hours apart.

bimatoprost A *prostaglandin analogue used in the treatment of chronic (open-angle) *glaucoma and raised blood pressure in the eye. Bimatoprost increases the outflow of aqueous fluid from the eye and thus reduces the pressure in the eye. It is available as eye drops on *prescription only.
Side effects: bimatoprost may increase the brown pigment in the iris, and people should be warned to notice any changes in eye colour. The eyes may become irritated, itchy, or bloodshot, the conjunctiva may become inflamed or swollen, and the eyelashes may become longer, darker, or thicker.
Precautions: bimatoprost should be used with caution in people with asthma and in women who are pregnant or breastfeeding.
Proprietary preparations: Lumigan; *Ganfort (combined with timolol maleate.

Binocrit (Sandoz) *See* ERYTHROPOIETIN.

BiNovum (Janssen-Cilag) A proprietary combination of *ethinylestradiol and *norethisterone used as an *oral contraceptive of the biphasic type. These tablets are packaged in two phases, which differ in the amounts of the active ingredients they contain. BiNovum is available on *prescription only.
Side effects, precautions, and interactions with other drugs: *see* ORAL CONTRACEPTIVES.

Biorphen (Alliance) *See* ORPHENADRINE.

biotin *See* VITAMIN B COMPLEX.

biphasic insulins *See* INSULIN.

bisacodyl A *stimulant laxative used to treat constipation and to clear the bowel before surgery, childbirth, or X-ray examination. It is available as *enteric-coated tablets and suppositories and can be obtained without a prescription, but only from pharmacies.
Side effects and precautions: *see* STIMULANT LAXATIVES.
Proprietary preparations: Dulcolax Suppositories; Dulcolax Suppositories for Children; Dulcolax Tablets.

bismuth oxide An *astringent that is used to relieve the discomfort of *haemorrhoids and the pain, soreness, or itching of other disorders of the anus or rectum. It is included as an ingredient in a variety of creams, ointments, and suppositories.
Proprietary preparations: *Anugesic-HC (combined with hydrocortisone acetate, zinc oxide, pramocaine hydrochloride, Peru balsam, and benzyl benzoate); *Anugesic-HC Suppositories (combined with benzyl benzoate, pramocaine hydrochloride, hydrocortisone acetate, zinc oxide, Peru balsam, and bismuth subgallate); *Anusol (combined with bismuth subgallate, Peru balsam, and zinc oxide); *Anusol-HC (combined with hydrocortisone acetate, benzyl benzoate, bismuth subgallate, Peru balsam, and zinc oxide); *Hemocane (combined with zinc oxide, benzoic acid, cinnamic acid, and lidocaine).

bismuth subgallate An *astringent that is used to relieve the discomfort of *haemorrhoids and the pain, soreness, or itching of other disorders of the anus or rectum. It is included as an ingredient in a variety of creams, ointments, and suppositories.
Proprietary preparations: *Anusol (combined with bismuth oxide, Peru balsam, and zinc oxide); *Anusol-HC (combined with hydrocortisone acetate, benzyl benzoate, bismuth oxide, Peru balsam, and zinc oxide); *Anugesic-HC Suppositories (combined with benzyl benzoate, pramocaine hydrochloride, hydrocortisone acetate, zinc oxide, Peru balsam, and bismuth oxide).

bismuth subsalicylate An insoluble salt of bismuth used for the treatment of diarrhoea, stomach upsets, nausea, and indigestion (*see* ANTACIDS). It is available as a suspension and can be obtained without a prescription, but only from pharmacies.
Side effects: bismuth subsalicylate causes blackening of the stools. If large quantities are taken, salicylate may be absorbed and produce the adverse effects associated with *salicylates.
Proprietary preparation: Pepto-Bismol.

Bisodol Antacid Powder (Forest Laboratories) A proprietary combination of *sodium bicarbonate and *magnesium carbonate, used for the relief of upset stomach, heartburn, indigestion, and trapped wind (*see* ACID-PEPTIC DISEASES). It is freely available *over the counter.
Side effects and interactions with other drugs: *see* ANTACIDS.
Precautions: this powder is not recommended for children.

Bisodol Antacid Tablets, Bisodol Extra Strong Mint (Forest

Laboratories) Proprietary combinations of *sodium bicarbonate, *calcium carbonate, and *magnesium carbonate, used for the relief of upset stomach, heartburn, indigestion, and trapped wind (*see* ACID-PEPTIC DISEASES). They are freely available *over the counter in the form of chewable tablets.
Side effects and interactions with other drugs: *see* ANTACIDS.
Precautions: these tablets are not recommended for children.

Bisodol Extra Tablets (Forest Laboratories) A proprietary combination of *sodium bicarbonate, *calcium carbonate, and *magnesium carbonate (antacids) and activated *dimeticone (an antifoaming agent), used for the relief of upset stomach, heartburn, indigestion, and trapped wind (*see* ACID-PEPTIC DISEASES). It is freely available *over the counter.
Side effects and interactions with other drugs: *see* ANTACIDS.
Precautions: these tablets are not recommended for children.

bisoprolol fumarate A cardioselective *beta blocker used for the treatment of *angina, *hypertension, and heart failure. It is available as tablets on *prescription only.
Side effects and precautions: *see* BETA BLOCKERS.
Interactions with other drugs:
Rifampicin: reduces the plasma concentration of bisoprolol.
For other interactions, *see* BETA BLOCKERS.
Proprietary preparation: Cardicor.

bisphosphonates A group of drugs that prevent the loss of calcium from bone and its transfer to the bloodstream. They are used to strengthen the bones in the treatment of Paget's disease (in which the bones become deformed and fracture easily), to lower high concentrations of calcium in the blood in patients with bone cancer, and to treat or prevent osteoporosis. *See* ALENDRONIC ACID; DISODIUM ETIDRONATE; DISODIUM PAMIDRONATE; IBANDRONIC ACID; RISEDRONATE SODIUM; SODIUM CLODRONATE; TILUDRONIC ACID; ZOLEDRONIC ACID.

bivalirudin An *analogue of hirudin, an anticoagulant produced by leeches. It is used in the treatment of people who have had angina and a heart attack and are waiting for urgent surgical treatment; it should be given with *aspirin and *clopidogrel. Bivalirudin is available as an intravenous injection on *prescription only.
Side effects: bleeding is the most common side effect.
Precautions: this medicine should be used with caution during pregnancy and breastfeeding. Patients should be monitored carefully for bleeding during treatment; the risk of bleeding is increased by the use of other anticoagulants.
Proprietary preparation: Angiox.

Bleo-Kyowa (Kyowa Hakko) *See* BLEOMYCIN.

bleomycin A *cytotoxic antibiotic that is injected into a vein or a muscle for the treatment of lymphomas, certain solid tumours, and squamous cell carcinoma (a form of skin cancer). It can be injected directly into the chest or

abdomen to treat metastases in accumulations of fluid caused by certain *cancers. It is available as a form for injection on *prescription only.
Side effects: bleomycin causes little *bone marrow suppression. The most likely side effects are increased pigmentation of the skin, especially between the toes and fingers, inside the elbows and knees, and in the groin, hard swellings beneath the skin, and inflammation of the mucous membranes. Allergic reactions, including chills and fevers, are common a few hours after administration of bleomycin. These can be treated with corticosteroids (such as hydrocortisone), antihistamines, and/or antipyretics. Fibrosis (thickening) of the lung tissue, which can have effects on breathing, may occur with long-term use. *See also* CYTOTOXIC DRUGS.
Precautions: *see* CYTOTOXIC DRUGS. Bleomycin is irritant to skin and must be handled with caution.
Interactions with other drugs:
Clozapine: there is an increased risk of agranulocytosis (a serious blood disorder), and therefore this drug should not be taken with bleomycin.
Proprietary preparation: Bleo-Kyowa.

Blistex Relief Cream (DDD) A proprietary combination of strong *ammonia solution, aromatic ammonia solution, and *phenol solution, used for the relief of cold sores and cracked or chapped lips. It is freely available *over the counter.
Precautions: if cold sores become recurrent, medical advice should be sought.

Bolamyn SR (Teva UK) *See* METFORMIN HYDROCHLORIDE.

Bondronat (Roche Products) *See* IBANDRONIC ACID.

Bonefos (Bayer) *See* SODIUM CLODRONATE.

bone marrow suppression A reduction in the activity of the bone marrow, the tissue contained within the internal cavities of the bones that produces blood cells. Many drugs, especially *cytotoxic drugs, suppress the activity of this tissue, resulting in a decrease in the number of white cells, red cells, and platelets in the blood. A loss of white blood cells leaves the individual susceptible to infection; decreased numbers of red blood cells causes *anaemia and tiredness; loss of platelets causes spontaneous bruising and prolonged bleeding after injury. Bone marrow suppression is usually reversible once the drug responsible is stopped, but it may take a couple of weeks for the bone marrow to return to its normal activity.

Bonjela (Reckitt Benckiser) A proprietary combination of *cetalkonium chloride (an antiseptic) and *choline salicylate (a local analgesic), used for the relief of pain and discomfort of mouth ulcers, cold sores, sores caused by dentures, and teething problems. It is freely available *over the counter.
Precautions: Bonjela is not recommended for children under four months old. *See also* CETALKONIUM CHLORIDE; CHOLINE SALICYLATE.

Bonviva (Roche Products) *See* IBANDRONIC ACID.

Boots Allergy Relief Antihistamine Tablets (Boots) *See* CHLORPHENAMINE MALEATE.

Boots Anaesthetic & Antibiotic Throat Lozenges (Boots) A proprietary combination of *benzocaine (a local anaesthetic) and *tyrothricin (an antibiotic), used for the relief of sore throats. It is available as tablets without a prescription, but only from Boots pharmacies.
Precautions: this medicine is not recommended for children under 12 years old.

Boots Anti-Dandruff Ketoconazole Shampoo (Boots) *See* KETOCONAZOLE.

Boots Antifungal Cream (Boots) *See* CLOTRIMAZOLE.

Boots Antiseptic Gel (Boots) *See* CETYLPYRIDINIUM CHLORIDE.

Boots Antiseptic Nappy Rash Cream (Boots) A proprietary combination of *cetrimide (an antiseptic) and *dimeticone (a water repellent), used as a *barrier preparation for the treatment of napkin rash and pressure sores. It is available *over the counter, but only from Boots stores.

Boots Antiseptic Sore Mouth Pastilles (Boots) *See* DICHLOROBENZYL ALCOHOL.

Boots Antiseptic Wound Wash (Boots) *See* CETRIMIDE.

Boots Avert (Boots) *See* ACICLOVIR.

Boots Bite and Sting Antihistamine Cream (Boots) *See* MEPYRAMINE.

Boots Bite & Sting Hydrocortisone Cream (Boots) *See* HYDROCORTISONE.

Boots Bronchial Cough Mixture (Boots) A proprietary combination of ammonium carbonate, *ammonium chloride, and *guaifenesin (all *expectorants), used for the relief of productive coughs with congestion. It is available as a syrup without a prescription, but only from Boots.
Side effects and precautions: *see* GUAIFENESIN.

Boots Catarrh Cough Syrup (Boots) A proprietary combination of *codeine (an analgesic and cough suppressant) and creosote (an antiseptic), used for the relief of productive coughs and congestion. It is available without a prescription, but only from Boots.
Side effects, precautions, and interactions with other drugs: *see* CODEINE; COUGH SUPPRESSANTS; OPIOIDS.

Boots Catarrh Syrup for Children (Boots) A proprietary combination of *diphenhydramine (a sedative antihistamine) and *pseudoephedrine (a decongestant), used for the relief of congestion associated with colds and hay fever in children. It is available without a prescription, but only from Boots.
Side effects, precautions, and interactions with other drugs: *see* ANTIHISTAMINES; DECONGESTANTS; EPHEDRINE.

Boots Chilblain Cream (Boots) A proprietary combination of *benzyl alcohol and *eucalyptus oil, used to soothe and heal broken and unbroken chilblains. It is available *over the counter, but only from Boots stores.

Boots Children's 1 Year Plus Night Time Cough Syrup (Boots) A proprietary combination of *diphenhydramine (a sedative antihistamine) and *pholcodine (a cough suppressant), used for the relief of dry irritating coughs in children. It is available without a prescription, but only from Boots.
Side effects, precautions, and interactions with other drugs: *see* ANTIHISTAMINES; PHOLCODINE; COUGH SUPPRESSANTS.

Boots Cold and 'Flu Relief Tablets (Boots) A proprietary combination of *paracetamol (an analgesic and antipyretic), *caffeine (a stimulant), *phenylephrine (a decongestant), and ascorbic acid (*vitamin C), used to relieve the symptoms of colds and influenza. It is available without a prescription, but only from Boots.
Side effects and precautions: *see* PARACETAMOL; CAFFEINE; PHENYLEPHRINE.
Interactions with other drugs: *see* PHENYLEPHRINE.

Boots Cold Relief Hot Blackcurrant, Boots Cold Relief Hot Lemon (Boots) *See* PARACETAMOL.

Boots Cold Relief Hot Lemon with Decongestant (Boots) A proprietary combination of *paracetamol (an analgesic and antipyretic) and *phenylephrine (a decongestant), used to relieve the symptoms of colds, including fever and nasal congestion. **Boots Cold Relief Hot Blackcurrant with Decongestant** is a similar preparation. Both are powders to be dissolved in hot water; they are available *over the counter, but only from Boots.
Side effects and precautions: *see* PARACETAMOL; PHENYLEPHRINE.
Interactions with other drugs: *see* PHENYLEPHRINE.

Boots Congestion Relief Capsules (Boots) *See* PHENYLEPHRINE.

Boots Constipation Relief 1 Year Plus (Boots) A proprietary combination of *senna and figs, used as a *stimulant laxative for the treatment of constipation. It is available without a prescription, but only from Boots.
Side effects and precautions: *see* STIMULANT LAXATIVES.

Boots Constipation Relief Suppositories (Boots) *See* GLYCERIN.

Boots Corn Removal Plasters (Boots) *See* SALICYLIC ACID.

Boots Cough and Decongestant Syrup 2 Years Plus (Boots) A proprietary combination of *guaifenesin (an expectorant) and *pseudoephedrine (a decongestant), used to relieve the symptoms of chest infections accompanied by a productive cough in children aged 2–12 years. It is available as a syrup and can be obtained without a prescription, but only from Boots pharmacies.
Side effects and interactions with other drugs: *see* EPHEDRINE HYDROCHLORIDE; GUAIFENESIN.
Precautions: *see* EPHEDRINE HYDROCHLORIDE.

Boots Cough Syrup 3 Months Plus (Boots) *See* GLYCERIN.

Boots Cradle Cap Cream from Birth (Boots) A proprietary combination of *almond oil and *lanolin (both emollients), used for the treatment of cradle cap. It is freely available as a cream *over the counter, but only from Boots stores.
Side effects: *see* LANOLIN.

Boots Cystitis Relief (Boots) *See* SODIUM CITRATE.

Boots Day Cold Comfort (Boots) A proprietary combination of *paracetamol (an analgesic and antipyretic), *pseudoephedrine (a decongestant), and *pholcodine (a cough suppressant), used to relieve the symptoms of colds and influenza. It is available as capsules without a prescription, but only from Boots.
Side effects and precautions: *see* PARACETAMOL; EPHEDRINE HYDROCHLORIDE; DECONGESTANTS; CODEINE.
Interactions with other drugs: *see* EPHEDRINE HYDROCHLORIDE; OPIOIDS.

Boots Daytime Cough Relief (Boots) *See* PHOLCODINE.

Boots Decongestant Tablets (Boots) *See* PSEUDOEPHEDRINE.

Boots Decongestant Tablets with Paracetamol (Boots) A proprietary combination of *paracetamol (an analgesic) and *pseudoephedrine (a decongestant), used to relieve the symptoms of colds and influenza, including feverishness, aches and pains, headache, and nasal and sinus congestion. It is available as tablets without a prescription, but only from Boots pharmacies.
Side effects and interactions with other drugs: *See* EPHEDRINE HYDROCHLORIDE; DECONGESTANTS.
Precautions: this medicine should not be taken by children under six years old. *See also* PARACETAMOL; DECONGESTANTS; EPHEDRINE HYDROCHLORIDE.

Boots Diareze (Boots) *See* LOPERAMIDE HYDROCHLORIDE.

Boots Dual Action Athlete's Foot Cream (Boots) A proprietary combination of *tolnaftate (an antifungal drug) and *benzalkonium (an antiseptic), used for the treatment of athlete's foot. It is also effective for treating other fungal infections, such as fungal groin infection. It is available *over the counter, but only from Boots stores.

Boots Dual Action Athlete's Foot Powder (Boots) A proprietary combination of *tolnaftate (an antifungal drug) and *chlorhexidine (an antiseptic), used for the treatment of athlete's foot. It is also effective for treating other fungal infections, such as fungal groin infection. It is available *over the counter, but only from Boots stores.

Boots Dual Action Athlete's Foot Spray (Boots) *See* TOLNAFTATE.

Boots Dual Action Cold Sore Lotion (Boots) A proprietary combination of *dichlorobenzyl alcohol (an *antiseptic, *menthol, *camphor (a cooling agent), and *benzyl alcohol (an antimicrobial preservative), used for the relief

of cold sores. It is freely available as a lotion *over the counter but only at Boots stores.
Side effects: *see* BENZYL ALCOHOL.

Boots Dual Action Diarrhoea Relief (Boots) A proprietary preparation consisting of capsules of *loperamide hydrochloride (an opioid) and sachets containing a combination of *sodium chloride, *potassium chloride, *sodium citrate, and *citric acid to be dissolved in water. It is used to treat the symptoms of acute diarrhoea and replace associated fluid and electrolyte loss. It is freely available *over the counter, but only from Boots stores.
Side effects: *see* LOPERAMIDE HYDROCHLORIDE; POTASSIUM.
Precautions: *see* LOPERAMIDE HYDROCHLORIDE; POTASSIUM; SODIUM CITRATE.
Interactions with other drugs: *see* POTASSIUM.

Boots Fever and Pain Relief 6 Months Plus Ibuprofen (Boots) *See* IBUPROFEN.

Boots First Aid Antiseptic Liquid (Boots) *See* CETYLPYRIDINIUM CHLORIDE.

Boots Glycerin and Blackcurrant Soothing Cough Syrup (Boots) *See* GLYCERIN.

Boots Gripe Mixture 1 Month Plus (Boots) *See* SODIUM BICARBONATE.

Boots Haemorrhoid Suppositories (Boots) *See* ALLANTOIN.

Boots Hayfever and Allergy Relief (Boots) *See* CETIRIZINE HYDROCHLORIDE.

Boots Hayfever Relief Eye Drops (Boots) *See* SODIUM CROMOGLICATE.

Boots IBS Relief (Boots) *See* MEBEVERINE HYDROCHLORIDE.

Boots Ibuprofen Pain Relief 6 Months Plus (Boots) *See* IBUPROFEN.

Boots Indigestion Relief Tablets Fruit (Boots) *See* CALCIUM CARBONATE.

Boots Infant Pain Relief (Boots) *See* PARACETAMOL.

Boots Lip and Cold Sore Cream (Boots) A proprietary combination of *cetrimide (an antiseptic), *dimeticone (a water repellent silicone), *urea (a hydrating agent), and *chlorocresol (a disinfectant), used for the relief of cracked lips and occasional cold sores. It is available *over the counter, but only from Boots stores.
Precautions: if cold sores become recurrent, medical advice should be sought.

Boots Maximum Strength Cold & Flu Relief Direct Dose Lemon/Blackcurrant (Boots) Proprietary combinations of *paracetamol (an analgesic and antipyretic) and *phenylephrine (a decongestant), used to relieve symptoms of the common cold and influenza, including aches and pains, sore throat, headache, fatigue and drowsiness, nasal congestion, and

high temperature. Powders to be dissolved in water, they are freely available *over the counter, but only at Boots stores.
Side effects and interactions with other drugs: *see* PHENYLEPHRINE.
Precautions: *see* PARACETAMOL; PHENYLEPHRINE.

b

Boots Max Strength Cold & Flu Capsules (Boots) A proprietary combination of *paracetamol (an analgesic and antipyretic), *caffeine (a stimulant), and *phenylephrine (a decongestant), used to relieve symptoms of the common cold and influenza, including aches and pains, sore throat, headache, fatigue and drowsiness, nasal congestion, and high temperature. It is freely available as capsules *over the counter, but only from Boots stores.
Side effects and precautions: *see* PARACETAMOL; CAFFEINE; PHENYLEPHRINE.
Interactions with other drugs: *See* PHENYLEPHRINE.

Boots Max Strength Sinus Relief Capsules (Boots) A proprietary combination of *paracetamol (an analgesic and antipyretic), *caffeine (a stimulant), and *phenylephrine (a decongestant), used to relieve the symptoms associated with sinus blockages. It is freely available as capsules *over the counter, but only at Boots stores.
Side effects and precautions: *see* PARACETAMOL; CAFFEINE; PHENYLEPHRINE.
Interactions with other drugs: *see* PHENYLEPHRINE.

Boots Mild Vapour Rub 3 Months Plus (Boots) A proprietary combination of *camphor (a rubefacient), *menthol, and *eucalyptus oil (an aromatic oil with cooling effects), used for the relief of head colds, stuffy nose, cough, and chest colds. It is available as an ointment *over the counter, but only from Boots stores.
Precautions: the ointment should not be applied to children under three months old.

Boots Muscular Pain Relief Gel (Boots) *See* KETOPROFEN.

Boots Nasal Spray (Boots) *See* OXYMETAZOLINE.

Boots Natural Senna Tablets (Boots) *See* SENNA.

Boots NicAssist (Boots) *See* NICOTINE.

Boots Night Cold Comfort (Boots) A proprietary combination of *paracetamol (an analgesic and antipyretic), *pseudoephedrine (a decongestant), *diphenhydramine (a sedative antihistamine), and *pholcodine (a cough suppressant), taken at night to relieve the symptoms of colds and influenza. It is available as tablets without a prescription, but only from Boots.
Side effects and precautions: *see* PARACETAMOL; EPHEDRINE HYDROCHLORIDE; ANTIHISTAMINES; CODEINE.
Interactions with other drugs: *see* EPHEDRINE HYDROCHLORIDE; ANTIHISTAMINES; OPIOIDS.

Boots Night-time Cough Relief Syrup 2 Years Plus (Boots) A proprietary combination of *diphenhydramine (a sedative antihistamine) and

*pholcodine (a cough suppressant), used for the relief of dry coughs that interfere with sleep. It is available as a syrup without a prescription, but only from Boots.
Side effects, precautions, and interactions with other drugs: *see* ANTIHISTAMINES; PHOLCODINE; OPIOIDS.
Precautions: the syrup should not be taken by children under 2 years old. *See also* ANTIHISTAMINES; CODEINE.

Boots Nirolex Chesty Cough & Congestion Relief Linctus (Boots) A proprietary combination of *guaifenesin (an expectorant) and *pseudoephedrine (a decongestant), used for the relief of chesty coughs, nasal congestion, and catarrh. It is available *over the counter, but only from Boots stores.
Side effects: may include restlessness, irritability, confusion, tremor, insomnia, palpitations, hypertension (high blood pressure), tachycardia (fast heart rate), stomach upsets, urinary retention, headache, and skin rashes.
Precautions: the linctus should not be taken by people with severe hypertension or severe coronary artery disease, overactivity of the thyroid gland, or glaucoma. It should be avoided by people with kidney disease.
Interactions with other drugs:
Monoamine oxidase inhibitors: may cause a rise in blood pressure and should therefore be avoided.
Tricyclic antidepressants: may cause a rise in blood pressure and should therefore be avoided.

Boots Nirolex Chesty Cough Relief Linctus (Boots) *See* GUAIFENESIN.

Boots Nirolex Dry Cough Relief Linctus (Boots) *See* GLYCERIN.

Boots Nirolex Night Time Cough Relief Linctus (Boots) A proprietary combination of *diphenhydramine (a sedative antihistamine) and *pholcodine (a cough suppressant), used for the relief of dry irritating coughs in children. It is available without prescription, but only from Boots *pharmacies.
Side effects, and precautions, interactions with other drugs: *see* ANTIHISTAMINES; PHOLCODINE; COUGH SUPPRESSANTS.

Boots Oral Antiseptic (Boots) *See* CETYLPYRIDINIUM CHLORIDE.

Boots Pain Relief Warming Spray (Boots) A proprietary combination of *camphor, *ethyl nicotinate, and *methyl salicylate, used as a *rubefacient for the relief of muscular and rheumatic pains and stiffness, including backache, sciatica, lumbago, fibrositis, and sprains. It is available *over the counter, but only from Boots.
Side effects and precautions: *see* RUBEFACIENTS; SALICYLATES.

Boots Paracetamol and Codeine Extra Capsules (Boots) A proprietary combination of *paracetamol (a non-opioid analgesic), *caffeine (a stimulant), and *codeine (an opioid analgesic), used for the relief of migraine

b

headaches. It is available as tablets and can be bought without a prescription, but only from Boots *pharmacies.
Side effects and precautions: *see* PARACETAMOL; CODEINE.
Interactions with other drugs: *see* OPIOIDS.

Boots Paracetamol Capsules/Suspension (Boots) *See* PARACETAMOL.

Boots Pharmacy Anaesthetic Throat Spray (Boots) *See* LIDOCAINE.

Boots Pharmacy Antibiotic Eye Drops (Boots) *See* CHLORAMPHENICOL.

Boots Skin Therapy Emollient Cream (Boots) A proprietary combination of *almond oil and *lanolin (both emollients), used for the relief of dry skin conditions (such as chapping caused by weather or water), nappy soreness, dry eczema, and sunburn. It is available *over the counter, but only from Boots stores.

Boots Sleepeaze Tablets (Boots) *See* DIPHENHYDRAMINE.

Boots Soothing Eye Drops (Boots) A proprietary combination of *cetrimide (an antiseptic) and *hamamelis (an astringent), used for the relief of minor eye irritations. It is available *over the counter, but only from Boots stores.

Boots Sore Throat Relief Dual Action Lozenges (Boots) *See* HEXYLRESORCINOL.

Boots Sore Throat Relief Lozenges (Boots) *See* AMYLMETACRESOL.

Boots Teething Gel 3 Months + (Boots) A proprietary combination of *lidocaine (a local anaesthetic) and *cetylpyridinium chloride (an antiseptic), used to relieve teething troubles. It is freely available *over the counter, but only from Boots stores.

Boots Tension Headache Relief (Boots) A proprietary combination of *paracetamol and *codeine (analgesics), *caffeine (a stimulant), and *doxylamine (an antihistamine), used for the relief of headaches brought on by stress. It is available as tablets and can be obtained without a prescription, but only from Boots.
Side effects and precautions: *see* PARACETAMOL; CAFFEINE; CODEINE; ANTIHISTAMINES.
Interactions with other drugs: *see* OPIOIDS; ANTIHISTAMINES.

Boots Thrush 1% Cream (Boots) *See* CLOTRIMAZOLE.

Boots Travel Calm Tablets (Boots) *See* HYOSCINE HYDROBROMIDE.

Boots Vapour Chest Rub (Boots) A proprietary combination of *eucalyptus oil, *menthol, and *camphor, used to relieve the symptoms of head colds, stuffy noses, coughs, and chest colds. **Boots Vapour Inhalant Oil** has the additional ingredient of *peppermint oil and is used to relieve the same symptoms. Both preparations are available without a prescription, but only from Boots stores.

Boots Verruca Removal Gel (Boots) A proprietary combination of *salicylic acid (a keratolytic) and *camphor, used for the treatment of warts and verrucas. It is available *over the counter, but only from Boots stores.
Precautions: this preparation is not recommended for children.

Boots Wind Relief Tablets (Boots) A proprietary combination of *aluminium hydroxide and *magnesium hydroxide (antacids) and simeticone (activated dimeticone; an antifoaming agent), used to relieve discomfort associated with painful wind, indigestion, heartburn, and excess acidity. It is freely available *over the counter, but only from Boots stores.
Side effects, precautions, and interactions with other drugs: *see* ANTACIDS.

bortezomib A drug used for the treatment of multiple myeloma, a cancer of the antibody-producing cells of the bone marrow. It works by affecting the ability of these cells to interact with the bone marrow. It is given by intravenous injection and is available on *prescription only.
Side effects: include nausea, vomiting, diarrhoea or constipation, dehydration, fever, loss of appetite, dizziness, muscle cramps, peripheral neuropathy (causing numbness and tingling of the limbs), and a fall in blood pressure on standing. *See also* CYTOTOXIC DRUGS.
Precautions: bortezomib should be used with caution or not taken by people with liver disease, heart disease, lung disease, or kidney disease. It should not be taken by women who are pregnant or breastfeeding. *See also* CYTOTOXIC DRUGS.
Interactions with other drugs:
Clozapine: should not be taken with bortezomib as this combination increases the risk of agranulocytosis (a blood disorder).
Proprietary preparation: Velcade.

bosentan A potent *vasodilator used in the treatment of pulmonary arterial hypertension (raised blood pressure in the vessels supplying the lungs) and ulcers of the fingers in people with systemic sclerosis (a disease of connective tissue). It blocks receptors for endothelin, a hormone that stimulates constriction of blood vessels. Bosentan is available as tablets on *prescription only.
Side effects: include nausea and vomiting, abdominal pain, dry mouth, flushing, low blood pressure, palpitations, chest pain, breathlessness, dizziness, back and leg pain, and allergic reactions (rash, itching).
Precautions: bosentan should be used with caution in people with impaired liver function. Liver function tests should be carried out before and during treatment, which should be stopped if signs of liver disease develop. Bosentan should not be taken by people with porphyria or by women who are pregnant or breastfeeding.
Interactions with other drugs:
Ciclosporin: increases the plasma concentration of bosentan and should not be taken with it.
Fluconazole: increases the plasma concentration of bosentan and should not be taken with it.

b

Glibenclamide: increases the risk of liver damage and should not be taken with bosentan.
Oral contraceptives: their effect may be reduced.
Rifampicin: causes a decrease in bosentan plasma levels and should not be taken with it.
Proprietary preparation: Tracleer.

Botox (Allergan) *See* BOTULINUM TOXIN TYPE A.

botulinum toxin type A A biological product used in minute doses as a *muscle relaxant for the treatment of hand, arm or foot spasticity, blepharospasm (a tight contraction of the eyelids), one-sided facial spasms, torticollis (twisting of the neck), and excessive sweating of the armpits. It is administered by local injection by specialists trained in its use; as its duration of action is only 8–12 weeks, repeated injections are usually necessary. Botulinum toxin is available on *prescription only.
Side effects: there may be weakness and pain in the injected muscle and some jitter in other muscles; a transient burning sensation can occur after injection and a rash may develop. Reduced response may occur after repeated injections due to the formation of antibodies against botulinum toxin.
Precautions: botulinum toxin should not be used in people who have myasthenia gravis or in women who are pregnant or breastfeeding.
Proprietary preparations: Azzalure; Botox; Dysport; Vistabel; Xeomin.

botulinum toxin type B A biological product used in minute amounts as a *muscle relaxant for the treatment of torticollis (twisting of the neck caused by muscle spasm). It is given under specialist supervision by intramuscular injection and is available on *prescription only.
Side effects: include dry mouth, blurred vision, difficulty in swallowing, and neck pain. There may be some jigger in distant muscles.
Precautions: botulinum toxin type B must not be given to patients with neuromuscular disease (e.g. myasthenia gravis) or to women who are pregnant or breastfeeding.
Proprietary preparation: NeuroBloc.

bowel-cleansing solutions Preparations used to evacuate the bowel before exploratory procedures, surgery, or radiography. Containing osmotic or stimulant *laxatives, they are available as solutions, or powders to be dissolved in water, and are taken by mouth at regular intervals until the bowel effluent does not contain any solid material.
Side effects: include nausea, bloating, and (less commonly) abdominal cramps and vomiting.
Precautions: bowel-cleansing solutions should not be taken by people with gastrointestinal obstruction or ulceration and should be used with caution in pregnant women and in people with heart disease, ulcerative colitis, diabetes mellitus, or reflux oesophagitis.
Proprietary preparations: Citramag (*see* MAGNESIUM CITRATE); *CitraFleet (sodium picosulfate laxatives, magnesium citrate, and citric acid); *Fleet

Phospho-soda (phosphate laxatives); *Klean-Prep (macrogol '3340' and salts); *Picolax (sodium picosulfate and magnesium citrate).

Bradosol (Novartis) *See* BENZALKONIUM CHLORIDE.

Bramitob (Chiesi) *See* TOBRAMYCIN.

bran The fibrous outer layers of cereal grain. Wheat or oat bran is an effective *bulk-forming laxative. Wheat bran is freely available *over the counter in the form of a powder.
Side effects and precautions: *see* ISPAGHULA HUSK.

Brasivol (Stiefel Laboratories) *See* ALUMINIUM OXIDE.

breath-activated inhaler (**breath-acuated inhaler**) *See* INHALER.

Brevibloc (Baxter Healthcare) *See* ESMOLOL HYDROCHLORIDE.

Brevinor (Pharmacia) A proprietary combination of *ethinylestradiol and *norethisterone used as an *oral contraceptive. It is available as tablets on *prescription only.
Side effects, precautions, and interactions with other drugs: *see* ORAL CONTRACEPTIVES.

Brevoxyl Cream (Stiefel Laboratories) *See* BENZOYL PEROXIDE.

Bricanyl (AstraZeneca) *See* TERBUTALINE SULPHATE.

brimonidine tartrate A *sympathomimetic drug, similar to *apraclonidine, that stimulates alpha *adrenoceptors. It is used primarily in the treatment of *glaucoma, in which it is thought to act by reducing the amount of fluid produced in the eye and also by aiding the drainage of the fluid from the eye. It may be used in conjunction with a *beta blocker. Brimonidine is available as eye drops on *prescription only.
Side effects: include bloodshot eyes, stinging, itching, allergic reactions, dry mouth, headache, fatigue, and drowsiness.
Precautions: brimonidine is not recommended for children. It should be used with caution in people with severe heart disease, depression, Raynaud's syndrome, or impaired kidney or liver function and in women who are pregnant or breastfeeding. People who wear soft contact lenses should wait at least 15 minutes after applying the drops before inserting their lenses.
Interactions with other drugs:
MAOIs: should not be used with brimonidine.
Tricyclic antidepressants: should not be used with brimonidine.
Proprietary preparations: Alphagan; *Combigan (combined with timolol maleate).

brinzolamide A *carbonic anhydrase inhibitor used to reduce the pressure inside the eye in the treatment of chronic (open-angle) *glaucoma and raised blood pressure in the eye. It is used either alone, to treat people who have not responded to *beta-blockers or in whom beta-blockers should not be used, or

in combination with beta-blockers or *prostaglandin analogues. Brinzolamide is available as eye drops on *prescription only.
Side effects: include taste disturbance, headache, inflammation of the eyelid, blurred vision, eye irritation, eye pain or itching, dry eye, eye discharge, and dry mouth.
Precautions: brinzolamide should not be used by people who have severe kidney disease.
Proprietary preparations: Azopt; *Azarga (combined with timolol maleate).

BritLofex (sanofi-aventis) *See* LOFEXIDINE HYDROCHLORIDE.

Brochlor (sanofi-aventis) *See* CHLORAMPHENICOL.

Broflex (Alliance) *See* TRIHEXYPHENIDYL HYDROCHLORIDE.

Brolene (sanofi-aventis) *See* PROPAMIDINE ISETHIONATE.

bromocriptine A drug that stimulates dopamine receptors in the brain (i.e. it is a *dopamine receptor agonist) and is used for the treatment of parkinsonism (*see* ANTIPARKINSONIAN DRUGS). As it is longer acting than *levodopa, bromocriptine may be useful for patients who have early-morning disability. However, it should only be used when treatment with levodopa (with benserazide or carbidopa) has failed. Bromocriptine inhibits the secretion of prolactin and is therefore also used to treat disorders associated with overproduction of this hormone, including prolactinoma (a tumour of the prolactin-secreting cells in the pituitary gland), as well as to prevent or suppress lactation in women who do not wish to breastfeed and to treat certain types of infertility in both men and women. It also inhibits the release of *growth hormone and is used to treat acromegaly (enlargement of the hands, feet, and face due to overproduction of this hormone). A *prescription only medicine, bromocriptine is available as tablets or capsules.
Side effects: include nausea, vomiting, constipation, headache, dizziness, suddenly falling asleep, and low blood pressure on standing. High doses of bromocriptine can cause confusion, excitation, hallucinations, involuntary abnormal movements, dry mouth, leg cramps, and fluid on the lungs (in which case treatment may need to be stopped). In rare cases bromocriptine can cause stomach ulcers.
Precautions: bromocriptine should not be taken during or shortly after childbirth by women with high blood pressure, coronary artery disease, or a serious psychiatric disorder or by people with heart-valve disease. It should be used with caution in people with a history of peptic ulcer or psychiatric illness and in those with cardiovascular disease. Women should undergo regular gynaecological assessment. Any breathing or lung problems should be reported to a doctor. Alcohol should be avoided as it increases the likelihood of bromocriptine causing adverse effects.
Interactions with other drugs:
Antiemetics: metoclopramide and domperidone reduce the effect of bromocriptine in inhibiting prolactin secretion.

Antipsychotics: reduce the effects of bromocriptine in treating parkinsonism and overproduction of prolactin.
Erythromycin: increases the plasma concentration of bromocriptine (and therefore its potential for toxicity).
Sympathomimetic drugs: there is an increased risk of adverse effects when phenylpropanolamine or isometheptene are taken with bromocriptine.
Proprietary preparation: Parlodel.

bronchodilators Drugs that cause widening of the airways by relaxing bronchial smooth muscle. *Sympathomimetic drugs that stimulate beta *adrenoceptors, such as *salbutamol, *terbutaline, and *salmeterol, are potent bronchodilators used for the relief of *asthma and chronic bronchitis. These drugs are often administered in aerosols to give rapid relief, but in high doses they may stimulate the heart, increasing heart rate. Other drugs used as bronchodilators are the *antimuscarinic drugs *ipratropium and *tiotropium and the *xanthines, including *theophylline.

See also BAMBUTEROL HYDROCHLORIDE; FORMOTEROL FUMARATE; FENOTEROL HYDROBROMIDE; ORCIPRENALINE SULPHATE.

Brufen, Brufen Retard (Abbott) *See* IBUPROFEN.

Brulidine Cream (Manx) *See* DIBROMPROPAMIDINE ISETHIONATE.

buccal Relating to the mouth or mouth cavity. Buccal tablets are designed to be dissolved in the mouth – between the upper lip and gum.

Buccastem (Forum Health Products) *See* PROCHLORPERAZINE.

buclizine hydrochloride An *antihistamine that is used as an *antiemetic in preparations for the treatment of *migraine.
Side effects, precautions, and interactions with other drugs: *see* ANTIHISTAMINES.
Proprietary preparation: *Migraleve (pink tablets: combined with paracetamol and codeine phosphate).

Budelin Novolizer (Meda Pharmaceuticals) *See* BUDESONIDE.

Budenofalk (Dr. Falk Pharma UK Ltd) *See* BUDESONIDE.

budesonide A *corticosteroid used for the prevention of *asthma attacks and the treatment of rhinitis (including hay fever). It is given by inhalation or nasal spray and may be used in conjunction with *bronchodilators and/or *sodium cromoglicate. Budesonide is also used to treat inflammatory bowel disease, being given by mouth for the treatment of Crohn's disease and rectally for ulcerative colitis. All preparations are available on *prescription only.
Side effects: when taken by inhalation or nasally, the most common side effects are hoarseness (due to weakness of the vocal muscles) and fungal (*Candida*) infections of the mouth or throat. For side effects when taken orally or rectally, *see* CORTICOSTEROIDS.
Precautions: budesonide inhalers or nasal sprays should not be used by

people who have untreated nasal infections or have had nasal surgery or by people who have (or have had) tuberculosis. For precautions when taken orally or rectally, *see* CORTICOSTEROIDS.
Proprietary preparations: Budelin Novolizer (powder for use with an inhalaler); Budenofalk (rectal foam, capsules, and oral solution); Entocort CR (modified-release capsules); Entocort Enema; Pulmicort Inhaler; Pulmicort Turbohaler (disks of powder, of varying strengths, for use with an inhaler); Pulmicort Respules (ampoules for use with a nebulizer); Rhinocort Aqua (nasal spray); *Symbicort (combined with formoterol).

bulk-forming laxatives (**bulking agents**) *Laxatives that act by absorbing water, increasing the bulk and softening the consistency of the stools. They consist either of plant fibre (e.g. *bran, *ispaghula husk, *sterculia) or of a synthetic agent (e.g. *methylcellulose). Bulking agents are usually effective 12–24 hours after being taken, but it can take some days for their full effect to develop. They are useful for encouraging bowel movements in people with a colostomy, ileostomy, haemorrhoids, or anal fissure and for treating chronic diarrhoea in people with irritable bowel syndrome or diverticular disease, when their ability to absorb water in the gut is exploited to decrease the liquidity of the stools.

Bulk-forming laxatives that swell in water should always be swallowed with plenty of water and should not be taken immediately before going to bed.

bumetanide A *loop diuretic used to treat *oedema resulting from congestive heart failure, kidney disease, or cirrhosis of the liver. It can be injected in emergencies to relieve pulmonary oedema (fluid in the spaces of the lungs causing breathing difficulties). Bumetanide is usually given with a *potassium supplement or a *potassium-sparing diuretic. A *prescription only medicine, it can be taken orally as tablets or a liquid and is also available as a solution for injection.
Side effects, precautions, and interactions with other drugs: *see* LOOP DIURETICS.
Proprietary preparation: Burinex.
See also DIURETICS.

bupivacaine *See* LOCAL ANAESTHETICS.

buprenorphine An *opioid analgesic used for the treatment of moderate to severe pain, including pain relief before and during surgery, and also for the treatment of people who are physically dependent on opioids, in whom it may lessen the symptoms of opioid withdrawal. Buprenorphine is a *controlled drug; it is available as tablets to be dissolved under the tongue, as skin patches, and as an injection.
Side effects and precautions: *see* MORPHINE. Buprenorphine may give rise to mild withdrawal symptoms in people who are regularly taking other opioids since it antagonizes their action.
Interactions with other drugs: *see* OPIOIDS.
Proprietary preparations: BuTrans (skin patches); Subutex (tablets);

Temgesic (tablets); Transtec (skin patches); *Suboxone (combined with naloxone hydrochloride).

bupropion hydrochloride A drug used to help smokers give up the habit. It is available as tablets on *prescription only.
Side effects: include dry mouth, nausea, vomiting, headache, dizziness, fever, and rash.
Precaution: bupropion should not be taken by people with a history of seizures, eating disorders, or bipolar disorder, by people with brain tumours, or by women who are pregnant or breastfeeding.
Interactions with other drugs: bupropion should be used with caution by people taking drugs that increase the risk of seizures; these include antidepressants, antipsychotics, sedating antihistamines, and quinolone antibiotics. A doctor should be consulted before taking any other drugs with bupropion.
Ritonavir: alters the plasma concentration of bupropion.
Tamoxifen: its metabolism may be inhibited by bupropion and the two drugs should not be taken together.
Proprietary preparation: Zyban.

Burinex (Leo Pharmaceuticals) *See* BUMETANIDE.

Burneze Spray (SSL International) *See* BENZOCAINE.

Buscopan (Boehringer Ingelheim) *See* HYOSCINE BUTYLBROMIDE.

buserelin An analogue of *gonadorelin used to treat *endometriosis and to suppress the release of gonadotrophins by the pituitary gland before inducing ovulation in women undergoing fertility treatment. It is also used to reduce concentrations of testosterone in the treatment of advanced prostate cancer that requires testosterone for growth (*see* LEUPRORELIN). Buserelin is available, on *prescription only, as a nasal spray or a solution for injection.
Side effects: include hot flushes, loss of libido, headache, and depression; the spray may cause transient nasal irritation. In women there may also be vaginal dryness, emotional upset, changes in breast size, breast tenderness, and ovarian cysts; men may rarely experience enlargement of the breasts.
Precautions: buserelin should not be taken by women who are pregnant or breastfeeding or who have undiagnosed vaginal bleeding; a nonhormonal method of contraception should be used during treatment. The drug should be used with caution in people with osteoporosis or depression.
Proprietary preparations: Suprecur (nasal spray or injection for endometriosis or infertility); Suprefact (nasal spray or injection for prostate cancer).

Busilvex (Pierre Fabre) *See* BUSULFAN.

Buspar (Bristol-Myers Squibb) *See* BUSPIRONE.

buspirone An *anxiolytic drug used for the short-term treatment of anxiety. Although some beneficial effects may be seen during the first week, the

response to buspirone treatment can take up to two weeks. It produces less sedation than the *benzodiazepines and less dependence and potential for abuse. If benzodiazepines are being replaced by buspirone, treatment with the benzodiazepine needs to be tapered off gradually, since buspirone will not alleviate the withdrawal symptoms associated with stopping benzodiazepines. Buspirone is available as tablets on *prescription only.
Side effects: include nausea, dizziness, headache, nervousness, light-headedness, excitement, and (rarely) a fast heart rate, palpitations, chest pain, drowsiness, confusion, dry mouth, fatigue, and sweating.
Precautions: buspirone should not be taken by people with epilepsy, severe liver or kidney disease, or by women who are pregnant or breastfeeding. Alcohol enhances the sedative effect of buspirone.
Interactions with other drugs: the sedative effect of buspirone is increased by a number of drugs, including anaesthetics, opioid analgesics, antidepressants, antihistamines, and antipsychotic drugs.

Erythromycin: increases the plasma concentration (and therefore adverse effects) of buspirone.
MAOIs: should not be taken with buspirone.
Ritonavir: increases the plasma concentration of buspirone, whose dosage will therefore need to be reduced.

Proprietary preparation: Buspar.

busulfan <**busulphan**> An *alkylating drug given by mouth for the treatment of chronic myeloid leukaemia (*see* CANCER) and given by mouth or intravenous infusion before blood-forming stem cell transplantation. It is available as tablets and a form for infusion on *prescription only.
Side effects: include *bone marrow suppression and increased pigmentation of the skin. *See also* CYTOTOXIC DRUGS.
Precautions: *see* CYTOTOXIC DRUGS.
Interactions with other drugs:

Clozapine: there is an increase in the risk of agranulocytosis (a blood disorder), and this drug should therefore not be taken with busulfan.
Metronidazole: increases the plasma concentration (and adverse effects) of busulfan.

Proprietary preparations: Busilvex (infusion); Myleran (tablets).

busulphan *See* BUSULFAN.

butobarbital <**butobarbitone**> An intermediate-acting *barbiturate used for the short-term treatment of severe insomnia in patients who are already taking barbiturates. A *controlled drug, it is available as tablets.
Side effects, precautions, and interactions with other drugs: *see* BARBITURATES.
Proprietary preparation: Soneryl.

butobarbitone *See* BUTOBARBITAL.

BuTrans (Napp Pharmaceuticals) *See* BUPRENORPHINE.

Buttercup Max Strength Sore Throat Lozenges (Chefaro UK) *See* HEXYLRESORCINOL.

Buttercup Syrup Traditional (Chefaro UK) *See* SQUILL.

Byetta (Eli Lilly & Co) *See* EXENATIDE.

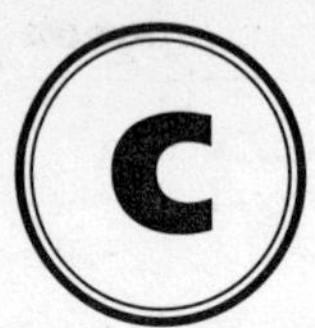

cabergoline A *dopamine agonist, very similar to *bromocriptine, that is used as an *adjunct to *levodopa (with carbidopa or benserazide) in the treatment of Parkinson's disease (*see* ANTIPARKINSONIAN DRUGS). It is also used to reduce high concentrations of the hormone prolactin in certain types of infertility. It is available as tablets on *prescription only.
Side effects: include dizziness, vertigo, nausea, constipation, headache, fatigue, suddenly falling asleep, breast pain, gastrointestinal upsets, hot flushes, and depression.
Precautions: cabergoline should not be taken by women who are pregnant or breastfeeding; it should be discontinued for one month before trying to conceive. It should not be taken by people with heart-valve disease or a history of breathing or lung problems and should be used with caution in those with severely impaired liver function.
Interactions with other drugs:
Antiemetics: metoclopramide and possibly domperidone reduce the effect of cabergoline in inhibiting prolactin secretion.
Antipsychotics: reduce the effects of cabergoline.
Erythromycin: increases the plasma concentration of cabergoline (and therefore its potential for toxicity).
Proprietary preparation: Dostinex.

Cacit (Procter & Gamble) *See* CALCIUM CARBONATE.

Cacit D3 (Procter & Gamble) A proprietary combination of *calcium carbonate and *colecalciferol (vitamin D_3), used to treat *vitamin D deficiency and as an *adjunct in the treatment of osteoporosis. It is available as effervescent granules and can be obtained without a prescription, but only from pharmacies.
Side effects: nausea, vomiting, and other stomach upsets may occur. *See* VITAMIN D.
Precautions: this medicine should be taken with caution by people with kidney disease or a history of kidney stones.
Interactions with other drugs:
Antiepileptic drugs: carbamazepine, phenobarbital, phenytoin, and primidone reduce the effects of Cacit D3.
Thiazide diuretics: increase the risk of high concentrations of calcium in the blood; *see* VITAMIN D.

cade oil (**juniper tar**) An oil extracted from the wood of *Juniperus oxycedrus*, a species of juniper. It is an ingredient of several topical preparations for the treatment of scaling conditions of the scalp, such as *psoriasis.

Proprietary preparations: *Polytar (combined with tar, coal tar extract, and other ingredients); *Polytar AF (combined with tar, coal tar extract, and other ingredients).

cadexomer iodine An antibacterial substance (*see* ANTIBIOTICS) used to absorb the liquid that exudes from ulcers and infected wounds. It is available as a paste, powder, or ointment on *prescription only.
Precautions: cadexomer iodine should not be used by women who are pregnant or breastfeeding or by people with diseases of the thyroid gland.
Proprietary preparations: Iodoflex (paste); Iodosorb (powder or ointment).

Caelyx (Schering-Plough) *See* DOXORUBICIN.

Cafergot (Alliance) *See* ERGOTAMINE TARTRATE.

caffeine A mild *stimulant that is found in tea and coffee. It is often included, in small doses, in analgesic preparations, and is claimed to increase analgesic effects. However, there is considerable scepticism as to whether it actually contributes to pain control.
Side effects and precautions: the alerting effect of caffeine in analgesic preparations may not always be wanted, and the caffeine may worsen a headache. Overconsumption of caffeine can cause feelings of anxiety and restlessness, and very large doses, or sudden withdrawal, can cause headaches.
Proprietary preparations: *Alka-Seltzer XS (combined with aspirin and paracetamol); *Anadin (combined with aspirin); *Anadin Extra, Anadin Extra Soluble (combined with aspirin and paracetamol); *Beechams Flu-Plus Caplets (combined with paracetamol and phenylephrine); *Beechams Powders (combined with aspirin); *Beechams Powders Capsules (combined with paracetamol and phenylephrine); *Boots Cold and 'Flu Relief Tablets (combined with paracetamol, phenylephrine, and ascorbic acid); *Boots Max Strength Cold & Flu Capsules (combined with paracetamol and phenylephrine); *Boots Max Strength Sinus Relief Capsules (combined with paracetamol and phenylephrine); *Boots Paracetamol and Codeine Extra Capsules (combined with paracetamol and Codeine); *Hedex Extra (combined with paracetamol); *Lemsip Cold & Flu Capsules (combined with paracetamol and phenylephrine); *Non-Drowsy Sudafed Congestion and Headache Capsules (combined with paracetamol and phenylephrine); *Panadol Extra (combined with paracetamol); *Solpadeine Headache (combined with paracetamol); *Solpadeine Plus (combined with paracetamol and codeine); *Syndol (combined with paracetamol, codeine, and doxylamine); *Veganin (combined with paracetamol and aspirin); *Yeast-Vite (combined with nicotinamide, riboflavin, and thiamine).

cajuput oil An aromatic oil distilled from the leaves of *Melaleuca cajuputi*, a tree native to southeast Asia and Australia. It is mildly antiseptic and acts as a *rubefacient, being included as an ingredient in preparations for the relief of muscular aches and pains. It is also included in inhalations to relieve the congestion associated with colds and catarrh.

Proprietary preparations: *Olbas Oil (combined with menthol, eucalyptus oil, clove oil, and juniper berry oil); *Tiger Balm (combined with camphor, clove oil, peppermint oil, and menthol).

C

calamine A preparation of zinc carbonate, coloured with ferric oxide. It is used in the form of a lotion or cream as a mild *astringent to relieve itching. It is also an ingredient of other skin preparations. Preparations containing calamine can be obtained without a prescription.
Proprietary preparation: *Vasogen Cream (combined with zinc oxide and dimeticone).

Calceos (Galen Limited) A proprietary combination of *calcium carbonate and *colecalciferol (vitamin D_3), used to treat *vitamin D deficiency and as an *adjunct in the treatment of osteoporosis. It is available as chewable tablets and can be obtained without a prescription, but only from pharmacies.
Side effects: nausea, vomiting, and other stomach upsets may occur. *See* VITAMIN D.
Precautions: this medicine should be taken with caution by people with kidney disease or a history of kidney stones.
Interactions with other drugs:
Antiepileptic drugs: carbamazepine, phenobarbital, phenytoin, and primidone reduce the effects of Calceos.
Thiazide diuretics: increase the risk of high concentrations of calcium in the blood; *see* VITAMIN D.

Calcicard CR (IVAX) *See* DILTIAZEM HYDROCHLORIDE.

Calcichew (Shire Pharmaceuticals) *See* CALCIUM CARBONATE.

Calcichew-D_3 (Shire Pharmaceuticals) A proprietary combination of *calcium carbonate and *colecalciferol (vitamin D_3), used for the treatment of *vitamin D deficiency and as an *adjunct in the treatment of osteoporosis. **Calcichew-D_3 Forte** is a similar preparation but contains twice as much colecalciferol. Both preparations are available as chewable tablets and can be obtained from pharmacies without a prescription.
Side effects: include constipation and flatulence. *See also* VITAMIN D.
Precautions and interactions with other drugs: *see* VITAMIN D.

calciferol A high-strength formulation of *colecalciferol or *ergocalciferol that is used to treat vitamin D deficiency caused by poor absorption of calcium from the intestines or liver disease. It is available as tablets, which can be obtained without a prescription, but only from pharmacies, or as a solution for injection, which is available on *prescription only.
Side effects, precautions, and interactions with other drugs: *see* VITAMIN D.

Calcijex (Abbott) *See* CALCITRIOL.

calcipotriol An *analogue of *vitamin D that is used in the treatment of *psoriasis. It acts by slowing down the division of skin cells whose overgrowth

causes the formation of scaly patches seen in this disease. Calcipotriol is available, on *prescription only, as an ointment, a cream, or a scalp lotion.
Side effects: calcipotriol may irritate the skin, causing itching or reddening; rarely, it may cause a rash on the face or around the mouth.
Precautions: calcipotriol should not be used by people with disorders of calcium metabolism and it should not be applied to the face. It should be used with caution by people with peeling psoriasis and by pregnant women.
Proprietary preparations: Dovonex Cream; Dovonex Scalp Lotion; *Dovobet (combined with betamethasone); *Xamiol (combined with betamethasone).

calcitonin (salmon) <salcatonin> A synthetic or genetically engineered form of **calcitonin**, a hormone secreted by the thyroid gland that lowers circulating concentrations of calcium by promoting the uptake of calcium into bone. It is used to reduce abnormally high concentrations of calcium in the blood, especially in people with cancer, to relieve pain in Paget's disease (in which the bones become deformed and fracture easily), and to reduce the risk of spinal fractures in the treatment and prevention of osteoporosis in postmenopausal women. Calcitonin (salmon) is available as an injection or nasal spray on *prescription only.
Side effects: include nausea, vomiting, and flushing (which diminish with use); the nasal spray may cause nose and throat irritation. Less common side effects are tingling of hands, an unpleasant taste, rash, and inflammation at the injection site.
Precautions: some people are allergic to calcitonin (salmon) and a scratch test may be necessary before taking the drug. It should be used with caution in women who are pregnant or breastfeeding.
Proprietary preparation: Miacalcic.

calcitriol A *vitamin D derivative used to prevent and treat the bone disease that may occur in kidney dialysis patients and to treat postmenopausal osteoporosis. It is also used for the topical treatment of mild to moderately severe *psoriasis. It is available as capsules, an injection, or an ointment on *prescription only.
Side effects, precautions, and interactions with other drugs: *see* VITAMIN D.
Proprietary preparations: Calcijex (injection); Rocaltrol (capsules); Silkis (ointment).

calcium A metallic element essential for the normal development and functioning of the body. It is required for many metabolic processes, including nerve function, muscle contraction, and blood clotting, and it is an important constituent of bones and teeth. Calcium is maintained at the correct concentration in the blood by the action of hormones (*see* CALCITONIN (SALMON); PARATHYROID HORMONE). The uptake of calcium from the gut and its deposition in bone is facilitated by *vitamin D; deficiency of this vitamin may therefore result in bone disorders, such as rickets in children and osteoporosis or osteomalacia in adults. Deficiency of calcium in the blood leads to tetany (spasm and twitching of the muscles). Conversely, high plasma concentrations of calcium may lead to the deposition of calcium in soft tissues and cause 'hardening' of the tissues (calcification).

Calcium supplements are given to prevent or treat calcium deficiency. Extra calcium may be required by growing children, pregnant or breastfeeding women, women who have reached the menopause, and elderly people; it reduces bone loss in people with osteoporosis. Supplementary calcium may also be required by people who cannot tolerate milk. Oral calcium supplements are available as a variety of calcium salts, including *calcium carbonate, *calcium gluconate, *calcium lactate, *calcium lactate gluconate, *calcium phosphate, **calcium glubionate**, and **calcium lactobionate**, which are readily absorbed. They are often packaged with *vitamin D. Calcium gluconate and *calcium chloride can be given intravenously. Calcium salts are also used in *antacid preparations.

Side effects: include constipation and flatulence. Injections may cause slowing of the heart rate, irregular heartbeat, and irritation.

Precautions: calcium supplements should not be taken by people with conditions associated with high plasma calcium concentrations or tissue calcification (including some forms of cancer and kidney disease) or by those who are immobile for long periods (since prolonged immobilization causes resorption of calcium from bone and high plasma calcium concentrations).

Interactions with other drugs:

Antibiotics: the absorption of tetracyclines and ciprofloxacin is reduced by calcium salts.

Bisphosphonates: their absorption is reduced by calcium salts.

Digoxin and digitoxin: calcium given by intravenous injection can cause irregular heartbeats.

Thiazide diuretics: the risk of high blood calcium concentrations is increased.

Calcium 500 (Martindale Pharmaceuticals) *See* CALCIUM CARBONATE.

calcium acetate A salt of *calcium that is used as a *phosphate-binding agent and is an ingredient of an antacid preparation. It is available as tablets and can be obtained without a prescription.

Precautions: calcium acetate should not be taken by people with low concentrations of phosphate in the blood or high concentrations of calcium in the blood or urine. Plasma *electrolytes and albumin may therefore need to be monitored.

Interactions with other drugs: *see* CALCIUM.

Proprietary preparations: Phosex; PhosLo; *Osvaren (combined with magnesium carbonate).

calcium antagonists Drugs that inhibit the influx of calcium into heart muscle and the smooth muscle of blood vessels. They are also called **calcium-channel blockers** (which is a more correct description of their action). Muscles need calcium to contract; these drugs therefore reduce the force of heart-muscle contractions and cause *vasodilatation in the blood vessels. Some of them also slow the passage of nerve signals through the heart, which

can be helpful in correcting certain types of abnormal heartbeat (*see* ARRHYTHMIA). Dilating the blood vessels decreases the work done by the heart and so relieves the strain on the heart that gives rise to *angina. Calcium antagonists are classified into three groups (I, II, and III) depending on the way in which they act. Class I drugs (e.g. *verapamil hydrochloride) act mainly on the heart, reducing the force of contractions and the conduction of nerve impulses. Class II drugs (e.g. *nifedipine, *nimodipine, *amlodipine, *felodipine, *isradipine, *lacidipine, *lercanidipine, *nicardipine) have actions mainly on the blood vessels and not on the heart. They are used for various cardiovascular disorders, such as *angina, and *hypertension, but have little anti-arrhythmic activity. They may be used in conjunction with *beta blockers, which prevent the reflex increase in heart rate that they cause, but they are also useful for people who cannot tolerate beta blockers. Class III drugs (e.g. *diltiazem) have actions mainly on the coronary arteries.
Side effects: dizziness and sometimes fainting, headaches at the start of treatment, and flushing of the face are quite common. Palpitations and ankle *oedema may occur with class II drugs.
Precautions: people taking calcium antagonists (except amlodipine and diltiazem) should avoid grapefruit juice, as this interferes with their metabolism by increasing their plasma concentrations.
Interactions with other drugs:

Anaesthetics: the general anaesthetic isoflurane increases the effect of the class II calcium antagonists in lowering blood pressure.
Antihypertensive drugs: their effects in lowering blood pressure are increased by calcium antagonists.
Beta blockers: should not be used with class I drugs (verapamil) as this combination causes severe hypotension (low blood pressure) and can precipitate heart failure. This is less likely to happen with class II drugs, which can be given with beta blockers if monitored closely.
Ritonavir: may increase the plasma concentrations of calcium antagonists.
For other interactions, see entries for individual drugs.

calcium carbonate A *calcium salt with a variety of uses. It is taken as a calcium supplement, and is often packaged with *vitamin D for the treatment of osteoporosis. It is used as a *phosphate-binding agent in people with kidney failure, especially if they are on dialysis. Calcium carbonate is a common ingredient in *antacid preparations, for the relief of indigestion, heartburn, and similar conditions, and is also included in some *antidiarrhoeal preparations. Calcium carbonate is available as chewable tablets, effervescent tablets, or granules and can be obtained without a prescription, but only from pharmacies. Antacid preparations containing calcium carbonate are usually freely available *over the counter.
Side effects, precautions, and interactions with other drugs: *see* CALCIUM.
Proprietary preparations: Adcal (chewable tablets); Boots Indigestion Relief Tablets Fruit; Cacit (effervescent tablets); Calcichew (chewable tablets); Calcichew Forte (chewable tablets); Calcium 500 (tablets); Tums (antacid); Remegel (antacid); Rennie Rap-Eze (antacid); *Actonel Combi (sachets:

combined with colecalciferol); *Adcal-D_3 (combined with vitamin D_3); *Andrews Antacid (combined with magnesium carbonate); *Bisodol Antacid Tablets (combined with sodium bicarbonate and magnesium carbonate); *Bisodol Extra Tablets (combined with sodium bicarbonate, magnesium carbonate, and simeticone); *Cacit D3 (combined with vitamin D_3); *Calceos (combined with vitamin D_3); *Calcichew-D_3, Calcichew-D_3 Forte (combined with vitamin D_3); *Gaviscon Double Action (combined with sodium alginate and sodium bicarbonate); *Gaviscon Liquid (combined with sodium alginate and sodium bicarbonate); *J Collis Browne's Tablets (combined with kaolin and morphine); *Kao-C (combined with kaolin); *Natecal D3 (combined with colecalciferol); *Peppermint Indigestion Tablets (combined with sodium bicarbonate, magnesium trisilicate, and magnesium carbonate); *PepcidTwo (combined with famotidine and magnesium sulphate); *Peptac (combined with alginic acid and sodium bicarbonate); *Rennie (combined with magnesium carbonate); *Rennie Deflatine (combined with simeticone and magnesium carbonate); *Sandocal 400 and Sandocal 1000 (combined with calcium lactate gluconate); *Sandocal + D 600 (combined with calcium lactate gluconate and colecalciferol).

calcium-channel blockers *See* CALCIUM ANTAGONISTS.

calcium chloride A *calcium salt that is given intravenously to resuscitate patients who have suffered a heart attack associated with high levels of *potassium in the blood. It is also included as an ingredient in artifical saliva preparations and in *balanced salt solution for washing out the eyes. Calcium chloride injection is available on *prescription only.
Side effects, precautions, and interactions with other drugs: *see* CALCIUM.
Proprietary preparation: Minijet Calcium Chloride.

calcium folinate *See* FOLINIC ACID.

calcium glubionate *See* CALCIUM; CALCIUM-SANDOZ.

calcium gluconate A *calcium salt used to treat calcium deficiency or to prevent osteoporosis. It is available as effervescent tablets, which can be obtained without a prescription from pharmacies, and as an injection (for treating tetany), which is available on *prescription only.
Side effects, precautions, and interactions with other drugs: *see* CALCIUM.

calcium lactate A *calcium salt used to correct calcium deficiency or to prevent osteoporosis. It is also combined with *ergocalciferol (as **calcium and ergocalciferol**) for the treatment of vitamin D deficiency. Calcium lactate is available as tablets and can be obtained without a prescription, but only from pharmacies.
Side effects, precautions, and interactions with other drugs: *see* CALCIUM.

calcium lactate gluconate A *calcium salt used to correct calcium deficiency or to prevent osteoporosis. It is available as effervescent tablets and can be obtained without a prescription, but only from pharmacies.
Side effects, precautions, and interactions with other drugs: *see* CALCIUM.

Proprietary preparations: *Sandocal 400 and Sandocal 1000 (combined with calcium carbonate); *Sandocal + D 600 (combined with calcium carbonate and colecalciferol).

calcium lactobionate *See* CALCIUM; CALCIUM-SANDOZ.

calcium leucovorin *See* FOLINIC ACID.

calcium levofolinate (**calcium levoleucovorin**) *See* FOLINIC ACID.

calcium phosphate A *calcium salt used to correct calcium deficiency or to prevent osteoporosis. It is also combined with *ergocalciferol (as **calcium and ergocalciferol**) for the treatment of vitamin D deficiency. Calcium phosphate is available as a powder to be dissolved in water and taken by mouth and can be obtained without a prescription, but only from pharmacies.
Side effects, precautions, and interactions with other drugs: *see* CALCIUM.
Proprietary preparation: *Calfovit D3 (combined with vitamin D_3).

calcium polystyrene sulphonate A resin that exchanges potassium ions for calcium ions in the intestine when it is taken by mouth or by enema. It is used to reduce high concentrations of potassium in blood associated with failure of the kidneys to produce sufficient urine or in patients on dialysis (*see* ELECTROLYTE). It is available as a powder and can be obtained without a prescription, but only from pharmacies.
Side effects: include high plasma calcium concentrations, low plasma potassium concentrations, loss of appetite, nausea and vomiting, constipation, and diarrhoea. If constipation occurs, treatment should be stopped and magnesium-containing laxatives avoided. Intestinal obstruction has been occasionally reported.
Precautions: calcium polystyrene sulphonate should not be taken by people with overactive parathyroid glands (*see* PARATHYROID HORMONE), myeloma (cancer of the bone marrow), metastatic cancer (secondaries) involving kidney failure, or obstructive bowel disease. It should be used with caution in women who are pregnant or breastfeeding. Plasma electrolytes may need to be monitored.
Proprietary preparation: Calcium Resonium.

Calcium Resonium (sanofi-aventis) *See* CALCIUM POLYSTYRENE SULPHONATE.

Calcium-Sandoz (Alliance) A proprietary combination of the salts calcium glubionate and calcium lactobionate, used as a *calcium supplement. It is available as a syrup and can be obtained without a prescription, but only from pharmacies.
Side effects, precautions, and interactions with other drugs: *see* CALCIUM.

Calcold (McNeil Ltd) A proprietary combination of *paracetamol (an antipyretic and analgesic) and *diphenhydramine (a sedative antihistamine), used for the treatment of mild to moderate pain in children aged 6–12 years, including headache and sore throat, and to relieve the symptoms of influenza and feverish colds. It is available *over the counter as an oral solution.

Side effects and interactions with other drugs: *see* ANTIHISTAMINES.
Precautions: *see* PARACETAMOL.

Calcort (sanofi-aventis) *See* DEFLAZACORT.

Calcough Six Plus (McNeil Ltd) *See* GUAIFENESIN.

Calcough Tickly (McNeil Ltd) *See* GLYCERIN.

Calfovit D3 (A. Menarini Pharma UK S.R.L.) A proprietary combination of *colecalciferol (vitamin D_3) and *calcium phosphate, used to correct calcium and *vitamin D deficiency and as an *adjunct to treatment for osteoporosis. It is available, on *prescription only, as an oral powder to be dissolved in water.
Side effects, precautions, and interactions with other drugs: *see* VITAMIN D.

Calgel (McNeil Ltd) A proprietary combination of *cetylpyridinium chloride (an antiseptic) and *lidocaine hydrochloride (a local anaesthetic) in the form of a gel, used to relieve teething pain and soothe the gums. It is freely available *over the counter.
Precautions: Calgel is not recommended for babies under three months old.

Califig California Syrup of Figs (Merck Consumer Health) A proprietary combination of *senna and figs, used as a *stimulant laxative for the treatment of constipation. It is freely available *over the counter.
Precautions: this syrup should not be taken by children under one year old. *See* STIMULANT LAXATIVES.

Calmurid (Galderma) A proprietary combination of *urea (a moisturizing agent) and *lactic acid (a keratolytic and antibiotic), used for the treatment of chronic dry and itching skin conditions. It is available as a cream and can be obtained without a prescription, but only from pharmacies.

Calmurid HC (Galderma) A proprietary combination of *hydrocortisone (a corticosteroid), *urea (a hydrating agent), and *lactic acid (a keratolytic and antibiotic), used for the treatment of dry *eczema and similar skin conditions. It is available as a cream on *prescription only.
Side effects and precautions: *see* TOPICAL STEROIDS.

Calpol (McNeil Ltd) *See* PARACETAMOL.

Calprofen (McNeil Ltd) *See* IBUPROFEN.

Calsalettes (Torbet Laboratories) *See* ALOIN.

CAM (Shire Pharmaceuticals) *See* EPHEDRINE HYDROCHLORIDE.

Camcolit (Norgine) *See* LITHIUM CARBONATE.

camphor An aromatic substance obtained from the wood of a southeast Asian tree (*Cinnamomum camphora*) or manufactured synthetically. When applied to the skin it produces a cooling effect. Camphor is used in *rubefacient preparations to relieve the pain of sprains and strains, backache, rheumatic pains, and neuralgia. It is also used in some *emollient skin

preparations to relieve the itching associated with such conditions as eczema. Camphor is also an ingredient in cough remedies, ear drops, and preparations for the removal of corns and verrucas.
Proprietary preparations: *Balmosa (combined with menthol, methyl salicylate, and capsicum oleoresin); *Benadryl Skin Allergy Relief Cream (combined with diphenhydramine and zinc oxide); *Boots Dual Action Cold Sore Lotion (combined with dichlorobenzyl alcohol, benzylalcohol, and levomenthol); *Boots Vapour Chest Rub (combined with eucalyptus oil and levomenthol); *Boots Pain Relief Warming Spray (combined with ethyl nicotinate and methyl salicylate); *Corn and Callus Removal Liquid (combined with salicylic acid); *Earex Ear Drops (combined with arachis oil and almond oil); *Non-Drowsy Sudafed Inhalant Oil (combined with eucalyptus oil, menthol, and peppermint oil); *PR Heat Spray (combined with methyl salicylate and ethyl nicotinate); *Seal and Heal Verruca Removal Gel (combined with salicylic acid); *Tiger Balm (combined with cajuput oil, clove oil, peppermint oil, and menthol); *Vicks Vaporub (combined with eucalyptus oil, turpentine oil, and menthol).

Campral EC (Merck Serono) *See* ACAMPROSATE CALCIUM.

Campto (Pfizer) *See* IRINOTECAN.

cancer Any one of a group of diseases characterized by unregulated cell division that gives rise to malignant tumours. Such tumours invade and destroy the tissues in which they originate and can spread to other parts of the body via the blood or lymphatic system or across a body cavity, such as the abdomen or chest. These secondary tumours, or **metastases**, are usually the cause of death, not the primary tumour. Tumours may be classified as solid tumours (usually occurring in an organ, such as the lung, stomach, or ovary), soft-tissue tumours (occurring in such tissue as muscle), **leukaemias** (cancers of the blood-producing tissue in the bone marrow characterized by overproduction of abnormal or immature forms of white blood cells), and **lymphomas** (cancers of the lymphatic system). Leukaemias are further classified according to the rate of progression of the disease (acute or chronic) and the type of white cell involved (e.g. hairy cell leukaemia, lymphoblastic leukaemia). Lymphomas are divided into Hodgkin's disease and non-Hodgkin's lymphomas, according to their appearance under the microscope.

Cancer can occur at any age, but the incidence of most cancers rises sharply after the age of 60 years. In the Western world the most common cancers are those of the lung, breast, skin, gut, and prostate gland. Cancer is treated by a combination of surgery, radiotherapy, and/or chemotherapy (*see* CYTOTOXIC DRUGS), depending on the site and type of tumour.

Cancidas (Merck Sharp & Dohme) *See* CASPOFUNGIN.

candesartan cilexetil An *angiotensin II inhibitor used in the treatment of *hypertension. It is available as tablets on *prescription only.
Side effects: include infections of the upper respiratory tract, influenza-like symptoms, and (less commonly) back pain, fluid retention, and nausea.

Precautions: candesartan should not be taken during pregnancy or by people with severe liver disease or some types of jaundice. It should be used with caution in people with kidney disease and some types of heart disease.
Interactions with other drugs: *see* ACE INHIBITORS.
Proprietary preparation: Amias.

C

candidiasis *See* ANTIFUNGAL DRUGS.

Canesten (Bayer) *See* CLOTRIMAZOLE.

Canesten-Combi (Bayer) *See* CLOTRIMAZOLE.

Canesten HC (Bayer) A proprietary combination of *hydrocortisone (a corticosteroid), and *clotrimazole (an antifungal drug), used for the treatment of fungal infections of the skin accompanied by inflammation. It is available as a cream on *prescription only.
Side effects, precautions, and interactions with other drugs: *see* TOPICAL STEROIDS; CLOTRIMAZOLE.

Canusal (CP Pharmaceuticals) *See* HEPARIN.

Capasal (Dermal Laboratories) A proprietary combination of *salicylic acid and *coal tar (both keratolytics), used for the treatment of seborrhoeic *eczema (including cradle cap in babies) and *psoriasis of the scalp. It is available as a shampoo and can be obtained without a prescription, but only from pharmacies.
Side effects and precautions: *see* SALICYLIC ACID.

Capastat (King) *See* CAPREOMYCIN.

capecitabine A drug that is broken down into *fluorouracil in the body; it is used for the treatment of advanced breast, colorectal, and stomach *cancers, either alone or in combination with other *cytotoxic drugs. Capecitabine available as tablets on *prescription only.
Side effects: *see* CYTOTOXIC DRUGS. There may in addition to diarrhoea and changes in the electrical activity of the heart.
Precautions: *see* CYTOTOXIC DRUGS. Capecitabine should not be taken by people with liver or severe kidney disease or by women who are breastfeeding. It should be used with caution in people with heart or cardiovascular disease or *arrhythmias.
Interactions with other drugs: *see* FLUOROURACIL.
Proprietary preparation: Xeloda.

Caplenal (APS-Berk) *See* ALLOPURINOL.

Capoten (E.R. Squibb & Sons) *See* CAPTOPRIL.

Capozide (E.R. Squibb & Sons) A proprietary combination of *captopril (an ACE inhibitor) and *hydrochlorothiazide (a thiazide diuretic), used in the treatment of mild to moderate *hypertension. It is available as tablets on *prescription only. **Capozide LS** is a similar preparation half the strength of Capozide.

Side effects, precautions, and interactions with other drugs: *see* ACE INHIBITORS; THIAZIDE DIURETICS.

See also ANTIHYPERTENSIVE DRUGS; DIURETICS.

capreomycin An *antibiotic reserved for treating *tuberculosis resistant to first-line antituberculosis drugs. It is available as an injection on *prescription only.
Side effects: include itching and rash, kidney impairment, and hearing loss with tinnitus and vertigo.
Precautions: capreomycin should be used with caution in patients who have liver, kidney, or hearing impairment and in women who are pregnant or breastfeeding.
Proprietary preparation: Capastat.

Caprin (Pinewood) *See* ASPIRIN.

capsaicin The active ingredient of *capsicum oleoresin; it is the chemical in chillies and peppers that is responsible for their 'hot' taste. Capsaicin is used as a *rubefacient to relieve the pain that follows an attack of shingles (it should not be applied until the rash has healed) and the pain associated with nerve damage in people with diabetes. It is also used in the treatment of osteoarthritis. Capsaicin is available as a cream on *prescription only.
Side effects and precautions: *see* RUBEFACIENTS.
Proprietary preparations: Axsain; Zacin (for osteoarthritis).

capsicin *See* CAPSICUM OLEORESIN.

capsicum oleoresin (**capsicin**) A resinous extract from sweet peppers and chillies that contains the active ingredient *capsaicin. It is used in the form of an ointment as a *rubefacient for the relief of muscular aches, pains, and stiffness, such as backache, sciatica, lumbago, and rheumatism. It is also an ingredient of various other ointments and creams. Preparations containing capsicum oleoresin are usually freely available *over the counter.
Side effects and precautions: *see* RUBEFACIENTS.
Proprietary preparations: Fiery Jack Ointment; *Balmosa (combined with camphor, menthol, and methyl salicylate); *Fiery Jack Cream (combined with diethylamine salicylate, glycol salicylate, and methyl nicotinate); *Ralgex Cream (combined with glycol monosalicylate and methyl nicotinate).

capsule A soluble case, usually made of gelatin, containing a drug (usually in powdered form) for oral administration.

captopril An *ACE inhibitor used as an adjunct to *diuretics for the treatment of *heart failure. It is also used to treat *hypertension, and kidney disease in people with insulin-dependent (type I) diabetes. Captopril is available as tablets on *prescription only.
Side effects, precautions, and interactions with other drugs: *see* ACE INHIBITORS.

Proprietary preparations: Acepril; Capoten; Kaplon; *Capozide and Capozide LS (combined with hydrochlorothiazide).

See also ANTIHYPERTENSIVE DRUGS.

Carace Plus (Bristol-Myers Squibb) A proprietary combination of *lisinopril (an ACE inhibitor) and *hydrochlorothiazide (a thiazide diuretic), used in the treatment of mild to moderate *hypertension. A *prescription only medicine, it is available as tablets of two strengths: **Carace 20 Plus** is twice the strength of **Carace 10 Plus**.
Side effects, precautions, and interactions with other drugs: *see* ACE INHIBITORS; THIAZIDE DIURETICS.

See also ANTIHYPERTENSIVE DRUGS; DIURETICS.

Caramet CR (Teva UK) *See* CO-CARELDOPA.

Carbalax (Forest Laboratories) A proprietary combination of *sodium acid phosphate (an osmotic laxative) and *sodium bicarbonate (which provides effervescence), used for the treatment of constipation or to evacuate the bowel before investigative procedures or surgery. It is freely available *over the counter in the form of suppositories.
Precautions: Carbalax is not recommended for children. *See also* PHOSPHATE LAXATIVES.

carbamazepine An *anticonvulsant drug used for the treatment of most types of epilepsy except absence seizures. It is also used to relieve the stabbing pains that may occur along the course of certain nerves, especially trigeminal neuralgia (a searing pain in the face) and phantom limb pain, and to treat bipolar disorder resistant to *lithium. It is available, on *prescription only, as tablets, *modified-release tablets, or a liquid for oral use and as *suppositories.
Side effects: include dizziness, drowsiness, nausea and vomiting, double vision, headache, and unsteady gait. Mild allergic skin reactions occur quite frequently; less common side effects are blood disorders, jaundice, hepatitis, kidney failure, depression, and impotence.
Precautions: carbamazepine should be used with caution in people who have liver, kidney, or heart disease and in women who are breastfeeding; women who are planning to become pregnant, or who are already pregnant, should seek specialist advice.
Interactions with other drugs:

Antibacterials: the effects of doxycycline and telithromycin are reduced; the concentration of carbamazepine in the blood is increased by clarithromycin, erythromycin, and isoniazid.
Anticoagulants: the effects of warfarin and acenocoumarol are reduced; dosages of these drugs may need to be adjusted.
Anticonvulsants: taking two or more anticonvulsants together may increase their adverse effects.
Antidepressants: reduce the anticonvulsant effect of carbamazepine.
Antipsychotics: reduce the anticonvulsant effect of carbamazepine;

carbamazepine reduces the plasma concentrations of haloperidol, olanzapine, and sertindole.
Calcium antagonists: diltiazem and verapamil increase the effect of carbamazepine.
Cimetidine: may increase the effects of carbamazepine.
Cytotoxic drugs: the plasma concentrations of imatinib and lapatinib are reduced by carbamazepine and these drugs should not be used with it.
Eplerenone: its plasma concentration is reduced by carbamazepine and the two drugs should not be used together.
Oral contraceptives: carbamazepine may reduce the effect of oral contraceptives; an alternative form of contraception may be required.
Voriconazole: its plasma concentration is reduced by carbamazepine and the two drugs should not be used together.
Proprietary preparations: Tegretol; Tegretol Retard (modifed-release tablets); Teril CR (modified-release tablets).

Carbellon (Torbet Laboratories) A proprietary combination of *magnesium hydroxide (an antacid), charcoal (*see* ACTIVATED CHARCOAL), and *peppermint oil (an antispasmodic), used for the relief of indigestion and flatulence. It is available as tablets that can be obtained without a prescription, but only from pharmacies.
Side effects and precautions: *see* MAGNESIUM SALTS.
Interactions with other drugs: *see* ANTACIDS.

carbetocin A drug used to restore normal elasticity to the uterus following Caesarean section under epidural or spinal anaesthesia. It works by binding to *oxytocin receptors in the smooth muscle of the uterus and stimulating uterine contraction. Carbetocin is given as a single intravenous injection, immediately after delivery of the baby and preferably preceding the removal of the placenta, and is available on *prescription only.
Side effects: include anaemia, dizziness, chest pain, breathlessness, vomiting, and back pain.
Precautions: carbetocin should not be given to women with pre-eclampsia, eclampsia, epilepsy, liver or kidney disease, or severe heart disease.
Proprietary preparation: Pabal.

carbidopa A drug that inhibits the enzyme that breaks down *levodopa (an antiparkinsonian drug) to *dopamine in the peripheral tissues. Given in combination with levodopa (*see* CO-CARELDOPA), it increases the amount of levodopa available to cross into the brain and also helps to minimize the side effects of vomiting and low blood pressure seen with levodopa therapy.

carbimazole An antithyroid drug that blocks the synthesis of *thyroid hormones. It is used for the long-term treatment of thyrotoxicosis (overproduction of thyroid hormones) and may also be given to decrease hormone concentrations before surgery to remove part of an overactive thryroid gland. Carbimazole is available as tablets on *prescription only.
Side effects: include rashes, nausea, stomach upsets, headache, joint pain,

hair loss, and suppression of blood-cell production by the bone marrow (increasing the risk of infection). A sore throat, mouth ulcers, or fever should be reported to a doctor immediately, as these may indicate a serious effect on blood cells.
Precautions: carbimazole should not be taken by people with severe blood disorders and should be used with caution in people with a large goitre or liver disorders and in women who are pregnant or breastfeeding.
Proprietary preparation: Neo-Mercazole.

carbocisteine A *mucolytic drug that reduces the viscosity of bronchial secretions by liquefying mucus and is used to relieve congestion of the airways. Carbocisteine is available, on *prescription only, as capsules or a syrup. It cannot be prescribed on the NHS unless it is to be used by children under 18 years old with a tracheostomy.
Side effects: include stomach and bowel upsets, nausea, and rash.
Precautions: carbocisteine should not be taken by people with an active peptic ulcer and should be used with caution in those with a history of peptic ulcers and in pregnant women.
Proprietary preparations: Mucodyne; Mucodyne Paediatric.

Carbo-Dome (Sandoz) *See* COAL TAR.

carbomer (**polyacrylic acid**) An agent used in the treatment of dry eyes to thicken and strengthen the natural film of tears that covers the eyes. It is available as a liquid gel in eye drops and can be obtained without a prescription, but only from pharmacies.
Side effects: there may be transient irritation and blurred vision on application.
Precautions: carbomer should not be used with soft contact lenses.
Proprietary preparations: GelTears; Liposic; Liquivisc; Viscotears.

Carbomix (Beacon Pharmaceuticals) *See* ACTIVATED CHARCOAL.

carbonic anhydrase inhibitors Drugs that inhibit the action of carbonic anhydrase, an enzyme in the red blood cells that controls the formation of carbonic acid or bicarbonate from carbon dioxide and is therefore important in maintaining the acid-base balance of the blood. Carbonic anhydrase inhibitors include *acetazolamide, *dorzolamide, and *brinzolamide; they have a weak *diuretic action but are used mainly in the treatment of *glaucoma.

carboplatin A *cytotoxic drug that is an *analogue of *cisplatin but is less toxic. It is active against the types of *cancer that are sensitive to cisplatin, including ovarian cancer and a form of lung cancer, but is less effective than cisplatin for treating testicular cancer. A *prescription only medicine, it is given by intravenous infusion in specialist oncology centres.
Side effects: the main side effect is *bone marrow suppression. Other adverse effects are those of *cisplatin, including nausea and vomiting, kidney damage, and hearing loss, but these are much less severe than with cisplatin.
Precautions and interactions with other drugs: *see* CISPLATIN; CYTOTOXIC DRUGS.

carboprost A *prostaglandin used to control the bleeding that occurs after delivery of a baby if the mother's uterus fails to contract normally. It is given by deep intramuscular injection by a doctor and is available on *prescription only.
Side effects: include nausea, vomiting, diarrhoea, high body temperature and flushing, and constriction of the airways; less frequently, pain at the injection site, raised blood pressure, breathlessness, chills, headache, and dizziness may occur.
Precautions: carboprost should not be given to women with acute pelvic inflammatory disease or heart, kidney, lung, or liver disease. It should be used with caution in women with a history of glaucoma, asthma, high or low blood pressure, anaemia, jaundice, diabetes, or epilepsy.
Proprietary preparation: Hemabate.

carboxymethylcellulose *See* CARMELLOSE.

Cardene, Cardene SR (Astellas Pharma Ltd) *See* NICARDIPINE.

cardiac glycosides A group of drugs used in the treatment of congestive *heart failure and *arrhythmias. Also known as **digitalis drugs**, they were originally extracted from the foxglove plant. These drugs slow down the heart so that each beat is more effective in pumping blood. They are also used to help reduce tiredness, breathlessness, and fluid retention in heart failure. *See* DIGOXIN.

Cardicor (Merck Serono) *See* BISOPROLOL FUMARATE.

Cardioplen XL (Chiesi) *See* FELODIPINE.

Cardioxane (Novartis) *See* DEXRAZOXANE.

Cardura (Pfizer) *See* DOXAZOSIN.

carmellose A substance used as an agent in which to suspend active ingredients, as an emulsifying and thickening agent, and as a coating for tablets. It is also used to make artificial saliva solutions, for the relief of dry mouth caused by such treatments as radiotherapy and *antimuscarinic drugs, and artificial tears, for the relief of dry eyes. Carmellose is an ingredient of protective agents used in the fitting of ileostomy or colostomy appliances (*see* STOMA and a component of thick pastes that adhere to the lining of the mouth to provide protection from mechanical damage. It is also an ingredient of *laxative preparations. Carmellose is available, in the form of **carmellose sodium** or **carmellose calcium** (also called **carboxymethylcellulose**), without a prescription.
Proprietary preparations: Celluvisc (carmellose sodium; artificial tears); *Glandosane (combined with electrolytes); *Optive (combined with glycerin); *Orabase (combined with pectin and gelatin); *Xerotin (combined with electrolytes).

carmustine (**BCNU**; **bis-chloroethylnitrosourea**) An *alkylating drug used for the treatment of myeloma (cancer of the plasma cells of the bone marrow),

lymphoma, and brain tumours (*see* CANCER). It is available as an injection and as *implants on *prescription only.
Side effects: include nausea and vomiting, which may be moderately severe, and pain at the injection site. *See also* CYTOTOXIC DRUGS.
Precautions: *see* CYTOTOXIC DRUGS.
Interactions with other drugs:
Clozapine: there is an increased risk of agranulocytosis (a serious blood disorder), and this drug should therefore not be taken with carmustine.
Proprietary preparation: Gliadel (implants).

Carnation Corn Caps, Carnation Verruca Care (Cuxson, Gerrard & Co) *See* SALICYLIC ACID.

carteolol hydrochloride A *beta blocker used for the treatment of chronic (open-angle) *glaucoma and some secondary types of glaucoma. It is available as eye drops on *prescription only.
Side effects: include irritation, stinging, burning, and pain in the eye, blurred vision, and bloodshot or dry eyes. The drops can trickle into the back of the nose and be swallowed, causing *systemic effects and possibly interactions with other drugs (*see* BETA BLOCKERS).
Precautions: carteolol should not be used by people who wear soft contact lenses, by pregnant women, or by people with heart failure or asthma.
Interactions with other drugs:
Beta blockers: other beta blockers taken by mouth can enhance the effect of these eye drops. *See also* BETA BLOCKERS.
Proprietary preparation: Teoptic.

carvedilol A combined *alpha and *beta blocker used in the treatment of *hypertension and angina. It is also used, under hospital supervision, in the treatment of some forms of chronic heart failure. Carvedilol is available as tablets on *prescription only.
Side effects: include low blood pressure on standing, dizziness, headache, fatigue, gastrointestinal upsets, and a slow heart rate. *See also* BETA BLOCKERS.
Precautions and interactions with other drugs: *see* BETA BLOCKERS.
Proprietary preparation: Eucardic.
See also ANTIHYPERTENSIVE DRUGS.

cascara A powerful *stimulant laxative extracted from the bark of the tree *Rhamnus purshiana*. It is usually active 6–8 hours after administration. Although no longer recommended as a laxative, it is still included as an ingredient of various *over the counter preparations for the treatment of constipation.
Side effects and precautions: *see* STIMULANT LAXATIVES.

Casodex (AstraZeneca) *See* BICALUTAMIDE.

caspofungin An *antifungal drug used for treating generalized candidiasis and aspergillosis. It is given by intravenous injection and is available on *prescription only.

Side effects: include anaemia, low levels of potassium in the blood, headache, breathlessness, nausea, diarrhoea, vomiting, rash, itching, flushing, sweating, fever, and chills.
Precautions: this medicine should not be used in women who are breastfeeding. It should be used with caution in people with severe liver disease and the dosage should be reduced in those with moderate liver disease.
Interactions with other drugs:
Antiepileptics: the plasma concentration of caspofungin may be reduced by phenytoin and carbamazepine.
Antivirals: the plasma concentration of caspofungin may be reduced by efavirenz and nevirapine.
Dexamethasone: the plasma concentration of caspofungin may be reduced.
Rifampicin: may reduce the plasma concentration of caspofungin.
Proprietary preparation: Cancidas.

C

Catapres (Boehringer Ingelheim) *See* CLONIDINE HYDROCHLORIDE.

cathartics *See* LAXATIVES.

caustics *See* KERATOLYTICS.

Caverject (Pharmacia) *See* ALPROSTADIL.

CCNU (medac GmbH) *See* LOMUSTINE.

Ceanel Concentrate (Ferndale) A proprietary combination of *cetrimide (an antiseptic), phenylethyl alcohol (an antibiotic), and *undecenoic acid (an antifungal agent), used as a shampoo for the treatment of psoriasis and seborrhoea of the scalp and dandruff; it may be applied directly to treat psoriasis of the trunk and limbs. Ceanel is available as a liquid without a *prescription, but only from pharmacies.
Precautions: the liquid should not be allowed to come into contact with the eyes.

cefaclor A second-generation *cephalosporin used for the treatment of infections of the urinary tract, respiratory tract, skin, and soft tissues. It is available, on *prescription only, as capsules, *modified-release tablets, or a suspension.
Side effects: diarrhoea and, rarely, antibiotic-associated inflammation of the colon may occur (both are more likely with higher doses); other possible side effects are nausea and vomiting, abdominal discomfort, headache, blood disorders, nervousness, sleep disturbances, confusion, and dizziness. Allergic reactions include rashes, itching, fever, and muscle aches.
Precautions: cefaclor should not be taken by people who are allergic to cephalosporins and should be used with caution in those who are allergic to penicillins.
Proprietary preparations: Distaclor; Distaclor MR (modified-release tablets).

C

cefadroxil A first-generation *cephalosporin used for the treatment of infections of the urinary tract, respiratory tract, skin, and soft tissues. It is available, on *prescription only, as capsules or a suspension.
Side effects and precautions: *see* CEFACLOR.
Proprietary preparation: Baxan.

cefalexin <cephalexin> A first-generation *cephalosporin used for the treatment of infections of the urinary tract, respiratory tract, skin, and soft tissues, and gonorrhoea. It is available, on *prescription only, as capsules, tablets, a suspension, or a syrup.
Side effects and precautions: *see* CEFACLOR.
Proprietary preparations: Ceporex; Keflex.

cefixime A third-generation *cephalosporin used for the treatment of infections of the urinary tract, respiratory tract, skin, and soft tissues. It is available, on *prescription only, as tablets or as a suspension for children.
Side effects and precautions: *see* CEFACLOR.
Proprietary preparation: Suprax.

cefotaxime A third-generation *cephalosporin used for the treatment of infections of the urinary tract, respiratory tract, skin, and soft tissues. It is also used to treat meningitis. Cefotaxime is given by intramuscular or intravenous injection and is available on *prescription only.
Side effects and precautions: *see* CEFACLOR.

cefpodoxime A third-generation *cephalosporin used for the treatment of infections of the respiratory tract, pharyngitis, and tonsillitis. Cefpodoxime is usually reserved for infections that are chronic, recurrent, or resistant to other antibiotics. It is available, on *prescription only, as tablets or an oral suspension.
Side effects and precautions: *see* CEFACLOR.
Proprietary preparation: Orelox.

cefradine <cephradine> One of the original (first-generation) *cephalosporins, used for the treatment of infections of the urinary and respiratory tracts, skin and soft tissues, bones, and joints. It is also used to prevent infections after surgery. Cefradine is available, on *prescription only, as capsules or a syrup for oral use and as an injection.
Side effects and precautions: *see* CEFACLOR.
Proprietary preparation: Velosef.

ceftazidime A third-generation *cephalosporin used for the treatment of infections of the urinary tract, respiratory tract, skin, and soft tissues. It is given by *intramuscular or *intravenous injection or intravenous infusion and is available on *prescription only.
Side effects and precautions: *see* CEFACLOR.
Proprietary preparations: Fortum; Kefadim.

ceftriaxone A third-generation *cephalosporin used for the treatment of pneumonia, septicaemia, meningitis, infections of bones, skin, and soft

tissues, and gonorrhoea. It is also used to prevent infections after surgery. It is given by *intramuscular or *intravenous injection or intravenous infusion and is available on *prescription only.
Side effects: *see* CEFACLOR.
Precautions: *see* CEFACLOR. In addition, ceftriaxone should be used with caution in patients with liver disease.
Proprietary preparation: Rocephin.

C

cefuroxime A second-generation *cephalosporin used for the treatment of infections of the urinary tract, respiratory tract, skin, and soft tissues, meningitis, and gonorrhoea. It is also used to prevent infections after surgery. Cefuroxime sodium is given by *intramuscular or *intravenous injection or intravenous infusion; cefuroxime axetil can be taken by mouth as tablets or a suspension. Cefuroxime is available on *prescription only.
Side effects and precautions: *see* CEFACLOR.
Proprietary preparations: Zinacef; Zinnat.

Celance (Eli Lilly & Co) *See* PERGOLIDE.

Celebrex (Pharmacia) *See* CELECOXIB.

celecoxib A COX-2 inhibitor (*see* NSAIDs) used to relieve pain and inflammation in the treatment of osteoarthritis, rheumatoid arthritis, and ankylosing spondylitis (a type of arthritis affecting the spine). It is available as capsules on *prescription only.
Side effects: *see* NSAIDs.
Precautions: *see* NSAIDs. In addition, celecoxib should not be taken by people with inflammatory bowel disease, heart failure, coronary artery disease, peripheral artery disease, or cerebrovascular disease. It should be used with caution in people with hypertension.
Interactions with other drugs:
Antihypertensive drugs: celecoxib may reduce the effects of diuretics, ACE inhibitors, and angiotensin II inhibitors.
See also NSAIDs.
Proprietary preparation: Celebrex.

Celectol (Winthrop Pharmaceuticals) *See* CELIPROLOL HYDROCHLORIDE.

Celevac (Amdipharm) *See* METHYLCELLULOSE.

celiprolol hydrochloride A cardioselective *beta blocker that also has some *vasodilator action on peripheral blood vessels. It is used to treat mild to moderate *hypertension. It is available as tablets on *prescription only.
Side effects, precautions, and interactions with other drugs: *see* BETA BLOCKERS.
Proprietary preparation: Celectol.
See also ANTIHYPERTENSIVE DRUGS.

CellCept (Roche Products) *See* MYCOPHENOLATE MOFETIL.

Celluvisc (Allergan) *See* CARMELLOSE.

Celsentri (Pfizer) *See* MARAVIROC.

cephalexin *See* CEFALEXIN.

C

cephalosporins A group of broad-spectrum beta-lactam *antibiotics. They have a similar action to *penicillins in that they inhibit bacterial cell wall formation and are also susceptible to degradation by enzymes produced by bacteria (penicillinases or beta-lactamases). The drug *probenecid may be given with cephalosporins to prevent their excretion by the kidneys and thus increase their concentrations in the body. Cephalosporins are used for the treatment of septicaemia, pneumonia, meningitis, biliary-tract infections, peritonitis, and urinary-tract infections. All act against the same types of bacteria, although individual drugs have differing activity against specific organisms. The principal side effects are allergic reactions; about 10% of people who are allergic to penicillins will also be allergic to cephalosporins. Modification of the chemical structure of cephalosporins has produced the second- and third-generation cephalosporins, which have activity against a wider range of bacteria. The older (first generation) cephalosporins include *cefradine, *cefalexin, and *cefadroxil; second-generation cephalosporins include *cefuroxime and *cefaclor. Third-generation drugs include *cefotaxime, *ceftazidime, *ceftriaxone, *cefixime, and *cefpodoxime.

cephradine *See* CEFRADINE.

Ceporex (Galen) *See* CEFALEXIN.

Cerazette (Organon Laboratories) *See* DESOGESTREL.

Cerezyme (Genzyme Therapeutics) *See* IMIGLUCERASE.

Cerumol (Thornton & Ross) A proprietary combination of *arachis oil, *chlorobutanol (an antiseptic), and paradichlorobenzene (which reduces the viscosity of the preparation so that it penetrates better), used for the softening and removal of earwax. It is available as ear drops and can be obtained without a *prescription, but only from pharmacies.
Precautions: Cerumol should not be used by people with otitis externa (inflammation of the outer ear), a perforated eardrum, dermatitis, or an allergy to peanuts. It should be used for a maximum of three days.

C1-esterase inhibitor A substance derived from human plasma that is used to treat acute attacks of hereditary angioedema, a severe inherited allergic condition that involves swelling of the lips, eyes, tongue, and throat. It works by inhibiting one of the pathways involved in the allergic response. C1-esterase inhibitor is available as an intravenous injection on *prescription only.
Side effects: include high temperature, reactions at the injection site, and allergic reactions.
Proprietary preparation: Berinert.

cetalkonium chloride An *antiseptic similar to *benzalkonium chloride. It is used in a variety of *topical preparations for the treatment of minor

infections of the eye, mouth, and throat; most of these preparations are freely available *over the counter.
Precautions: cetalkonium should not be swallowed as it can cause nausea and vomiting, and strong solutions can cause damage to the oesophagus (gullet). Very large doses can depress breathing, which can be dangerous.
Proprietary preparation: *Bonjela (combined with choline salicylate).

Cetavlex (AstraZeneca) *See* CETRIMIDE.

cetirizine hydrochloride One of the newer (non-sedating) *antihistamines, used to relieve the symptoms of such allergic conditions as hay fever and urticaria. It is available as an oral solution or syrup and as tablets and may be purchased from pharmacies without a prescription.
Side effects, precautions, and interactions with other drugs: *see* ANTIHISTAMINES.
Proprietary preparations: Benadryl Allergy Oral Syrup; Benadryl for Children Allergy Solution; Benadryl One A Day; Boots Hayfever and Allergy Relief; Piriteze Allergy Syrup; Piriteze Allergy Tablets; Pollenshield Hayfever (tablets); Pollenshield Hayfever Relief (tablets); Zirtek.
See also ANTIHYPERTENSIVE DRUGS.

Cetraben Emollient Bath Additive (Genus Pharmaceuticals) *See* LIQUID PARAFFIN.

Cetraben Emollient Cream (Genus Pharmaceuticals) A proprietary combination of *white soft paraffin and *liquid paraffin (both emollients), used for the relief of red, inflamed, damaged, dry, or chapped skin. It is freely available *over the counter.

cetrimide (**cetrimonium bromide**) An *antiseptic with detergent properties and variable activity against different types of bacteria and some fungi. It is used alone or in combination with *chlorhexidine for cleansing and disinfecting the skin and for treating minor wounds, burns, and napkin rash. A very dilute solution is applied topically for the relief of sore gums. It is also used as an ingredient of shampoos for treating seborrhoea and psoriasis. Cetrimide liquid or cream is freely available *over the counter, but some combined preparations can only be bought from pharmacies.
Side effects: cetrimide may cause local irritation or allergic reactions; if swallowed, it may cause nausea and vomiting.
Proprietary preparations: Boots Antiseptic Wound Wash; Cetavlex; *Boots Antiseptic Nappy Rash Cream (combined with dimeticone); *Boots Lip and Cold Sore Cream (combined with dimeticone, urea, and chlorocresol); *Boots Soothing Eye Drops (combined with hamamelis); *Ceanel Concentrate (combined with phenylethyl alcohol and undecenoic acid); *Savlon Antiseptic Cream, Savlon Antiseptic Liquid (combined with chlorhexidine); *Tisept, Tisept Concentrate (combined with chlorhexidine); *Travasept 100 (combined with chlorhexidine).

cetrorelix A drug that antagonizes the action of *gonadotrophin-releasing

hormone and thus inhibits the release of *gonadotrophins. It is used to prevent premature ovulation in women undergoing controlled stimulation of the ovaries during assisted reproduction techniques. Cetrorelix is available as a subcutaneous injection on *prescription only.
Side effects: include reactions at the injection site, nausea, and headache.
Precautions: cetrorelix should not be given to women who are pregnant or breastfeeding, postmenopausal women, or women with moderate or severe kidney disease.
Proprietary preparation: Cetrotide.

Cetrotide (Merck Serono) *See* CETRORELIX.

cetuximab A *monoclonal antibody that inhibits epidermal growth factor receptor, a protein that is present in increased amounts in tumour cells and binds to epidemal growth factor, which causes proliferation of these cells. It is used in the treatment of advanced colorectal cancer, either alone – if alternative treatments have failed – or in combination with other chemotherapy drugs. It is also licensed for the treatment of certain cancers of the head and neck in combination with radiotherapy or other chemotherapy drugs. Cetuximab is available as a form for intravenous infusion on *prescription only.
Side effects: include allergic and other reactions after infusion (e.g. rash, fever, breathlessness), diarrhoea, nausea, vomiting, conjunctivitis, dehydration, and loss of appetite.
Precautions: because of the risk of infusion-related reactions, an antihistamine should be given before the first infusion. Cetuximab should not be given to women who are pregnant or breastfeeding and should be used with caution in people with heart or lung disease.
Proprietary preparation: Erbitux.

cetylpyridinium chloride An antiseptic used alone or in combination with other drugs for cleansing the mouth and treating minor throat or mouth infections and teething problems. Used alone, cetylpyridinium is freely available *over the counter in the form of a solution or lozenges, but some combined preparations can only be bought from pharmacies.
Proprietary preparations: Boots Antiseptic Gel; Boots First Aid Antiseptic Liquid; Boots Oral Antiseptic; Merocet (gargle or mouthwash); Merocets (lozenges); *Anbesol (combined with chlorocresol and lidocaine); *Boots Teething Gel 3 Months + (combined with lidocaine); *Calgel (combined with lidocaine); *Dentinox Teething Gel (combined with lidocaine); *Junior Meltus Chesty Coughs with Catarrh (combined with guaifenesin); *Merocaine (combined with benzocaine).

Champix (Pfizer) *See* VARENICLINE.

charcoal *See* ACTIVATED CHARCOAL.

Charcodote (Teva UK) *See* ACTIVATED CHARCOAL.

chemotherapy *See* CYTOTOXIC DRUGS.

Chemydur 60XL (Sovereign Medical) *See* ISOSORBIDE MONONITRATE.

Chloractil (DDSA Pharmaceuticals) *See* CHLORPROMAZINE HYDROCHLORIDE.

chloral betaine *See* CLORAL BETAINE.

chloral hydrate A *hypnotic drug used for the short-term treatment of insomnia. It is available, on *prescription only, as a mixture (oral solution) and as an elixir for children.
Side effects: include nausea and vomiting, abdominal distension, flatulence, vertigo, shaky movements and unsteady gait, excitement, nightmares, headache, light-headedness, and allergic rashes.
Precautions: chloral hydrate should not be taken by people with heart disease, gastritis (inflammation of the stomach), or liver or kidney disease, or by women who are pregnant or breastfeeding. It should be used with caution in people with respiratory diseases and by those with a history of drug or alcohol abuse. Prolonged use can lead to *dependence and should be avoided; treatment should be stopped gradually. *See also* HYPNOTIC DRUGS.
Interactions with other drugs: the sedative effects of chloral hydrate are increased by a number of other drugs, including anaesthetics, opioid analgesics, antidepressants, antihistamines, and antipsychotic drugs.
Proprietary preparation: Welldorm Elixir.

chlorambucil An *alkylating drug that is used mainly for the treatment of chronic lymphocytic leukaemia, non-Hodgkin's lymphoma, Hodgkin's disease, and ovarian cancer (*see* CANCER). It is available as tablets on *prescription only.
Side effects: *bone marrow suppression is the most common side effect. Occasionally a widespread severe rash develops: if this occurs, the prescribing doctor should be informed and treatment stopped. *See also* CYTOTOXIC DRUGS.
Precautions: chlorambucil should not be taken by people with porphyria or by women who are pregnant or breastfeeding. *See also* CYTOTOXIC DRUGS.
Proprietary preparation: Leukeran.

chloramphenicol A potent *antibiotic that is effective against many microorganisms but is reserved for the treatment of life-threatening *systemic infections, such as bacterial meningitis and typhoid, because it has serious side effects when given systemically. However, it may be used safely as a topical treatment for local infections of the eyes or ears. A *prescription only medicine, it is available as eye drops or ointment, ear drops, capsules, or a solution for *intravenous injection or infusion; some low-strength topical preparations are available from *pharmacies without a prescription.
Side effects: when given by mouth or injection, chloramphenicol may cause blood disorders, inflammation of peripheral or optic nerves, nausea, vomiting, diarrhoea, and sore mouth. Topical preparations may sting.
Precautions (apply only to systemic preparations): chloramphenicol should not be taken by women who are pregnant or breastfeeding or by people with porphyria. It should be used with caution in people with liver or kidney

disease. Repeated courses or prolonged administration should be avoided, and regular blood counts should be carried out.
Interactions with other drugs (with systemic preparations only):
Anticoagulants: the effects of warfarin and acenocoumarol are enhanced.
Clozapine: there is an increased risk of agranulocytosis (a blood disorder) and this drug should not be taken with chloramphenicol.
Phenobarbital: reduces the effect of chloramphenicol.
Phenytoin: the effect of this antiepileptic drug is enhanced.
Rifampicin: reduces the effect of chloramphenicol.
Tacrolimus: its plasma concentration may be increased by chloramphenicol.
Tolbutamide: the effects of this and other oral antidiabetic drugs are enhanced.
Proprietary preparations: Boots Pharmacy Antibiotic Eye Drops; Brochlor (eye drops and ointment); Chloromycetin (eye drops or ointment); Kemicetine (injection); Minims Chloramphenicol (single-dose eye drops).

ChloraPrep (Enturia) *See* CHLORHEXIDINE.

chlordiazepoxide A long-acting *benzodiazepine used for the short-term treatment of anxiety. It is also used to relieve the symptoms of alcohol withdrawal. It is available as tablets or capsules on *prescription only. Proprietary preparations cannot be prescribed on the NHS.
Side effects and precautions: *see* DIAZEPAM; BENZODIAZEPINES.
Interactions with other drugs: *see* BENZODIAZEPINES.
Proprietary preparations: Librium; Tropium.

chlorhexidine An antiseptic and disinfectant that is widely used for dressing minor skin wounds and burns to prevent infection and in oral preparations for treating sore gums and mouth ulcers, cleansing the mouth, and preventing the formation of plaque on teeth. It is used before surgery and obstetrical procedures to cleanse and disinfect the skin of the patient and the hands of the surgeon. Chlorhexidine is also used for washing out catheters and may be instilled into the bladder for treating bladder infections. It is used in the form of gluconate, acetate, or hydrochloride, either alone or in combination with other drugs, and is available as a liquid, mouthwash, dental gel, spray, cream, or powder. Preparations in which it is the sole ingredient are usually freely available *over the counter, but some combined preparations can only be bought from pharmacies.
Side effects: very rarely chlorhexidine may cause local irritation or allergic reactions. Dental preparations may cause local discoloration, taste disturbances, and bleeding of the gums.
Proprietary preparations: Acriflex Cream; ChloraPrep; Chlorohex; Corsodyl; Corsodyl Mint Mouthwash; Corsodyl Dental Gel; CX Powder; HiBi Liquid Hand Rub; Hibiscrub; Hibitane Cream; Hibitane Obstetric; Hydrex; Periogard; Savlon Antiseptic Wound Wash; Unisept; Uriflex C (solution for catheters); Uro-Tainer Chlorhexidine (solution for catheters); *Boots Dual Action Athlete's Foot Powder (combined with tolnaflate); *Dermol (combined with

liquid paraffin, isopropyl myristate, and benzalkonium chloride); *Eludril Mouthwash (combined with chlorobutanol); *Germolene Antiseptic Cream (combined with phenol); *Instillagel (combined with lidocaine hydrochloride); *Naseptin (combined with neomycin sulphate); *Nystaform (combined with nystatin); *Nystaform-HC (combined with nystatin and hydrocortisone); *Savlon Antiseptic Cream, Savlon Antiseptic Liquid (combined with cetrimide); *Tisept, Tisept Concentrate (combined with cetrimide); *Travasept 100 (combined with cetrimide).

chlormethiazole *See* CLOMETHIAZOLE.

chlorobutanol <**chlorbutol**> An *antiseptic that is active against bacteria and fungi and is used in preparations for the treatment of mouth ulcers. It is also used as a preservative in solutions for injection, eye drops, and ear drops. Chlorobutanol is available without a prescription, but some preparations can only be obtained from pharmacies.
Proprietary preparations: *Cerumol (combined with arachis oil and paradichlorobenzene); *Eludril Mouthwash (combined with chlorhexidine); *Frador (combined with menthol, styrax, and balsamic benzoin); *Karvol (combined with aromatic oils).

chlorocresol An *antiseptic and disinfectant active against a wide range of bacteria and fungi. It is used in various preparations for disinfecting skin and wounds and as a preservative in many creams, lotions, and solutions for injection.

Chlorohex (Colgate-Palmolive) *See* CHLORHEXIDINE.

Chloromycetin (Goldshield) *See* CHLORAMPHENICOL.

chloroquine A drug used for the treatment of benign *malarias, although resistance to it has developed in some areas, and for the prevention of malaria (when it may be used in conjunction with *proguanil hydrochloride). It is also used in the long-term treatment of active rheumatoid arthritis, to slow down the progress of the disease; it may take 4–6 months to have a full effect. Chloroquine can also be used for the eradication of the parasites causing amoebic hepatitis. It is available, on *prescription only, as tablets or a syrup.
Side effects: include nausea, diarrhoea, abdominal pain, headache, and (more rarely) rash, blurred vision, loss of pigmentation in the hair, and hair loss. Occasionally, with long-term use, irreversible damage to the retina may occur.
Precautions: eye examinations should be performed regularly in people taking chloroquine on a long-term basis. The drug should be used with caution in people who have liver or kidney disease and in women who are pregnant or breastfeeding. It can exacerbate psoriasis and neurological disorders and should not be used for the prevention of malaria in anyone with epilepsy. It may aggravate myasthenia gravis and severe gastrointestinal disorders.
Interactions with other drugs:

Amiodarone: increases the risk of abnormal heartbeats and should not be taken with chloroquine.
Antacids: reduce the absorption of chloroquine.
Antiepileptics: chloroquine reduces their anticonvulsant effect.
Antimalarials: there is a risk of convulsions with mefloquine.
Ciclosporin: the likelihood of toxic effects of ciclosporin is increased.
Cimetidine: increases plasma concentrations of chloroquine.
Digoxin: its plasma concentration is increased by chloroquine.
Droperidol: increases the risk of abnormal heartbeats and should not be taken with chloroquine.
Moxifloxacin: increases the risk of abnormal heartbeats and should not be taken with chloroquine.

Proprietary preparations: Avloclor; Nivaquine; *Paludrine/Avloclor (packaged with proguanil).

chloroxylenol A *disinfectant with antibacterial activity. It is used diluted as an *antiseptic for treating minor wounds, bites, stings, etc., and is included as an ingredient in many preparations for treating minor skin conditions (its activity may be enhanced by edetic acid). Chloroxylenol is freely available *over the counter.

Side effects: chloroxylenol may rarely cause local allergic reactions.

Proprietary preparations: Dettol Liquid; *Dettol Antiseptic Cream (combined with triclosan and edetic acid); *Rinstead Adult Gel (combined with benzocaine); *Rinstead Sugar Free Pastilles (combined with menthol); *TCP Antiseptic Cream (combined with triclosan and TCP Antiseptic Liquid); *ZeaSORB (combined with aldioxa).

chlorphenamine maleate <**chlorpheniramine maleate**> One of the original (sedating) *antihistamines, used to relieve the symptoms of such allergic conditions as hay fever and urticaria. It is also used for the emergency treatment of anaphylactic shock (an extreme and potentially life-threatening allergic reaction). It is also an ingredient in many cough medicines and decongestants. Chlorphenamine is available as tablets or syrup from pharmacies without a prescription or as an injection on *prescription only.

Side effects, precautions, and interactions with other drugs: *see* ANTIHISTAMINES.

Proprietary preparations: ALLERcalm Allergy Relief Tablets; Boots Allergy Relief Antihistamine Tablets; Piriton; *Haymine (combined with ephedrine); *Tixylix Cough & Cold (combined with pholcodine and pseudoephedrine).

chlorpromazine hydrochloride A phenothiazine *antipsychotic drug used for the treatment of schizophrenia and other psychoses. It has a pronounced sedative effect and is effective in calming violent or agitated patients. Chlorpromazine is also used as an *antiemetic for controlling nausea and vomiting in patients who are terminally ill and have not responded to other antiemetics, and is occasionally used for the treatment of severe hiccups. It is available, on *prescription only, as tablets, an oral solution, an injection, or suppositories.

Side effects: include marked drowsiness and apathy, pallor, nightmares, insomnia, depression, antimuscarinic effects (such as dry mouth, difficulty in passing urine, constipation, and blurred vision), *extrapyramidal reactions, nasal stuffiness, low blood pressure, hypothermia, a fast heart rate, and abnormal heartbeats (*arrhythmias). Other side effects can include weight gain, enlargement of the breasts, menstrual changes, jaundice, blood disorders, sensitivity to sunlight, dermatitis, and (with prolonged high dosage) eye changes.

Precautions: chlorpromazine should not be given to comatose patients, to people whose bone marrow function is impaired, or to people with phaeochromocytoma (a tumour of the adrenal gland). It should be used with caution in people with disorders of circulation affecting the heart or brain, chest diseases, parkinsonism, epilepsy, an underactive thyroid gland, an enlarged prostate gland, glaucoma, liver disease or a history of jaundice, kidney disease, or myasthenia gravis. It should be used with care in elderly people (especially in very hot or very cold weather) and in women who are pregnant or breastfeeding. Drowsiness can affect driving or the performance of other skilled tasks and is increased by alcohol.

Interactions with other drugs:

Anaesthetics: their effect in lowering blood pressure is enhanced.

Anti-arrhythmic drugs: amiodarone and disopyramide increase the risk of arrhythmias; amiodarone should not be taken with chlorpromazine.

Antidepressants: there is an increased risk of antimuscarinic effects and arrhythmias if chlorpromazine is taken with tricyclic antidepressants.

Antiepileptic drugs: their anticonvulsant effects are antagonized by chlorpromazine.

Beta blockers: the risk of arrhythmias is increased if sotalol is taken with chlorpromazine; if propranolol is taken with chlorpromazine, the plasma concentrations of both drugs may be increased.

Methadone: increases the risk of arrhythmias.

Moxifloxacin: increases the risk of arrhythmias and should not be taken with chlorpromazine.

Pentamidine: increases the risk of arrhythmias.

Ritonavir: may increase the effects of chlorpromazine.

Sedatives: the sedative effects of chlorpromazine are increased if it is taken with anxiolytic or hypnotic drugs, or any other drug that causes sedation.

Sibutramine: there is an increased risk of damage to the central nervous system if it is taken with chlorpromazine.

Proprietary preparations: Chloractil; Largactil.

chlortalidone <**chlorthalidone**> A thiazide-like diuretic (*see* THIAZIDE DIURETICS) used for the treatment of *hypertension and *oedema associated with heart failure, liver disease, or kidney disease. It is available as tablets on *prescription only.

Side effects, precautions, and interactions with other drugs: see THIAZIDE DIURETICS.

Proprietary preparations: Hygroton; *Kalspare (combined with triamterene); Tenoret 50 (*see* CO-TENIDONE); Tenoretic (*see* CO-TENIDONE).

See also ANTIHYPERTENSIVE DRUGS; DIURETICS.

C

chlortetracycline A tetracycline antibiotic used, in combination with a corticosteroid, for the treatment of severe inflammatory skin conditions. It is available, on *prescription only, as an ointment.
Side effects, precautions, and interactions with other drugs: *see* TETRACYCLINES.
Proprietary preparation: *Aureocort (combined with triamcinolone).

chlorthalidone *See* CHLORTALIDONE.

cholecalciferol *See* COLECALCIFEROL.

Cholestagel (Genzyme Therapeutics) *See* COLESEVELAM HYDROCHLORIDE.

cholesterol A complex molecule that has a core structure similar to that of a *steroid molecule; it is attached to a fatty acid to form cholesterol ester. Cholesterol is vital to life, being an essential component of all animal cell membranes (plants do not contain cholesterol), and is required to make bile acids (needed for fat absorption), adrenal hormones *corticosteroids, sex hormones (*androgens, *oestrogens), and *vitamin D. Cholesterol forms part of the diet and is also synthesized in the body, mainly in the liver. It is carried in the blood by *lipoproteins. Too much cholesterol in the bloodstream (**hypercholesterolaemia**: *see* HYPERLIPIDAEMIA) can lead to deposits (plaques) on the inner wall of the arteries, giving rise to *atherosclerosis. In the advanced stage, usually when a vessel is more than 50% blocked, atherosclerosis can result in thrombosis, causing a stroke or heart attack. A high circulating concentration of low-density lipoprotein (LDL) cholesterol is one of the most important risk factors for developing coronary heart disease. It enhances the adverse effects of other risk factors, such as smoking, *obesity, *hypertension, and *diabetes. Reducing circulating cholesterol lowers the incidence of heart attacks and other events related to coronary artery disease. Cholesterol reduction is achieved by dietary modification (reducing the intake of saturated fats and increasing consumption of fibre, oats, and pulses), which is the usual first-line treatment, or by *lipid-lowering drugs. It is important that other cardiovascular risk factors are also addressed.

cholestyramine *See* COLESTYRAMINE.

cholinergic drugs Drugs whose actions resemble those of *acetylcholine. Because they have the effect of stimulating the *parasympathetic nervous system they are also called **parasympathomimetic drugs**. These effects include stimulating secretions of the salivary glands, tear ducts, and bronchi, slowing the heart rate, increasing movements of the bowel, contracting the bladder, and constricting the iris of the eye and thus reducing the size of the pupil. Cholinergic drugs produce their effects in various ways and with varying intensity, which determines which conditions they are used to treat. Cholinergic drugs include alkaloids (such as *pilocarpine), *anticholinesterases (such as neostigmine and pyridostigmine), and choline esters (such as *bethanechol).

choline salicylate An *analgesic used in *topical preparations for the relief of pain in ear infections, mouth ulcers, cold sores, and denture irritation. It is available, in the form of solutions or gels, without a prescription, but some preparations can only be obtained from pharmacies.
Precautions: frequent applications should be avoided, since this could give rise to salicylate poisoning (*see* SALICYLATES).
Proprietary preparations: *Bonjela (combined with cetalkonium chloride); *Earex Plus Ear Drops (combined with glycerin).

Choragon (Ferring Pharmaceuticals) *See* HUMAN CHORIONIC GONADOTROPHIN.

chorionic gonadotrophin *See* HUMAN CHORIONIC GONADOTROPHIN.

chromones A group of anti-allergic drugs that are thought to act by preventing the release of *histamine, an important mediator of the allergic response; they also inhibit the release of other body chemicals that promote the allergic response. Because they act in this way (unlike the *antihistamines, which antagonize the action of histamine once it has been released), chromones are best used to prevent an attack before contact with the allergen occurs. When used to treat hay fever it is often necessary to continue taking the chromone even during symptom-free days. Chromones can be used regularly to prevent recurrent *asthma or exercise-induced asthma (but not to treat asthma attacks) and allergic conditions in the lungs, nose, eyes (including vernal keratoconjunctivitis), and intestines (e.g. food allergies). The main chromones are *sodium cromoglicate and *nedocromil sodium.

Cialis (Eli Lilly & Co) *See* TADALAFIL.

ciclesonide A glucocorticoid (*see* CORTICOSTEROIDS) that is used to control persistent *asthma. It is available as an aerosol inhaler on *prescription only.
Side effects: may include fungal infections of the mouth, headache, difficulty in speaking, and cough.
Precautions: ciclesonide should be used with caution in people who have (or have had) tuberculosis.
Proprietary preparation: Alvesco.

ciclosporin **<cyclosporin>** An *immunosuppressant drug used to limit rejection after organ or bone-marrow transplant surgery. It is also used for the treatment of active rheumatoid arthritis and certain skin conditions, including atopic *eczema and *psoriasis. Unlike many immunosuppressants, it does not affect the blood-cell-producing capacity of the bone marrow, but it can damage the kidneys. It is available, on *prescription only, as capsules or a solution for oral use and as a form for intravenous infusion.
Side effects: the most common side effects are nausea, gum swelling, excessive hair growth, and tremor; liver and kidney function may be impaired. Other side effects may include diarrhoea, headache, high blood pressure, fluid

retention, fatigue, muscle weakness or cramps, burning sensations in the hands and feet, rashes, and itching.

Precautions: kidney function must be monitored closely; liver function and blood pressure should also be monitored. Grapefruit juice can increase the plasma concentration of ciclosporin and therefore increase its toxic effects.

Interactions with other drugs:

Aliskiren: its plasma concentration is increased and it should not be used with ciclosporin.
Antibacterial drugs: increase plasma concentrations of ciclosporin.
Antiepileptics: reduce plasma concentrations of ciclosporin.
Antifungal drugs: amphotericin increases the risk of toxic effects on the liver; itraconazole, ketoconazole, posaconazole, and voriconazole increase plasma concentrations of ciclosporin; the plasma concentration of caspofungin is increased.
Antihypertensive drugs: ACE inhibitors and angiotensin II antagonists increase the risk of high concentrations of *potassium in the blood.
Antiviral drugs: atazanavir, indinavir, nelfinavir, ritonavir, and saquinavir increase plasma concentrations of ciclosporin.
Bosentan: its plasma concentration is increased by ciclosporin and the two drugs should not be used together.
Calcium antagonists: increase plasma concentrations of ciclosporin; lercanidipine should not be used with ciclosporin.
Carvedilol: increases the plasma concentration of ciclosporin.
Chloroquine: increases plasma concentrations of ciclosporin (and the risk of toxic effects).
Cimetidine: may increase plasma concentrations of ciclosporin.
Colchicine: increases plasma concentrations of ciclosporin (and the risk of toxic effects on the kidneys and muscles).
Cytotoxic drugs: there is an increased risk of toxic effects with methotrexate, doxorubicin, and melphalan.
Danazol: increases plasma concentrations of ciclosporin.
Digoxin: its plasma concentration (and the risk of toxic effects) are increased by ciclosporin.
Methylprednisolone: increases plasma concentrations of ciclosporin.
Metoclopramide: increases plasma concentrations of ciclosporin.
Modafinil: reduces plasma concentrations of ciclosporin.
NSAIDs: increase the risk of toxic effects on the kidneys and liver; cyclosprorin increases plasma concentrations of diclofenac.
Potassium-sparing diuretics and potassium salts: increase the risk of high concentrations of potassium in the blood.
Progestogens: increase plasma concentrations of ciclosporin.
Sitaxentan: its plasma concentrations are increased by ciclosporin and the two drugs should not be used together.
Statins: increase the risk of muscle weakness; rosuvastin should not be taken with ciclosporin.

St John's wort: reduces plasma concentrations of ciclosporin and should not be used with it.

Tacrolimus: increases the risk of toxic effects and should not be taken with ciclosporin.

Proprietary preparations: Deximune; Neoral; Sandimmun (available for named patients only).

cidofovir An *antiviral drug that inhibits DNA polymerase, the enzyme within human cells that is required by the virus to replicate itself. Cidofovir is used for the treatment of cytomegalovirus retinitis (a serious eye infection that can cause blindness) in AIDS patients when other drugs are unsuitable. It is given in combination with *probenecid to prevent its adverse effects on the kidneys. Cidofovir is available as a solution for intravenous infusion on *prescription only.
Side effects: include protein in the urine, a low white-blood-cell count, fever, hair loss, nausea, vomiting, and rash.
Precautions: cidofovir should not be given to people with kidney disease or to women who are pregnant or breastfeeding. Women should avoid becoming pregnant during treatment and for a month after treatment stops; men should not father a child during, or for three months after, treatment. Cidofovir should be used with caution in diabetics. Blood tests to monitor kidney function may be necessary.
Interactions with other drugs:

Zidovudine: interacts with probenecid, which may be given with cidofovir; zidovudine may therefore be stopped, or its dosage reduced, before treatment with cidofovir and probenecid.

Proprietary preparation: Vistide.

Cidomycin (sanofi-aventis) *See* GENTAMICIN.

cilastatin An agent that inhibits the activity of an enzyme in the kidneys that partially breaks down the antibiotic *imipenem. It is used in combination with imipenem to enhance the activity of this antibiotic.
Proprietary preparation: Primaxin (*see* IMIPENEM).

cilazapril An *ACE inhibitor used as an adjunct to *diuretics for the treatment of *heart failure. It is also used to treat essential *hypertension. It is available as tablets on *prescription only.
Side effects, precautions, and interactions with other drugs: *see* ACE INHIBITORS.
Proprietary preparation: Vascace.

See also ANTIHYPERTENSIVE DRUGS.

Cilest (Janssen-Cilag) A proprietary combination of *ethinylestradiol and *norgestimate used as an *oral contraceptive. It is available as tablets on *prescription only.
Side effects, precautions, and interactions with other drugs: *see* ORAL CONTRACEPTIVES.

cilostazol A *phosphodiesterase inhibitor with *antiplatelet activity. It is used for the treatment of the symptoms of severe intermittent claudication, in which poor circulation in the legs gives rise to cramping pain on exercise. Cilostazol is available as tablets on *prescription only.
Side effects: include headache, diarrhoea, nausea, vomiting, easy bruising, anxiety, dizziness, palpitations, angina, rhinitis, and rash.
Precautions: cilostazol should not be taken by people with severe liver or kidney disease, heart failure, or *arrhymias; by people with a predisposition to bleeding (e.g. because of peptic ulcers, a recent stroke, or hypertension); or by women who are pregnant or breastfeeding. Cilostazol may cause dizziness and should be used with caution by people intending to drive or operate machinery. It should also be used with caution by people taking anticoagulants (e.g. warfarin) as it inhibits the activity of platelets, which are involved in blood clotting.
Interactions with other drugs: cilostazol is extensively metabolized by several enzyme systems in the liver. Therefore any drug affecting these systems will alter cilostazol plasma concentrations and should either not be used with it or used with caution. A doctor should be consulted before taking cilostazol with any other drug.
Proprietary preparation: Pletal.

Ciloxan (Alcon Laboratories) *See* CIPROFLOXACIN.

cimetidine An *H_2-receptor antagonist used in the treatment of gastric and duodenal ulcers, reflux oesophagitis, Zollinger-Ellison syndrome, and all other types of *acid-peptic disease. It is available, as tablets or a syrup, on *prescription only; packs containing no more than two weeks' supply of tablets, for the relief of indigestion and heartburn in people over 16 years old, can be obtained from pharmacies without a prescription.
Side effects: side effects, which are uncommon, include diarrhoea, dizziness, rash, tiredness, and reversible liver damage; rarely, reversible confusion, blood disorders, and muscle or joint pain may occur. In high doses cimetidine can cause breast pain and enlargement in men.
Precautions: cimetidine should be used with caution in people with poor kidney or liver function and in women who are pregnant or breastfeeding.
Interactions with other drugs: cimetidine can inhibit the metabolism (and therefore may increase the effects) of a number of drugs, most importantly the following:

Anti-arrhythmic drugs: cimetidine increases the plasma concentrations of amiodarone, flecainide, lidocaine, and propafenone.
Anticoagulants: cimetidine enhances the anticoagulant properties of warfarin and acenocoumarol.
Antiepileptic drugs: cimetidine increases the plasma concentrations of carbamazepine, phenytoin, and valproate.
Ciclosporin: cimetidine increases the plasma concentration of ciclosporin.
Theophylline and aminophylline: cimetidine increases the plasma concentrations of these drugs.

In addition:
Sertindole: increases the risk of irregular heartbeats and should not be given with cimetidine.
Proprietary preparation: Tagamet.

cinacalcet A drug used to reduce excessive secretion of *parathyroid hormone, which causes high levels of calcium in the blood. This may occur in people with kidney disease who are on dialysis or in people with cancer of the parathyroid gland. Cinacalcet works by mimicking the effects of calcium on tissues. It is available as tablets on *prescription only.
Side effects: include nausea, vomiting, loss of appetite, dizziness, 'pins and needles', and loss of strength.
Precautions: cinacalcet should not be taken by women who are breastfeeding and should be used with caution in people with liver disease and in pregnant women.
Proprietary preparation: Mimpara.

cinchocaine hydrochloride A *local anaesthetic that is included in creams, ointments, and suppositories for the relief of *haemorrhoids and other painful or itching anorectal conditions.
Proprietary preparations: *Proctosedyl (combined with hydrocortisone); *Scheriproct (combined with prednisolone hexanoate); *Ultraproct (combined with fluocortolone); *Uniroid-HC (combined with hydrocortisone).

cineole *See* EUCALYPTUS OIL.

cinnarizine An *antihistamine used for the treatment of nausea and vomiting, especially that associated with disorders of the ear (such as Ménière's disease) and motion sickness. Cinnarizine is available as tablets and can be obtained from pharmacies without a prescription.
Side effects: include drowsiness and allergic skin reactions; *see also* ANTIHISTAMINES.
Precautions and interactions with other drugs: *see* ANTIHISTAMINES.
Proprietary preparations: Stugeron; *Arlevert (combined with dimenhydrinate.

Cipralex (Lundbeck) *See* ESCITALOPRAM.

Cipramil (Lundbeck) *See* CITALOPRAM.

ciprofibrate A *fibrate used for the treatment of a wide variety of *hyperlipidaemias that have not responded to dietary modification and other appropriate measures. It is available as tablets on *prescription only.
Side effects and precautions: *see* FIBRATES.
Interactions with other drugs: *see* BEZAFIBRATE.

ciprofloxacin A *quinolone antibiotic used for the treatment of infections of the respiratory and urinary tracts and of the gastrointestinal system, typhoid, gonorrhoea, and septicaemia. It is also used to treat corneal ulcers. It

is used to prevent infections after gastrointestinal surgery. Ciprofloxacin is available, on *prescription only, as tablets, a suspension, an intravenous infusion, or eye drops or ointment.
Side effects: *see* QUINOLONES. Local irritation may occur with eye drops or ointment.
Precautions and interactions with other drugs: *see* QUINOLONES.
Proprietary preparations: Ciloxan (eye drops or ointment); Ciproxin.

C

Ciproxin (Bayer) *See* CIPROFLOXACIN.

Circadin (Lundbeck) *See* MELATONIN.

cis-diamminedichloroplatinum *See* CISPLATIN.

cisplatin (**cisplatinum; cis-diamminedichloroplatinum**) A platinum-containing compound that is a powerful *cytotoxic drug: it acts by binding to DNA and thus preventing cell replication. It is highly effective in the treatment of testicular *cancer, usually in combination with *vinblastine and *bleomycin. It is also used for the treatment of cancer of the ovary and bladder, lymphomas, a form of lung cancer, and some cancers of the head and neck. It is, however, highly toxic (see side effects below) and this limits its use. A *prescription only medicine, cisplatin is given by intravenous infusion in specialist oncology units.
Side effects: cisplatin causes severe nausea and vomiting that may persist for several days. It also has adverse effects on the kidneys and when given in high doses must be accompanied by large volumes of fluid to prevent kidney damage. It can damage the nerves to the ears, resulting in some hearing loss and tinnitus (the sensation of noises in the ears), and the nerves in the arms and legs, causing numbness and tingling in the fingers and toes. Other side effects include *bone marrow suppression (which is not severe) and a reduction in magnesium concentrations in the blood. *See also* CYTOTOXIC DRUGS.
Precautions: cisplatin should not be given to people with kidney disease or to women who are pregnant or breastfeeding. *See also* CYTOTOXIC DRUGS.
Interactions with other drugs:
Antibiotics: aminoglycosides, colistin, and capreomycin increase the risk of damage to the kidneys and possibly hearing.
Clozapine: there is an increased risk of agranulocytosis (a blood disorder) and the two drugs should not be used together.
Cytotoxic drugs: bleomycin and methotrexate increase the risk of lung damage.
Diuretics: increase the risk of damage to the kidneys and possibly to hearing.

citalopram An *antidepressant drug of the *SSRI group that is used for the treatment of depressive illness and panic disorder. It is available as tablets or oral drops on *prescription only.
Side effects, precautions, and interactions with other drugs: *see* SSRIs.
Proprietary preparation: Cipramil.

Citanest (AstraZeneca) *See* PRILOCAINE.

CitraFleet (Laboratorios Casen Fleet S.L.U) A proprietary combination of *sodium picosulfate (a stimulant laxative), *magnesium citrate (an osmotic laxative), and *citric acid, used to evacuate the bowel before radiological procedures, investigation, or surgery. It is available as an oral powder to be dissolved in water and can be obtained without a prescription, but only from *pharmacies.
Side effects, precautions, and interactions with other drugs: *see* BOWEL-CLEANSING SOLUTIONS.

Citramag (Sanochemia) *See* MAGNESIUM CITRATE.

citric acid An acid found in citrus fruits that is included in pharmaceutical preparations to produce effervescent formulations (e.g. tablets or granules). Preparations containing citric acid are also used to dissolve small kidney stones, to treat cystitis and other infections of the urinary tract, or to prevent the encrustation of urinary catheters. Citric acid is also included in some anticoagulant preparations and in preparations used for the relief of gastrointestinal upsets.
Proprietary preparations: *Boots Dual Action Diarrhoea Relief (sachets: combined with sodium chloride, potassium chloride, and sodium citrate); *Cymalon (combined with sodium bicarbonate, sodium carbonate, and sodium citrate); *Eno (combined with sodium bicarbonate and sodium carbonate); *Resolve (combined with paracetamol, potassium bicarbonate, sodium bicarbonate, sodium carbonate, and vitamin C); *Uriflex G (combined with sodium bicarbonate, magnesium oxide, and disodium edetate).

cladribine A potent but rather toxic *antimetabolite that is used for the treatment of hairy cell leukaemia and for treating chronic lymphocytic leukaemia (*see* CANCER) that has not responded to *alkylating drugs. It is available, on *prescription only, as a solution for intravenous infusion or subcutaneous injection.
Side effects: *see* CYTOTOXIC DRUGS: *bone marrow suppression may be severe and nerve damage may occur rarely.
Precautions: *see* CYTOTOXIC DRUGS.
Proprietary preparations: Leustat (infusion); LITAK (injection).

Clarelux Cutaneous Foam (Pierre Fabre) *See* CLOBETASOL PROPIONATE.

Clariteyes (Schering-Plough) *See* SODIUM CROMOGLICATE.

clarithromycin A *macrolide antibiotic, similar to *erythromycin, that is used for the treatment of respiratory-tract infections and mild to moderate skin and soft-tissue infections and to eradicate causative bacteria in the treatment of duodenal ulcers (*see* ACID-PEPTIC DISEASES). It is available, on *prescription only, as tablets, granules, *modified-release tablets, a suspension for children, and a form for intravenous *infusion.
Side effects and precautions: *see* ERYTHROMYCIN.
Interactions with other drugs:

Antiviral drugs: the plasma concentrations of etravirine, maraviroc, and tipranavir are increased by clarithromycin and its plasma concentration is increased by ritonavir and tipranavir. Clarithromycin reduces the absorption of zidovudine.
Eplerenone: its plasma concentration is increased and it should not be used with clarithromycin.
Sirolimus: its plasma concentration is increased and it should not be used with clarithromycin.
For other interactions, *see* ERYTHROMYCIN.
Proprietary preparations: Klaricid; Klaricid XL (modifed-release tablets).

Clasteon (Beacon Pharmaceuticals) *See* SODIUM CLODRONATE.

clavulanic acid An agent that inhibits the activity of beta-lactamases, enzymes that are produced by bacteria and destroy *penicillins. It is given in combination with some penicillins to prevent their destruction. *See* CO-AMOXICLAV; TIMENTIN.

Clearasil Max 10 (Reckitt Benckiser) *See* BENZOYL PEROXIDE.

Clearasil Treatment Cream Regular (Reckitt Benckiser) A proprietary combination of the antiseptics *triclosan and *sulphur, used for the treatment and prevention of spots and acne. It is freely available *over the counter.

clemastine One of the original (sedating) *antihistamines, used to relieve the symptoms of such allergic conditions as hay fever and urticaria. It is available as tablets from pharmacies without a prescription.
Side effects, precautions, and interactions with other drugs: *see* ANTIHISTAMINES.
Proprietary preparation: Tavegil.

Clenil Modulite (Chiesi) *See* BECLOMETASONE DIPROPIONATE.

Clexane (sanofi-aventis) *See* ENOXAPARIN.

Climagest (Novartis) A proprietary preparation of *estradiol tablets and *norethisterone tablets used as sequential combined *hormone replacement therapy for the relief of menopausal symptoms in women who have not had a hysterectomy. The tablets, which are available on *prescription only, must be taken in the prescribed order.
Side effects, precautions, and interactions with other drugs: *see* HORMONE REPLACEMENT THERAPY.

Climanor (ReSource Medical) *See* MEDROXYPROGESTERONE.

Climaval (Novartis) *See* ESTRADIOL; HORMONE REPLACEMENT THERAPY.

Climesse (Novartis) A proprietary combination of *estradiol and *norethisterone used as continuous combined *hormone replacement therapy for the relief of menopausal symptoms and prevention of osteoporosis in women who have not had a hysterectomy and who have not had a period for a year. It is available as tablets on *prescription only.

Side effects, precautions, and interactions with other drugs: *see* HORMONE REPLACEMENT THERAPY.

clindamycin An *antibiotic used for the treatment of infections of the bones, joints and soft tissue, including those caused by meticillin-resistant *Staphylococcus aureus* (MRSA). It is also applied topically to treat bacterial infections of the vagina and *acne. It is available, on *prescription only, as capsules, a solution for intravenous *infusion or *intramuscular injection, and as a cream, gel, or lotion. Because of its serious side effects clindamycin is not widely used.
Side effects: clindamycin can cause overgrowth of the microbes normally found in the gut resulting in pseudomembranous colitis, a condition associated with severe diarrhoea that can in extreme cases be fatal. This complication is most common in middle-aged and elderly women, especially following surgery. Any signs of diarrhoea, particularly if accompanied by blood, should be reported to a doctor and treatment discontinued. Other possible side effects are abdominal discomfort, nausea, vomiting, rash, and jaundice. There may be a local reaction after intramuscular injection.
Precautions: clindamycin should be used with caution in people who have liver or kidney disease and in women who are pregnant or breastfeeding.
Proprietary preparations: Dalacin (cream); Dalacin C (capsules); Dalacin T (lotion); Zindaclin (gel); *Duac Once Daily (combined with benzoyl peroxide).

Clinitar Cream (CHS) *See* COAL TAR.

Clinitas (Altacor) *See* SODIUM HYALURONATE.

Clinorette (ReSource Medical) A propietary preparation of *estradiol tablets and combined estradiol/*norethisterone tablets, used as sequential combined *hormone replacement therapy for the relief of menopausal symptoms in women who have not had a hysterectomy. It is available on *prescription only.
Side effects, precautions, and interactions with other drugs: *see* HORMONE REPLACEMENT THERAPY.

clioquinol An *antibiotic with activity against fungi, used for the treatment of *Candida* infections of the skin and outer ear. It is combined with other drugs in creams, ointments, and ear drops that are available on *prescription only.
Side effects: local allergic reactions may occur; clioquinol stains skin and clothing.
Precautions: clioquinol should not be applied to perforated eardrums.
Proprietary preparations: *Betnovate-C (combined with betamethasone); *Locorten-Vioform (combined with flumetasone pivalate); *Synalar C (combined with fluocinolone acetonide).

Clipper (Chiesi) *See* BECLOMETASONE DIPROPIONATE.

clobazam A long-acting *benzodiazepine used in the treatment of epilepsy and for the short-term treatment of anxiety. It is available as tablets on *prescription only and cannot be prescribed on the NHS.

Side effects and precautions: *see* DIAZEPAM; BENZODIAZEPINES.
Interactions with other drugs: *see* BENZODIAZEPINES.
Proprietary preparation: Frisium.

clobetasol propionate A very potent *topical steroid used to treat *psoriasis, *eczema that is unresponsive to other treatments, and other inflammatory conditions of the skin. It is available, on *prescription only, as a cream, ointment, scalp application, or shampoo.
Side effects and precautions: *see* TOPICAL STEROIDS.
Proprietary preparations: Clarelux Cutaneous Foam (scalp application); Dermovate; Dermovate Scalp; Etrivex (shampoo); *Dermovate-NN (combined with nystatin and neomycin).

clobetasone butyrate A moderately potent *topical steroid used for the treatment of all types of *eczema and dermatitis. It is available, on *prescription only, as a cream or ointment.
Side effects and precautions: *see* TOPICAL STEROIDS.
Proprietary preparations: Eumovate; *Trimovate (combined with nystatin and oxytetracycline). *See also* CORTICOSTEROIDS.

clofarabine An *antimetabolite that is used for the treatment of people up to 21 years old with acute lymphoblastic lymphoma (*see* CANCER) in whom at least two previous chemotherapy treatments have failed. It is available as a form for intravenous infusion on *prescription only.
Side effects: *see* CYTOTOXIC DRUGS. In addition, there may be allergic reactions, fluid retention, peripheral neuropathy (causing numbness and tingling of the limbs), and pain in the muscles and joints.
Precautions: *see* CYTOTOXIC DRUGS. Clofarabine should not be given to patients with severely impaired liver or kidney function.
Proprietary preparation: Evoltra.

clofazimine An *antibiotic used for the treatment of leprosy. It is available as capsules on *prescription only.
Side effects: include nausea, vomiting, abdominal pain, headache, tiredness, and discoloration of skin exposed to light and also of hair, urine, faeces, and body fluids; discoloration of soft contact lenses may occur. Other possible side effects are rash, itching, acne-like eruptions, and loss of appetite.
Precautions: clofazimine should be used with caution in people with liver or kidney disease and in women who are pregnant or breastfeeding.

clomethiazole **<chlormethiazole>** A *hypnotic drug that does not have the hangover effects of *benzodiazepines and is therefore suitable for the treatment of insomnia in elderly people. However, it should only be taken in the short term as *dependence can occur. It is also used to treat the symptoms of alcohol withdrawal. Clomethiazole is available, on *prescription only, as capsules.
Side effects: include nasal congestion and irritation, conjunctival (eye) irritation, headache, and (rarely) paradoxical excitement, confusion,

dependence, nausea, vomiting, and rash. Excessive sedation can occur with high doses.
Precautions: clomethiazole should not be taken by people with severe lung disease or by those who are dependent on alcohol and continue drinking. It should be used with caution in people with heart or lung disease, a history of drug abuse, or marked personality disorder. The sedative effects of clomethiazole are enhanced by alcohol. *See also* HYPNOTIC DRUGS.
Interactions with other drugs: the sedative effects of clomethiazole are increased by a number of drugs, including anaesthetics, opioid analgesics, antidepressants, antihistamines, antipsychotics, cimetidine, and possibly ritonavir.
Proprietary preparation: Heminevrin.

Clomid (sanofi-aventis) *See* CLOMIFENE CITRATE.

clomifene citrate <**clomiphene citrate**> An *oestrogen antagonist used for the treatment of infertility in women caused by failure of the ovaries to produce egg cells; it acts by stimulating the secretion of *gonadotrophins by the pituitary gland. Clomifene, which is sometimes used in conjunction with *human chorionic gonadotrophin, is available as tablets on *prescription only.
Side effects: the most common are hot flushes and abdominal discomfort; more rare side effects are ovarian enlargement and hyperstimulation (the uncontrolled production of large numbers of follicles in the ovaries), visual disturbances (in which case treatment should be stopped), nausea, vomiting, depression, insomnia, breast tenderness, headache, weight gain, and hair loss. There is a risk of multiple pregnancy, cysts in the ovaries, fibroids, ectopic pregnancy, and convulsions.
Precautions: clomifene should not be used during pregnancy or by women who have liver disease, ovarian cysts, hormone-dependent tumours, or undiagnosed vaginal bleeding.
Proprietary preparation: Clomid.

clomipramine hydrochloride A *tricyclic antidepressant drug used for the treatment of depressive illness, phobias, and obsessional states and as an adjunct for treating narcolepsy (an extreme tendency to fall asleep). It is available, on *prescription only, as capsules or *modified-release tablets.
Side effects, precautions, and interactions with other drugs: *see* AMITRIPTYLINE HYDROCHLORIDE; TRICYCLIC ANTIDEPRESSANTS.
Proprietary preparations: Anafranil; Anafranil SR (modified-release tablets).

clonazepam A *benzodiazepine used for the treatment of all forms of epilepsy (*see* ANTICONVULSANT DRUGS) and muscle spasms. It is available, on *prescription only, as tablets for oral use and as a form for injection or infusion for treating status epilepticus. Intravenous infusion of clonazepam may be hazardous and should only be performed in specialist centres where intensive care facilities are available.
Side effects: include drowsiness, fatigue, dizziness, lack of coordination, and

behavioural changes, such as paradoxical aggression and irritability (*see also* BENZODIAZEPINES). There is increased salivation in babies.
Precautions: clonazepam should not be taken by patients with severe lung problems and should be used with caution in people who have liver or kidney disease and in women who are pregnant or breastfeeding; women who are planning to become pregnant should seek specialist advice. Dosage of the drug should be reduced gradually at the end of treatment (*see* BENZODIAZEPINES).
Interactions with other drugs: *see* BENZODIAZEPINES.
Proprietary preparation: Rivotril.

clonidine hydrochloride An alpha stimulant (*see* SYMPATHOMIMETIC DRUGS) that acts centrally (on receptors in the brain). It is used in the treatment of all grades of *hypertension, sometimes in combination with *diuretics, and may also be used to prevent *migraine attacks and to treat hot flushes associated with menopause. Clonidine is available, on *prescription only, as tablets or a solution for injection.
Side effects: include drowsiness, dry mouth, dizziness, and fluid retention.
Precautions: abrupt withdrawal of clonidine can cause severe hypertension; treatment must therefore be stopped gradually. Drowsiness may affect driving ability and may be increased by alcohol.
Interactions with other drugs:

Antidepressants: tricyclic antidepressants may reduce the effects of clonidine and increase the risk of rebound hypertension if clonidine is stopped.

Beta blockers: the risk of hypertension is increased if beta blockers are stopped suddenly.

Sympathomimetic drugs: adrenaline and noradrenaline may increase the risk of hypertension; adverse effects may occur if methylphenidate is taken with clonidine.

Proprietary preparations: Catapres; Dixarit (for migraine prophylaxis).
See also ANTIHYPERTENSIVE DRUGS.

clopamide *See* VISKALDIX.

clopidogrel An *antiplatelet drug used to prevent strokes or heart attacks occurring in people at risk, particularly in those who have had a previous stroke or heart attack. It is available as tablets on *prescription only.
Side effects: bleeding from the stomach, intestines, or elsewhere can occur; other side effects may include nausea, vomiting, abdominal discomfort, constipation, diarrhoea, headache, dizziness, and rashes.
Precautions: clopidogrel should not be taken by people with bleeding peptic ulcers or bleeding from other sites or by women who are breastfeeding, and it is not recommended for people with severe angina or for those who have had coronary-artery surgery. It should be used with caution in pregnant women and in people with liver or kidney disease.
Interactions with other drugs:

Anticoagulants: their effects are enhanced by clopidogrel; warfarin should not be used with clopidogrel.
NSAIDS (including aspirin): may increase the risk of gastrointestinal bleeding.
Proton pump inhibitors: may reduce the effect of clopidogrel and should not be taken with it.
Proprietary preparations: Grepid; Plavix.

Clopixol, Clopixol Acuphase, Clopixol Conc. (Lundbeck) *See* ZUCLOPENTHIXOL.

cloral betaine <**chloral betaine**> A *hypnotic drug that is a derivative of *chloral hydrate and is used for the short-term treatment of insomnia. It is available as tablets on *prescription only.
Side effects, precautions, and interactions with other drugs: *see* CHLORAL HYDRATE.
Proprietary preparation: Welldorm.

Clotam Rapid (Galen Ltd) *See* TOLFENAMIC ACID.

clotrimazole An imidazole *antifungal drug used for the treatment of candidiasis (thrush) of the vagina and tinea (ringworm) of the ear, skin, and nails. It is available as a solution, cream, pessaries, powder, or spray for topical application and can be obtained without a prescription, but only from pharmacies (compound preparations containing corticosteroids are *prescription only medicines).
Side effects: local mild burning or irritation is the most common side effect.
Proprietary preparations: Boots Antifungal Cream; Boots Thrush 1% Cream; Canesten; Canesten 10% (vaginal cream); Canesten AF (cream or powder for athlete's foot); Canesten Cream; Canesten Pessaries (Canesten 1); Canesten Powder; Canesten Spray; Canesten-Combi (pessaries and cream); Mycil Gold (cream); *Canesten HC (combined with hydrocortisone); *Lotriderm (combined with betamethasone).

clove oil An oil produced from the distillation of cloves. It can produce local anaesthesia when applied topically and is used as a home remedy for toothache. It is also an ingredient of mixtures used for the treatment of flatulent colic, of preparations to relieve the congestion of colds and catarrh, and of *rubefacient preparations for the relief of minor muscular aches and pains. Preparations containing clove oil are freely available *over the counter.
Proprietary preparations: *Olbas Oil (combined with eucalyptus oil, menthol, cajuput oil, and juniper berry oil); *Olbas Pastilles (combined with eucalyptus oil, menthol, peppermint oil, juniper berry oil, and oil of wintergreen); *Tiger Balm (combined with cajuput oil, camphor, peppermint oil, and menthol).

clozapine An atypical *antipsychotic drug used for the treatment of schizophrenia in patients who have not responded to or cannot tolerate conventional antipsychotic drugs. Because it can cause a severe deficiency of certain white blood cells, people taking clozapine must be registered with the Clozaril Patient Monitoring Service. Clozapine is available as tablets or a suspension on *prescription only.

Side effects: include headache, dizziness, weight gain, low blood pressure on standing, increased salivation, urinary incontinence and retention, fever, and a decrease in the number of white blood cells. Less frequently it can cause sedation and *extrapyramidal reactions (which are usually mild and transient).

Precautions: clozapine should not be taken by people who have bone marrow disorders or who have previously had low white cell counts due to drug treatment, or by people with severe heart failure, liver disease, severe kidney disease, psychosis due to alcohol or drugs, or uncontrolled epilepsy, or by women who are pregnant or breastfeeding. It should be used with caution in people with kidney disease, acute glaucoma, or an enlarged prostate gland and in those with a history of bowel disease or who are taking drugs that may cause constipation (e.g. antimuscarinic drugs). Therapy should be started in hospital and blood counts must be monitored regularly (weekly at the start of treatment).

Interactions with other drugs: clozapine should not be used with drugs that cause *bone marrow suppression, especially carbamazepine, co-trimoxazole, chloramphenicol, sulphonamides, azapropazone, penicillamine, cytotoxic drugs, or antipsychotic drugs given by *depot injection.

Anaesthetics: their effect in lowering blood pressure is enhanced.

Antidepressants: fluoxetine, fluvoxamine, sertraline, and venlafaxine may increase the plasma concentration of clozapine; the effects of MAOIs on the central nervous system may be increased by clozapine.

Antiepileptic drugs: their anticonvulsant effects are antagonized by clozapine; the effects of clozapine are reduced by carbamazepine and phenytoin.

Erythromycin: may possibly increase the plasma concentration of clozapine and the risk of convulsions.

Phenytoin: reduces the effects of clozapine.

Ritonavir: increases the plasma concentration (and the risk of adverse effects) of clozapine: the two drugs should therefore not be taken together.

Sedatives: the sedative effects of clozapine are increased if it is taken with anxiolytic or hypnotic drugs, or any other drug that causes sedation.

Proprietary preparations: Clozaril; Denzapine; Zaponex.

Clozaril (Novartis) *See* CLOZAPINE.

coal tar A complex mixture of substances obtained from the distillation of coal. Crude coal tar is potent but may be irritating and stains clothing; coal tar extract is usually milder and more acceptable. Coal tar is a *keratolytic that also relieves inflammation and itching and has *antiseptic properties. It also has a photosensitizing action (i.e. it makes skin more susceptible to the effects of sunlight). Coal tar is used for the treatment or relief of a variety of skin disorders, including *psoriasis (in which it also stops proliferation of skin

cells), *eczema, and dandruff. It is an ingredient of many lotions, creams, and shampoos and is usually freely available *over the counter, but some combined preparations can only be obtained from pharmacies.
Side effects: include local irritation and an acne-like rash; the skin may become more sensitive to sunlight.
Precautions: coal tar should not be applied to broken or inflamed skin and should not come into contact with the eyes; it should be used with caution on the face and genitals. It may stain the skin and clothing.
Proprietary preparations: Alphosyl 2-in-1 Shampoo; Carbo-Dome (cream); Clinitar Cream; Exorex (lotion); Neutrogena T/Gel Therapeutic Shampoo; Pentrax (shampoo); Psoriderm (cream and scalp lotion); T/Gel (shampoo); *Alphosyl HC (combined with allantoin and hydrocortisone); *Capasal (combined with salicylic acid and coconut oil); *Cocois (combined with sulphur and salicylic acid); *Polytar (combined with tar, cade oil, oleyl alcohol, and polypeptide); *Polytar AF (combined with arachis oil, cade oil, pine tar, and pyrithione zinc); *Polytar Plus (combined with arachis oil, cade oil, oleyl alcohol, and hydrolysed animal protein).

co-amilofruse A mixture of *furosemide (a loop diuretic) and *amiloride hydrochloride (a potassium-sparing diuretic), used for the treatment of *oedema (fluid retention) associated with cirrhosis of the liver, heart failure, or other conditions. It is available as tablets on *prescription only.
Side effects, precautions, and interactions with other drugs: *see* LOOP DIURETICS; THIAZIDE DIURETICS.
Proprietary preparations: Frumil; Frumil LS.

co-amilozide A mixture of *hydrochlorothiazide (a thiazide diuretic) and *amiloride hydrochloride (a potassium-sparing diuretic), used for the treatment of *oedema and *hypertension. It is available as tablets or an oral solution on *prescription only.
Side effects, precautions, and interactions with other drugs: *see* THIAZIDE DIURETICS; POTASSIUM-SPARING DIURETICS.
Proprietary preparations: Amil-Co; Moduretic.

co-amoxiclav A mixture of *amoxicillin (a penicillin) and *clavulanic acid (a beta-lactamase inhibitor). It is used for the treatment of infections of the respiratory tract, ear, nose, throat, skin and soft tissues, bones, joints, and the urinary tract and for dental infections. It is available, on *prescription only, as tablets, dispersible tablets, and a syrup for oral use and as an injection.
Side effects: *see* AMPICILLIN. Additional side effects may include jaundice and hepatitis.
Precautions: co-amoxiclav should not be taken by those who are allergic to penicillins. It should be used with caution in people with liver or kidney disease and in pregnant women.
Interactions with other drugs: *see* AMPICILLIN.
Proprietary preparation: Augmentin.

CoAprovel (Bristol-Myers Squibb) A proprietary combination of *irbesartan

(an angiotensin II inhibitor) and *hydrochlorothiazide (a thiazide diuretic), used in the treatment of *hypertension in people whose blood pressure is not adequately controlled by irbesartan alone. It is available as tablets on *prescription only.
Side effects and precautions: *see* IRBESARTAN; THIAZIDE DIURETICS; ANTIHYPERTENSIVE DRUGS.
Interactions with other drugs: *see* ACE INHIBITORS; THIAZIDE DIURETICS; ANTIHYPERTENSIVE DRUGS.

Cobalin-H (Archimedes Pharma) *See* HYDROXOCOBALAMIN.

co-beneldopa A combination of *levodopa and *benserazide hydrochloride, used for the treatment of Parkinson's disease (*see* ANTIPARKINSONIAN DRUGS). It is available as capsules, *modified-release capsules, or dispersible tablets on *prescription only.
Side effects, precautions, and interactions with other drugs: *see* LEVODOPA.
Proprietary preparations: Madopar; Madopar CR (modified-release capsules).

cocaine A drug that stimulates the central nervous system and produces a feeling of euphoria or exhilaration. It is addictive and is a commonly used drug of abuse. Cocaine is a *controlled drug; in clinical medicine it is now used only as a *local anaesthetic in ear, nose, and throat operations, being applied in the form of a solution or paste to the mucous membranes of the nasal passages (which it readily penetrates) before surgery. Because it constricts small blood vessels at the site of application (which prolongs its action), cocaine does not need to be given with adrenaline (*see* LOCAL ANAESTHETICS). Care must be used when it is applied since it can cause *arrhythmias if absorbed. Cocaine is now little used in eye surgery, because it has toxic effects on the cornea. Formerly cocaine was used as an ingredient of soothing and painkilling mixtures for the terminally ill, but this practice has been discontinued.

co-careldopa A combination of *levodopa and *carbidopa used for the treatment of Parkinson's disease (*see* ANTIPARKINSONIAN DRUGS). It is available, on *prescription only, as tablets, *modified-release tablets, or a gel delivered to the intestine via a pump.
Side effects, precautions, and interactions with other drugs: *see* LEVODOPA.
Proprietary preparations: Caramet CR (modified-release tablets); Duodopa (gel); Half Sinemet CR (modified-release tablets); Sinemet; Sinemet CR (modified-release tablets); Sinemet LS; Sinemet Plus; *Stalevo (combined with entacapone).

co-codamol A mixture of *paracetamol (a non-opioid analgesic) and *codeine phosphate (an opioid analgesic), used for the relief of mild to moderate pain. **Co-codamol 8/500** contains 8 mg of codeine and is available as tablets, capsules, or dispersible (effervescent) tablets; it is a *prescription only medicine, but under certain circumstances can be obtained from pharmacies without a prescription. Preparations containing a higher dosage

of codeine are **co-codamol 30/500** and **co-codamol 60/1000** (which also contains a higher dosage of paracetamol). They are available on *prescription only.
Side effects and precautions: *see* CODEINE; PARACETAMOL. Higher strength preparations are not recommended for children and the dosage should be reduced for elderly people.
Interactions with other drugs: *see* OPIOIDS.
Proprietary preparations: Codipar (tablets); Kapake (higher strength tablets and capsules); Paracetamol and Codeine Caplets; Paracodol (capsules and effervescent tablets); Solpadol (higher strength); Tylex (higher strength).

co-codaprin A mixture of *aspirin (a non-opioid analgesic) and *codeine phosphate (an opioid analgesic), used for the relief of mild to moderate pain. It is available as tablets or dispersible tablets and can be obtained without a prescription provided that packs contain no more than 32 (or exceptionally 100) tablets; larger quantities are available on *prescription only.
Side effects, precautions, and interactions with other drugs: *see* ASPIRIN; CODEINE; OPIOIDS.

Cocois (UCB Pharma) A proprietary combination of *coal tar, *sulphur, and *salicylic acid (all keratolytics), used in the form of an ointment for treating *psoriasis and *eczema of the scalp and dandruff. It is freely available *over the counter.
Side effects and precautions: *see* COAL TAR; SALICYLIC ACID.

Codalax, Codalax Forte (Napp Pharmaceuticals) *See* CO-DANTHRAMER.

co-danthramer A mixture of *dantron (a stimulant laxative) and poloxamer '188' (a *faecal softener). It is used for the treatment of constipation produced by analgesic drugs in the terminally ill. Co-danthramer is available as a suspension or capsules on *prescription only.
Side effects: *see* DANTRON.
Precautions: co-danthramer should not be taken by people with gastrointestinal obstruction or acute painful conditions of the abdomen or by babies in napkins.
Proprietary preparations: Codalax (suspension); Codalax Forte (a strong suspension); Danlax (suspension); Strong Co-danthramer (capsules or a suspension).

co-danthrusate A mixture of *dantron and *docusate sodium, used as a stimulant laxative and faecal softener for the treatment of constipation caused by analgesics in terminally ill patients. Co-danthrusate is available as capsules or a suspension on *prescription only.
Side effects: *see* DANTRON.
Precautions: co-danthrusate should not be taken by people with intestinal obstruction and should be used with caution by women who are pregnant or breastfeeding.
Proprietary preparation: Normax.

codeine A weak *opioid that is usually used for the relief of mild to moderate pain and is an ingredient in many *analgesic medications. It is also used as a *cough suppressant, being included in many cough medicines. Codeine slows down the movements of the intestines, causing constipation, and is therefore used as an *antidiarrhoeal drug. Codeine hydrochloride and codeine phosphate are available as tablets, a linctus, or a solution for injection. At lower dosages codeine is available without a prescription, but only from pharmacies; at higher dosages and as a form for injection it is available on *prescription only. *See also* CO-CODAMOL; CO-CODAPRIN.
Side effects: constipation is the most common side effect. In therapeutic doses codeine is unlikely to produce the other adverse effects associated with opioids, such as nausea, vomiting, and drowsiness, although respiratory depression can occur in sensitive individuals. Dependence is unusual.
Precautions: cough suppressants and antidiarrhoeal preparations are generally not recommended for children. Cough suppressants should be used with caution by people with asthma, and antidiarrhoeal preparations should not be used in acute conditions or when abdominal distension is present.
Interactions with other drugs: *see* OPIOIDS.
Proprietary preparations: Galcodeine and Galcodeine Paediatric (liquids); *Boots Catarrh Cough Syrup (combined with creosote); *Boots Paracetamol and Codeine Extra Capsules (combined with paracetamol and caffeine); *Boots Tension Headache Relief (combined with paracetamol, caffeine, and doxylamine); *Codis 500 (combined with aspirin); *Famel Original (combined with creosote); Kapake (*see* CO-CODAMOL); *Migraine Relief (combined with paracetamol); *Migraleve (combined with buclizine hydrochloride and/or paracetamol); Panadeine (*see* CO-CODAMOL); *Panadol Ultra (combined with paracetamol); Paracodol (*see* CO-CODAMOL); *Pulmo Bailly (combined with guaiacol); *Solpadeine Max (combined with paracetamol); *Solpadeine Migraine Ibuprofen & Codeine (combined with ibuprofen); *Solpadeine Plus (combined with caffeine and paracetamol); Solpadol (*see* CO-CODAMOL); *Syndol (combined with caffeine, doxylamine, and paracetamol); Tylex (*see* CO-CODAMOL); *Veganin (combined with aspirin and paracetamol).

Co-Diovan (Novartis) A proprietary combination of *valsartan (an angiotensin II inhibitor), and *hydrochlorothiazide (a thiazide diuretic), used in treatment of people whose blood pressure is poorly controlled by valsartan alone. It is available as tablets on *prescription only.
Side effects, and precautions: *see* ANGIOTENSIN II INHIBITORS; THIAZIDE DIURETICS; ANTIHYPERTENSIVE DRUGS.
Interactions with other drugs: *see* ACE INHIBITORS; THIAZIDE DIURETICS; ANTIHYPERTENSIVE DRUGS.

Codipar (Goldshield) *See* CO-CODAMOL.

Codis 500 (Reckitt Benckiser) A proprietary combination of *aspirin (an analgesic and antipyretic) and *codeine (an opioid analgesic), used for the treatment of mild to moderate pain (including headache, neuralgia, toothache, and period pains) and fever and to relieve the symptoms of

influenza and colds. It is freely available *over the counter as dispersible tablets.
Side effects: *see* ASPIRIN; CODEINE.
Precautions: these tablets should not be given to children, except on medical advice. *See also* ASPIRIN; OPIOIDS.
Interactions with other drugs: *see* ASPIRIN; OPIOIDS.

co-dydramol A mixture of *paracetamol (a non-opioid analgesic) and *dihydrocodeine tartrate (a weak opioid analgesic), used for the relief of mild to moderate pain. It is available as tablets on *prescription only.
Side effects and precautions: *see* PARACETAMOL; MORPHINE. Co-dydramol is not recommended for children.
Interactions with other drugs: *see* OPIOIDS.

co-fluampicil A mixture of *ampicillin and *flucloxacillin (both broad-spectrum *antibiotics), used for the treatment of infections caused by more than one type of bacterium (e.g. skin infections) when the exact type of bacterium is unknown. It is available, on *prescription only, as capsules, a syrup, and as a solution for injection.
Side effects, precautions, and interactions with other drugs: *see* AMPICILLIN; FLUCLOXACILLIN.
Proprietary preparations: Flu-Amp; Magnapen.

co-flumactone A mixture of *spironolactone (a potassium-sparing diuretic) and *hydroflumethiazide (a thiazide diuretic), used to treat congestive *heart failure. It is available as tablets on *prescription only.
Side effects, precautions, and interactions with other drugs: *see* POTASSIUM-SPARING DIURETICS; THIAZIDE DIURETICS.
Proprietary preparations: Aldactide 25; Aldactide 50 (higher-strength tablets).

Colazide (Almirall) *See* BALSALAZIDE SODIUM.

colchicine A drug that is used for the treatment of acute attacks of gout and to prevent attacks of gout in people who are taking *allopurinol. It is usually given to people who have been unable to tolerate *NSAIDs. Unlike NSAIDs, colchicine does not cause fluid retention, and can therefore be taken by people with heart failure. However, its use is limited because it has toxic effects at higher dosages (see below). Colchicine is available as tablets on *prescription only.
Side effects: nausea, vomiting, and abdominal pain are the most common effects; high doses can cause profuse diarrhoea, gastrointestinal bleeding, rashes, and damage to the kidneys and liver.
Precautions: colchicine should not be taken by women who are pregnant or breastfeeding and should be used with caution in the elderly and in people with heart, liver, or kidney disease.
Interactions with other drugs:

Antibiotics: the risk of adverse effects is increased if clarithromycin or erythromycin are taken with colchicine.

Ciclosporin: the risk of kidney and muscle damage is increased if ciclosporin is taken with colchicine.
Statins: the risk of muscle damage may be increased if these drugs are taken with colchicine.

C

colecalciferol <**cholecalciferol**> (vitamin D_3) One of the D vitamins (*see* VITAMIN D), which is used for the treatment of simple vitamin D deficiency, such as that caused by lack of sunlight. Combined with *calcium carbonate or *calcium phosphate, it is available as tablets without a prescription, but only from pharmacies; a solution for injection is available on *prescription only (*see* CALCIFEROL).
Side effects, precautions, and interactions with other drugs: *see* VITAMIN D.
Proprietary preparations: *Actonel Combi (sachets: combined with calcium carbonate); *Adcal-D_3 (combined with calcium carbonate); *Cacit D3 (combined with calcium carbonate); *Calceos (combined with calcium carbonate); *Calcichew-D_3 (combined with calcium carbonate); *Calfovit D3 (combined with calcium phosphate); *Fosavance (combined with alendronic acid); *Natecal D3 (combined with calcium carbonate); *Sandocal + D 600 (combined with calcium carbonate and calcium lactate gluconate).

colesevelam hydrochloride A *bile-acid sequestrant used as an *adjunct to dietary measures to lower plasma *cholesterol (*see* HYPERLIPIDAEMIA), either alone or in combination with a *statin. It is available as tablets on *prescription only.
Side effects: *see* BILE-ACID SEQUESTRANTS. In addition, colesevelam may cause headache.
Precautions: colesevelam should not be taken by people with obstruction to the bowel or bile duct. It should be used with caution by people with difficulties in swallowing, inflammatory bowel disease, or liver failure.
Interactions with other drugs: *see* BILE-ACID SEQUESTRANTS.
Proprietary preparation: Cholestagel.

Colestid (Pharmacia) *See* COLESTIPOL.

colestipol A *bile-acid sequestrant that is used to lower plasma *cholesterol in the treatment of certain types of *hyperlipidaemia. It is available, on *prescription only, as granules or a powder to be dissolved in liquid.
Side effects, precautions, and interactions with other drugs: *see* BILE-ACID SEQUESTRANTS.
Proprietary preparation: Colestid.

colestyramine A *bile-acid sequestrant used to lower plasma *cholesterol in *hyperlipidaemia and for the prevention of coronary heart disease in men with high plasma cholesterol concentrations that are unresponsive to diet and other appropriate measures. It is also used for the relief of diarrhoea associated with surgical removal of part of the small intestine, Crohn's disease, or radiation and of itching associated with bile duct disease. A *prescription only medicine, it is available as a powder to be dissolved in liquid.
Side effects and precautions: *see* BILE-ACID SEQUESTRANTS.

Interactions with other drugs:

Acarbose: its effect in lowering blood sugar is increased by colestyramine.

Paracetamol: absorption of these analgesics is reduced by colestyramine.

Vancomycin: its effect is antagonized by colestyramine.

Warfarin: its anticoagulant effect may be reduced or increased.

See also BILE-ACID SEQUESTRANTS.

Proprietary preparations: Questran; Questran Light.

Colifoam (Meda Pharmaceuticals) *See* HYDROCORTISONE.

colistin An *antibiotic that is given by intravenous injection to treat serious infections that are resistant to other antibiotics. It is not absorbed from the gut but may be taken orally in the form of tablets or a syrup to treat gut infections and to sterilize the bowel before surgery. It can also be inhaled via a *nebulizer as an *adjunct to standard antibiotics by people with cystic fibrosis. Colistin is available on *prescription only.

Side effects: include numbness around the mouth, vertigo, muscle weakness, breathlessness, and kidney damage. Rare side effects are slurred speech, visual disturbances, and confusion.

Precautions: colistin should not be taken by people with myasthenia gravis or by women who are pregnant or breastfeeding. It should be used with caution in people who have kidney disease or porphyria.

Interactions with other drugs: *see* GENTAMICIN.

Proprietary preparations: Colomycin; Promixin (injection and nebulizer solution).

collodion A syrupy solution of nitrocellulose in a mixture of alcohol and ether. When applied to the surface of the body it evaporates to leave a thin clear transparent skin, useful for the protection of minor wounds. Flexible collodion also contains camphor and castor oil, which allow the skin to stretch a little more.

Colofac (Solvay Healthcare) *See* MEBEVERINE HYDROCHLORIDE.

Colomycin (Forest Laboratories) *See* COLISTIN.

Colpermin (McNeil Ltd) *See* PEPPERMINT OIL.

co-magaldrox A mixture of *aluminium hydroxide and *magnesium hydroxide, used as an *antacid for the relief of digestive disorders (*see* ACID-PEPTIC DISEASES). It is freely available *over the counter in the form of a suspension.

Side effects and interactions with other drugs: *see* ANTACIDS.

Precautions: *see* ALUMINIUM HYDROXIDE; MAGNESIUM SALTS.

Proprietary preparations: Maalox (sugar-free suspension); Mucogel (sugar-free suspension).

Combigan (Allergan) A proprietary combination of *brimonidine tartrate (an alpha stimulant) and *timolol maleate (a beta blocker), used to reduce the pressure inside the eye in people with chronic (open-angle) glaucoma or

raised blood pressure in the eye who have not responded to beta blockers alone. It is available as eye drops on *prescription only.
Side effects, precautions, and interactions with other drugs: *see* BETA BLOCKERS; BRIMONIDINE TARTRATE.

C

Combivent (Boehringer Ingelheim) A proprietary combination of the bronchodilators *salbutamol (a sympathomimetic drug) and *ipratropium bromide (an antimuscarinic drug), used to relieve constriction of the airways associated with chronic bronchitis or emphysema. It is available as a solution for use in a *nebulizer on *prescription only.
Side effects, precautions, and interactions with other drugs: *see* SALBUTAMOL; IPRATROPIUM BROMIDE.

Combivir (GlaxoSmithKline) A proprietary combination of the antiviral drugs *zidovudine and *lamivudine, used to delay the progression of disease in *HIV-infected patients. It is available as tablets on *prescription only.
Side effects, precautions, and interactions with other drugs: *see* ZIDOVUDINE; LAMIVUDINE.

Competact (Takeda) A proprietary combination of *pioglitazone and *metformin hydrochloride (both oral hypoglycaemic drugs), used in the treatment of people with type 2 *diabetes mellitus, particularly those who are overweight, whose blood-glucose levels are not controlled by metformin alone. It is available as tablets on *prescription only.
Side effects, precautions, and interactions with other drugs: *see* METFORMIN HYDROCHLORIDE; PIOGLITAZONE.

Comtess (Orion Pharma) *See* ENTACAPONE.

Concerta XL (Janssen-Cilag) *See* METHYLPHENIDATE HYDROCHLORIDE.

Condyline (Ardern Healthcare) *See* PODOPHYLLOTOXIN.

congestive heart failure *See* HEART FAILURE.

Conotrane (Astellas Pharma) A proprietary combination of *benzalkonium chloride (an antiseptic) and *dimeticone (a water repellent), used in the form of a cream as a *barrier preparation for the treatment of napkin rash and pressure sores. It is freely available *over the counter.

Contac (GlaxoSmithKline) *See* PSEUDOEPHEDRINE.

Contac CoughCaps (GlaxoSmithKline) *See* DEXTROMETHORPHAN.

continuous-release preparation *See* MODIFIED-RELEASE PREPARATION.

contraceptives *See* DEPOT CONTRACEPTIVES; ORAL CONTRACEPTIVES.

controlled drugs Drugs that can only be prescribed under the guidelines of the Misuse of Drugs Act (1971) and Regulations (1997, 2001). These are usually drugs that have the potential for *dependence and abuse and they are divided into three classes; the most serious drugs of addiction (class A) include *cocaine, *diamorphine (heroin), *morphine, and the synthetic *opioids. The

Regulations specify the categories of persons who may supply these drugs and lay down rules for writing prescriptions (including the requirement that the prescription must be in the prescriber's own handwriting). There are also regulations relating to manufacture, supply, and record keeping.

Convulex (Pharmacia) *See* VALPROIC ACID.

Copaxone (Teva Pharmaceuticals) *See* GLATIRAMER ACETATE.

Copegus (Roche Products) *See* RIBAVIRIN.

co-phenotrope A mixture of diphenoxylate hydrochloride (an *opioid that reduces gut motility) and *atropine sulphate (an antispasmodic drug), used for the treatment of diarrhoea (*see* ANTIDIARRHOEAL DRUGS). It is available as tablets on *prescription only.
Side effects: include allergic skin reactions and abdominal cramp and bloating. *See also* ANTIMUSCARINIC DRUGS; OPIOIDS.
Precautions: co-phenotrope should not be used by people with intestinal obstruction, acute ulcerative colitis, antibiotic-induced colitis, or jaundice. It should not be taken until severe dehydration or *electrolyte imbalance has been corrected.

Coppertone (Schering-Plough) A proprietary *sunscreen preparation consisting of a cream containing ethylhexyl *p*-methoxycinnamate, oxybenzone, and padimate-O. It protects against both UVA and UVB (SPF 23) and can be prescribed on the NHS or obtained without a prescription.

co-proxamol A mixture of *paracetamol (a non-opioid analgesic) and dextropropoxyphene hydrochloride (a weak opioid analgesic), used for the relief of mild to moderate pain. It is available as tablets on *prescription only.
Side effects and precautions: overdosage with co-proxamol can cause respiratory depression and heart failure (due to dextropropoxyphene) and liver damage (due to paracetamol), which requires rapid emergency treatment. Co-proxamol should therefore not be given to those who are suicidal or otherwise at risk. It is not recommended for children, and the dosage should be reduced for elderly people.
Interactions with other drugs: *see* OPIOIDS.

Coracten SR, Coracten XL (UCB Pharma) *See* NIFEDIPINE.

Cordarone X (sanofi-aventis) *See* AMIODARONE.

Cordilox (Dexcel Pharma) *See* VERAPAMIL HYDROCHLORIDE.

Corgard (sanofi-aventis) *See* NADOLOL.

Corlan (UCB Pharma) *See* HYDROCORTISONE.

Corn and Callus Removal Liquid (SSL International) A proprietary combination of *salicylic acid (a keratolytic) and *camphor, used for the treatment of corns and calluses. It is freely available *over the counter.
Precautions: this preparation is not recommended for children.

Corn Removal Pads, Corn Removal Plasters (SSL International) *See* SALICYLIC ACID.

Coro-Nitro Pump Spray (Ayrton Saunders) *See* GLYCERYL TRINITRATE.

Corsodyl (GlaxoSmithKline) *See* CHLORHEXIDINE.

corticosteroids Steroid hormones that are secreted by the outer layer (cortex) of the adrenal glands, or semisynthetic substances that closely resemble the natural products. There are two main types of corticosteroids: **mineralocorticoids** and **glucocorticoids**. Mineralocorticoids (e.g. aldosterone) assist in the maintenance of salt and water balance. Glucocorticoids (e.g. cortisol, cortisone) affect the metabolism of glucose, protein, and fat and inhibit inflammation.

Synthetic mineralocorticoids (e.g. *fludrocortisone acetate) are used for replacement therapy in people who lack the natural hormone as a result of disease or surgical removal of the adrenal glands. Drugs with glucocorticoid activity (e.g. *hydrocortisone, *betamethasone, *prednisolone) may be used as replacement therapy but are more commonly employed for their anti-inflammatory activity. They are used to treat a wide range of inflammatory conditions, including asthma, rheumatoid arthritis, inflammatory bowel disease (e.g. Crohn's disease, ulcerative colitis), and connective tissue disorders (such as systemic lupus erythematosus). They are also included in the therapy for some cancers and to prevent the rejection of organ and tissue transplants (*see* IMMUNOSUPPRESSANTS). Corticosteroids may be given by mouth or intravenous injection. They can be applied topically for the treatment of inflammatory conditions of the skin, eyes, ears, and nose (*see* TOPICAL STEROIDS). They may also be administered in enemas, by direct injection into joints or around tendons, or by inhalation. Inhaled steroids are used for the prevention of *asthma attacks; they must be inhaled regularly, even when no symptoms are present.

Because the concentration of corticosteroids required to produce anti-inflammatory activity is higher than that normally present in the body, corticosteroid therapy can have adverse effects on metabolism. When given in high doses or during long-term treatment, *systemic corticosteroids are associated with a number of side effects (see below). Steroids administered locally or topically have, in general, fewer and less serious side effects: the severity of these will depend on the strength of the steroid, the area of the body that is exposed to the steroid, and the duration of treatment. Long-term use of systemic corticosteroids leads to adrenal suppression, in which the adrenal glands fail to produce the normal amount of hormones. For this reason, withdrawal of treatment after long-term use must always be gradual; sudden withdrawal can lead to severe lowering of the blood pressure and may even be fatal. Increased amounts of corticosteroids are normally produced by the adrenal glands in response to stress (e.g. injury, surgery, or infection). Because normal production is suppressed in those taking long-term corticosteroid therapy, increased doses must be given to cope with episodes of stress.

See also BECLOMETASONE DIPROPIONATE; BUDESONIDE; DEFLAZACORT; DEXAMETHASONE; FLUNISOLIDE; FLUTICASONE PROPIONATE; METHYLPREDNISOLONE; TRIAMCINOLONE ACETONIDE.

Side effects: long-term use of systemic corticosteroids in high doses can lead to decreased activity of the immune system and susceptibility to infection; the inflammatory response is reduced, which can mask signs of infection. Disturbance in calcium metabolism results in loss of bone tissue, which can retard growth in children and exacerbate osteoporosis in adults. Salt and water balance is affected, especially with mineralocorticoids, resulting in retention of *sodium and water (and loss of *potassium), with consequent fluid retention and high blood pressure. Glucocorticoids also affect protein metabolism, causing muscle weakness and thinning of the skin, with delayed wound healing and stretch marks (striae); glucose metabolism, resulting in diabetes mellitus; and the metabolism of fat, which is deposited in the face ('moon face'), on the shoulders ('buffalo hump'), and in the abdomen. These signs of excess glucocorticoids are sometimes called 'Cushingoid features'. Long-term use of steroids leads to adrenal suppression, in which the response to stress is reduced (see above). Other side effects include indigestion (which is common) and possibly peptic ulceration; increased appetite and weight gain; acne; increased growth of facial and body hair; mood changes, ranging from euphoria to depression and paranoia; insomnia; and menstrual irregularities. Inhaled steroids commonly cause hoarseness or huskiness of the voice, due to weakening of the vocal muscles, and a sore throat, due to fungal (*Candida*) infection. Rinsing the mouth out after each inhaled dose helps to prevent the latter complication. *See also* TOPICAL STEROIDS.

Precautions: people taking steroids should always mention this fact to their doctor, dentist, or chiropodist when undergoing other treatment. People taking corticosteroids by mouth for more than one month are advised to carry a warning card; higher doses may be required during periods of illness or stress. Withdrawal of treatment after long-term use should be gradual (see above). Corticosteroids should not be taken by people with systemic infections unless active treatment of the infection is given at the same time. People taking systemic corticosteroids for purposes other than replacement therapy should avoid contact with those suffering from chickenpox or shingles while taking the steroids and up to three months after treatment; anyone taking systemic steroids who has been in close contact with someone suffering from chickenpox should see a doctor. People taking high doses of corticosteroids systemically should not be given vaccinations with live vaccines. High doses of systemic corticosteroids have been associated with psychiatric symptoms (including depression and suicidal thoughts) and should be given with caution to people with a history of psychiatric illness. Corticosteroids reduce the effect of insulin and care must be taken by people with diabetes. Dosage may need to be reduced in the elderly, in whom side effects may be more pronounced. Corticosteroids should be used with caution during pregnancy.

Interactions with other drugs (systemic corticosteroids):
Amphotericin: increases the risk of reduced potassium concentrations in the plasma and should not be given with corticosteroids.
Antidiabetic drugs: their effect is reduced to a small extent.
Antiepileptics: carbamazepine, phenobarbital, phenytoin, and primidone reduce the effects of corticosteroids.
Antihypertensive drugs: their effect in lowering blood pressure is antagonized.
Barbiturates: reduce the effects of corticosteroids.
Digoxin: there is an increased risk of toxicity from digoxin if plasma potassium concentrations fall.
Diuretics: there is an increased risk of reduced plasma potassium concentrations, and steroids (especially mineralocorticoids) tend to cause water retention.
Methotrexate: increases the risk of blood disorders if given with corticosteroids.
Rifampicin: reduces the effects of corticosteroids.
Warfarin: its anticoagulant effect is increased by high doses of corticosteroids.

cortisol *See* CORTICOSTEROIDS; HYDROCORTISONE.

cortisone acetate A *corticosteroid that has been used as replacement therapy when the adrenal glands are functioning poorly or have been surgically removed, but *hydrocortisone (to which it is converted in the liver) is now preferred. It is available as tablets on *prescription only.
Side effects, precautions, and interactions with other drugs: *see* CORTICOSTEROIDS.

co-simalcite *See* ALTACITE PLUS.

Cosmegen Lyovac (Ovation) *See* DACTINOMYCIN.

CosmoFer (Vitaline Pharmaceuticals) *See* IRON DEXTRAN.

Cosopt (Merck Sharp & Dohme) A proprietary combination of *dorzolamide (a carbonic anhydrase inhibitor) and *timolol maleate (a beta blocker), used for the treatment of chronic (open-angle) *glaucoma that has not responded to beta blockers alone. It is available as eye drops on *prescription only.
Side effects, precautions, and interactions with other drugs: *see* DORZOLAMIDE; BETA BLOCKERS.

Cosuric (DDSA Pharmaceuticals) *See* ALLOPURINOL.

co-tenidone A mixture of *atenolol (a cardioselective beta blocker) and *chlortalidone (a thiazide diuretic), used for the treatment of *hypertension. It is available as tablets on *prescription only.
Side effects, precautions, and interactions with other drugs: *see* BETA BLOCKERS; THIAZIDE DIURETICS.

Proprietary preparations: Atenix-Co; Tenoret 50; Tenoretic (contains twice the amount of atenolol as Tenoret 50).

See also ANTIHYPERTENSIVE DRUGS; DIURETICS.

C

co-trimoxazole A mixture of *trimethoprim (an antibacterial drug) and sulfamethoxazole (a *sulphonamide antibiotic) in the proportions 1:5; the effect of this combination is greater than the sum of the effects of its two constituent drugs given singly. It is the drug of choice for treating pneumonia caused by *Pneumocystis jirovecii* (*carinii*); it is also used to treat toxoplasmosis (a protozoal disease that can cause blindness and mental retardation in a fetus) and nocardiasis (a bacterial infection of the lungs, skin, and brain, causing abscesses). Co-trimoxazole is available, on *prescription only, as tablets, a suspension, or a paediatric syrup for oral use and as a solution for intravenous infusion.

Side effects: include nausea, vomiting, rash, and blood disorders; if the last two effects occur, the treatment should be discontinued immediately. More rarely, allergic reactions, diarrhoea, sore mouth, loss of appetite, and muscle and joint pains may occur.

Precautions: co-trimoxazole should not be taken by patients with liver or kidney failure or porphyria, and it should be used with caution in those who have impaired liver or kidney function or blood disorders and in women who are pregnant or breastfeeding.

Interactions with other drugs:

Amiodarone: there is an increased risk of ventricular *arrhythmias and aminodarone should not be given with co-trimoxazole.

Anticoagulants: the effects of warfarin and acenocoumarol are increased.

Azathioprine: there is an increased risk of blood disorders.

Ciclosporin: there is an increased risk of adverse effects on the kidneys.

Clozapine: there is an increased risk of agranulocytosis (a serious blood disorder) and the two drugs should not be used together.

Cytotoxic drugs: there is an increased risk of blood disorders if mercaptopurine or methotrexate are given with co-trimoxazole.

Phenytoin: the plasma concentration of this drug is increased.

Pyrimethamine: there is an increased risk of folate deficiency, which may lead to megaloblastic anaemia.

Sulphonylureas: the effects of these oral antidiabetic drugs are enhanced.

Proprietary preparations: Fectrim; Fectrim Forte; Septrin.

cough suppressants (**antitussives**) Drugs that act on the brain to suppress the cough reflex; they do not treat the underlying cause of the coughing. Cough suppressants are used to relieve dry persistent coughs. The most commonly used drugs are *dextromethorphan, *codeine, and *pholcodine, all of which are *opioids; they tend to cause constipation. *See also* EXPECTORANTS; DEMULCENTS.

counterirritants *See* RUBEFACIENTS.

Coversyl Arginine (Servier Laboratories) *See* PERINDOPRIL.

Coversyl Arginine Plus (Servier Laboratories) A proprietary combination of *perindopril (an ACE inhibitor) and *indapamide (a thiazide-like diuretic), used for the treatment of hypertension not controlled by perindopril alone. It is available as tablets on *prescription only.
Side effects and precautions: *see* INDAPAMIDE; ACE INHIBITORS.
Interactions with other drugs: *see* ACE INHIBITORS; THIAZIDE DIURETICS.

Covonia Bronchial Balsam (Thornton & Ross) A proprietary combination of *dextromethorphan (a cough suppressant) and *menthol, used for the relief of dry coughs, such as those associated with colds and bronchitis. It is available as a syrup without a prescription, but only from pharmacies.
Side effects and interactions with other drugs: *see* DEXTROMETHORPHAN; OPIOIDS.
Precautions: this medicine is not recommended for children under six years old. *See also* OPIOIDS.

Covonia Night Time Formula (Thornton & Ross) A proprietary combination of *dextromethorphan (a cough suppressant) and *diphenhydramine (a sedative antihistamine), used to relieve dry coughs that interfere with sleep. It is available as a syrup without a prescription, but only from pharmacies.
Side effects and interactions with other drugs: *see* DEXTROMETHORPHAN; OPIOIDS.
Precautions: this medicine is not recommended for children. *See also* OPIOIDS.

COX-2 inhibitors *See* NSAIDs.

Cozaar (Merck Sharp & Dohme) *See* LOSARTAN POTASSIUM.

Cozaar-Comp (Merck Sharp & Dohme) A proprietary combination of *losartan potassium (an angiotensin II inhibitor) and *hydrochlorothiazide (a thiazide diuretic), used in the treatment of *hypertension. It is available as tablets on *prescription only.
Side effects, precautions, and interactions with other drugs: *see* ANGIOTENSIN II INHIBITORS; THIAZIDE DIURETICS.
See also ANTIHYPERTENSIVE DRUGS; DIURETICS.

Crampex (Thornton & Ross) A proprietary combination of *nicotinic acid, vitamin D_3 (*see* COLECALCIFEROL), and *calcium gluconate, used for the relief of muscle cramps at night. It is available as tablets that can be obtained without a prescription, but only from pharmacies.
Precautions: Crampex is not recommended for children.

cream A medicinal preparation consisting of an oil-in-water emulsion that is applied to the skin. Less greasy than *ointments and easier to apply, creams are usually readily absorbed into the skin. *See* EMOLLIENTS.

Creon, Creon 10 000, Creon 25 000, Creon 40 000, Creon Micro (Solvay Healthcare) *See* PANCREATIN.

Crestor (AstraZeneca) *See* ROSUVASTATIN.

cretinism *See* THYROID HORMONES.

Crinone (Serono) *See* PROGESTERONE.

crisantaspase An enzyme preparation (asparaginase) used as a *cytotoxic drug for the treatment of acute lymphoblastic leukaemia (*see* CANCER). It is given by intramuscular, intravenous, or subcutaneous injection in specialist units and is available on *prescription only.
Side effects: include nausea, vomiting, depression of central nervous system activity, and changes in liver function and blood lipids (fats); severe allergic reactions (*see* ANAPHYLAXIS) may occur. *See also* CYTOTOXIC DRUGS.
Precautions: tests for liver function, blood lipids, and concentrations of glucose in the urine should be performed throughout treatment. *See also* CYTOTOXIC DRUGS.
Proprietary preparation: Erwinase.

Crixivan (Merck Sharp & Dohme) *See* INDINAVIR.

cromoglicate *See* SODIUM CROMOGLICATE.

crotamiton A drug that is used to relieve itching, including that associated with *scabies. It is freely available *over the counter in the form of a cream or lotion.
Precautions: crotamiton should not be used to treat weeping skin conditions. It should not be used near the eyes or on broken skin.
Proprietary preparations: Eurax; Eurax Lotion.

Crystacide (GP Pharma) *See* HYDROGEN PEROXIDE.

crystal violet (**gentian violet**) A purple dye that has *antiseptic properties. Diluted in purified water, it is used to disinfect unbroken skin in the treatment of burns, boils, and minor bacterial or fungal infections. It is also used to cleanse the skin before surgery. Crystal violet is available as a paint that can be obtained without a prescription, but only from pharmacies.
Side effects and precautions: crystal violet should not be applied to mucous membranes (because it causes ulceration) or to open wounds. It stains skin and clothing.

Crystapen (Genus Pharmaceuticals) *See* BENZYLPENICILLIN.

Cubicin (Novartis) *See* DAPTOMYCIN.

Cuplex (Crawford Pharmaceuticals) A proprietary combination of *salicylic acid and *lactic acid (keratolytics) and copper acetate (an astringent), used for the treatment of warts, verrucas, corns, and calluses. It is available as a gel and can be obtained without a prescription, but only from pharmacies.
Side effects and precautions: *see* SALICYLIC ACID.

Cuprofen, Cuprofen Gel, Cuprofen Maximum Strength (SSL International) *See* IBUPROFEN.

Curanail Nail Lacquer (Galderma) *See* AMOROLFINE.

Curatoderm (Almirall) *See* TACALCITOL.

Curosurf (Chiesi) *See* PORACTANT ALFA.

Cutivate (GlaxoSmithKline) *See* FLUTICASONE PROPIONATE.

Cuxson Gerrard Belladonna Plasters (Cuxson, Gerrard & Co) *See* BELLADONNA EXTRACT.

CX Powder (Adams Healthcare) *See* CHLORHEXIDINE.

cyanocobalamin A form of vitamin B_{12} (*see* VITAMIN B COMPLEX) that is used to treat or prevent deficiency of this vitamin (such as occurs in strict vegetarians). For treating pernicious anaemia, cyanocobalamin has been replaced by *hydroxocobalamin. Cyanocobalamin is available as tablets or a liquid, which can be obtained from pharmacies without a prescription, or as an injection, which is available on *prescription only.
Side effects: cyanocobalamin may rarely cause allergic reactions.
Proprietary preparations: Cytacon; Cytamen (injection).

Cyclimorph (Amdipharm) A proprietary combination of *morphine tartrate (an opioid analgesic) and *cyclizine tartrate (an antiemetic antihistamine). It is used for the treatment of moderate to severe pain; the cyclizine is included to prevent the nausea and vomiting associated with opioids. Cyclimorph is available as an injection; it is a *controlled drug.
Side effects: include drowsiness, dry mouth, blurred vision, and dependence (*see* MORPHINE).
Precautions: Cyclimorph is not recommended for terminally ill patients. In people who have had a heart attack it may aggravate severe heart failure.
Interactions with other drugs: *see* ANTIHISTAMINES; OPIOIDS.

cyclizine An *antihistamine used for the treatment of nausea, vomiting, vertigo, motion sickness, and disorders of the inner ear affecting balance. When used alone, it is available as tablets without a prescription or as an injection, which is a *prescription only medicine.
Side effects: drowsiness is the most common side effect; dry mouth and blurred vision may occasionally occur (*see* ANTIHISTAMINES).
Precautions and interactions with other drugs: *see* ANTIHISTAMINES.
Proprietary preparations: Valoid; *Cyclimorph (combined with morphine); *Diconal (combined with dipipanone); *Migril (combined with ergotamine).

Cyclogest (Actavis) *See* PROGESTERONE.

cyclopenthiazide A *thiazide diuretic used for the treatment of *hypertension and *oedema associated with heart failure, liver disease, or kidney disease. It is available as tablets on *prescription only.
Side effects, precautions, and interactions with other drugs: *see* THIAZIDE DIURETICS.
Proprietary preparations: Navidrex; *Trasidrex (combined with oxprenolol).
See also ANTIHYPERTENSIVE DRUGS; DIURETICS.

cyclopentolate hydrochloride An *antimuscarinic drug that is applied to the eye before examination of the interior in order to dilate the pupil and paralyse the ciliary muscles (which control the focusing ability of the eye). It is particularly useful for examining the eyes of young children. Cyclopentolate is available as eye drops on *prescription only.

Side effects: cyclopentolate may cause transient stinging and an increase in pressure in the eye; with prolonged use, local irritation and conjunctivitis can occur. Systemic effects may occur in very young children and elderly people (*see* ANTIMUSCARINIC DRUGS).
Precautions and interactions with other drugs: *see* ANTIMUSCARINIC DRUGS.
Proprietary preparations: Mydrilate; Minims Cyclopentolate (single-dose eye drops).

cyclophosphamide An *alkylating drug used to treat a wide variety of *cancers. In the body it is converted to phosphoramide mustard (the active agent) and a substance called acrolein. Acrolein can cause irritation and bleeding in the bladder. Cyclophosphamide is therefore often given with *mesna, an agent that binds to acrolein and prevents this problem. Fluid intake must also be increased to reduce the time acrolein is present in the bladder. Cyclophosphamide may be given intravenously or as tablets and is available on *prescription only.
Side effects: include nausea and vomiting (which are more severe when the drug is given intravenously), hair loss, *bone marrow suppression, blood in the urine, lack of periods in women, and decreased fertility in men. Cyclophosphamide can also have adverse effects on the heart. *See also* CYTOTOXIC DRUGS.
Precautions: cyclophosphamide should not be taken by people who are already passing blood in their urine, by those who have a urinary-tract infection or porphyria, or by women who are pregnant or breastfeeding. *See also* CYTOTOXIC DRUGS.
Interactions with other drugs:
Clozapine: there is an increased risk of agranulocytosis (a serious blood disorder) and the two drugs should not be used together.
Pentostatin: adverse effects are increased and the two drugs should not be used together.

Cyclo-Progynova (Meda Pharmaceuticals) A proprietary preparation of *estradiol and combined estradiol/*levonorgestrel tablets used as sequential combined *hormone replacement therapy for the relief of menopausal symptoms in women who have not had a hysterectomy. It also provides protection against osteoporosis. A *prescription only medicine, the tablets must be taken in the prescribed order.
Side effects, precautions, and interactions with other drugs: *see* HORMONE REPLACEMENT THERAPY.

cycloserine (King) A drug that is used in combination with other drugs for the treatment of *tuberculosis that is resistant to the standard therapy. It is available as capsules on *prescription only.

Side effects: include headache, dizziness, vertigo, drowsiness, tremor, convulsions, confusion, depression, rashes, and megaloblastic *anaemia.
Precautions: cycloserine should not be taken by people with kidney disease, epilepsy, depression, severe anxiety, psychotic illness, or alcohol dependence (alcohol increases the risk of convulsions).
Interactions with other drugs:

Isoniazid: increases the risk of adverse effects on the nervous system.
Phenytoin: cycloserine may increase the plasma concentration of phenytoin and therefore the risk of side effects associated with it.

cyclosporin *See* CICLOSPORIN.

Cyklokapron (Meda Pharmaceuticals) *See* TRANEXAMIC ACID.

Cymalon (Actavis) A proprietary combination of *sodium citrate, *sodium bicarbonate, sodium carbonate, and *citric acid, used for the treatment of cystitis in adult females. It is freely available *over the counter as granules to make an oral solution.
Side effects: see SODIUM BICARBONATE.
Precautions: see SODIUM BICARBONATE; SODIUM CITRATE.

Cymalon Cranberry Liquid (Actavis) *See* POTASSIUM CITRATE.

Cymbalta (Eli Lilly & Co) *See* DULOXETINE.

Cymevene (Roche Products) *See* GANCICLOVIR.

cyproheptadine hydrochloride One of the original (sedating) *antihistamines, used to relieve the symptoms of such allergic conditions as hay fever and urticaria (nettle rash). Cyproheptadine also antagonizes the action of *serotonin and is used for the prevention of *migraine attacks in people who have not responded to other prophylactic treatments. It is available as tablets from pharmacies without a prescription.
Side effects: see ANTIHISTAMINES. Additional side effects may include weight gain, an increase in appetite, and fatigue.
Precautions and interactions with other drugs: see ANTIHISTAMINES.
Proprietary preparation: Periactin.

Cyprostat (Bayer) *See* CYPROTERONE ACETATE.

cyproterone acetate An *anti-androgen used to treat hypersexuality and sexual deviation in men; it is also used in the treatment of cancer of the prostate. Cyproterone produces a temporary infertility. Combined with ethinylestradiol, it is used to treat severe acne in women. It is available, on *prescription only, as tablets.
Side effects: include fatigue and lassitude (which may impair driving and other skilled tasks), breathlessness, weight changes, reduced sebum production, changes in hair pattern, and breast enlargement. High-dose treatment (for prostate cancer) may cause liver damage (jaundice, hepatitis).
Precautions: cyproterone should not be taken by people with liver disease, severe diabetes, sickle-cell anaemia, wasting disease, severe depression, or a

history of thromboembolism or by boys under 18 years old (except when used for treating prostate cancer).
Proprietary preparations: Androcur; Cyprostat; *Acnocin (combined with ethinylestradiol); *Dianette (combined with ethinylestradiol).

Cystadane (Orphan Europe) *See* BETAINE.

Cystrin (sanofi-aventis) *See* OXYBUTYNIN HYDROCHLORIDE.

Cytacon (Goldshield) *See* CYANOCOBALAMIN.

Cytamen (UCB Pharma) *See* CYANOCOBALAMIN.

cytarabine An *antimetabolite that is used predominantly for the treatment of acute myeloblastic leukaemia but is also used to treat leukaemias and lymphoma (*see* CANCER). It is available, on *prescription only, as a solution for subcutaneous or intravenous injection or as a lipid formulation for injection into the meninges of the spinal cord.
Side effects and precautions: *see* CYTOTOXIC DRUGS.
Interactions with other drugs:
Clozapine: there is an increased risk of agranulocytosis (a serious blood disorder), and therefore this drug should not be taken with cytarabine.
Proprietary preparation: DepoCyte (lipid formulation).

cytoprotectant Describing the action of certain drugs in protecting the lining of the stomach. Such drugs act by various mechanisms to form a barrier between the stomach wall and the acid contents of the stomach, which relieves the symptoms or prevents the formation of gastric ulcers. They may increase the secretion of protective mucus in the stomach, or they may coat the ulcer and thus prevent contact with stomach acid. Drugs with cytoprotectant actions include *sucralfate, *misoprostol, and salts of bismuth (including *tripotassium dicitratobismuthate).

Cytotec (Pharmacia) *See* MISOPROSTOL.

cytotoxic antibiotics A group of antibiotics that are used for the treatment of *cancer because they interfere with DNA replication and protein synthesis (*see* CYTOTOXIC DRUGS). They mimic the action of radiation and should not be used together with radiotherapy. The common cytotoxic antibiotics are *bleomycin, *dactinomycin, *daunorubicin, *doxorubicin, *epirubicin, *idarubicin, *mitomycin, and *mitoxantrone. With the exception of bleomycin and mitoxantrone, these antibiotics are derived or synthesized from *Streptomyces* bacteria and are known as **anthracyclines**.

cytotoxic drugs A group of drugs that are toxic to cells and cause cell death or prevent cell replication. These drugs are used mainly to treat *cancer, although some have other uses. Cancer treatment with cytotoxic drugs is known as **chemotherapy** and has a variety of purposes. The drugs may be used to shrink a tumour before surgery (neoadjuvant chemotherapy); they may be used after the primary tumour has been treated with surgery or radiotherapy to prevent the spread and growth of secondary tumours (adjuvant chemotherapy), or they may be the main treatment for the disease. Chemotherapy may be given to cure the disease or, if cure is not possible, to control its symptoms (palliative chemotherapy). Not every type of cancer responds to cytotoxic drugs, and some cancers are unresponsive to them (e.g. pancreatic cancer). Because cytotoxic drugs also attack healthy cells they can cause a variety of adverse effects, and a balance has to be struck between the likely benefit and the severity of the adverse effects (see below).

The main classes of cytotoxic drugs are: *alkylating drugs, *antimetabolites, *vinca alkaloids, *cytotoxic antibiotics, and a miscellaneous group, which includes platinum compounds (e.g. *carboplatin), *taxanes, *topoisomerase inhibitors, *tyrosine kinase inhibitors, *procarbazine, *crisantaspase, and *hydroxycarbamide. Several *monoclonal antibodies have also been developed for treating cancer. Sex hormones are also used to treat cancer. Tumours of the prostate gland are often stimulated by male sex hormones (the androgens) and so these cancers may be treated with *oestrogens (to oppose the androgens) or with *anti-androgens. Analogues of gonadorelin, such as *buserelin, *goserelin, *leuprorelin, and *triptorelin, are also used. Some breast cancers are stimulated by oestrogens; such cancers respond to the *oestrogen antagonists *tamoxifen and *toremifene or to *aromatase inhibitors. Cytotoxic drugs are usually only prescribed by cancer specialists (oncologists) and administered in a hospital. They may be taken by mouth or given by injection or infusion, by specially trained nurses or doctors. Quite often a combination of two, three, or more drugs will be given. The effects of cytotoxic drugs are carefully monitored and blood tests are carried out regularly.
Side effects: the cells most susceptible to the actions of cytotoxic drugs are those that are rapidly dividing: the cells lining the gut, the cells of the mucous membranes, and the cells of the bone marrow and the hair follicles. The resultant side effects are: nausea and vomiting; inflammation and soreness of the mucous membranes (mucositis), especially the mouth; *bone marrow suppression, which will make the patient extremely susceptible to infection (due to loss of white cells) and bleeding (due to loss of platelets); and hair loss. With some drugs, nausea and vomiting can be particularly severe and can last for several days, which may cause patients to refuse further treatment. Some people experience these symptoms when going for their treatment, even before the drugs are administered. It is important, therefore, that people who are likely to be sick are given *antiemetics and have antiemetics to take after they have left hospital. Some drugs, especially the vinca alkaloids, can cause pain and local tissue damage if they leak out (extravasation) during intravenous infusion.
Precautions: most cytotoxic drugs can cause malformations in a fetus and should not be given during pregnancy, although severe circumstances may make this unavoidable. Contraception should be used during treatment by both men and women. Treatment with some drugs may result in irreversible infertility; counselling is necessary, and the possibility of storing sperm or eggs to allow the patient to try to have children at a later date may be discussed. Most cytotoxic drugs should not be used by breastfeeding women.

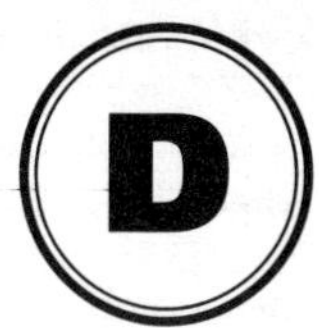

dabigatran etexilate An *anticoagulant used for the prevention of thromboembolism (*see* THROMBOSIS) following hip and knee surgery. It works by inhibiting thrombin, a substance that is involved in the formation of blood clots. Dabigatran is available as capsules on *prescription only.
Side effects: include bleeding (including major bleeding) and anaemia.
Precautions: dabigatran etexilate should not be taken by people with severely impaired liver or kidney function, by people who are actively bleeding (e.g. from a peptic ulcer) or are at risk of bleeding (see also Interactions below), or by women who are pregnant or breastfeeding.
Interactions with other drugs:
Anti-arrhythmic drugs: the plasma concentration of dabigatran is increased by amiodarone and its dose should therefore be reduced.
Anticoagulants: should not be taken at the same time as dabigatran etexilate because of a risk of bleeding.
NSAIDs: increase the risk of bleeding; diclofenac and ketorolac should not be taken with dabigatran.
Proprietary preparation: Pradaxa.

dacarbazine A *cytotoxic drug used for the treatment of melanoma (a type of skin cancer) and cancers of soft tissue (e.g. muscle). In combination with doxorubicin, bleomycin, and vinblastine, it is also used to treat Hodgkin's disease (*see* CANCER). Dacarbazine is available as a form for intravenous injection on *prescription only.
Side effects: the main side effects are severe nausea and vomiting and *bone marrow suppression. Dacarbazine is irritant to skin and other tissues. *See also* CYTOTOXIC DRUGS.
Precautions: dacarbazine should not be given to people with severely impaired liver or kidney function; the dosage may need to be reduced in people with lesser degrees of impairment. *See also* CYTOTOXIC DRUGS.

dactinomycin (**actinomycin D**) A *cytotoxic antibiotic used for the treatment of cancers in children. It is available as a form for intravenous injection on *prescription only.
Side effects: similar to those of *doxorubicin, except that dactinomycin does not have adverse effects on the heart.
Precautions: *see* CYTOTOXIC DRUGS.
Proprietary preparation: Cosmegen Lyovac.

Daktacort (Janssen-Cilag) A proprietary combination of *miconazole (an antifungal drug) and *hydrocortisone (a mild topical steroid), used for the

treatment of fungal and bacterial infections accompanied by inflammation. It is available as a cream or ointment on *prescription only.
Side effects, precautions, and interactions with other drugs: *see* MICONAZOLE; TOPICAL STEROIDS.

Daktarin (Janssen-Cilag) *See* MICONAZOLE.

d

Daktarin Gold (Janssen-Cilag) *See* KETOCONAZOLE.

Dalacin, Dalacin C, Dalacin T (Pharmacia) *See* CLINDAMYCIN.

dalfopristin *See* SYNERCID.

Dalivit (LPC) A proprietary combination of *vitamin A, vitamins of the B group (*see* VITAMIN B COMPLEX), *vitamin C, and *vitamin D, used as a multivitamin supplement. It is freely available *over the counter in the form of drops.

Dalmane (Valeant) *See* FLURAZEPAM.

dalteparin sodium A *low molecular weight heparin used for the prevention and treatment of deep-vein *thrombosis and in the treatment of unstable *angina. It is also used in patients undergoing kidney dialysis, in order to prevent the formation of blood clots. Dalteparin is available as a solution for subcutaneous or intravenous injection on *prescription only.
Side effects, precautions, and interactions with other drugs: *see* HEPARIN.
Proprietary preparation: Fragmin.

danaparoid sodium A *heparinoid used for the prevention of deep-vein *thrombosis in patients undergoing surgery. It may also be used in place of *heparin in those patients who develop low platelet counts as a side effect of heparin therapy. Danaparoid is available as a solution for subcutaneous or intravenous injection on *prescription only.
Side effects, precautions, and interactions with other drugs: *see* HEPARIN.
Proprietary preparation: Orgaran.

danazol A drug that inhibits the release of *gonadotrophins from the pituitary gland and therefore reduces the secretion of oestrogen and progesterone by the ovaries. It is used for the treatment of *endometriosis and severe breast pain associated with breast cysts when other treatments have failed, but is now little used because of the severity of its side effects. It has also been used for the treatment of hereditary angioedema (*see* ANAPHYLAXIS), although it does not have a *licence for this use. Danazol is available as capsules on *prescription only.
Side effects: include nausea, dizziness, rashes or other skin reactions, fluid retention and weight gain, acne, unusual hair growth or hair loss, voice changes, mood changes, reduction in breast size, backache, flushing, muscle spasm, menstrual disturbances, headache, and emotional upset.
Precautions: danazol should not be taken by women who are pregnant (it must be stopped if pregnancy occurs) or breastfeeding or by women who have severe liver, kidney, or heart disease.

Interactions with other drugs:
Anticoagulants: the effects of warfarin and acenocoumarol are enhanced.
Carbamazepine: its side effects are increased.
Ciclosporin: its side effects are increased.
Simvastatin: the risk of muscle damage may be increased.
Proprietary preparation: Danol.

Danlax (Sovereign Medical) *See* CO-DANTHRAMER.

Danol (sanofi-aventis) *See* DANAZOL.

danthron *See* DANTRON.

Dantrium (Spepharm UK) *See* DANTROLENE SODIUM.

dantrolene sodium A *muscle relaxant used in the form of capsules for the treatment of chronic severe spasms of voluntary muscles. It is given by intravenous injection for the treatment of malignant hyperthermia, a dangerous rise in body temperature that may occur as a complication of anaesthesia. Danolene is a *prescription only medicine.
Side effects: include transient drowsiness, dizziness, weakness, malaise, fatigue, diarrhoea (treatment should be stopped if this is severe), loss of appetite, nausea, headache, and rash.
Precautions: drowsiness may impair the performance of skilled tasks, and this is exacerbated by alcohol. Dantrolene should not be taken by people with liver disease or acute muscle spasms or by woman who are pregnant or breastfeeding and should be used with caution in those with heart or lung disease. It may cause severe liver damage; liver function tests should be carried out before and during treatment, which should be stopped if symptoms of liver disease (e.g. nausea, itching, dark-coloured urine) develop.
Proprietary preparations: Dantrium (capsules); Dantrium Intravenous (injection).

dantron <**danthron**> A *stimulant laxative that is used for the prevention and treatment of constipation in terminally ill patients caused by analgesics, especially *opioids. Dantron is no longer widely used since animal studies have indicated that it has a potential for causing cancer. A *prescription only medicine, it is available (combined with other laxatives) in the form of capsules or a suspension (*see* CO-DANTHRAMER; CO-DANTHRUSATE).
Side effects: dantron may cause abdominal cramps and colour the urine red; prolonged contact with the skin (for example in incontinent patients) may cause irritation.
Precautions: *see* CO-DANTHRAMER; CO-DANTHRUSATE; STIMULANT LAXATIVES.
Proprietary preparations: Codalax (*see* CO-DANTHRAMER); Danlax (*see* CO-DANTHRAMER); Normax (*see* CO-DANTHRUSATE).

dapsone An *antibiotic used for the treatment of leprosy and dermatitis herpetiformis (an itchy blistering rash). It is also used in treating pneumonia caused by *Pneumocystis jirovecii,* for which it is given in combination with

*trimethoprim, although it does not have a *licence for this. A *prescription only medicine, dapsone is available as tablets.
Side effects: include blood disorders, rashes, gastrointestinal upset, headache, and psychiatric disturbances.
Precautions: dapsone should be used only under specialist supervision and should not be taken by people with severe anaemia or porphyria. It should be used with caution in women who are breastfeeding, and folate supplements should be taken during pregnancy. Symptoms of blood disorders (e.g. fever, rash, bruising, bleeding) should be reported to a doctor.
Interactions with other drugs:
Probenecid: increases the risk of side effects of dapsone.
Rifampicin: reduces plasma concentrations of dapsone.

daptomycin An antibiotic that is used for the treatment of complicated skin and soft-tissue infections and endocarditis (inflammation of the lining of the heart cavity) caused by the bacterium *Staphylococcus aureus*, including meticillin-resistant *Staphylococcus aureus* (MRSA). It is available as an intravenous infusion on *prescription only.
Side effects: include headache, nausea, vomiting, diarrhoea, fungal infections, rash, and reactions at the infusion site. Rarely, muscular pain, weakness, and inflammation may occur.
Precautions: daptomycin should be used with caution in people with impaired kidney of liver function. Breastfeeding should be discontinued during treatment.
Proprietary preparation: Cubicin.

Daraprim (GlaxoSmithKline) *See* PYRIMETHAMINE.

darbepoetin *See* ERYTHROPOIETIN.

darifenacin An *antimuscarinic drug that reduces the frequency of bladder contractions and is used to treat incontinence and increased frequency and urgency in passing urine. It is available as tablets on *prescription only.
Side effects: include dry mouth, constipation, altered taste, blurred vision, dry eyes, drowsiness, difficulty in passing urine, headache, restlessness, disorientation, dry skin, and rash.
Precautions: darifenacin should not be taken by children under 18 years of age, pregnant women, or people with obstruction of the gut, severe ulcerative colitis, glaucoma, or obstruction of the outlet of the bladder. It should be used with caution in frail elderly people, breastfeeding women, and people with liver or kidney disease, some types of heart disease, or an overactive thyroid gland.
Proprietary preparation: Emselex.

darunavir A protease inhibitor used, in combination with other antiretroviral medicines (*see* ANTIVIRAL DRUGS), for the treatment of *HIV infection. It is taken as tablets under expert supervision and is available on *prescription only.

Side effects: include rash, nausea, vomiting, abdominal pain, diarrhoea, raised blood lipids, headache, insomnia, fatigue, and altered heart rate.
Precautions: darunavir should not be taken by women who are breastfeeding, by people with porphyria, or by children under 6 years of age. Darunavir should be used with caution in pregnant women and in people with liver disease, diabetes, or haemophilia.

Interactions with other drugs: darunavir is extensively metabolized by several enzyme systems in the liver. Therefore any drug affecting these systems will alter darunavir plasma concentrations and should be used with caution. A doctor should be consulted before taking darunavir with any other drug.
Kaletra: darunavir should not be taken with Kaletra as this will significantly reduce its therapeutic effect.
Rifampicin: should not be taken with darunavir.
Rosuvastin: should not be taken with darunavir as this increases the risk of muscle damage.
St John's wort: reduces the plasma concentration of darunavir and should not be taken with it.
Proprietary preparation: Prezista.

dasatinib A *tyrosine kinase inhibitor used for the treatment of myeloid leukaemia and lymphoblastic leukaemia (*see* CANCER) that has not responded to other therapy (including *imatinib). It is available as tablets on *prescription only.
Side effects: *see* CYTOTOXIC DRUGS. Additional side effects may include skin rashes, headache, loss of appetite, tinnitus, visual disturbance, palpitations, heart problems, bleeding, breathlessness, and cough.
Precautions: dasatinib should not be taken by breastfeeding women and should be used with caution by people susceptible to arrhythmias and by those with liver disease.
Interactions with other drugs:
Clozapine: increases the risk of agranulocytosis (a blood disorder) and should not be taken with dasatinib.
Rifampicin: reduces the plasma concentration of dasatinib and should not be taken with it.
Proprietary preparation: Sprycel.

daunorubicin A *cytotoxic antibiotic that is similar to *doxorubicin. It is used for the treatment of acute leukaemias (*see* CANCER) and advanced AIDS-related Kaposi's sarcoma (a tumour of blood vessels in the skin). A *prescription only medicine, it is available as a solution for intravenous infusion; a lipid formulation, which enhances its uptake by the tumour cells, is used for the treatment of Kaposi's sarcoma.
Side effects and precautions: *see* DOXORUBICIN; CYTOTOXIC DRUGS.
Proprietary preparation: DaunoXome (lipid formulation).

DaunoXome (Diatos) *See* DAUNORUBICIN.

Day and Night Nurse (GlaxoSmithKline) A proprietary combination of

*paracetamol (an analgesic and antipyretic), *pholcodine and *dextromethorphan (cough suppressants), *pseudoephedrine (a decongestant), and *promethazine hydrochloride (a sedating antihistamine), taken at day or night to relieve the symptoms of colds and influenza. It is available as capsules and can be obtained without a prescription, but only from pharmacies.
Side effects: *see* ANTIHISTAMINES; CODEINE; DEXTROMETHORPHAN; EPHEDRINE HYDROCHLORIDE.
Precautions: this medicine is not recommended for children under six years old. *See also* ANTIHISTAMINES; CODEINE; EPHEDRINE HYDROCHLORIDE; PARACETAMOL.
Interactions with other drugs: *see* ANTIHISTAMINES; EPHEDRINE HYDROCHLORIDE; OPIOIDS.

Day Nurse (GlaxoSmithKline) A proprietary combination of *paracetamol (an analgesic and antipyretic), *pseudoephedrine (a decongestant), and *pholcodine (a cough suppressant), used to relieve the symptoms of colds and influenza, including nasal congestion, cough, and running nose. It is available as capsules or a liquid (the liquid is twice the strength of the capsules) and can be obtained without a prescription, but only from pharmacies.
Side effects: *see* CODEINE; EPHEDRINE HYDROCHLORIDE.
Precautions: Day Nurse is not recommended for children under six years old. *See also* PARACETAMOL; EPHEDRINE HYDROCHLORIDE; CODEINE.
Interactions with other drugs: *see* EPHEDRINE HYDROCHLORIDE; OPIOIDS.

DDAVP, DDAVP Melt (Ferring Pharmaceuticals) *See* DESMOPRESSIN.

Deca-Durabolin (Organon Laboratories) *See* NANDROLONE DECANOATE.

De-capeptyl SR (Ipsen) *See* TRIPTORELIN.

decongestants Drugs that are administered to relieve or reduce congestion of the airways and the nose. Nasal decongestants are used for the treatment of colds. They may be applied locally, in the form of nose drops or sprays, or given orally; they are a common ingredient in proprietary cold remedies. Decongestants may also be used to relieve congestion due to hay fever and similar allergic reactions, but *antihistamines are usually preferred for treating these conditions. Most decongestants are *sympathomimetic drugs that act by constricting the blood vessels in the membranes lining the nose and airways. This reduces the swelling associated with congestion and therefore improves drainage. However, when given by mouth these drugs also act on other blood vessels and the heart, increasing heart rate and blood pressure. In addition, most sympathomimetic drugs interact with *monoamine oxidase inhibitors (a class of antidepressants) to cause a dangerous rise in blood pressure. For these reasons medicines containing sympathomimetic drugs should be used with caution by people with heart disease, high blood pressure, an overactive thyroid gland, or diabetes mellitus. Nasal drops and sprays are less likely to cause these adverse effects because little of the drug is absorbed into the body. However, if drops or sprays are used for more than a few days nasal congestion can increase (rebound congestion) as the effect of the drug wears off. *See also* EPHEDRINE HYDROCHLORIDE; PHENYLEPHRINE; PSEUDOEPHEDRINE; XYLOMETAZOLINE.

Deep Freeze Cold Gel (The Mentholatum Co) *See* MENTHOL.

Deep Heat Massage Liniment (The Mentholatum Co) A proprietary combination of *menthol and *methyl salicylate, used as a rubefacient for the relief of muscular and rheumatic pains and stiffness, including backache, sciatica, lumbago, and fibrositis. **Deep Heat Maximum Strength** is a stronger cream formulation. Both preparations are freely available *over the counter.
Side effects and precautions: *see* RUBEFACIENTS; SALICYLATES.

Deep Heat Maximum Strength (The Mentholatum Co) *See* DEEP HEAT MASSAGE LINIMENT.

Deep Heat Rub (The Mentholatum Co) A proprietary combination of *menthol, *turpentine oil, *eucalyptus oil, and *methyl salicylate in the form of a cream, used as a rubefacient for the relief of muscular and rheumatic aches, pains, and stiffness (including backache, sciatica, lumbago, and fibrositis), bruises, sprains, and chilblains. It is freely available *over the counter.
Side effects and precautions: *see* RUBEFACIENTS.

Deep Heat Spray (The Mentholatum Co) A proprietary combination of *methyl salicylate, *methyl nicotinate, *ethyl salicylate, and *glycol salicylate, used as a rubefacient for the relief of muscular and rheumatic aches and pains, including fibrositis, lumbago, and sciatica. It is freely available *over the counter.
Side effects and precautions: *see* RUBEFACIENTS; SALICYLATES.

Deep Relief (The Mentholatum Co) A proprietary combination of *ibuprofen (an NSAID) and *menthol, applied to the skin for the relief of rheumatic pain, muscular pain, strains, and sprains. It is available as a gel and can be obtained from pharmacies without a prescription.
Side effects and precautions: *see* NSAIDs.

DEET *See* DIETHYLTOLUAMIDE.

deferasirox A drug that binds to iron and is used to reduce levels of iron in the body in people over the age of six who are receiving repeated blood transfusions for the genetic blood disorder thalassaemia major. People who receive frequent blood transfusions are at risk of excessive iron deposition in their organs. It is also used to treat people who are receiving multiple blood transfusions for other reasons and *desferrioxamine cannot be given or is not adequate. Deferasirox is available as dispersible tablets on *prescription only.
Side effects: include headache, diarrhoea, constipation, vomiting, nausea, abdominal pain, abdominal distension, indigestion, rash, and itching.
Precautions: deferasirox is not recommended for people with moderate to severe kidney disease or for women who are pregnant or breastfeeding. Eye

and ear examinations should be carried out before and at yearly intervals during treatment. Liver function tests should be carried out before and at frequent intervals during treatment.
Interactions with other drugs:
Repaglinide: its plasma concentration is increased by defasirox.
Rifampicin: its plasma concentration is reduced by defasirox.
Proprietary preparation: Exjade.

d

deferiprone A drug that binds to iron and is used to reduce the amount of iron in the body of people with the genetic blood disorder thalassaemia major who are receiving repeated blood transfusions and for whom *desferrioxamine therapy is not appropriate or inadequate. It is available as tablets or an oral solution on *prescription only.
Side effects: include nausea, abdominal pain, vomiting, diarrhoea, headache, increased appetite, fatigue, and a red-brown discoloration of the urine.
Precautions: deferiprone should not be taken by women who are pregnant or breastfeeding, and women capable of bearing children should use contraception during treatment because there is a risk of damaging the fetus. The drug may cause agranulocytosis, a blood disorder marked by a deficiency of neutrophils (a type of white blood cell); neutrophil counts should be done weekly and treatment stopped if signs of agranulocytosis develop. Deferiprone should be used with caution in people with liver or kidney disease.
Proprietary preparation: Ferriprox.

deferoxamine mesilate *See* DESFERRIOXAMINE MESILATE.

deflazacort A *corticosteroid used for the treatment of inflammatory and allergic conditions. It is available as tablets on *prescription only.
Side effects, precautions, and interactions with other drugs: *see* CORTICOSTEROIDS.
Proprietary preparation: Calcort.

degarelix A drug that blocks the action of *gonadotrophin-releasing hormone and is used to treat advanced testosterone-dependent prostate cancer. It acts by reducing the production of testosterone within the body and therefore reduces the growth of the cancer, which is driven by testosterone. Degarelix is available as a form for subcutaneous injection on *prescription only.
Side effects: include insomnia, dizziness, headache, nausea, sweating, weight gain, fatigue, and influenza-like symptoms.
Precautions: degarelix can cause *arrhythmias in susceptible people; other drugs that may cause arrhythmias should be avoided during treatment. Degarelix should be used with caution in people with liver or kidney disease.
Proprietary preparation: Firmagon.

Delph (Fenton) A proprietary combination of avobenzone, octinoxate, oxybenzone, and *titanium dioxide, used as a *sunscreen preparation for protection against UVA and UVB radiation. It is available as a lotion without a prescription.

Deltacortril (Alliance) *See* PREDNISOLONE.

Deltastab (Sovereign Medical) *See* PREDNISOLONE.

demeclocycline hydrochloride A tetracycline antibiotic used for the treatment of chronic bronchitis, brucellosis, chlamydial infections, infections caused by mycoplasmas and rickettsias, severe gum disease, and acne (*see* TETRACYCLINES). It is also used to treat low plasma concentrations of sodium in people with high plasma levels of *vasopressin as it blocks the effect of vasopressin in the kidneys. Demeclocycline is available as capsules on *prescription only.
Side effects, precautions, and interactions with other drugs: *see* TETRACYCLINES.
Proprietary preparation: Ledermycin.

demulcents Soothing preparations that protect mucous membranes and relieve irritation. Demulcents are included in proprietary medicines for relieving dry irritating coughs and in mouthwashes and gargles, as they protect and soothe the membranes lining the throat and mouth. They include *glycerin, syrup, and **simple linctus** (citric acid monohydrate).

De-Noltab (Astellas Pharma) *See* TRIPOTASSIUM DICITRATOBISMUTHATE.

Dentinox Cradle Cap Shampoo (DDD) A proprietary combination of sodium lauryl ether sulphosuccinate and sodium lauryl ether sulphate (detergents and foaming agents), used for the treatment of infant cradle cap and general care of the infant scalp and hair. It is available without a prescription, but only from pharmacies.
Precautions: the shampoo may cause irritation of the scalp.

Dentinox Infant Colic Drops (DDD) *See* DIMETICONE.

Dentinox Teething Gel (DDD) A proprietary combination of *cetylpyridinium chloride (an antiseptic) and *lidocaine hydrochloride (a local anaesthetic), used to relieve teething pain and soothe the gums. It is suitable for use from birth onwards and is freely available *over the counter.

Dentomycin (Blackwell) *See* MINOCYCLINE.

Denzapine (Merz Pharma) *See* CLOZAPINE.

Depakote (Sanofi-aventis) *See* VALPROIC ACID.

dependence The physical and/or psychological effects produced by the habitual taking of certain drugs, characterized by a compulsive need for the drug. In **physical dependence** withdrawal of the drug causes specific symptoms (**withdrawal symptoms**), such as sweating, vomiting, or tremors, that are reversed by further doses. Drugs that induce physical dependence include alcohol, morphine, diamorphine (heroin), and cocaine. **Psychological**

dependence is the condition in which repeated use of a drug induces reliance on it for a state of well-being and contentment, but there are no physical withdrawal symptoms if use of the drug is stopped. Psychological dependence is produced by such drugs as nicotine (in tobacco), cannabis, and amphetamines. The term **addiction** is used synonymously with dependence, although some would argue that addiction should refer to the state in which both physical and psychological dependence are present.

Depixol (Lundbeck) *See* FLUPENTIXOL.

DepoCyte (Napp Pharmaceuticals) *See* CYTARABINE.

Depodur (Flynn Pharma) *See* MORPHINE.

Depo-Medrone (Pharmacia) *See* METHYLPREDNISOLONE.

Depo-Medrone with Lidocaine (Pharmacia) A proprietary combination of *methylprednisolone (a corticosteroid) and *lidocaine hydrochloride (a local anaesthetic), which is injected into a joint to relieve pain and increase mobility in the treatment of rheumatoid arthritis and other inflammatory diseases of joints. It is available on *prescription only.
Side effects, precautions, and interactions with other drugs: *see* CORTICOSTEROIDS.

Deponit (UCB Pharma) *See* GLYCERYL TRINITRATE.

Depo-Provera (Pfizer) *See* MEDROXYPROGESTERONE.

depot contraceptives Preparations of synthetic *progestogens that are designed to release the hormone over a prolonged period (which may range from weeks to years) to provide long-term reversible contraception. Formulations given by intramuscular injection are Depo-Provera (*see* MEDROXYPROGESTERONE), which provides contraceptive cover for up to three months, and Noristerat (*see* NORETHISTERONE), which lasts up to eight weeks. *Levonorgestrel is available as an intrauterine system (Mirena) and *etonogestrel as an implant (Implanon), both of which last for up to three years. Etonogestrel, combined with an oestrogen, is also available in the form of a vaginal ring (*NuvaRing), which remains in place for three weeks.

depot injection A formulation of a drug that is injected into a muscle, where it resides and releases the active ingredient(s) slowly over a period of days, weeks, or years. Depot injection is most often used to deliver hormones for long-term contraception (*see* DEPOT CONTRACEPTIVES).

depression *See* ANTIDEPRESSANT DRUGS.

Dequacaine (Crookes Healthcare) A proprietary combination of *dequalinium chloride (an antiseptic) and *benzocaine (a local anaesthetic), used for the relief of sore throats. It is available as lozenges and can be obtained without a prescription, but only from pharmacies.

Dequadin (Crookes Healthcare) *See* DEQUALINIUM CHLORIDE.

dequalinium chloride A mild *antiseptic with weak antifungal properties, used for the treatment of bacterial or fungal infections of the mouth and throat. It is available as lozenges and can be obtained without a prescription, but only from pharmacies.
Precautions: dequalinium chloride is not usually given to children under 10 years old.
Proprietary preparations: Dequadin; *Dequacaine (combined with benzocaine).

Derbac-M (SSL International) *See* MALATHION.

Dermacort (Sankyo Pharma) *See* HYDROCORTISONE.

Dermalo (Dermal Laboratories) A proprietary combination of wood alcohols and *liquid paraffin in the form of a bath oil, used an an *emollient for the relief of contact dermatitis (an allergic skin condition), dry skin, and itching. It is freely available *over the counter.

Dermamist (Alliance) A proprietary combination of *white soft paraffin and *liquid paraffin (both emollients), used to relieve *eczema and dry skin conditions, including those associated with itching. It is available as a spray and can be obtained without a prescription, but only from pharmacies.
Precautions: Dermamist should not be used on broken skin.

dermatitis *See* ECZEMA.

Dermax Therapeutic Shampoo (Dermal Laboratories) A proprietary combination of *benzalkonium chloride (a detergent antiseptic) and sodium lauryl ether sulphate (a detergent and a foaming agent), used for the treatment of pityriasis and other scalp conditions where scaling and dandruff are present. It is available without a prescription, but only from pharmacies.

Dermidex (Actavis) A proprietary combination of *lidocaine (a local anaesthetic), *chlorobutanol and *cetrimide (antiseptics), and aluminium chlorhydroxyallantoinate (an astringent; a derivative of *allantoin), used to relieve the pain of stings, grazes, and dermatitis. It is available as a cream that can be obtained without a prescription, but only from pharmacies.
Precautions: Dermidex should not be used for longer than seven days and should not be applied to mucous membranes; it is not recommended for children under four years old.

Dermol (Dermal Laboratories) A proprietary combination of the antiseptics *benzalkonium chloride and *chlorhexidine hydrochloride and the emollients *liquid paraffin and *isopropyl myristate, used as a lotion for the relief of dry and itching skin conditions, such as eczema. **Dermol 200 Shower Emollient** may be applied to the skin or used in the shower. **Dermol 600 Bath Emollient** is added to a bath of warm water. Dermol preparations may be bought without a *prescription, but only from pharmacies.
Precautions: Dermol preparations should not be used in or around the eyes.

Dermovate, Dermovate Scalp (GlaxoSmithKline) *See* CLOBETASOL PROPIONATE.

Dermovate-NN (Chemidex Pharma) A proprietary combination of *clobetasol propionate (a very potent topical steriod), *neomycin sulphate (an antibiotic), and *nystatin (an antifungal agent), used for the treatment of psoriasis, eczema that is unresponsive to other treatments and other inflammatory conditions of the skin when infection is present. It is available as a cream or an ointment on *prescription only.
Side effects and precautions: *see* TOPICAL STEROIDS.

Deseril (Alliance) *See* METHYSERGIDE.

Desferal (Novartis) *See* DESFERRIOXAMINE MESILATE.

desferrioxamine mesilate (**deferoxamine mesilate**) A drug that binds to iron and is used to treat iron poisoning, which most commonly occurs in children as a result of accidental ingestion and causes nausea, vomiting, abdominal pain, diarrhoea, and rectal bleeding. Desferrioxamine can also be used to bind to excessive amounts of iron in the body that can occur in patients with certain types of anaemias as a result of repeated blood transfusions, and it may be used for treating haemochromatosis (iron-storage disease), in which there is excessive absorption and storage of iron. Desferrioxamine is available in a form for infusion on *prescription only.
Side effects: include generalized allergic reactions, low blood pressure (if given too rapidly), dizziness, convulsions, disturbances of hearing or vision, and pain at the injection site.
Precautions: desferrioxamine should be used with caution in people with kidney disease. Eye and ear examinations may be necessary before treatment and at three-monthly intervals during treatment.
Interactions with other drugs:
Prochlorperazine: should not be taken with desferrioxamine.
Proprietary preparation: Desferal.

desloratadine A nonsedating *antihistamine used to relieve the symptoms of hay fever and urticaria. It is available as tablets and an oral solution on *prescription only.
Side effects: include fatigue, dry mouth, and headache.
Precautions: desloratadine should not be taken by women who are pregnant or breastfeeding. *See also* ANTIHISTAMINES.
Interactions with other drugs: *see* ANTIHISTAMINES.
Proprietary preparation: NeoClarityn.

DesmoMelt (Ferring Pharmaceuticals) *See* DESMOPRESSIN.

desmopressin An analogue of *vasopressin that has a longer duration of action than vasopressin and does not cause constriction of blood vessels. It is used for the treatment of diabetes insipidus and for those who have problems with bedwetting, including people with multiple sclerosis. It is also used for the treatment of haemophilia and von Willebrand's disease (*see* VON

WILLEBRAND FACTOR). Desmopressin is available, on *prescription only, as tablets, tablets to be dissolved under the tongue (sublingual), an injection, or a nasal spray.
Side effects: include abdominal cramps, nausea, an urge to defecate, and headache; nasal congestion and irritation may occur with use of a nasal spray.
Precautions: *see* VASOPRESSIN.
Interactions with other drugs:
Carbamazepine: may increase the effect of desmopressin.
Indometacin: increases the effect of desmopressin.
Loperamide increases the effect of desmopressin taken by mouth.
Proprietary preparations: DDAVP; DDAVP Melt (sublingual tablets); Desmotabs (tablets); Desmospray (nasal spray) DesmoMelt (sublingual tablets); Nocutil (nasal spray); Octim (nasal spray).

Desmospray (Ferring Pharmaceuticals) *See* DESMOPRESSIN.

Desmotabs (Ferring Pharmaceuticals) *See* DESMOPRESSIN.

desogestrel A synthetic *progestogen used as an ingredient in combined *oral contraceptives. It is also used alone as a progestogen-only contraceptive pill. There is a higher risk of thromboembolism with this progestogen than with certain others. It is available on *prescription only.
Side effects and interactions with other drugs: *see* ORAL CONTRACEPTIVES.
Precautions: desogestrel should not be taken by women who are at risk of developing thromboembolism, for example because they are very overweight or have varicose veins or a history of thrombosis. It should therefore only be taken by women who cannot tolerate other brands and who are prepared to accept the increased risk. *See also* ORAL CONTRACEPTIVES.
Proprietary preparations: Cerazette; *Marvelon (combined with ethinylestradiol); *Mercilon (combined with ethinylestradiol).

Destolit (Norgine) *See* URSODEOXYCHOLIC ACID.

Detrunorm, Detrunorm XL (Amdipharm) *See* PROPIVERINE HYDROCHLORIDE.

Detrusitol, Detrusitol XL (Pharmacia) *See* TOLTERODINE TARTRATE.

Dettol Antiseptic Cream (Reckitt Benckiser) A proprietary combination of *triclosan and *chloroxylenol (both antiseptics) and edetic acid (an agent that enhances the activity of chloroxylenol), used for the treatment of cuts, bites, stings, and abrasions. It is freely available *over the counter.

Dettol Liquid (Reckitt Benckiser) *See* CHLOROXYLENOL.

dexamethasone A *corticosteroid with anti-inflammatory activity. It is used for the treatment of inflammatory conditions (including rheumatic disease) and nausea and vomiting associated with cancer chemotherapy and it is injected intravenously to treat shock and cerebral oedema (swelling of the brain). Dexamethasone is also used in the diagnosis of Cushing's disease. A *prescription only medicine, it is available as tablets or an oral solution, as a

solution for intravenous injection or local injection into joints or around tendons, as eye drops or ointment, and as ear drops.
Side effects: *see* CORTICOSTEROIDS. In addition, perineal or scrotal irritation and pain can occur if intravenous injections are given too rapidly.
Precautions and interactions with other drugs: *see* CORTICOSTEROIDS.
Proprietary preparations: Dexsol (oral solution); Maxidex (eye drops); Minims Dexamethasone (single-dose eye drops); *Maxitrol (combined with neomycin, polymyxin B sulphate, and hypromellose); *Otomize (combined with acetic acid and neomycin sulphate); *Sofradex (combined with framycetin sulphate and gramicidin); *Tobradex (combined with tobramycin).

dexamfetamine sulphate **<dexamphetamine sulphate>** A drug that acts directly on the brain as a *stimulant (*see* AMPHETAMINES). In adults it is used to treat narcolepsy (an extreme tendency to fall asleep). Paradoxically it has a sedative effect in children and can be used to treat attention deficit hyperactivity disorder. A *controlled drug, it is available as tablets and is potentially addictive.
Side effects: include insomnia, irritability, restlessness, night terrors, euphoria, tremor, dizziness, headache, loss of appetite and stomach upsets, and raised blood pressure and a fast heart rate. Growth restriction may occur in children.
Precautions: *tolerance to the effects of dexamfetamine develops with prolonged use, and *dependence can occur. Dexamfetamine should only be given to children under specialist supervision, owing to its effects on growth and lack of knowledge of its effects with long-term use. It should not be taken by people with heart disease, high blood pressure, thyroid disease, glaucoma, or liver or kidney disease; by those with states of hyperexcitability or with a history of drug or alcohol abuse; or by women who are pregnant or breastfeeding. It may affect driving ability.
Interactions with other drugs:
MAOIs: there is a risk of a dangerous rise in blood pressure.
Proprietary preparation: Dexedrine.

Dexedrine (UCB Pharma) *See* DEXAMFETAMINE SULPHATE.

dexibuprofen An *NSAID used to relieve the pain and inflammation of osteoarthritis and to relieve period pains, pain in muscles and joints, and toothache. It is available as tablets on *prescription only.
Side effects, precautions, and interactions with other drugs: *see* NSAIDs.
Proprietary preparation: Seractil.

Deximune (Dexcel) *See* CICLOSPORIN.

dexketoprofen An *NSAID used for the relief of mild to moderate pain, including dysmenorrhoea (period pains). It is available as tablets on *prescription only.
Side effects, precautions, and interactions with other drugs: *see* NSAIDs.
Proprietary preparation: Keral.

Dexomon SR, Dexomon Retard 100 (Hillcross Pharmaceuticals) *See* DICLOFENAC SODIUM.

dexrazoxane A drug used during anticancer treatment to prevent the adverse effects on the heart and the local tissue damage caused by leakage from veins that may result from infusion of the anthracyclines *doxorubicin or epirubicin. It is available as an intravenous infusion on *prescription only.
Side effects: include nausea and vomiting, *bone-marrow suppression, and inflammation of the mouth.
Precautions: dexrazoxane should not be given to women who are pregnant (unless clearly necessary) or breastfeeding. It should be used with caution in people with kidney or liver disease. The combination of dexrazoxane with chemotherapy may lead to an increased risk of thromboembolism (*see* THROMBOSIS).
Proprietary preparations: Cardioxane; Savene.

Dexsol (Rosemont Pharmaceuticals) *See* DEXAMETHASONE.

dextran A carbohydrate that strengthens the natural film of tears that covers the eyes and is used as an ingredient of eye drops to treat dry eyes. It is also used in intravenous infusions to increase blood volume in some conditions of shock.
Proprietary preparation: *Tears Naturale (combined with hypromellose).

dextranomer A substance used to absorb the liquid that exudes from ulcers and infected wounds. It is available as beads or a paste and can be obtained without a prescription, but only from pharmacies.

dextromethorphan An *opioid that acts as a *cough suppressant; it has no analgesic or sedative properties. Dextromethorphan is used for the relief of dry irritating persistent coughs, either alone or in combination with other drugs in linctuses, syrups, and lozenges. It can be bought from pharmacies without a prescription.
Side effects: side effects, such as dizziness, drowsiness, constipation, nausea, and vomiting, are rare and there is no evidence of dependence. Confusion and depression of breathing may occur after overdosage. *See also* OPIOIDS.
Precautions and interactions with other drugs: *see* OPIOIDS.
Proprietary preparations: Benylin Dry Coughs Non Drowsy (liquid); Contac CoughCaps (*modified-release capsules); Robitussin Dry Cough; Robitussin Junior Persistent Cough; Vicks Cough Lozenges with Honey; *Benylin Children's Coughs and Colds (combined with triprolidine); *Benylin Dry Coughs Original (combined with diphenhydramine and menthol); *Covonia Bronchial Balsam (combined with menthol); *Covonia Night Time Formula (combined with diphenhydramine); *Day and Night Nurse (combined with paracetamol, promethazine hydrochloride, pseudoephedrine, and pholcodine); *Junior Meltus Dry Coughs with Congestion (combined with pseudoephedrine); *Meltus Dry Cough (combined with pseudoephedrine); *Multi-Action Actifed Dry Coughs (combined with pseudoephedrine and tripolidine); *Night Nurse (combined with paracetamol and promethazine);

*Non-Drowsy Sudafed Linctus (combined with pseudoephedrine); *Vicks Cold & Flu Care Medinite Complete (combined with doxylamine, ephedrine, and paracetamol).

DF 118 Forte (Martindale Pharmaceuticals) *See* DIHYDROCODEINE TARTRATE.

d

D-GAM (Bio Products Laboratory) *See* ANTI-D (RH_0) IMMUNOGLOBULIN.

DHC Continus (Napp Pharmaceuticals) *See* DIHYDROCODEINE TARTRATE.

diabetes insipidus *See* VASOPRESSIN.

diabetes mellitus A disease in which glucose (sugar) is not adequately taken up from the bloodstream by the cells of the body and therefore cannot be metabolized to produce energy or stored in the liver. It is caused by an abnormality in the synthesis and secretion of the hormone *insulin. Diabetes mellitus is characterized by high concentrations of glucose in the blood (**hyperglycaemia**) and in the urine, with symptoms of thirst, loss of weight, tiredness, and an excessive production of urine.

People affected with **insulin-dependent** (or **type I**) **diabetes mellitus** have little or no ability to produce the hormone and depend on daily injections of insulin. This type of diabetes can also be referred to as **juvenile-onset diabetes** because it usually starts during childhood or adolescence. The dosage of insulin must be carefully controlled and matched to the dietary intake of glucose. If cells receive insufficient glucose, fats may be used as an alternative source of energy, which can lead to alteration of the acidity of the blood, the accumulation of ketones (formed when fats are metabolized) in the bloodstream (**ketoacidosis**), and eventually to diabetic coma. **Type II** (**noninsulin-dependent** or **maturity-onset**) **diabetes mellitus** develops in adults, usually over 40 years old, because of a decrease in the production of natural insulin, although the pancreas still functions to some extent; alternatively, the body becomes resistant to the effect of insulin. This condition occurs more often in people who are overweight; it is usually treated by diet, weight reduction, and *oral hypoglycaemic drugs, but some patients may need insulin instead.

All people with diabetes, regardless of which type, must pay attention to their diet, in which the amount of carbohydrate should be carefully controlled to suit their body's needs, and be aware of the importance of monitoring blood glucose concentrations. Very low blood glucose (*hypoglycaemia) may be caused by excessive dosage of insulin or some oral antidiabetic drugs or by missing a meal. Good control of blood sugar is necessary to prevent such long-term consequences of diabetes as atherosclerosis (giving rise to heart disease), poor circulation in the extremities (causing foot ulcers), impairment of eyesight, and kidney damage.

Diacomit *See* STIRIPENTOL.

Dialar (Lagap Pharmaceuticals) *See* DIAZEPAM.

Diamicron, Diamicron MR (Servier Laboratories) *See* GLICLAZIDE.

diamorphine hydrochloride (**heroin hydrochloride**) An *opioid analgesic that is used to treat acute pain, such as that associated with a heart attack, or long-term chronic pain, such as that caused by advanced cancer. It is also used in the treatment of pulmonary *oedema and heart attacks. Diamorphine is a *controlled drug; it is available as tablets or a form for injection and is usually administered in a hospital.
Side effects and precautions: *see* MORPHINE.
Interactions with other drugs: *see* OPIOIDS.

Diamox, Diamox SR (Goldshield) *See* ACETAZOLAMIDE.

Dianette (Bayer) A proprietary combination of *ethinylestradiol (a synthetic oestrogen) and *cyproterone acetate (an anti-androgen), used for the treatment of severe *acne in women that has not responded to prolonged antibiotic therapy. It is also used to treat hirsutism (abnormal growth of facial and body hair in women). Dianette acts as an *oral contraceptive in women taking it. It is available as tablets on *prescription only.
Side effects: include breast enlargement, fluid retention with a bloated feeling, weight gain, cramps and pains in the legs, headache, nausea, depression, vaginal discharge, skin changes (including brown patches on the face), and breakthrough bleeding. There may be changes in libido, depression, and irritation from contact lenses. The occurrence of a migraine-like headache for the first time, frequent severe headaches, or visual disturbance should be reported immediately to a doctor.
Precautions: Dianette should not be taken by women who are pregnant or have a history of thrombosis. For other precautions, *see* ORAL CONTRACEPTIVES.
Interactions with other drugs: *see* ORAL CONTRACEPTIVES.

diarrhoea *See* ANTIDIARRHOEAL DRUGS.

Diazemuls (Actavis) *See* DIAZEPAM.

diazepam A long-acting *benzodiazepine used for the short-term treatment of anxiety and insomnia. It is also used to relieve the symptoms of alcohol withdrawal and to treat status epilepticus (repeated epileptic seizures), convulsions associated with fever in children, and chronic muscle spasm. Diazepam is also used to relax patients before operations or uncomfortable diagnostic procedures. It is available, on *prescription only, as tablets, an oral solution, an injection, suppositories, or a rectal solution. Some proprietary preparations of diazepam cannot be prescribed on the NHS.
Side effects: include drowsiness, light-headedness, confusion, shaky movements, and unsteady gait (especially in elderly people), amnesia, dependence, and paradoxical overexcitedness (*see* BENZODIAZEPINES). Rare side effects include headache, vertigo, gastrointestinal upsets (such as nausea or constipation), blurred vision, changes in libido, difficulty in passing urine, rashes, and a fall in blood pressure.
Precautions: diazepam should not be taken by people who have respiratory depression, severe breathing problems, or severe liver disease, and it should not be used for treating depression, chronic psychosis, phobias, or

obsessional states. Diazepam should be used with caution in people who have lung disease or a history of alcohol or drug abuse and by women who are pregnant or breastfeeding. *See also* BENZODIAZEPINES.

Interactions with other drugs:

Antipsychotic drugs: increase the sedative effects of diazepam.

Rifampicin: reduces the effects of diazepam.

Ritonavir: increases the plasma concentration of diazepam, causing profound sedation; these drugs should therefore not be taken together.

Sodium oxybate: its effects are enhanced by diazepam and these drugs should therefore not be taken together.

See also BENZODIAZEPINES.

Proprietary preparations: Dialar (oral solution); Diazemuls (injection); Diazepam Rectubes (rectal solution); Rimapam (tablets); Stesolid (rectal solution); Tensium (tablets).

Diazepam Rectubes (Wockhardt UK) *See* DIAZEPAM.

diazoxide A drug that has two separate actions and uses. When given by intravenous injection it causes *vasodilatation of the small arteries and consequently rapid lowering of blood pressure; it is therefore sometimes used as an emergency treatment of *hypertension. Diazoxide also increases the concentration of glucose in the bloodstream and is taken orally to treat chronic *hypoglycaemia (low blood glucose) resulting from excessive secretion of insulin (for example, by an insulin-secreting tumour in the pancreas). It is not used to treat acute hypoglycaemia resulting from insulin overdosage in people with diabetes. Diazoxide is available as an injection or tablets on *prescription only.

Side effects: include loss of appetite, nausea, vomiting, low blood pressure, a fast heart rate, sweating, abnormal heart rhythms, and *extrapyramidal reactions.

Precautions: diazoxide should be used with caution in people with heart disease or severe kidney disease. Growth and development of children must be monitored.

Interactions with other drugs:

Anaesthetics: their effects in lowering blood pressure are increased.

Antihypertensive drugs: their effects in lowering blood pressure are enhanced.

Diuretics: their effects in lowering blood pressure are enhanced.

Proprietary preparation: Eudemine.

Dibenyline (Goldshield) *See* PHENOXYBENZAMINE HYDROCHLORIDE.

dibrompropamidine isethionate An antibiotic used for the treatment of minor skin infections (bacterial and fungal), burns, scalds, and abrasions, infections of the outer ear, and nappy rash. It is freely available *over the counter as a cream.

Proprietary preparation: Brulidine Cream.

dichlorobenzyl alcohol An *antiseptic used as an ingredient of lozenges for the treatment of minor infections of the mouth and throat.
Proprietary preparations: Boots Antiseptic Sore Mouth Pastilles; *Boots Dual Action Cold Sore Lotion (combined with benzyl alcohol, camphor, and levomenthol).

diclofenac sodium An *NSAID used for the treatment of pain and inflammation in rheumatoid arthritis (including arthritis in children) and other disorders of the muscles and joints; it is also used to treat acute gout and postoperative pain. Diclofenac is applied to the skin for the treatment of sprains and strains. It is also applied to the eye to inhibit constriction of the pupil during eye surgery and to reduce inflammation and pain after surgery. It is available, on *prescription only, as tablets, dispersible tablets, *modified-release capsules and tablets, an injection, suppositories, eye drops, and as a gel or solution for topical application.
Side effects: *see* NSAIDs. Suppositories may cause local irritation.
Precautions: *see* NSAIDs.
Interactions with other drugs: *see* NSAIDs. In addition:
Anticoagulants: should not be used with injections of diclofenac as the risk of bleeding is increased.
Ciclosporin: increases the plasma concentration of diclofenac, whose dosage will therefore need to be halved.
Proprietary preparations: Dexomon SR, Dexomon Retard 100 (modified-release tablets); Dicloflex; Dicloflex SR, Dicloflex Retard (modified-release tablets); Diclomax SR, Diclomax Retard (modified-release capsules); Dyloject (solution for injection); Econac; Fenactol; Flexotard MR 75, Flexotard MR 100 (modified-release tablets); Mobigel Spray; Motifene 75 mg (modified-release capsules); Pennsaid (topical solution); Rhumalgan CR (modified-release tablets); Slofenac SR (modified-release tablets); Solaraze (gel); Volsaid Retard (modified-release tablets); Voltarol; Voltarol Emulgel (gel); Voltarol Gel Patch; Voltarol Ophtha (single-use eye drops); Voltarol Ophtha Multidose (eye drops); Voltarol Rapid (diclofenac potassium tablets); Voltarol 75 mg SR, Voltarol Retard (modified-release tablets); *Arthrotec (combined with misoprostol).

Dicloflex, Dicloflex Retard, Dicloflex SR (Dexcel Pharma) *See* DICLOFENAC SODIUM.

Diclomax Retard, Diclomax SR (Galen) *See* DICLOFENAC SODIUM.

dicobalt edetate A drug used for the treatment of poisoning by cyanides. It is given by intravenous injection and is available on *prescription only.
Side effects: include low blood pressure, a fast heart rate, and vomiting.
Precautions: because it is toxic, dicobalt edetate should only be given to patients who are unconscious or about to become unconscious.

Diconal (Amdipharm) A proprietary combination of *cyclizine hydrochloride (an antiemetic antihistamine) and *dipipanone hydrochloride (a strong opioid analgesic), used for the relief of moderate to severe pain;

cyclizine is included to prevent the nausea and vomiting associated with opioids. Diconal is available as tablets; it is a *controlled drug.
Side effects: include drowsiness, dry mouth, blurred vision, and dependence (*see* MORPHINE).
Precautions: Diconal is not recommended for children or terminally ill patients. *See also* MORPHINE; OPIOIDS.
Interactions with other drugs: *see* ANTIHISTAMINES; OPIOIDS.

dicyclomine hydrochloride *See* DICYCLOVERINE HYDROCHLORIDE.

dicycloverine hydrochloride **<dicyclomine hydrochloride>** An *antimuscarinic drug used for the treatment of irritable bowel syndrome and other conditions marked by spasms of the gut (*see* ANTISPASMODICS). Dicycloverine is available as tablets or a syrup on *prescription; packs of tablets in which the maximum single dose is 10 mg and the maximum daily dose is 60 mg can be obtained from pharmacies without a prescription.
Side effects and precautions: *see* ANTIMUSCARINIC DRUGS.
Proprietary preparations: Merbentyl (10 mg); Merbentyl 20 (20 mg); *Carbellon (combined with magnesium hydroxide and charcoal); *Kolanticon Gel (combined with aluminium hydroxide, magnesium hydroxide, and dimeticone).

Dicynene (sanofi-aventis) *See* ETAMSYLATE.

didanosine An antiretroviral drug (*see* ANTIVIRAL DRUGS): it is a nucleoside analogue that inhibits the action of reverse transcriptase. Didanosine is used, in combination with other antiretroviral agents, to treat *HIV infection. It is available as tablets or *enteric-coated capsules on *prescription only.
Side effects: include diarrhoea, nausea, vomiting, damage to peripheral nerves (causing weakness and numbness in the limbs), pancreatitis, blood disorders, and (rarely) liver failure and visual disturbances.
Precautions: didanosine should be used with caution by those with a history of pancreatitis, disease of the peripheral nerves, gout, or impaired kidney or liver function and by pregnant women. It should not be taken by women who are breastfeeding.
Interactions with other drugs:

Allopurinol: increases the plasma concentration (and therefore the risk of toxic effects) of didanosine and these two drugs should not be used together.

Antiviral drugs: ribavirin and tenofovir increase the the risk of toxic effects of didanosine and should not be used with it; stavudine increases the risk of side effects of didanosine.

Hydroxycarbamide: increases the risk of toxic effects and should therefore not be used with didanosine.

Proprietary preparations: Videx (tablets); Videx EC (capsules).

Didronel (Procter & Gamble) *See* DISODIUM ETIDRONATE.

Didronel PMO (Procter & Gamble) *See* DISODIUM ETIDRONATE.

dienogest *See* QLAIRA.

diethylamine salicylate A *salicylate that is applied to the skin for the relief of muscular aches and pains, including backache, sciatica, lumbago, and sprains. It is available as an ingredient of *rubefacient preparations that are freely available *over the counter.
Side effects and precautions: *see* RUBEFACIENTS.
Proprietary preparations: *Fiery Jack Cream (combined with capsicum oleoresin, glycol salicylate, and methyl nicotinate); *Transvasin Heat Spray (combined with 2-hydroxyethyl salicylate, and methyl nicotinate).

diethylstilbestrol <**stilboestrol**> A synthetic *oestrogen sometimes used for the treatment of breast cancer in postmenopausal women and prostate cancer in men. Diethylstilbestrol is available as tablets on *prescription only.
Side effects: *see* ETHINYLESTRADIOL; OESTROGENS. There may also be thrombosis.
Precautions: diethylstilbestrol should not be taken by people with liver disease. *See also* ETHINYLESTRADIOL.
Interactions with other drugs: *see* ETHINYLESTRADIOL.

diethyltoluamide (**DEET**) A chemical used as an insect repellent. It is an ingredient of various lotions, sprays, and roll-on sticks that are applied to the skin for repelling mosquitoes, midges, and other bloodsucking insects. Preparations containing DEET are effective but their action lasts only a few hours; they are freely available *over the counter.
Side effects and precautions: preparations may occasionally cause skin irritation. They should not be applied to the lips, eyes, or broken skin, and prolonged use in young children should be avoided.

Differin (Galderma) *See* ADAPALENE.

Difflam (Meda Pharmaceuticals) *See* BENZYDAMINE HYDROCHLORIDE.

Diflucan (Pfizer) *See* FLUCONAZOLE.

diflucortolone valerate A potent *topical steroid used for the treatment of a variety of severe skin disorders (including eczema and psoriasis). It is available, on *prescription only, as a cream, an oily cream, or an ointment.
Side effects and precautions: *see* TOPICAL STEROIDS.
Proprietary preparations: Nerisone; Nerisone Forte (a stronger preparation).

Digibind (GlaxoSmithKline) A proprietary preparation of antibodies to *digoxin, used for the rapid treatment of overdosage of digoxin and other cardiac glycosides. It is given by injection and is available on *prescription only.

digitalis drugs *See* CARDIAC GLYCOSIDES; DIGOXIN.

digitoxin A digitalis drug having the same effects as *digoxin, but with a much longer duration of action. It is available as tablets on *prescription only.
Side effects, precautions, and interactions with other drugs: *see* DIGOXIN.

digoxin A *cardiac glycoside (digitalis drug). It is used to treat congestive *heart failure and supraventricular *arrhythmias (particularly atrial fibrillation). The effective dose of digoxin can also be the dose at which side effects become common, so treatment must be monitored carefully. Digoxin is available on *prescription only as a solution for infusion, as tablets, or as an elixir.
Side effects: include nausea, vomiting, loss of appetite, diarrhoea, confusion, visual disturbance, and arrhythmias.
Precautions: side effects must be observed and reported to the doctor, since thay can be a sign of too high a dosage.
Interactions with other drugs:

Anti-arrhythmic drugs: amiodarone and propafenone increase the plasma concentration of digoxin; the dosage of digoxin should be halved.
Calcium antagonists: diltiazem, lercanidipine, nicardipine, and nifedipine increase the plasma concentration of digoxin; verapamil increases the plasma concentration of digoxin and slows the heart rate.
Diuretics: because digoxin is more toxic if potassium is depleted, a potassium-sparing diuretic should be added if patients are taking other diuretics with digoxin.
Itraconazole: increases the plasma concentration of digoxin.
Spironolactone: enhances the effect of digoxin.
St John's wort: reduces the plasma concentration of digoxin and should not be taken with it.

Proprietary preparations: Lanoxin; Lanoxin-PG.

dihydrocodeine tartrate An *opioid analgesic, similar to codeine in its pain-relieving effects, used for the treatment of mild to severe pain (depending on the dosage). It is also used in combination with paracetamol (*see* CO-DYDRAMOL). Dihydrocodeine is available as tablets, *modified-release tablets, or an oral solution on *prescription only; an injection of dihydrocodeine is a *controlled drug.
Side effects and precautions: *see* MORPHINE.
Interactions with other drugs: *see* OPIOIDS.
Proprietary preparations: DF 118 Forte (high-strength tablets); DHC Continus (high-strength modified-release tablets); *Remedeine (combined with paracetamol).

dihydrotachysterol An *analogue of *vitamin D used for the treatment of tetany, spasm and twitching of the muscles caused by low plasma calcium concentrations due to underworking of the parathyroid glands (*see* PARATHYROID HORMONE). It is available as an oral solution that contains *arachis oil (and should therefore not be used by people who are allergic to peanuts). Dihydrotachysterol can be obtained without a prescription, but only from pharmacies.
Side effects, precautions, and interactions with other drugs: *see* VITAMIN D.
Proprietary preparation: AT 10.

Dilcardia SR (Generics) *See* DILTIAZEM HYDROCHLORIDE.

dill seed oil An oil distilled from the seeds of the dill plant (*Anethum graveolens*). It is included, as dill water, as an ingredient in a preparation to relieve flatulence and wind pains.
Proprietary preparation: *Woodward's Gripe Water (combined with sodium bicarbonate).

diloxanide furoate A drug used for the treatment of chronic infections of the intestine by the amoeba *Entamoeba histolytica*, which causes amoebic dysentry. It is available as tablets on *prescription only.
Side effects: include flatulence and (rarely) vomiting and itching.
Precautions: diloxanide should not be taken by women who are pregnant or breastfeeding.

diltiazem hydrochloride A class III *calcium antagonist used for the prevention and treatment of most forms of *angina. Longer-acting formulations are also used for the treatment of *hypertension. A *prescription only medicine, it is available as capsules or tablets in short-acting or *modified-release formulations.
Side effects: *see* CALCIUM ANTAGONISTS.
Precautions: diltiazem should not be taken by people with severe bradycardia (slow heart rate) or some other forms of heart disease, or by women who are pregnant or breastfeeding. *See also* ANTIHYPERTENSIVE DRUGS.
Interactions with other drugs:

Alpha blockers: there is an increased blood-pressure-lowering effect if these drugs are taken with diltiazem.
Amiodarone: diltiazem increases the risk of amiodarone having adverse effects on the heart.
Antiepileptic drugs: phenytoin reduces the effects of diltiazem, which itself increases the plasma concentration of phenytoin; diltiazem enhances the effects of carbamazepine.
Atazanavir: increases the effects of diltiazem, whose dosage should therefore be reduced.
Beta blockers: the risk of bradycardia (slow heart rate) is increased if beta blockers are taken with diltiazem.
Ciclosporin: its plasma concentration is increased by diltiazem.
Cilostazol: its plasma concentration is increased by diltiazem and these two drugs should not be used together.
Digoxin: its plasma concentration is increased by diltiazem.
Ivabradine: reduces the effect of diltiazem.
Rifampicin: reduces the effect of diltiazem.
Sirolimus: its plasma concentration is increased by diltiazem.
Tacrolimus: its plasma concentration is increased by diltiazem.
Theophylline: its effects are enhanced by diltiazem.
See also CALCIUM ANTAGONISTS.

Proprietary preparations: Adizem-SR (modified-release tablets or capsules); Adizem-XL (modified-release capsules); Angitil SR, Angitil XL (modified-release capsules); Calcicard CR (modified-release tablets); Dilcardia SR (modified-release capsules); Dilzem SR (modified-release capsules); Dilzem XL (high-strength modified-release capsules); Slozem (modified-release capsules); Tildiem LA (modified-release capsules); Tildiem Retard (low-strength modified-release tablets); Viazem XL (modified-release capsules); Zemtard (modified-release capsules).

Dilzem SR, Dilzem XL (Cephalon) *See* DILTIAZEM HYDROCHLORIDE.

dimenhydrinate *See* ARLEVERT.

dimercaprol (**BAL**) A drug that is used as an antidote to poisoning by metals, such as antimony, arsenic, bismuth, gold, and mercury (but not iron, cadmium, or selenium). Dimercaprol is available as an injection on *prescription only.
Side effects: include low blood pressure, a fast heart rate, general malaise, nausea, vomiting, increased production of saliva, tears, and sweat, a burning sensation in the mouth, throat, and eyes, a feeling of constriction in the chest and throat, headache, muscle spasms, and (in children) fever.
Precautions: dimercaprol should not be given to people with severely impaired liver function (unless this is caused by arsenic poisoning). It should be used with caution in people with high blood pressure or impaired kidney function, elderly people, and women who are pregnant or breastfeeding.

dimethicone *See* DIMETICONE.

dimethyl sulfoxide (<**dimethyl sulphoxide**>; **DMSO**) A drug that is used to relieve the pain and other symptoms of a form of cystitis that is associated with an ulcer in the wall of the bladder. It is instilled into the bladder and then voided. Dimethyl sulfoxide is available as a solution for instillation on *prescription only. DMSO may also be combined with other drugs in preparations that are applied topically as it improves their absorption.
Side effects: dimethyl sulfoxide may cause bladder spasms and allergic reactions.
Precautions: prolonged use of dimethyl sulfoxide requires six-monthly monitoring of its effects on the eyes, liver, and kidneys.
Proprietary preparations: Rimso-50; Herpid (combined with *idoxuridine).

dimeticone <**dimethicone**> A water-repellent silicone used in *barrier preparations, for example for the treatment of napkin rash, pressure sores, eczema, and head lice. Activated dimeticone (**simeticone**) is used to relieve wind, gripes, and colic in babies and is also included in *antacid and antidiarrhoeal preparations to disperse gas in the stomach and gut. Dimeticone is available without a prescription, but some combined preparations can only be obtained from pharmacies.
Proprietary preparations: Dentinox Infant Colic Drops; Hedrin (lotion for headlice); Infacol (liquid for colic and wind); Wind-eze (capsules and chewable tablets); *Altacite Plus (combined with hydrotalcite, aluminium hydroxide, and magnesium hydroxide); *Asilone Suspension (combined with aluminium hydroxide and magnesium hydroxide); *Bisodol Extra Tablets

(combined with sodium bicarbonate, calcium carbonate, and magnesium carbonate); *Boots Antiseptic Nappy Rash Cream (combined with cetrimide); *Boots Lip and Cold Sore Cream (combined with cetrimide, urea, and chlorocresol); *Boots Wind Relief Tablets (combined with aluminium hydroxide and magnesium hydroxide); *Conotrane (combined with benzalkonium chloride); *Imodium Plus (combined with loperamide); *Kolanticon Gel (combined with dicycloverine hydrochloride, aluminium hydroxide, and magnesium oxide); *Maalox Plus (combined with aluminium hydroxide and magnesium hydroxide); *Rennie Deflatine (combined with calcium carbonate and magnesium carbonate); *Siopel (combined with cetrimide); *Sprilon (combined with zinc oxide); *Timodine (combined with nystatin, hydrocortisone, and benzalkonium chloride); *Vasogen Cream (combined with zinc oxide and calamine).

dinoprostone A *prostaglandin used to induce labour, to soften the cervix before labour, and (rarely) to induce abortion. It is available as a vaginal gel, pessaries, vaginal tablets, or a solution for intravenous infusion or injection into the amniotic sac. A *prescription only medicine, dinoprostone should only be used under direct medical supervision.
Side effects: include nausea, vomiting, diarrhoea, high body temperature and flushing, and constriction of the airways; less frequently raised blood pressure, breathlessness, chills, headache, and dizziness may occur.
Precautions: dinoprostone should not be given to women with acute pelvic inflammatory disease or heart, kidney, lung, or liver disease. It should be used with caution in women with a history of glaucoma, asthma, high or low blood pressure, anaemia, jaundice, diabetes, or epilepsy.
Proprietary preparations: Propess (pessaries); Prostin E2 Vaginal Tablets; Prostin E2 Solution; Prostin E2 Vaginal Gel.

Diocalm Dual Action (SSL International) A proprietary combination of *morphine hydrochloride (which reduces gut motility) and *attapulgite (an antidiarrhoeal drug), used for the treatment of occasional diarrhoea and associated discomfort or pain. It is available as tablets and can be obtained without a prescription, but only from pharmacies.
Side effects and interactions with other drugs: *see* MORPHINE; OPIOIDS.
Precautions: this medicine should not be given to children under six years old.

Diocalm Ultra (SSL International) *See* LOPERAMIDE HYDROCHLORIDE.

Dioctyl (UCB Pharma) *See* DOCUSATE SODIUM.

dioctyl sodium sulphosuccinate *See* DOCUSATE SODIUM.

Dioderm (Dermal Laboratories) *See* HYDROCORTISONE.

Dioralyte Natural, Blackcurrent and Citrus GSL (sanofi-aventis) A proprietary combination of glucose, *sodium chloride, *potassium chloride, and *disodium hydrogen citrate, used for the replacement of *electrolytes in people with diarrhoea (*see* ORAL REHYDRATION THERAPY). It is available as a

powder to be dissolved in water and can be obtained without a prescription, but only from pharmacies.
Precautions: Dioralyte Natural should not be taken by people with kidney disease or intestinal obstruction.

Dioralyte Relief (sanofi-aventis) A proprietary combination of *sodium chloride, *potassium chloride, *sodium citrate, and precooked rice powder (a carbohydrate), used for the treatment of diarrhoea (*see* ORAL REHYDRATION THERAPY). It is available as a powder to be dissolved in water and can be obtained without a prescription, but only from pharmacies.
Precautions: Dioralyte Relief should not be taken by people with kidney disease or intestinal obstruction.

Diovan (Novartis) *See* VALSARTAN.

Dipentum (UCB Pharma) *See* OLSALAZINE SODIUM.

diphenhydramine An *antihistamine used, in the form of the citrate or hydrochloride, mainly as an ingredient in many cough and cold preparations. As it has marked sedative properties, it is also used for the relief of temporary insomnia. Diphenhydramine is also included in preparations for treating irritating skin conditions. It is available as tablets, capsules, syrups, a cream, or a lotion and may be bought from pharmacies without a prescription.
Side effects: sedation is common and *extrapyramidal reactions have been reported. *See also* ANTIHISTAMINES.
Precautions and interactions with other drugs: *see* ANTIHISTAMINES.
Proprietary preparations: Boots Sleepeaze Tablets; Medinex (liquid for insomnia); Nytol (tablets for insomnia); *Benadryl Skin Allergy Relief Cream (combined with zinc oxide and camphor); *Benylin Chesty Coughs Original (combined with ammonium chloride and menthol); *Benylin Children's Night Coughs (combined with menthol); *Benylin Day & Night Tablets (night tablets; combined with paracetamol); *Benylin Dry Coughs Original (combined with dextromethorphan and menthol); *Benylin Four Flu (combined with paracetamol and phenylephrine); *Benylin Mucus Cough Night (combined with guaifenesin and levomenthol); *Boots Catarrh Syrup for Children (combined with pseudoephedrine); *Boots Children's 1 Year Plus Night Time Cough Syrup (combined with pholcodine); *Boots Night Cold Comfort (combined with paracetamol, pholcodine, and pseudoephedrine); *Boots Night-time Cough Relief Syrup 2 Years Plus (combined with pholcodine); *Boots Nirolex Night Time Cough Relief Linctus (combined with pholcodine); *Calcold (combined with paracetamol); *Covonia Night Time Formula (combined with dextromethorphan); *Histalix (combined with ammonium chloride and menthol); *Panadol Night (combined with paracetamol).

diphenoxylate hydrochloride *See* CO-PHENOTROPE; OPIOIDS.

diphenylpyraline An *antihistamine that is not used alone but is included as an ingredient of some proprietary cold or cough remedies (capsules or

syrup). Preparations containing diphenylpyraline are available without a prescription, but usually only from pharmacies.
Side effects, precautions, and interactions with other drugs: *see* ANTIHISTAMINES.

dipipanone hydrochloride A strong *opioid analgesic that is used in combination with an antiemetic drug for the treatment of moderate to severe pain. Dipipanone is a *controlled drug.
Side effects and precautions: *see* MORPHINE.
Interactions with other drugs: *see* OPIOIDS.
Proprietary preparation: *Diconal (combined with cyclizine).

dipivefrine A *sympathomimetic drug used for the treatment of chronic (open-angle) *glaucoma. It acts in a similar way to *adrenaline, to which it is converted in the eye. Dipivefrine is available as eye drops on *prescription only.
Side effects: there may be transient stinging and allergic reactions.
Precautions: dipivefrine should not be used by people who wear soft contact lenses and should be used with caution by people with heart disease and high blood pressure (*hypertension). It should not be used to treat closed-angle glaucoma.
Proprietary preparation: Propine.

Diprobase (Schering-Plough) A proprietary combination of *liquid paraffin and *white soft paraffin (both emollients) in the form of a cream or ointment, used to soothe dry skin conditions. It is freely available *over the counter .

Diprobath (Schering-Plough) A proprietary combination of light *liquid paraffin and *isopropyl myristate, used as an emollient to relieve dry skin conditions. It is available as an emulsion to be added to the bath and can be obtained without a prescription, but only from pharmacies.

Diprosalic (Schering-Plough) A proprietary combination of *betamethasone (a corticosteroid) and *salicylic acid (a keratolytic), used as a potent topical steroid and skin softener for the treatment of *eczema that has not responded to less potent steroids and *psoriasis. A *prescription only medicine, it is available as an ointment and as a lotion for the scalp (**Diprosalic Scalp Application**).
Side effects, precautions, and interactions with other drugs: *see* TOPICAL STEROIDS; SALICYLIC ACID.

Diprosone (Schering-Plough) *See* BETAMETHASONE.

dipyridamole An *antiplatelet drug that is used as additional therapy (to oral *anticoagulants) for the prevention of thromboembolism (*see* THROMBOSIS). *Modified-release preparations are also used to prevent further strokes in people who have already had a stroke. Dipyridamole is available, on *prescription only, as tablets, a suspension, modified-release capsules, or an injection.

Side effects: include nausea, indigestion, headache, dizziness, muscle aches, low blood pressure, a fast heart rate, hot flushes, and allergic rashes.
Precautions: dipyridamole should be used with caution by people with severe angina, migraine, or low blood pressure, and by those who have had a recent heart attack.
Interactions with other drugs:
Adenosine: the anti-arrhythmic effects of adenosine are increased and prolonged by dipyridamole.
Antacids: may reduce the absorption of dipyridamole.
Anticoagulants: their effects are enhanced by dipyridamole.
Proprietary preparations: Persantin; Persantin Retard (modified-release capsules); *Asasantin Retard (combined with aspirin).

disease-modifying antirheumatic drugs (**DMARDs**) Any of various drugs used in the treatment of rheumatic disease: they affect the progression of the disease by suppressing the disease process. DMARDs include drugs affecting the immune response (immunomodulators), such as *immunosuppressants and **anti-TNF drugs**: these latter inhibit the action of tumour necrosis factor alpha (TNF-α), whose effects include mediating inflammation. Anti-TNF drugs include *adalimumab, *etanercept, and *infliximab. Other DMARDs include gold salts, *penicillamine, *sulfasalazine, and *hydroxychloroquine.

disinfectants Agents that destroy or remove bacteria and other microorganisms and are used to cleanse surgical instruments and other objects. Examples are cresol, *hexachlorophene, and *phenol. Dilute solutions of some disinfectants may be used as *antiseptics or as preservatives in solutions of eye drops or injections.

Disipal (Astellas Pharma) *See* ORPHENADRINE.

disodium edetate A compound included in many preparations as an antioxidant and preservative. It is also a chelating agent that binds free calcium, and is included in solutions for washing out urinary catheters.
Proprietary preparations: *Uriflex G (combined with citric acid, sodium bicarbonate, and magnesium oxide); *Uriflex R (combined with citric acid, magnesium carbonate, and gluconolactone); *Uro-Tainer Suby G (combined with citric acid, magnesium oxide, and sodium bicarbonate).

disodium etidronate A *bisphosphonate that is used to treat Paget's disease (in which the bones become deformed and fracture easily). Taken with *calcium carbonate, it is also used for the treatment and prevention of postmenopausal osteoporosis of the spine, especially in women for whom *hormone replacement therapy is unsuitable, and corticosteroid-induced osteoporosis. Etidronate is available, on *prescription only, as tablets and a form of infusion.
Side effects: include nausea and diarrhoea, and there may initially be increased bone pain in patients with Paget's disease (this usually disappears

as treatment continues); rare side effects are allergic skin reactions (itching or rash), abdominal pain, constipation, headache, and 'pins and needles'.
Precautions: etidronate should not be taken by people with liver or kidney disease or by women who are pregnant or breastfeeding. Food and certain drugs (see below) should be avoided for at least two hours before and after taking the tablets, since they bind to etidronate in the stomach and intestine and prevent its absorption.
Interactions with other drugs:
Aminoglycosides: in combination with etidronate, they may cause abnormally low concentrations of calcium in the plasma.
Antacids: reduce the absorption of etidronate tablets.
Calcium supplements: reduce the absorption of etidronate tablets.
Iron supplements: reduce the absorption of etidronate tablets.
Proprietary preparations: Didronel; Didronel PMO (packaged with effervescent tablets of calcium carbonate).

disodium folinate, disodium levofolinate *See* FOLINIC ACID.

disodium hydrogen citrate A salt of *sodium that has a clean sharp lemon taste. It is an ingredient of *electrolyte replacement solutions used in *oral rehydration therapy.
Proprietary preparation: *Dioralyte Natural, Blackcurrent and Citrus GSL (combined with glucose, sodium chloride, and potassium chloride).

disodium pamidronate A *bisphosphonate used to reduce high concentrations of calcium in the blood in the treatment of bone cancer, bone pain due to secondary tumours, and Paget's disease. It is available as an injection on *prescription only.
Side effects: include mild transient fever, influenza-like symptoms, local reactions at the injection site, and transient bone pain or muscle aches.
Precautions: people should not drive or operate machinery immediately after treatment. Pamidronate should not be given to women who are pregnant or breastfeeding and should be used with caution in people with kidney disease.
Interactions with other drugs:
Aminoglycosides: in combination with pamidronate, they may cause abnormally low concentrations of calcium in the plasma.
Proprietary preparation: Aredia.

disodium phosphate dodecahydrate *See* PHOSPHATE LAXATIVES.

disopyramide A class I *anti-arrhythmic drug used to treat superventricular arrhythmias or ventricular arrhythmias after a heart attack (*see* ARRHYTHMIA). It is available, on *prescription only, as capsules, *modified-release tablets, or an injection.
Side effects: include dry mouth, urinary retention, constipation, blurred vision, gastrointestinal upset, and hypotension (low blood pressure).
Precautions: disopyramide should not be given to people with untreated heart failure and should be used with caution during pregnancy and by

people with liver or kidney disease, heart failure, enlarged prostate, or glaucoma. *See also* ANTI-ARRHYTHMIC DRUGS.

Interactions with other drugs:

Other anti-arrhythmic drugs: amiodarone increases the risk of ventricular arrhythmias and should not be used with disopyramide; depression of heart function is increased if disopyramide is taken with any other anti-arrhythmic.

Antibiotics: the plasma concentration (and therefore effects) of disopyramide is increased by erythromycin (and possibly clarithromycin) and reduced by rifampicin. Moxifloxacin and Synercid increase the risk of ventricular arrhythmias and should not be taken with disopyramide.

Antipsychotic drugs: disopyramide should not be taken with amisulpride, droperidol, pimozide, sertindole, or zuclopenthixol as these drugs increase the risk of ventricular arrhythmias.

Atomoxetine: increases the risk of ventricular arrhythmias.

Beta blockers: sotalol increases the risk of ventricular arrhythmias and should not be taken with disopyramide; heart function is depressed if other beta blockers are taken with disopyramide.

Diuretics: increase toxicity to the heart through potassium depletion.

Ivabradine: increases the risk of ventricular arrhythmias.

Ketoconazole: increases the risk of ventricular arrhythmias and should not be taken with disopyramide.

Mizolastine: should not be taken with disopyramide as it increases the risk of ventricular arrhythmias.

Tolterodine: increases the risk of ventricular arrhythmias.

Tricyclic antidepressants: increase the risk of ventricular arrhythmias.

Verapamil: depression of heart function is increased if verapamil is taken with disopyramide.

Proprietary preparations: Rythmodan; Rythmodan Retard (modified-release tablets).

Disprin, Disprin Direct (Reckitt Benckiser) *See* ASPIRIN.

Disprin Extra (Reckitt Benckiser) A proprietary combination of *aspirin and *paracetamol (analgesics and antipyretics), used for the treatment of mild to moderate pain (including headache, neuralgia, toothache, and period pains) and fever and to relieve the symptoms of influenza and colds. It is freely available *over the counter in the form of soluble tablets.

Side effects and interactions with other drugs: *see* ASPIRIN.

Precautions: Disprin Extra should not be given to children, except on medical advice. *See also* ASPIRIN; PARACETAMOL.

Disprol (Reckitt Benckiser) *See* PARACETAMOL.

Distaclor, Distaclor MR (Flynn Pharma) *See* CEFACLOR.

Distamine (Alliance) *See* PENICILLAMINE.

distigmine bromide An *anticholinesterase drug used to treat urinary

retention, especially after surgery and in people with motor neuron disease. It is also used (rarely) for the treatment of myasthenia gravis. Distigmine is similar to *pyridostigmine and *neostigmine but has a longer duration of action. It is available as tablets on *prescription only.
Side effects: include nausea and vomiting, sweating, increased salivation, diarrhoea, abdominal cramps, and blurred vision.
Precautions: distigmine should not be taken by people with intestinal or urinary obstruction, by those in postoperative shock, or by those with asthma. It should be used with caution in people with low blood pressure, peptic ulcers, epilepsy, Parkinson's disease, or kidney disease.
Interactions with other drugs: *see* PYRIDOSTIGMINE.
Proprietary preparation: Ubretid.

disulfiram A drug used in the treatment of chronic alcohol dependence, but only under specialist supervision. It causes acetaldehyde, a breakdown product of alcohol, to accumulate in the blood, which results in extremely unpleasant reactions after consuming even a small amount of alcohol; these include flushing, a throbbing headache, palpitation, a fast heart rate, nausea, and vomiting. If large amounts of alcohol are consumed the reaction is severe: an abnormal heart rhythm (*see* ARRHYTHMIA), with low blood pressure and eventually collapse. It is essential for people to abstain from alcohol for at least 24 hours before starting treatment with disulfiram and that they understand the severity and possible dangers of the reaction between disulfiram and alcohol. Disulfiram is available as tablets on *prescription only.
Side effects: include drowsiness and fatigue at the start of the treatment, nausea, vomiting, bad breath, and decreased libido. Rarely, depression, paranoia, mania, allergic skin rashes, liver damage, and damage to peripheral nerves may occur.
Precautions: people taking disulfiram may be advised to carry a warning card, emphasizing the dangerous effects of alcohol taken with disulfiram. Even the small amounts of alcohol in some oral medicines may be sufficient to cause a reaction, and toiletries containing alcohol should be avoided. Disulfiram should not be taken by people who have heart failure, coronary artery disease, a history of stroke, high blood pressure, psychosis, or personality disorder. It should not be taken by women who are pregnant or breastfeeeding.
Interactions with other drugs:
Anticoagulants: the anticoagulant effects of warfarin and acenocoumarol are increased.
Phenytoin: the risk of phenytoin causing adverse effects is increased.
Proprietary preparation: Antabuse.

dithranol A drug used in the treatment of mild to moderately severe chronic *psoriasis. Since dithranol is irritant to healthy skin, care must be taken to apply it only to affected areas. Also, as some people are allergic to this drug, a small area of skin should be tested for sensitivity to dithranol before treatment starts. It is usual to start with a low concentration (0.1%), which is gradually built up to higher concentrations (1–3%). Preparations are washed off after each treatment. Dithranol is sometimes used in conjunction with *coal tar and UVB (ultraviolet-B) light. It is available as a cream, an ointment, or a paste (containing dithranol in *Lassar's paste). Preparations containing more than 1% dithranol are *prescription only medicines, but those with lower concentrations can be obtained from pharmacies without a prescription.

d

Side effects: dithranol commonly causes local irritation of the skin and a burning sensation; it stains skin, clothing, and other fabrics.

Precautions: dithranol should not be used to treat acute psoriasis. It should not come into contact with the eyes, face, mucous membranes, broken skin, or genitals. It should be used with caution by women who are pregnant or breastfeeding. Soaps or shampoos should not be used to remove the cream.

Proprietary preparations: Dithrocream (0.1–0.25%); Dithrocream Forte (0.5%); Dithrocream HP (1%); Dithrocream 2%; Micanol; *Psorin (combined with coal tar and salicylic acid); *Psorin Scalp Gel (combined with salicylic acid).

Dithrocream (Dermal Laboratories) *See* DITHRANOL.

Ditropan (sanofi-aventis) *See* OXYBUTYNIN HYDROCHLORIDE.

Diumide-K Continus (Teofarma) A proprietary combination of *furosemide (a loop diuretic) and *potassium chloride. Available on *prescription only, it is taken orally in the form of *modified-release tablets for the treatment of *oedema associated with congestive heart failure, liver disease, or kidney disease.

Side effects, precautions, and interactions with other drugs: *see* LOOP DIURETICS.

See also DIURETICS.

diuretics A class of drugs that increase the volume of urine (diuresis) by promoting the excretion of salts (especially sodium and potassium) and water via the kidneys. Diuretics are used to reduce the *oedema due to salt and water retention in disorders of the kidneys, heart, or liver. They are also used, alone or in combination with other drugs, in the treatment of high blood pressure (*see* HYPERTENSION). The use of diuretics can result in potassium deficiency; this is corrected by the simultaneous administration of a *potassium supplement or by adding another diuretic with a potassium-sparing effect, such as amiloride or triamterene. (Potassium is essential for the normal functioning of nerves and muscles; low concentrations of potassium cause weakness, confusion, and in severe cases abnormal heart rhythms.) The main classes of diuretics are the *loop diuretics, *thiazide diuretics, and *potassium-sparing diuretics.

Diurexan (Meda Pharmaceuticals) *See* XIPAMIDE.

Dixarit (Boehringer Ingelheim) *See* CLONIDINE HYDROCHLORIDE.

DMARDs *See* DISEASE-MODIFYING ANTIRHEUMATIC DRUGS.

dobutamine hydrochloride A drug that stimulates beta-adrenoceptors in the heart (*see* SYMPATHOMIMETIC DRUGS). It is used to increase blood pressure in patients who have had a heart attack or open heart surgery or in cases of shock. It may also be used for heart stress testing during diagnostic procedures. Available as an intravenous solution on prescription, it is only used in hospitals.
Side effects and precautions: a fast heart rate and a marked increase in blood pressure may indicate an overdose.
Interactions with other drugs:
Beta blockers: severe hypertension may result if these drugs are taken with dobutamine.
Entacapone: may enhance the effects of dobutamine.
Rasagiline: should not be used with dobutamine.

docetaxel A *taxane used for the treatment of breast *cancer, lung cancer, and some other cancers, either alone or in combination with other cytotoxic drugs. Docetaxel can cause fluid retention and (like *paclitaxel) severe allergic reactions: *dexamethasone is usually given before treatment to reduce these side effects. Docetaxel is available as a solution for intravenous infusion on *prescription only.
Side effects: include fluid retention causing swelling of the legs, allergic reactions, *bone marrow suppression, hair loss, and muscle pain. *See also* CYTOTOXIC DRUGS.
Precautions: docetaxel should not be given to women who are pregnant or breastfeeding and should be used with caution in people with liver disease. *See also* CYTOTOXIC DRUGS.
Interactions with other drugs:
Clozapine: there is a risk of agranulocytosis (a blood disorder), and clozapine should not be used with docetaxel.
Proprietary preparation: Taxotere.

docusate sodium (**dioctyl sodium sulphosuccinate**) A *stimulant laxative and *faecal softener that is used, alone or in combination with other laxatives, in the treatment of constipation and to clear the bowel before X-ray examination. It has a detergent action, which reduces surface tension, and is therefore also used to soften ear wax. Docusate is available as capsules, a solution, an enema, or ear drops and can be obtained without a prescription, but only from pharmacies. *See also* CO-DANTHRUSATE.
Side effects and precautions: *see* STIMULANT LAXATIVES.
Proprietary preparations: Dioctyl (capsules); Docusol (adult or paediatric solutions); DulcoEase (capsules); Molcer (ear drops); Norgalax Micro-enema; Waxsol (ear drops); Normax (*see* CO-DANTHRUSATE).

Docusol (Typharm) *See* DOCUSATE SODIUM.

Do-Do ChestEze (Novartis) A proprietary combination of *ephedrine (a decongestant), *theophylline (a bronchodilator), and *caffeine, used for the relief of bronchial coughs, wheezing, and breathlessness and to clear the chest

of mucus following infections of the upper airways. It is available as tablets without a prescription, but only from pharmacies.
Side effects and interactions with other drugs: *see* EPHEDRINE HYDROCHLORIDE; DECONGESTANTS; THEOPHYLLINE; XANTHINES.
Precautions: this medicine is not recommended for children under 12 years old except on medical advice. *See also* EPHEDRINE HYDROCHLORIDE; DECONGESTANTS; THEOPHYLLINE; XANTHINES.

Dolmatil (sanofi-aventis) *See* SULPIRIDE.

domiphen An *antiseptic used in solutions to disinfect the skin and in lozenges for the treatment of minor infections of the mouth and throat.

domperidone A drug that antagonizes the action of *dopamine. It is an *antiemetic used to prevent or treat nausea and vomiting, especially that associated with *cytotoxic drug therapy. Domperidone also stimulates gastric motility (*see* PROKINETIC DRUGS) and is used in the treatment of indigestion not due to peptic ulceration. It is available, on *prescription only, as tablets, a suspension, or suppositories; packs of 10 tablets for the relief of indigestion can be obtained from pharmacies without a prescription.
Side effects: these are rare: stomach cramps and breast enlargement may occur.
Precautions: domperidone should not be taken by people with prolactinoma (a tumour of the pituitary gland) or liver disease or by pregnant women. It should be used with caution by people with kidney disease and by women who are breastfeeding.
Proprietary preparations: Motilium (tablets and suppositories); Motilium 10 (tablets).

donepezil hydrochloride An *acetylcholinesterase inhibitor that increases the amounts of acetylcholine in the brain. It is used to treat the symptoms of mild to moderate dementia (including short-term memory loss) that occur in people with Alzheimer's disease and has been shown to have some success in slowing the progress of the disease. Donepezil is not effective in treating other forms of dementia or confusion. It is available as tablets and dispersible tablets on *prescription only, and treatment should be supervised by a specialist.
Side effects: include nausea, vomiting, diarrhoea, fatigue, insomnia, muscle cramps, and (less commonly) headache, dizziness, fainting, and slowing of the heart rate.
Precautions: donepezil should not be taken by women who are pregnant or breastfeeding and should be used with caution in people who have certain heart conditions, or who are likely to develop a peptic ulcer, or who have asthma or chronic bronchitis.
Interactions with other drugs:

Muscle relaxants: donepezil may either increase or reduce the effects of muscle relaxants used in surgery to paralyse muscles.

Proprietary preparations: Aricept (tablets); Aricept Evess (dispersible tablets).

Dopacard (Cephalon) *See* DOPEXAMINE.

dopamine A substance that transmits messages between nerve cells in the brain. Dopamine is also an intermediate product in the biochemical pathway that manufactures other neurotransmitters, noradrenaline and adrenaline. Dopamine also controls the secretion of the hormones prolactin and *growth hormone by exerting an inhibitory effect. Outside the brain, dopamine has effects on the heart and blood vessels and is used in the form of *dopamine hydrochloride to treat circulatory collapse.

Imbalance of dopamine concentrations in the brain causes a variety of conditions that may be treated by drugs that either increase dopamine levels or inhibit the action of dopamine. Drugs that stimulate dopamine receptors (leading to increased production of dopamine) or increase dopamine activity are known as **dopamine receptor agonists**. They include *amantadine, *bromocriptine, *cabergoline, *pramipexole, *quinagolide, and *ropinirole and are used to treat Parkinson's disease (*see* ANTIPARKINSONIAN DRUGS) and to relieve some hormone disorders.

Drugs that prevent the action of dopamine by competing with it to occupy and block dopamine receptor sites in the brain and elsewhere are called **dopamine receptor antagonists**. It is thought that psychoses may be associated with excessive dopamine activity in the brain, and some *antipsychotic drugs (e.g. the phenothiazines and butyrophenones) are dopamine antagonists. The antiemetic drugs *domperidone and *metoclopramide act partly by blocking the action of dopamine at the vomiting centre in the brain. Antagonism of dopamine action also produces a group of side effects known as *extrapyramidal reactions.

dopamine hydrochloride A preparation of *dopamine used to treat cardiogenic shock (collapse of the circulation) resulting from heart failure, heart attack, or heart surgery; it is thought to stimulate beta-receptors in the heart (*see* SYMPATHOMIMETIC DRUGS) and also dopamine receptors in blood vessels, particularly in the kidney. It is available, on *prescription only, as a solution for infusion.

Side effects: include nausea and vomiting, changes in heart rate and blood pressure, and constriction of the blood vessels in the fingers and toes.

Precautions: dopamine hydrochloride should not be given to patients with phaeochromocytoma (a tumour of the adrenal gland) or abnormal heart rhythms (*see* ARRHYTHMIA).

Interactions with other drugs:

MAOIs: there is a risk of a dangerous rise in blood pressure; dopamine should not be taken within two weeks of stopping MAOIs.

Rasagiline: should not be taken with dopamine.

Proprietary preparations: Dopamine Hydrochloride in Dextrose (Glucose) Injection; Select-A-Jet Dopamine.

dopexamine A beta-adrenoceptor stimulant (*see* SYMPATHOMIMETIC DRUGS) that also has some other pharmacological actions. It increases the output of the heart and increases blood flow to the kidneys and gut. It is used to maintain heart function during heart surgery. Available on *prescription only as a form for intravenous infusion, it is only used in hospitals.
Side effects: include a fast heartbeat; nausea, vomiting, anginal pain, tremor, and headache have also been reported.
Interactions with other drugs:
Adrenaline and noradrenaline: their effects may be increased by dopexamine.
MAOIs: a severe rise in blood pressure may occur if these drugs are taken with dopexamine.
Rasagiline: should not be used with dopexamine.
Proprietary preparation: Dopacard.

Dopram (Goldshield) *See* DOXAPRAM HYDROCHLORIDE.

Doralese (Chemidex Pharma) *See* INDORAMIN HYDROCHLORIDE.

Doribax (Janssen-Cilag) *See* DORIPENEM.

doripenem A broad-spectrum beta-lactam *antibiotic used to treat hospital-acquired pneumonia, complicated abdominal infections, and complicated urinary-tract infections. It is available as a form for intravenous infusion on *prescription only.
Side effects: include nausea, diarrhoea, headache, itching, and rash.
Precautions: there is a risk of allergic reactions. Doripenem is not recommended for pregnant or breastfeeding women and should be used with caution in people with kidney disease.
Proprietary preparation: Doribax.

dornase alfa A *mucolytic drug that breaks down mucus by cleaving DNA; it is a genetically engineered version of a natural human enzyme. Dornase alfa is used for the management of cystic fibrosis patients who accumulate large amounts of tenacious mucus. It is administered by inhalation using a jet nebulizer and is available on *prescription only.
Side effects: include sore throat, hoarseness, laryngitis, chest pain, conjunctivitis, and rash.
Precautions: dornase alfa should not be mixed with other drugs in the nebulizer. It should be used with caution in women who are pregnant or breastfeeding.
Proprietary preparation: Pulmozyme.

dorzolamide A *carbonic anhydrase inhibitor that is used to reduce the pressure inside the eye in the treatment of chronic (open-angle) *glaucoma and high blood pressure in the eye; it acts by reducing the production of aqueous fluid in the eye. Dorzolamide is used, either alone or in combination with a *beta blocker, to treat patients who have not responded to beta

blockers alone or in whom beta blockers should not be used. It is available as eye drops on *prescription only.
Side effects: include burning, stinging, and itching of the eye, a bitter taste in the mouth, blurred vision, increased production of tears, conjunctivitis, inflammation of the eyelid, headache, dizziness, tingling in the fingers, nausea, rash, and allergic reactions.
Precautions: dorzolamide should not be used in people with severe kidney disease or in women who are pregnant or breastfeeding. It should be used with caution in people with liver disease and in people with chronic disorders of the cornea or who have had previous eye surgery.
Interactions with other drugs:
Phenytoin: there is an increased risk of osteomalacia.
Proprietary preparations: Trusopt; Trusopt for Single Use; *Cosopt (combined with timolol maleate).

Dostinex (Pharmacia) *See* CABERGOLINE.

dosulepin hydrochloride <**dothiepin hydrochloride**> A *tricyclic antidepressant drug used for the treatment of depressive illness and anxiety with depression, especially when sedation is required. It should only be prescribed by specialists and is available as tablets or capsules.
Side effects, precautions, and interactions with other drugs: *see* TRICYCLIC ANTIDEPRESSANTS; AMITRIPTYLINE HYDROCHLORIDE.
Proprietary preparation: Prothiaden.

dothiepin hydrochloride *See* DOSULEPIN HYDROCHLORIDE.

Doublebase Emollient Bath Additive (Dermal Laboratories) *See* LIQUID PARAFFIN.

Doublebase Emollient Shower Gel (Dermal Laboratories) A proprietary combination of *liquid paraffin and *isopropyl myristate, used as an *emollient to treat and prevent dry skin conditions that may be also be itchy or inflamed. **Doublebase Emollient Wash Gel** is a similar preparation. Both are available without a prescription.

Dovobet (Leo Pharmaceuticals) A proprietary combination of *betamethasone (a corticosteroid) and *calcipotriol (a vitamin D analogue), used for the treatment of *psoriasis. It is available as an ointment on *prescription only.
Side effects and precautions: *see* CALCIPOTRIOL, TOPICAL STEROIDS.
Interactions with other drugs: *see* TOPICAL STEROIDS.

Dovonex (Leo Pharmaceuticals) *See* CALCIPOTRIOL.

Doxadura XL (Discovery Pharmaceuticals) *See* DOXAZOSIN.

doxapram hydrochloride A drug that stimulates breathing (i.e. it is a respiratory *stimulant). It may be used to reverse the inhibition of breathing (respiratory depression) caused by drugs during surgery. It can also be used to

treat acute respiratory failure. Doxapram is available as a form for intravenous injection or infusion on *prescription only.
Side effects: include warmth around the perineum, dizziness, sweating, and increases in blood pressure and heart rate.
Precautions: doxapram should not be used in people with severe asthma or hypertension, coronary artery disease, epilepsy, an overactive thyroid gland, or obstructed airways.
Interactions with other drugs:
MAOIs: may increase the effects of doxapram.
Sympathomimetic drugs: the risk of high blood pressure is increased if these drugs are given with doxapram.
Theophylline: stimulation of the central nervous system is increased.
Proprietary preparation: Dopram.

doxazosin An *alpha blocker used to treat *hypertension and to relieve the obstruction of urine flow that can occur in men with an enlarged prostate gland. It is available as tablets or *modified-release tablets on *prescription only.
Side effects, precautions, and interactions with other drugs: *see* ALPHA BLOCKERS.
Proprietary preparations: Cardura (tablets); Cardura XL (modified-release tablets); Doxadura XL (modified-release tablets).
See also ANTIHYPERTENSIVE DRUGS; VASODILATORS.

doxepin A *tricyclic antidepressant drug that is taken by mouth for the treatment of depressive illness and anxiety with depression, especially when sedation is required, and is applied to the skin for the relief of itching associated with *eczema. Doxepin is available, on *prescription only, as capsules or a cream.
Side effects: *see* AMITRIPTYLINE HYDROCHLORIDE. The cream can cause drowsiness and local burning, stinging, irritation, or rash.
Precautions: *see* TRICYCLIC ANTIDEPRESSANTS. Doxepin capsules should not to be taken by women who are breastfeeding; the cream should not be applied to large areas of skin.
Interactions with other drugs: *see* TRICYCLIC ANTIDEPRESSANTS.
Proprietary preparations: Sinepin (capsules); Xepin (cream).

doxorubicin One of the most widely used and effective *cytotoxic drugs. An anthracycline (*see* CYTOTOXIC ANTIBIOTICS), doxorubicin is administered intravenously for the treatment of acute leukaemias, lymphomas, and a variety of solid tumours (*see* CANCER) and is instilled directly into the bladder to treat bladder cancer. It is also used to treat AIDS-related Kaposi's sarcoma (a tumour of blood vessels in the skin), for which it is available as a lipid formulation for infusion; the lipid enhances its uptake by the tumour cells and may reduce the incidence of adverse effects on the heart. The lipid formulation may also be used to treat breast and ovarian cancer and myeloma. Doxorubicin is a *prescription only medicine.
Side effects: include moderate to severe nausea and vomiting, *bone marrow

suppression, hair loss, and inflammation of the mouth. High doses can have adverse effects on the heart. Leakage from the infusion tube can damage the surrounding tissue, and there can be infusion-related reactions with the lipid formulation (e.g. a painful red rash on the hands and feet). *See also* CYTOTOXIC DRUGS.

Precautions: doxorubicin should not be given to people with pre-existing heart disease, severe liver disease, or an inflamed bladder or to women who are pregnant or breastfeeding. It should be used with caution in elderly people and in anyone who has received radiation. Heart function should be closely monitored. Doxorubicin is irritant to the skin and must be handled carefully. *See also* CYTOTOXIC DRUGS.

Interactions with other drugs:

Ciclosporin: the risk of this drug causing nerve damage is increased.

Clozapine: there is a risk of agranulocytosis (a blood disorder), and this drug should not be used with doxorubicin.

Proprietary preparations: Caelyx (lipid formulation); Myocet (lipid formulation).

doxycycline A tetracycline antibiotic used for the treatment of chronic bronchitis, brucellosis, Lyme disease, chlamydial infections, and infections caused by mycoplasmas and rickettsias (*see* TETRACYCLINES). It is also used to treat mouth ulcers, gum disease, acne, prostatitis, sinusitis, and pelvic inflammatory disease. Doxycycline is also used as a prophylactic protection against malaria, especially in areas, such as southeast Asia, where the malarial parasites are resistant to mefloquine and in people who cannot take chloroquine or mefloquine. Unlike most other tetracyclines, doxycycline does not exacerbate kidney disease and may be taken by those with impaired kidney function. It is available, on *prescription only, as tablets, dispersible tablets, capsules, or *modified-release capsules.

Side effects and precautions: *see* TETRACYCLINES.

Interactions with other drugs:

Antiepileptics: carbamazepine, phenobarbital, phenytoin, and primidone reduce the plasma concentration of doxycycline.

See also TETRACYCLINES.

Proprietary preparations: Doxylar (capsules); Efracea (modified-release capsules); Periostat (tablets); Vibramycin Acne Pack; Vibramycin-D (dispersible tablets).

doxylamine An *antihistamine that is included as an ingredient of preparations to relieve headaches and treat colds.

Side effects, precautions, and interactions with other drugs: *see* ANTIHISTAMINES.

Proprietary preparations: *Boots Tension Headache Relief (combined with paracetamol, caffeine, and codeine); *Vicks Cold & Flu Care Medinite Complete (combined with dextromethorphan, pseudoephedrine, and paracetamol).

Doxylar (Sandoz) *See* DOXYCYCLINE.

Dozic (Rosemont Pharmaceuticals) *See* HALOPERIDOL.

Drapolene Cream (Chefaro UK) A proprietary combination of the antiseptics *benzalkonium chloride and *cetrimide in a base that includes *white soft paraffin and wool fat (*see* LANOLIN), used as a *barrier preparation for the prevention and treatment of napkin rash. It is freely available *over the counter.

Driclor (Stiefel Laboratories) *See* ALUMINIUM CHLORIDE.

droperidol A butyrophenone *antipsychotic drug used as an *antiemetic for controlling nausea and vomiting induced by cytotoxic drugs in cancer patients. Droperidol is available, on *prescription only, as a form for intravenous injection.
Side effects: the most common side effects are drowsiness and low blood pressure.
Precautions: droperidol should not be given to patients who have certain types of arrhythmia (abnormal heartbeats) or are taking drugs that cause arrhythmias (see below). *See also* CHLORPROMAZINE HYDROCHLORIDE.
Interactions with other drugs:

Anaesthetics: their effect in lowering blood pressure is enhanced.
Anti-arrhythmic drugs: there is an increased risk of arrhythmias if droperidol is taken with amiodarone, disopyramide, or sotalol.
Antidepressants: there is an increased risk of arrhythmias if droperidol is taken with tricyclic antidepressants or SSRIs.
Antiepileptic drugs: their anticonvulsant effects are antagonized by droperidol.
Antipsychotic drugs: there is an increased risk of arrhythmias if droperidol is taken with amisulpride, pimozide, sertindole, sulpride, or phenothiazines.
Moxifloxacin: there is an increased risk of arrhythmias if this drug is taken with droperidol.
Ritonavir: may increase the effects of droperidol.
Sedatives: the sedative effects of droperidol are increased if it is taken with anxiolytic or hypnotic drugs, or any other drug that causes sedation.
Tacrolimus: increases the risk of arrhythmias.
Tamoxifen: increases the risk of arrhythmias.

Proprietary preparation: Xomolix.

drospirenone *See* ANGELIQ; YASMIN.

drotrecogin alfa A genetically engineered form of activated protein C, which has a role in blood clotting. It is used as an *adjunct in the treatment of severe sepsis (blood poisoning) resulting from the failure of at least two organs to function. Drotrecogin is given by intravenous infusion and is available on *prescription only.
Side effects: include bleeding and headache.
Precautions: drotrecogin should not be given to people with internal bleeding, brain tumours, platelet deficiency, or severe liver disease.

Interactions with other drugs:

Heparin: high doses should not be used with drotrecogin as this increases the risk of bleeding.

Proprietary preparation: Xigris.

Duac Once Daily (Stiefel Laboratories) A proprietary combination of *benzoyl peroxide (a keratolytic) and *clindamycin (an antibiotic), used to treat mild to moderate *acne. It is available as a gel on *prescription only.
Side effects and precautions: *see* BENZOYL PEROXIDE; CLINDAMYCIN.

Dubam Cream (Norma Chemicals) A proprietary combination of *methyl salicylate, *menthol, and cineole (*see* TURPENTINE OIL), used as a *rubefacient for the relief of aches, pains, and stiffness in muscles, tendons, and joints, including backache, sciatica, lumbago, and fibrositis. It is freely available *over the counter.
Side effects and precautions: *see* RUBEFACIENTS; SALICYLATES.

Dubam Spray (Norma Chemicals) A proprietary combination of *methyl salicylate, *ethyl salicylate, *methyl nicotinate, and *glycol salicylate, used as a *rubefacient for the relief of aches, pains, and stiffness in muscles, tendons and joints, including backache, sciatica, lumbago, and fibrositis. It is freely available *over the counter.
Side effects and precautions: *see* RUBEFACIENTS; SALICYLATES.

DulcoEase (Boehringer Ingelheim) *See* DOCUSATE SODIUM.

Dulcolax (Boehringer Ingelheim) *See* BISACODYL.

Dulcolax Liquid, Dulcolax Perles (Boehringer Ingelheim) *See* SODIUM PICOSULFATE.

duloxetine An *antidepressant that is related to the *SSRI group; it inhibits the reuptake of *serotonin and *noradrenaline. It used for the treatment of moderate to severe depression, generalized anxiety disorder, and pain caused by nerve damage in people with diabetes. Duloxetine is also used to treat stress incontinence in women. It is available as capsules on *prescription only.
Side effects: include fatigue, decreased appetite and weight loss, blurred vision, tremor, anxiety, palpitations, insomnia, abnormal dreams, headache, somnolence, dizziness, tinnitus, flushing, nausea, constipation, diarrhoea, vomiting, indigestion, sweating, rash, and abdominal pain.
Precautions: duloxetine should not be taken by people with liver or kidney disease or uncontrolled hypertension or by women who are pregnant or breastfeeding. It should be used with caution in people with a history of mania or a diagnosis of bipolar disorder and in people with raised pressure inside the eye.

Interactions with other drugs:

Monoamine oxidase inhibitors: should not be taken with duloxetine.

Proprietary preparations: Cymbalta; Yentreve.

Duodopa (Solvay Healthcare) *See* CO-CARELDOPA.

Duofilm (Stiefel Laboratories) A proprietary combination of *salicylic acid and *lactic acid (both keratolytics), used for the treatment of verrucas. It is available as a paint and can be obtained without a prescription, but only from pharmacies.
Side effects and precautions: *see* SALICYLIC ACID.

DuoTrav (Alcon Laboratories) A proprietary combination of *timolol maleate (a beta blocker) and *travoprost (a prostaglandin analogue), used to reduce the pressure in the eye in the treatment of *glaucoma and raised blood pressure in the eye. It is used when a beta blocker or rostaglandin alone have failed to reduce the pressure and is available as eye drops on *prescription only.
Side effects and precautions: *see* BETA BLOCKERS; TRAVOPROST.
Interactions with other drugs: *see* BETA BLOCKERS.

Duovent (Boehringer Ingelheim) A proprietary combination of *fenoterol hydrobromide and *ipratropium bromide (both bronchodilators), used for the treatment of asthma. It is available as a nebulizer solution on *prescription only.
Side effects: *see* SALBUTAMOL; IPRATROPIUM BROMIDE. An additional side effect may be glaucoma.
Precautions: *see* IPRATROPIUM BROMIDE; SALBUTAMOL.
Interactions with other drugs: *see* SALBUTAMOL.

Duphalac (Solvay Healthcare) *See* LACTULOSE.

Duraphat (Colgate-Palmolive) *See* FLUORIDE.

Durogesic DTrans (Janssen-Cilag) *See* FENTANYL.

dutasteride An *anti-androgen that acts by inhibiting the enzyme testosterone 5α-reductase and thus prevents the conversion of testosterone to the more active dihydrotestosterone. It is used for the treatment of benign enlargement of the prostate and is available as capsules on *prescription only.
Side effects: *see* FINASTERIDE.
Precautions: *see* FINASTERIDE. In addition, dutasteride should not be taken by people with severely impaired liver function.
Interactions with other drugs:
Antifungal drugs: the plasma concentration of dutasteride may be increased by ketoconazole, fluconazole, and itraconazole.
Antiviral drugs: the plasma concentration of dutasteride may be increased by indinavir and ritonavir.
Calcium antagonists: the plasma concentration of dutasteride may be increased by diltiazem and verapamil.
Proprietary preparation: Avodart.

Dyazide (Goldshield) A proprietary combination of *triamterene (a potassium-sparing diuretic) and *hydrochlorothiazide (a thiazide diuretic), used for the treatment of *hypertension or *oedema associated with heart

failure, liver disease, or kidney disease. It is available as tablets on *prescription only.
Side effects, precautions, and interactions with other drugs: *see* POTASSIUM-SPARING DIURETICS; THIAZIDE DIURETICS.
See also ANTIHYPERTENSIVE DRUGS; DIURETICS.

dydrogesterone A *progestogen used in conjunction with oestrogens in *hormone replacement therapy (HRT). Dydrogesterone is available as tablets on *prescription only.
Side effects, precautions, and interactions with other drugs: *see* PROGESTOGENS.
Proprietary preparations: *Femapak 40 (packaged with estradiol); *Femoston 2/10 (combined with estradiol); *Femoston-conti (combined with estradiol).

Dyloject (Javelin Pharmaceuticals) *See* DICLOFENAC SODIUM.

Dynastat (Pfizer) *See* PARECOXIB.

dyspepsia *See* ACID-PEPTIC DISEASES.

Dysport (Ipsen) *See* BOTULINUM TOXIN TYPE A.

Dytac (Goldshield) *See* TRIAMTERENE.

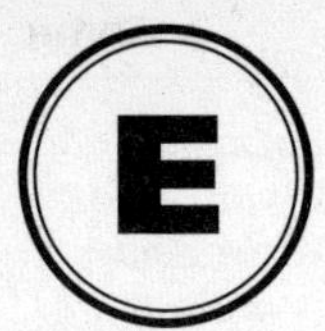

E45 Bath Oil (Forum Health Products) A proprietary combination of light *liquid paraffin (an emollient) and cetyl *dimeticone (a water repellent), used for the relief of *eczema and dry skin conditions. It is freely available *over the counter.

E45 Cream (Forum Health Products) A proprietary combination of *white soft paraffin, hypoallergenic *lanolin, and light *liquid paraffin (all emollients), used for the relief of *eczema and dry skin conditions. It is freely available *over the counter.

E45 Itch Relief Cream (Forum Health Products) A proprietary combination of *urea (an emollient) and *lauromacrogols (antipruritic agents), used to relieve itching and soothe irritated skin. It is freely available *over the counter.
Side effects: *see* LAUROMACROGOLS.
Precautionss: *see* UREA.

E45 Wash Cream (Forum Health Products) A proprietary combination of *zinc oxide (an astringent) and light *liquid paraffin (an emollient), used as a soap substitute for the relief of *eczema, dermatitis, and dry skin conditions (including ichthyosis and itching in the elderly). It is freely available *over the counter.

Earcalm Spray (GlaxoSmithKline) *See* ACETIC ACID.

Earex Ear Drops (SSL International) A proprietary combination of *arachis oil, *almond oil, and *camphor, used for the removal of earwax. It is freely available *over the counter.

Earex Plus Ear Drops (SSL International) A proprietary combination of *choline salicylate (an analgesic) and *glycerin, used for the removal of earwax and for the relief of irritation and inflammation of the outer ear. It is available from pharmacies without a prescription.
Precautions: frequent application should be avoided, and the drops should not be used in children under one year old.

Ebixa (Lundbeck) *See* MEMANTINE.

Ebufac (DDSA Pharmaceuticals) *See* IBUPROFEN.

Ecalta (Pfizer) *See* ANIDULAFUNGIN.

Eccoxolac (Meda Pharmaceuticals) *See* ETODOLAC.

Econac (Goldshield) *See* DICLOFENAC SODIUM.

econazole nitrate An imidazole *antifungal drug used for the treatment of candidiasis (thrush) of the vagina or penis, napkin rash infected with thrush, and fungal or bacterial skin infections (especially where skin surfaces touch, such as the groin, armpit, or between the toes). Available as *pessaries and as a cream for topical application, it can be obtained without a prescription, but only from pharmacies (Ecostatin pessaries and Gyno-Pevaryl are available on *prescription only).
Side effects: there may be local mild burning or irritation.
Precautions: the drug should not come in contact with the eyes or mucous membranes.
Interactions with other drugs:
Antipsychotic drugs: there is an increased risk of ventricular *arrhythmias if pimozide or sertindole are taken with econazole, and these drugs should not be used with it.
Ergotamine: its toxic effects are increased by econazole, and the two drugs should not be used together.
Reboxetine: should not be taken with econazole.
Tacrolimus: its plasma concentration may be increased by econazole.
Proprietary preparations: Gyno-Pevaryl 1 (cream or pessaries); Pevaryl (cream).

eculizumab A *monoclonal antibody used to reduce the destruction of red blood cells in people with paroxysmal nocturnal haemoglobinuria (a type of haemolytic *anaemia). To reduce the risk of meningococcal infection, all patients are vaccinated at least two weeks before treatment. Eculizumab is given by intravenous infusion and is available on *prescription only.
Side effects: include headache, dizziness, urinary and airways infections, nausea, vomiting, diarrhoea, and joint pain.
Precautions: eculizumab should not be given to breastfeeding women and should be used with caution during pregnancy and in people with active infections.
Proprietary preparation: Soliris.

eczema A common itchy skin disease characterized by reddening and vesicle formation, which may lead to weeping and crusting. It is endogenous, i.e. outside agents do not play a primary role, in contrast to **dermatitis**, in which similar symptoms result from contact with irritant substances. However, in some contexts the terms 'dermatitis' and 'eczema' are used interchangeably. There are several types of eczema, the most common of which is **atopic eczema**, which is usually associated with asthma and hay fever. **Seborrhoeic eczema** (or **dermatitis**) involves the scalp, eyelids, nose, and lips, and is associated with the presence of *Pityrosporum* yeasts. **Gravitational** (or **stasis**) **eczema**, incorrectly known as **varicose eczema**, is associated with poor circulation.

Treatment of eczema is with *topical steroids but *emollients are very important, especially in treating mild cases. Other treatments include *coal tar and *ichthammol. *Ciclosporin and *tacrolimus are reserved for severe atopic eczema that is resistant to other treatments. Severe eczema of the hands may be treated orally with *alitretinoin.

Edronax (Pharmacia) *See* REBOXETINE.

edrophonium A short-acting *anticholinesterase used for the diagnosis of myasthenia gravis. It acts by briefly increasing the level of interaction between nerves and muscles and can help distinguish between overdose and underdose of *cholinergic drugs used in the treatment of myasthenia. It is available as a form for injection on *prescription only.
Side effects and precautions: *see* NEOSTIGMINE.

efavirenz A non-nucleoside reverse transcriptase inhibitor (*see* ANTIVIRAL DRUGS) used, in combination with other antiretroviral drugs, in the treatment of HIV infection. It is available as capsules, tablets, and an oral solution on *prescription only.
Side effects: include rash, diarrhoea, nausea and vomiting, abdominal pain, anxiety, sleep disturbances, dizziness, headache, and lack of concentration.
Precautions: efavirenz should not be taken by breastfeeding women or by people with severe liver disease or porphyria. It should be used with caution in people with chronic hepatitis B or C, severe kidney disease, or a history of mental illness and in pregnant women.
Interactions with other drugs:
Antifungal drugs: efavirenz reduces plasma concentrations of itraconazole, posaconazole, and voriconazole (which increases the plasma concentration of efavirenz).
Antiviral drugs: efavirenz reduces plasma concentrations of several antivirals, including atazanavir, etravirine (which should not be taken with it), Kaletra, and maraviroc.
Ciclosporin: its plasma concentration may be reduced by efavirenz.
Ergotamine: its toxic effects are increased by efavirenz and the two drugs should not be taken together.
Midazolam: the risk of profound sedation is increased when it is taken with efavirenz; the two drugs should therefore not be taken together.
Pimozide: its plasma concentration and the risk of ventricular arrhythmias are increased; pimozide should therefore not be taken with efavirenz.
St John's wort: reduces plasma concentrations of efavirenz and should not be taken with it.
Proprietary preparations: Sustiva; *Atripla (combined with tenofovir disoproxil and emtricitabine).

Efcortesol (GlaxoSmithKline) *See* HYDROCORTISONE.

Effentora (Cephalon) *See* FENTANYL.

Effercitrate (Typharm) *See* POTASSIUM CITRATE.

Efient (Eli Lilly & Co) *See* PRASUGREL HYDROCHLORIDE.

eflornithine A drug used to reduce the growth of facial hair in women; it

works by inhibiting an enzyme in the hair follicles. Eflornithine is available as a cream on *prescription only.
Side effects: include acne, a stinging or burning sensation, itching, and rash.
Precautions: eflornithine should not be used by women who are pregnant or breastfeeding.
Proprietary preparation: Vaniqa.

eformoterol fumarate *See* FORMOTEROL FUMARATE.

Efracea (Galderma) *See* DOXYCYCLINE.

Efudix (Meda Pharmaceuticals) *See* FLUOROURACIL.

Elantan, Elantan LA (UCB Pharma) *See* ISOSORBIDE MONONITRATE.

Elaprase (Shire Pharmaceuticals) *See* IDURSULFASE.

Eldepryl (Orion Pharma) *See* SELEGILINE.

Eldisine (Baxter Healthcare) *See* VINDESINE SULPHATE.

Electrolade (Actavis) A proprietary combination of *sodium chloride, *potassium chloride, *sodium bicarbonate, and glucose, used to replace fluids and *electrolytes in cases of dehydration (*see* ORAL REHYDRATION THERAPY). It is freely available *over the counter as a flavoured powder to be dissolved in water.
Precautions: Electrolade should not be taken by people with kidney disease.

electrolyte A solution that produces ions (an ion is an atom or group of atoms that conduct electricity); for example, sodium chloride solution consists of free sodium and free chloride ions. In medical usage electrolyte usually means the ion itself; thus plasma electrolytes are the ions in the circulating blood, which include *sodium, *potassium, *calcium, chloride, bicarbonate, and phosphate. Electrolytes are essential for the normal functioning of cells: imbalances of electrolytes in the body can have serious consequences.

Measurement of plasma electrolytes forms part of a thorough medical examination. Concentrations of various electrolytes can be altered by many diseases in which electrolytes are lost from the body (as in vomiting or diarrhoea) or are not excreted and accumulate (as in kidney failure). Electrolyte depletion or retention can also be caused by drugs (e.g. *diuretics). When electrolyte concentrations are severely reduced they can be corrected by administering the appropriate substance by mouth or intravenously. Severe diarrhoea is also accompanied by dehydration: both fluids and electrolytes can be replaced by *oral rehydration therapy. Excess electrolytes in the blood can be removed by dialysis or by drugs, including special absorbent resins that are taken by mouth or by enema (*see* CALCIUM POLYSTYRENE SULPHONATE; SODIUM POLYSTYRENE SULPHONATE).

eletriptan An *$5HT_1$ agonist used to treat migraine headaches. It is available as tablets on *prescription only.

Side effects: include sensations of heaviness, pressure, heat, tingling, or tightness; if tightness in the chest or throat is severe, treatment should be stopped. Other side effects include flushing, fatigue, dizziness, abdominal pain, indigestion, dry mouth, headache, and drowsiness.
Precautions: eletriptan should not be taken by people who have previously had a stroke or a heart attack or by those with coronary artery disease, severe hypertension, arrhythmias, heart failure, peripheral artery disease, or severe liver or kidney disease. It should be used with caution in women who are pregnant or breastfeeding.
Interactions with other drugs:
Antibiotics: clarithromycin and erythromycin increase the plasma concentration of eletriptan and should not be taken with it.
Antifungal drugs: itraconazole and ketoconazole increase the plasma concentration (and adverse effects) of eletriptan and should not be used with it.
Antiviral drugs: indinavir, nelfinavir, and ritonavir increase the plasma concentration of eletriptan and should not be taken with it.
Ergotamine: its toxic effects are increased by eletriptan; ergotamine should not be started for 24 hours after stopping eletriptan, which should not be started for 24 hours after stopping ergotamine.
Proprietary preparation: Relpax.

Elidel (Novartis) *See* PIMECROLIMUS.

elixir A medicinal liquid preparation that is sweetened by the addition of alcohol or glycerin; these mask the taste of bitter or unpleasant drugs.

EllaOne (HRA Pharma) *See* ULIPRISTAL.

Elleste Duet (Meda Pharmaceuticals) A proprietary preparation of *estradiol tablets and *norethisterone tablets, used as sequential combined *hormone replacement therapy for the relief of menopausal symptoms in women who have not had a hysterectomy. The tablets, which are available on *prescription only, must be taken in the prescribed order.
Side effects, precautions, and interactions with other drugs: *see* HORMONE REPLACEMENT THERAPY.

Elleste Duet Conti (Meda Pharmaceuticals) A proprietary combination of *estradiol and *norethisterone, used as continuous combined *hormone replacement therapy for the relief of menopausal symptoms and prevention of osteoporosis in women who have not had a hysterectomy and who have not had a period for a year. It is available as tablets on *prescription only.
Side effects, precautions, and interactions with other drugs: *see* HORMONE REPLACEMENT THERAPY.

Elleste Solo, Elleste Solo MX (Meda Pharmaceuticals) *See* ESTRADIOL; HORMONE REPLACEMENT THERAPY.

Elliman's Universal Muscle Rub Lotion (Actavis) A proprietary combination of *acetic acid and *turpentine oil, used as a *rubefacient for the

relief of aches, pains, and stiffness of muscles, joints, and tendons, including backache, sciatica, lumbago, and fibrositis. It is freely available *over the counter.
Side effects and precautions: *see* RUBEFACIENTS.

Elocon (Schering-Plough) *See* MOMETASONE FUROATE.

Eloxatin (sanofi-aventis) *See* OXALIPLATIN.

Eltroxin (Goldshield) *See* LEVOTHYROXINE SODIUM.

Eludril Mouthwash (Pierre Fabre) A proprietary combination of the antiseptics *chlorobutanol and *chlorhexidine gluconate, used for the prevention and treatment of gingivitis (inflammation of the gums), mouth ulcers, *Candida* infections (thrush), and minor throat infections and for general oral hygiene. It is freely available *over the counter.
Precautions: this mouthwash is not recommended for children.

Eludril Spray (Pierre Fabre) A proprietary combination of *chlorhexidine gluconate (an antiseptic) and *tetracaine (a local anaesthetic), used for the treatment of mouth and throat conditions, such as gingivitis (inflammation of the gums), stomatitis (inflammation of the mouth lining), mouth ulcers, tonsillitis, and minor infections. It can be obtained from pharmacies without a prescription.
Precautions: Eludril Spray should not be used immediately before eating and is not suitable for children under 12 years old.

Elyzol (Colgate-Palmolive) *See* METRONIDAZOLE.

Emadine (Alcon Laboratories) *See* EMEDASTINE.

embrocation A lotion that is rubbed onto the body to treat sprains and strains. Embrocations usually include *rubefacients as ingredients.

Emcor, Emcor LS (Merck Serono) *See* BISOPROLOL FUMARATE.

emedastine An *antihistamine used to relieve the symptoms of seasonal allergic conjunctivitis. It is available as eye drops on *prescription only.
Side effects: include headache, eye irritation, and blurred vision.
Precautions: if blurring of vision occurs the eye drops should not be used while driving or operating heavy machinery.
Proprietary preparation: Emadine.

Emend (Merck Sharp & Dohlme) *See* APREPITANT.

Emeside (Chemidex Pharma) *See* ETHOSUXIMIDE.

emetics Drugs that induce vomiting. *Ipecacuanha was formerly used to empty the stomach after ingestion of a poisonous substance, although there is little evidence that it significantly reduces absorption of the poison. Apomorphine, solutions of common salt (sodium chloride), copper sulphate, and mustard are also emetics that should not be used in the treatment of poisoning.

Emflex (Merck Serono) *See* ACEMETACIN.

Emla (AstraZeneca) A proprietary combination of the local anaesthetics *lidocaine and *prilocaine, used for surface anaesthesia of the skin (for example, before taking blood samples) and of the genital area preparatory to removing genital warts. It is available as a cream without a *prescription, but only from pharmacies.
Side effects: include transient local pallor, redness, or swelling.
Precautions: Emla should not be applied to wounds or to mucous membranes other than the genital region and should not be used in children under one year old. It should be used with caution in people with anaemia (*see* PRILOCAINE).

e

emollients Agents that soothe and soften the skin. Emollients are oil-in-water emulsions (*creams) or greasy and insoluble in water (*ointments). They are used alone as moisturizers in the treatment of such conditions as *eczema and *psoriasis to lessen the need for, or complement, active drug therapy (such as corticosteroids) and in skin preparations as a base for a more active drug (such as an antibiotic). They either prevent water loss by forming a greasy layer to stop evaporation from the skin (e.g. *white soft paraffin) or improve the binding of water to the skin, in which case they are called **humectants** (e.g. *urea creams). *Liquid paraffin, *lanolin, and vegetable oils (such as *arachis oil, *almond oil, and *soya oil) are other commonly used emollients. Some emollients are applied directly to the skin; others are added to the bath or used in the shower, in some cases as a substitute for soap.

Emollin (CD Medical) A proprietary combination of *liquid paraffin and *white soft paraffin, used as an *emollient for treating dry skin conditions. It is available as a spray without a prescription.

Emselex (Novartis) *See* DARIFENACIN.

emtricitabine An antiretroviral drug (*see* ANTIVIRAL DRUGS) – a nucleoside reverse transcriptase inhibitor – used, in combination with other antiretroviral drugs, for the treatment of *HIV infection. It acts to prevent replication of HIV by blocking the action of the reverse transcriptase enzyme. Emtricitabine is available as capsules or an oral solution on *prescription only.
Side effects: include blood disorders, redistribution of body fat, insomnia, abnormal dreams, headache, dizziness, nausea, vomiting, diarrhoea, abdominal pain, disturbance of liver function, and itching.
Precautions: emtricitabine should be used with caution in people with chronic hepatitis B or C, impaired liver or kidney function, and during pregnancy. It should not be taken during breastfeeding or with *lamivudine.
Proprietary preparations: Emtriva; *Atripla (combined with tenofovir disoproxil and efavirenz); *Truvada (combined with tenofovir disoproxil).

Emtriva (Gilead Sciences) *See* EMTRICITABINE.

Emulsiderm (Dermal Laboratories) A proprietary combination of *liquid paraffin and *isopropyl myristate (both emollients) and *benzalkonium chloride (an antiseptic), used for the treatment of dry and itching skin conditions. It is freely available *over the counter in the form of a liquid to be rubbed into the skin or added to the bath.

emulsion A preparation in which fine droplets of one liquid (such as oil) are dispersed in another liquid (such as water). Medicines are prepared in the form of emulsions to disguise the taste of an oil, which is dispersed in a flavoured liquid.

enalapril maleate An *ACE inhibitor used as an adjunct to *diuretics for the treatment of *heart failure. It is also used to treat all grades of *hypertension. It is available, on *prescription only, as tablets.
Side effects, precautions, and interactions with other drugs: *see* ACE INHIBITORS.
Proprietary preparations: Innovace; *Innozide (combined with hydrochlorothiazide).

See also ANTIHYPERTENSIVE DRUGS.

Enbrel (Pfizer) *See* ETANERCEPT.

En-De-Kay, En-De-Kay Fluotabs (Manx) *See* FLUORIDE.

endometriosis The presence of tissue similar to the endometrium (lining of the uterus) at other sites in the pelvis, such as the wall of the uterus, the ovary, Fallopian tubes, or the peritoneum (membrane) lining the pelvis. This tissue undergoes the periodic changes similar to those of the endometrium and causes pelvic pain and painful periods. Drugs used in the treatment of endometriosis include *danazol, *gestrinone, some *gonadorelin analogues (including *leuprorelin, *nafarelin, and *triptorelin), and some progestogens (*see* MEDROXYPROGESTERONE; NORETHISTERONE).

enema A liquid infused into the rectum through a tube passed into the anus. Some drugs are administered in the form of enemas; for example, corticosteroids in the treatment of inflammatory bowel disease.

enfuvirtide An antiretroviral drug (*see* ANTIVIRAL DRUGS) used, in combination with other antiretroviral drugs, to treat *HIV infection when *first-line treatment has failed to achieve the desired response. It is available for subcutaneous injection on *prescription only.
Side effects: include sinusitis, ear infection, decreased appetite, weight loss, raised blood lipids, diabetes, anxiety, nightmares, irritability, peripheral neuropathy (causing numbness and tingling of the limbs), tremor, conjunctivitis, vertigo, and influenza-like symptoms.
Precautions: there is a risk of severe allergic reactions, including nausea, vomiting, chills, and low blood pressure; the treatment should be stopped if any symptoms develop. Enfuvirtide is not recommended for people with liver disease or for women who are pregnant or breastfeeding.
Proprietary preparation: Fuzeon.

Eno, Eno Lemon (GlaxoSmithKline) Proprietary combinations of *sodium

bicarbonate, sodium carbonate, and *citric acid used as an antacid for the relief of indigestion, flatulence, and nausea. They are freely available *over the counter in the form of effervescent powders.
Side effects, precautions, and interactions with other drugs: *see* ANTACIDS.

enoxaparin A *low molecular weight heparin used for the prevention and treatment of deep-vein *thrombosis and in the treatment of pulmonary embolism, heart attacks, and unstable coronary artery disease. It is also used in patients undergoing kidney dialysis, in order to prevent blood-clot formation. Enoxaparin is available as a solution for subcutaneous injection on *prescription only.
Side effects, precautions, and interactions with other drugs: *see* HEPARIN.
Proprietary preparation: Clexane.

enoximone A drug that acts on the heart muscles to strengthen the heartbeat and is used for the short-term treatment of congestive *heart failure. It is given by intravenous injection or infusion and is available on *prescription only.
Side effects: enoximone may cause abnormal heartbeats or (less commonly) low blood pressure, headache, insomnia, nausea, vomiting, and diarrhoea.
Precautions: enoximone should be used with caution in people with some types of heart disease (in whom heart and blood monitoring will be required during treatment) and in women who are pregnant or breastfeeding.
Interactions with other drugs:
Anagrelide: should not be taken with enoximone.

entacapone A *dopamine agonist that is used as an *adjunct to *levodopa (with carbidopa or benserazide) for treating Parkinson's disease when levodopa alone has become less effective in controlling symptoms. It is available as tablets on *prescription only.
Side effects: include nausea, vomiting, abdominal pain, constipation, diarrhoea, dry mouth, and abnormal involuntary movements; the urine may become reddish brown.
Precautions: entacapone should not be taken by women who are pregnant or breastfeeding or by people with liver disease or phaeochromocytoma (a tumour of the adrenal gland).
Interactions with other drugs:
Antidepressant drugs: tricyclic antidepressants, MAOIs, moclobemide, paroxetine, and venlafaxine should not be taken with entacapone.
Apomorphine: its effect may be increased by entacapone.
Iron: reduces the absorption of entacapone.
Methyldopa: its effect may be increased by entacapone.
Sympathomimetic drugs: the effects of adrenaline, noradrenaline, dobutamine, and dopamine may be increased by entacapone.
Warfarin: its anticoagulant effect is increased by entacapone.
Proprietary preparations: Comtess; *Stalevo (combined with co-careldopa); .

entecavir A nucleoside analogue (*see* ANTIVIRAL DRUGS) used in the

treatment of chronic hepatitis B infection. It is available as tablets or an oral solution on *prescription only.
Side effects: include headache, dizziness, somnolence, vomiting, diarrhoea, nausea, indigestion, fatigue, and insomnia.
Precautions: entecavir should not be taken by breastfeeding women. Liver function tests should be carried out in all patients every three months and the treatment stopped if liver function deteriorates. Entecavir should be used with caution in people with kidney disease and in pregnant women.
Proprietary preparation: Baraclude.

enteric-coated Describing tablets that are coated with a substance that enables them to pass through the stomach and into the intestine unchanged. Drugs contained in enteric-coated tablets may irritate the stomach, so that it is better for them to be released into the intestine (e.g. aspirin, prednisolone), or they may be destroyed by the acid contents of the stomach (e.g. pancreatin).

Entocort CR, Entocort Enema (AstraZeneca) *See* BUDESONIDE.

Epaderm (Mölnycke) A proprietary combination of *yellow soft paraffin, emulsifying wax, and *liquid paraffin in the form of an ointment, used as an *emollient and a soap substitute for the relief of dry skin conditions. It is freely available *over the counter.

Epanutin (Pfizer) *See* PHENYTOIN.

ephedrine hydrochloride A *sympathomimetic drug that relaxes smooth muscle and constricts blood vessels. It was formerly widely used as a *bronchodilator in the treatment of such conditions as asthma and chronic bronchitis, but has largely been replaced for treating these conditions by drugs that have fewer adverse effects. Its main use now is as a nasal *decongestant (alone or in combination with other drugs) and it is included as an ingredient in many medicines for treating colds and coughs. It is also used to reverse the low blood pressure induced by spinal or epidural anaesthesia. Ephedrine hydrochloride is available as tablets or an injection on *prescription only and as an *elixir or nose drops that can be bought from pharmacies without a prescription.
Side effects: with nose drops, side effects are rare; local irritation may occur. When taken by mouth fast heart rate, anxiety, restlessness, and insomnia are the most common side effects; the injection may cause nausea, vomiting, loss of appetite, dizziness, flushing, breathlessness, tremor, irregular heart rhythms, anxiety, and restlessness.
Precautions: when taken by mouth or given by injection, ephedrine should be used with caution in the elderly and in people with an overactive thyroid gland, diabetes mellitus, high blood pressure, heart disease, kidney disease, or an enlarged prostate gland. The injection should not be given to women who are breastfeeding.
Interactions with other drugs:
Antidepressant drugs: MAOIs and moclobemide may cause a dangerous rise in blood pressure.

Antihypertensive drugs: ephedrine may antagonize the effects of guanethidene and possibly other antihypertensive drugs in lowering blood pressure.

Rasagiline: should not be taken with ephedrine.

Proprietary preparations: CAM (sugar-free mixture); *Adult Meltus Chesty Coughs with Congestion (combined with guaifenesin); *Haymine (combined with chlorphenamine); *Vicks Cold & Flu Care Medinite Complete (combined with dextromethorphan, doxylamine, and paracetamol).

e

epilepsy *See* ANTICONVULSANT DRUGS.

Epilim (sanofi-aventis) *See* SODIUM VALPROATE.

Epilim Chrono (sanofi-aventis) A proprietary combination of *sodium valproate and valproic acid (anticonvulsants), used for the treatment of epilepsy. It is available for oral use as *modified-release tablets; a similar preparation, **Epilim Chronosphere**, is in the form of modified-release granules. Both preparations are *prescription only medicines.

Side effects, precautions, and interactions with other drugs: *see* SODIUM VALPROATE.

epinastine hydrochloride An *antihistamine used for the treatment of allergic conjunctivitis. It is available as eye drops on *prescription only.

Side effects: include a burning sensation, taste disturbance, and dry mouth.

Proprietary preparation: Relestat.

epinephrine *See* ADRENALINE.

Epipen (ALK) *See* ADRENALINE.

epirubicin A *cytotoxic antibiotic similar to *doxorubicin. It is given intravenously for the treatment of breast cancer and is instilled directly into the bladder to treat bladder cancer. Epirubicin is available as an injection on *prescription only.

Side effects and precautions: *see* DOXORUBICIN; CYTOTOXIC DRUGS.

Proprietary preparation: Pharmorubicin.

Episenta (Beacon Pharmaceuticals) *See* SODIUM VALPROATE.

Epivir (GlaxoSmithKline) *See* LAMIVUDINE.

eplerenone A *potassium-sparing diuretic that acts by inhibiting the activity of aldosterone, a hormone secreted by the adrenal gland that promotes potassium excretion and sodium retention by the kidneys. It is used as an *adjunct to control heart failure after a recent heart attack. Eplerenone is available as tablets on *prescription only.

Side effects: include raised blood levels of potassium, nausea, dizziness, low blood pressure, and rash.

Precautions: serum potassium levels must be monitored before and during treatment. This drug is not recommended for patients with severe liver or kidney disease.

Interactions with other drugs:
Antiepileptics: carbamazepine and phenytoin reduce the plasma concentration of eplerenone and should not be used with it.
Antifungal drugs: the plasma concentration of eplerenone is increased by itraconazole and ketoconazole, which should therefore not be used with it.
Antiviral drugs: the plasma concentration of eplerenone is increased by nelfinavir and ritonavir, which should therefore not be used with it.
Phenobarbital: reduces the plasma concentration of eplerenone and should not be used with it.
St John's wort: reduces the plasma concentration of eplerenone; the two drugs should not be used together.
Proprietary preparation: Inspra.

epoetin *See* ERYTHROPOIETIN.

epoprostenol An *antiplatelet drug that is used in patients undergoing kidney dialysis to prevent platelets aggregating and forming a blood clot; it may be given alone or with *heparin. Epoprostenol is also used, often with an anticoagulant, for tthe treatment of pulmonary hypertension (high blood pressure in the vessels supplying the lungs). It is available as a form for intravenous infusion on *prescription only.
Side effects: epoprostenol has a potent action in dilating blood vessels, causing headache, flushing, and low blood pressure; pallor, sweating, and slowing of the heart rate may occur with higher dosages.
Precautions: if epoprostenol is given with an anticoagulant, the clotting time of the patient's blood should be regularly monitored (*see* ANTICOAGULANTS).
Proprietary preparation: Flolan.

Eposin (medac GmbH) *See* ETOPOSIDE.

Eprex (Janssen-Cilag) *See* ERYTHROPOIETIN.

eprosartan An *angiotensin II inhibitor used for the treatment of essential *hypertension. It is available as tablets on *prescription only.
Side effects: include dizziness, joint pain, flatulence, and raised blood lipids.
Precautions: eprosartan should not be taken by women who are breastfeeding or pregnant or by people with severe liver disease.
Interactions with other drugs: *see* ACE INHIBITORS.
Proprietary preparation: Teveten.

Epsom salts *See* MAGNESIUM SULPHATE.

eptifibatide An *antiplatelet drug that is used to prevent heart attacks in people with unstable *angina who have had recent chest pain (within the preceding 24 hours). Eptifibatide is administered, under specialist supervision, as an intravenous injection followed by infusion. It is a *prescription only medicine.
Side effects and precautions: *see* TIROFIBAN.
Proprietary preparation: Integrilin.

Equasym, Equasym XL (Shire Pharmaceuticals) *See* METHYLPHENIDATE HYDROCHLORIDE.

Erbitux (Merck Serono) *See* CETUXIMAB.

erdosteine A *mucolytic drug that acts as an expectorant, used to relieve the symptoms of acute exacerbations of chronic bronchitis. It is available as capsules on *prescription only.
Precautions: erdosteine should not be taken by women who are breastfeeding. It is not recommended for people with severe kidney or liver disease or peptic ulcers or for pregnant women.
Proprietary preparation: Erdotin.

e

Erdotin (Galen) *See* ERDOSTEINE.

ergocalciferol (vitamin D_2) One of the D vitamins (*see* VITAMIN D), which is used for the treatment of simple vitamin D deficiency, such as that caused by lack of sunlight. Ergocalciferol is not available as plain tablets, so is usually given in combination with *calcium lactate and *calcium phosphate as **calcium and ergocalciferol** tablets, which are available without a prescription, but only from pharmacies. A form of ergocalciferol for injection is available on *prescription only (*see* CALCIFEROL).
Side effects, precautions, and interactions with other drugs: *see* VITAMIN D.

ergometrine maleate An *alkaloid that constricts blood vessels and also stimulates the uterus to contract. It is used in childbirth to bring about delivery of the placenta and, usually in conjunction with oxytocin, to stop bleeding due to an incomplete abortion. Ergometrine is also used to prevent or treat bleeding from the uterus after childbirth. For these purposes it is given by intravenous or intramuscular injection. Ergometrine is available, on *prescription only, as a solution for injection.
Side effects: include nausea, vomiting, headache, dizziness, tinnitus (the sensation of sounds in the ears), abdominal pain, chest pain, bouts of palpitation, breathlessness, a slow heart rate, and a temporary increase in blood pressure.
Precautions: ergometrine should not be given to women with severe heart or circulatory disease, severely impaired kidney or liver function, or very high blood pressure.
Interactions with other drugs:
Antiviral drugs: atazanavir and efavirenz increase the risk of ergometrine causing adverse effects and should not be used with it.
Proprietary preparation: *Syntometrine (combined with oxytocin).

ergotamine tartrate An alkaloid derived from the fungus ergot, used for the treatment of acute attacks of *migraine that have not responded to analgesics; it acts by constricting the arteries in the scalp. Because of the severity of its side effects, *$5HT_1$ agonists are usually preferred. Ergotamine is available, on *prescription only, as tablets or suppositories.
Side effects: include nausea, vomiting, abdominal pain, muscle cramps, and

(rarely) exacerbation of the headache. Ergotamine can cause vasospasm (constriction of the arteries) of the fingers and toes: if numbness or tingling of the fingers and toes develops, treatment should be stopped and a doctor informed.

Precautions: ergotamine should not be taken by people with heart disease, vascular disease (including Raynaud's syndrome), severe hypertension, liver or kidney disease, or an overactive thyroid gland, or by women who are pregnant or breastfeeding.

Interactions with other drugs:

Antibiotics: erythromycin, telithromycin, and possibly azithromycin increase the risk of ergot toxicity and should not be used with ergotamine.

Antiviral drugs: atazanavir, efavirenz, fosamprenavir, indinavir, nelfinavir, ritonavir, and saquinavir increase the risk of ergot toxicity and should not be taken with ergotamine.

Antifungal drugs: imidazoles and triazoles increase the risk of ergot toxicity and should not be taken with ergotamine.

Cimetidine: increases the risk of toxic effects of ergotamine and should not be used with it.

5HT$_1$ agonists: should not be taken with ergotamine since they increase the risk of vasospasm.

Proprietary preparations: Cafergot; *Migril (combined with cyclizine and caffeine).

erlotinib A *tyrosine kinase inhibitor that is used for the treatment of a type of lung *cancer that has not responded to previous chemotherapy and, in combination with *gemcitabine, for the treatment of pancreatic cancer. It is available as tablets on *prescription only.

Side effects: include rash, diarrhoea, fatigue, and loss of appetite. *See also* CYTOTOXIC DRUGS.

Precautions: erlotimib should not be taken by people with severe kidney disease or by women who are pregnant or breastfeeding. It should be used with caution in people with liver disease. *See also* CYTOTOXIC DRUGS.

Interactions with other drugs:

Clozapine: increases the risk of agranulocytosis (a blood disorder) and should not be taken with erlotinib.

NSAIDs: increase the risk of bleeding.

Warfarin: there is an increased risk of bleeding.

Proprietary preparation: Tarceva.

ertapenem sodium A beta-lactam *antibiotic used for the treatment of abdominal infections, community-acquired pneumonia, acute gynaecological infections, and foot infections in people with diabetes. It is available as a form for intravenous infusion on *prescription only.

Side effects: include headache, diarrhoea, nausea, vomiting, rash, itching, and a raised platelet count.

Precautions: there is a risk of *anaphylaxis, and ertapenem should not be given to people with a penicillin allergy. It is not recommended for pregnant or breastfeeding women and should be used with caution in the elderly and in people who have kidney disease or are liable to have seizures.

Interactions with other drugs:

Valproic acid: ertapenem may lower the plasma concentration of this drug.

Proprietary preparation: Invanz.

Erwinase (EUSA Pharma) *See* CRISANTASPASE.

Erymax (Cephalon) *See* ERYTHROMYCIN.

Erythrocin (Amdipharm) *See* ERYTHROMYCIN.

erythromycin The oldest and probably best known of the *macrolide antibiotics. A useful alternative to penicillins for treating patients who are allergic to these drugs, it is used to treat respiratory infections, whooping cough, syphilis, legionnaires' disease, gastrointestinal infections, and *acne. It is also effective against *Chlamydia* bacteria (which cause a variety of diseases, notably sexually transmitted conditions, parrot disease, and eye infections) and mycoplasmas (microorganisms that cause respiratory and genital infections). Erythromycin is also used with *neomycin to sterilize the gut before surgery. It is available, on *prescription only, as tablets, capsules, or a solution for oral use, an alcoholic solution or gel for topical application, or as a form for intravenous infusion.

Side effects: include nausea, vomiting, abdominal discomfort, diarrhoea, and rashes or other allergic reactions; reversible hearing loss may occur after large doses.

Precautions: erythromycin should be used with caution in those with liver impairment, kidney disease, heart conditions, or porphyria and in women who are pregnant or breastfeeding.

Interactions with other drugs:

Anti-arrhythmic drugs: erythromycin increases the risk of amiodarone causing arrhythmias and should not be used with it; plasma concentrations of disopyramide are increased, which may cause adverse effects.

Antipsychotic drugs: erythromycin increases the risk of amisulpride, pimozide, and zuclopenthixol causing *arrhythmias and should not be taken with them.

Atomoxetine: there is an increased risk of arrhythmias.

Carbamazepine: plasma concentrations of carbamazepine are increased.

Ciclosporin: plasma concentrations of ciclosporin are increased.

Cilostazol: its plasma concentration is increased and that of erythromycin reduced; the two drugs should therefore not be taken together.

Colchicine: its toxicity is increased.

Eletriptan: its plasma concentration is increased and it should not be taken with erythromycin.

Ergotamine: its risk of causing adverse effects is increased and it should not be taken with erythromycin.

Ivabradine: its risk of causing arrhythmias is increased and it should not be taken with erythromycin.

Midazolam: plasma concentrations of midazolam are increased, causing sedation.
Mizolastine: its plasma concentration may be increased and it should not be taken with erythromycin.
Moxifloxacin: there is an increased risk of arrhythmias and these two drugs should not be used together.
Pentamidine: there is an increased risk of arrhythmias.
Reboxetine: should not be taken with erythomycin.
Simvastatin: its risk of causing muscle damage is increased and it should not be taken with erythomycin.
Sirolimus: the plasma concentrations of both drugs are increased.
Tacrolimus: its plasma concentration is increased.
Theophylline: plasma concentrations of theophylline are increased.
Verapamil: its plasma concentration (and risk of causing adverse effects) is increased.
Vinblastine: its toxicity is increased and it should not be given with erythromycin.
Warfarin and acenocoumarol: plasma concentrations of these drugs are increased, which increases the risk of bleeding.

Proprietary preparations: Erymax; Erythrocin; Erythroped; Erythroped A; Stiemycin (topical solution); Tiloryth; *Aknemycin Plus (combined with tretinoin); *Zineryt (combined with zinc acetate).

Erythroped, Erythroped A (Amdipharm) *See* ERYTHROMYCIN.

erythropoietin A hormone produced naturally by the kidneys that stimulates the production of red blood cells by the bone marrow. Forms of erythropoietin (**epoetin alfa**, **beta**, and **zeta** and **darbepoetin**), produced by genetic engineering, and an erythropoietin receptor activator (**methoxy polyethylene glycol-epoetin beta**, or **pegzerepoetin alfa**) are used to treat *anaemia associated with chronic kidney failure and to shorten the period of anaemia in patients undergoing chemotherapy with platinum-containing drugs. They are given by subcutaneous or intravenous injection and are available on *prescription only.

Side effects: include diarrhoea, nausea, vomiting, raised blood pressure, headache, thrombosis, influenza-like symptoms, epileptic seizures, and rashes.

Precautions: erythropoietin should not be given to people with untreated high blood pressure. It should be used with caution in those with vascular disease, cancer, a history of epilepsy, or liver disease and in pregnant or breastfeeding women.

Proprietary preparations: Aranesp (darbepoetin alfa); Binocrit (epoetin alfa); Eprex (epoetin alfa); Mircera (pegzerepoetin alfa); NeoRecormon (epoetin beta); Retacrit (epoetin zeta).

escitalopram An *antidepressant drug of the *SSRI group: it is the active form of *citalopram. Escitalopram is used in the treatment of depressive

illness, anxiety and panic disorders, and obsessive-compulsive disorder. It is available as tablets and oral drops on *prescription only.
Side effects, and precautions: *see* SSRIs.
Interactions with other drugs: *see* CITALOPRAM.
Proprietary preparation: Cipralex.

esmolol hydrochloride A cardioselective *beta blocker used for the treatment and prevention of heart *arrhythmias and the treatment of *hypertension that occurs after surgery. It is available as a solution for intravenous infusion on *prescription only. Since it has a very short duration of action it is usually reserved for diagnostic use in the short term. After stabilization of the heart rate transition is usually made to oral medication.
Side effects, precautions, and interactions with other drugs: *see* BETA BLOCKERS.
Proprietary preparation: Brevibloc.

esomeprazole A *proton pump inhibitor used for the treatment of reflux oesophagitis, gastric and duodenal ulcers (including those associated with *Helicobacter pylori* infection and the use of *NSAIDs), and Zollinger-Ellison syndrome (*see* ACID-PEPTIC DISEASES). It is a *prescription only medicine, available as tablets, granules, and as a form for intravenous injection or infusion.
Side effects: *see* PROTON PUMP INHIBITORS. There may also be nausea, constipation, dizziness, itching, and allergic reactions, and the skin may become sensitive to sunlight.
Precautions: *see* PROTON PUMP INHIBITORS.
Interactions with other drugs:

Antiplatelet drugs: the effects of clopidrogel and prasugrel may be reduced and these drugs should not be taken with esomeprazole.
Phenytoin: its effect is enhanced by esomeprazole.
Tipranavir: reduces the plasma concentration of esomeprazole.
Warfarin: its effect may be enhanced by esomeprazole.

Proprietary preparation: Nexium.

Estracyt (Pharmacia) *See* ESTRAMUSTINE.

Estraderm MX, Estraderm TTS (Novartis) *See* ESTRADIOL; HORMONE REPLACEMENT THERAPY.

estradiol <**oestradiol**> One of the female sex hormones produced by the ovaries (*see* OESTROGENS). It is used mainly for *hormone replacement therapy (HRT), either alone or in combination with a *progestogen. Estradiol is available, on *prescription only, as tablets, a gel or patches to be applied to the skin, or as a vaginal ring or tablets.
Side effects, precautions, and interactions with other drugs: *see* HORMONE REPLACEMENT THERAPY.
Proprietary preparations: Climaval; Elleste Solo; Elleste Solo MX; Estraderm TTS, Estraderm MX; Estradiol Implants; Estradot; Estring; Evorel; Fematrix; FemSeven; Oestrogel; Progynova; Progynova TS; Sandrena; Vagifem;

Zumenon; *Angeliq (combined with drospirenone); *Climagest (packaged with norethisterone); *Climesse (combined with norethisterone); *Clinorette (combined with norethisterone); *Cyclo-Progynova (combined with levonorgestrel); *Elleste Duet (packaged with norethisterone); *Elleste Duet Conti (combined with norethisterone); *Evorel Conti (combined with norethisterone); *Evorel Sequi (combined with norethisterone); *Femapak 40 (packaged with dydrogesterone); *Femoston 2/10 (packaged with dydrogesterone); *Femoston-conti (packaged with dydrogesterone); *Hormonin (combined with estriol and estrone); *Indivina 1 mg/2.5 mg (combined with medroxyprogesterone); *Kliofem (combined with norethisterone); *Kliovance (combined with norethisterone); *Novofem (combined with norethisterone); *Qlaira (combined with dienogest); *Tridestra (packaged with medroxyprogesterone); *Trisequens (packaged with norethisterone). See table at *hormone replacement therapy.

Estradiol Implants (Organon) *See* ESTRADIOL; HORMONE REPLACEMENT THERAPY.

Estradot (Novartis) *See* ESTRADIOL; HORMONE REPLACEMENT THERAPY.

estramustine An oestrogenic *alkylating drug (a combination of chlormethine and an oestrogen) used for the treatment of prostate *cancer. It is available as capsules on *prescription only.
Side effects: include nausea and vomiting, impairment of liver function, enlargement of the breasts, and (rarely) angina. *See also* CYTOTOXIC DRUGS.
Precautions: estramustine should not be taken by people with peptic ulcers, severe liver disease, or severe heart disease. *See also* CYTOTOXIC DRUGS.
Interactions with other drugs:
Clozapine: increases the risk of agranulocytosis (a blood disorder) and therefore should not be taken with estramustine.
Sodium clodronate: increases the plasma concentration of estramustine.
Proprietary preparation: Estracyt.

Estring (Pharmacia) *See* ESTRADIOL; HORMONE REPLACEMENT THERAPY.

estriol <**oestriol**> One of the female sex hormones produced by the ovaries (*see* OESTROGENS). It is used in *hormone replacement therapy, mainly for the local relief of wasting or inflammation of the vagina, shrinkage or itching of the vulva (external genitals), or pain on intercourse, in menopausal and postmenopausal women. Estriol is available as pessaries or a cream on *prescription only.
Side effects, precautions, and interactions with other drugs: *see* OESTROGENS; HORMONE REPLACEMENT THERAPY.
Proprietary preparations: Gynest (cream); Ortho-Gynest (pessaries or cream); Ovestin (cream); *Hormonin (combined with estradiol and estrone); *Trisequens (combined with estradiol).

estrone <**oestrone**> One of the female sex hormones produced by the ovaries (*see* OESTROGENS). Combined with other oestrogens, it is used in

*hormone replacement therapy for the relief of menopausal symptoms and prevention of osteoporosis. It is available on *prescription only. *See also* ESTROPIPATE.
Side effects, precautions, and interactions with other drugs: *see* HORMONE REPLACEMENT THERAPY.
Proprietary preparation: *Hormonin (combined with estriol and estradiol).

estropipate A semisynthetic *oestrogen that is converted to *estrone in the body. It is used as *hormone replacement therapy to relieve menopausal symptoms and to prevent postmenopausal osteoporosis. Women who have not had a hysterectomy may also need to take *progestogen supplements. Estropipate is available as tablets on *prescription only.
Side effects, precautions, and interactions with other drugs: *see* HORMONE REPLACEMENT THERAPY.
Proprietary preparation: Harmogen.

etamsylate **<ethamsylate>** A *haemostatic drug that reduces bleeding in capillaries (very small blood vessels); it acts by improving the ability of platelets to stick together, which is part of the normal blood-clotting process. Etamsylate is taken for the short-term treatment of blood loss due to heavy periods. It is available, on *prescription only, as tablets.
Side effects: include nausea, headache, and rashes.
Precautions: etamsylate should not be given to people with porphyria.
Proprietary preparation: Dicynene.

etanercept A *disease-modifying antirheumatic drug (DMARD) used alone or in combination with other drugs to treat rheumatoid arthritis, psoriatic arthritis, juvenile arthritis, *psoriasis, and ankylosis spondylitis (a type of arthritis affecting the spine). It is available as a form for subcutaneous injection on *prescription only.
Side effects: include infections, allergic reactions, itching, nausea, abdominal pain, fever, headache, and blood disorders.
Precautions: etanercept should not be given to people with active infections or by pregnant or breastfeeding women. It should be used with caution in patients with tuberculosis.
Interactions with other drugs: *see* ADALIMUMAB.
Proprietary preparation: Enbrel.

ethambutol hydrochloride An *antibiotic that inhibits the growth of the bacterium that causes *tuberculosis. It is used in combination with other drugs to treat tuberculosis, especially when resistance to the common drugs is suspected, but it may cause visual damage, which limits its use. A *prescription only medicine, it is available as tablets.
Side effects: include inflammation of the optic nerve (causing blurred vision) and red/green colour blindness. Any visual changes should be reported to a doctor immediately.
Precautions: ethambutol should be used with caution in children under six

years old, who cannot report visual symptoms reliably, in people with kidney disease, and in women who are pregnant or breastfeeding.

ethamsylate *See* ETAMSYLATE.

ethanolamine oleate An irritant substance that is used in *sclerotherapy to treat varicose veins. It is available, on *prescription only, as a solution for slow injection into the affected vein.
Side effects: ethanolamine oleate may cause allergic reactions, and if it leaks out of the vein it may damage surrounding tissue.
Precautions: ethanolamine oleate should not be used in people who cannot walk, or have obese legs or acutely inflamed veins, or by women taking oral contraceptives.

e

Ethibide XL (Baxter Healthcare) *See* INDAPAMIDE.

ethinylestradiol <**ethinyloestradiol**> A synthetic *oestrogen that is used mainly in combination with *progestogens in *oral contraceptives. Alone, it is used to treat menstrual disorders, certain types of female infertility, oestrogen deficiency (in the short term), and prostate cancer and to prevent postmenopausal osteoporosis if other treatment cannot be used. A *prescription only medicine, ethinylestradiol in nonproprietary form is available as tablets.
Side effects: include nausea, fluid retention, and (in men) impotence and enlargement of the breasts. *See also* OESTROGENS; ORAL CONTRACEPTIVES.
Precautions: ethinylestradiol should be used with caution by people with cardiovascular disease or jaundice. *See also* OESTROGENS; ORAL CONTRACEPTIVES.
Interactions with other drugs: *see* OESTROGENS.
Proprietary preparations: *Acnocin (combined with cyproterone acetate); *BiNovum (combined with norethisterone); *Brevinor (combined with norethisterone); *Cilest (combined with norgestimate); *Dianette (combined with cyproterone acetate); *Evra (combined with norelgestromin); *Femodene (combined with gestodene); *Loestrin 20 and Loestrin 30 (combined with norethisterone); *Logynon (combined with levonorgestrel); *Marvelon (combined with desogestrel); *Mercilon (combined with desogestrel); *Microgynon 30 (combined with levonorgestrel); *Norimin (combined with norethisterone); *NuvaRing (combined with etonogestrel); *Ovranette (combined with levonorgestrel); *Ovysmen (combined with norethisterone); *Sunya 20/75 (combined with gestodene); *Synphase (combined with norethisterone); *Triadene (combined with gestodene); *TriNovum (combined with norethisterone); *Yasmin (combined with drospirenone). See table at *oral contraceptives.

ethosuximide An *anticonvulsant drug used for the treatment of absence seizures. It is available, on *prescription only, as capsules or a syrup.
Side effects: include gastrointestinal upsets, weight loss, drowsiness, dizziness, shaky movements, hiccups, headache, depression, and skin rashes.
Precautions: ethosuximide should be used with caution in people who have

liver or kidney disease and in women who are pregnant or breastfeeding; women who are planning to become pregnant should seek specialist advice. Fever, sore throat, mouth ulcers, or bruising should be reported to a doctor as they may indicate a blood disorder.

Interactions with other drugs:

Antidepressants: reduce the anticonvulsant effect of ethosuximide.

Antipsychotics: may reduce the anticonvulsant effect of ethosuximide.

Isoniazid: increases the plasma concentration (and risk of adverse effects) of ethosuximide.

Mefloquine: reduces the anticonvulsant effect of ethosuximide.

Phenytoin: may reduce the plasma concentration (and anticonvulsant effect) of ethosuximide and its own plasma concentration may be increased.

Proprietary preparations: Emeside; Zarontin.

ethyl nicotinate A drug that is used as a *rubefacient for the relief of muscular aches and pains. It is an ingredient of creams and sprays that are freely available *over the counter.

Side effects and precautions: *see* RUBEFACIENTS.

Proprietary preparations: *Boots Pain Relief Warming Spray (combined with methyl salicylate and camphor); *Pain Relief Balm (combined with glycol salicylate and nonylic acid vanillylamide); *PR Heat Spray (combined with methyl salicylate and camphor); *Transvasin Heat Rub (combined with hexyl nicotinate and tetrahydrofurfuryl salicylate).

ethyl salicylate A *salicylate that is used as an ingredient of several *rubefacient sprays for the relief of aches, pains, and stiffness in muscles, joints, and tendons. It is freely available *over the counter.

Side effects and precautions: *see* SALICYLATES.

Proprietary preparations: *Deep Heat Spray (combined with glycol salicylate, methyl salicylate, and methyl nicotinate); *Dubam Spray (combined with methyl salicylate, glycol salicylate, and methyl nicotinate).

ethynodiol diacetate *See* ETYNODIOL DIACETATE.

etidronate disodium *See* DISODIUM ETIDRONATE.

etodolac An *NSAID used to relieve pain and inflammation in rheumatoid arthritis and osteoarthritis. It is available as capsules and *modified-release tablets on *prescription only.

Side effects: *see* NSAIDs. There may also be palpitations, breathlessness, 'pins and needles', tremor, frequency in passing urine, and itching.

Precautions and interactions with other drugs: *see* NSAIDs.

Proprietary preparations: Eccoxolac (capsules); Etopan XL (modified-release tablets); Lodine SR (modified-release tablets).

etonogestrel A synthetic *progestogen used as a *depot contraceptive in the form of an implant and (in combination with an oestrogen) a vaginal ring. The implant is a flexible rod that is inserted under the skin of the upper arm

between days 1 and 5 of the menstrual cycle. It can remain in place for three years. Etonogestrel is available on *prescription only.
Side effects, precautions, and interactions with other drugs: *see* PROGESTOGENS.
Proprietary preparations: Implanon; *NuvaRing (combined with ethinylestradiol).

Etopan XL (Taro) *See* ETODOLAC.

Etopophos (Bristol-Myers Squibb) *See* ETOPOSIDE.

etoposide A *cytotoxic drug, derived from an extract of the American mandrake plant, that is similar to the *vinca alkaloids. It acts by causing breaks in DNA so that cell replication cannot take place. Etoposide is used for the treatment of lymphomas, some forms of lung cancer, testicular cancer, acute leukaemias, and brain tumours (*see* CANCER). It is available, on *prescription only, as capsules or a form for intravenous infusion.
Side effects: include hair loss, *bone marrow suppression, nausea, and vomiting; there may be pain and irritation at the injection site. *See also* CYTOTOXIC DRUGS.
Precautions: etoposide should not be taken by women who are pregnant or breastfeeding or by people with severe liver disease.
Interactions with other drugs:

Anticoagulants: the effects of warfarin and acenocoumarol may be enhanced.

Clozapine: increases the risk of agranulocytosis (a blood disorder) and therefore should not be taken with etoposide.

Proprietary preparations: Eposin; Etopophos; Vepesid.

etoricoxib A COX-2 inhibitor (*see* NSAIDs) used to relieve pain and inflammation in the treatment of osteoarthritis, rheumatoid arthritis, ankylosing spondylitis (a type of arthritis of the spine), and acute gout. It is available as tablets on *prescription only.
Side effects: *see* NSAIDs.
Precautions: *see* NSAIDs. In addition, etoricoxib should not be taken by people with inflammatory bowel disease, heart failure, poorly controlled hypertension, coronary artery disease, peripheral artery disease, or cerebrovascular disease.
Interactions with other drugs: *see* NSAIDs; CELECOXIB.
Proprietary preparation: Arcoxia.

etravirine A non-nucleoside antiretroviral drug (*see* ANTIVIRAL DRUGS) that inhibits reverse transcriptase by binding directly to the enzyme, thus blocking the synthesis of retroviral DNA and preventing viral replication. It is used, in combination with other antiretroviral drugs, in the treatment of *HIV infection that has not responded to other non-nucleoside reverse transcriptase inhibitors (NNRTIs) or protease inhibitors. It is available as tablets on *prescription only.
Side effects: include rash, regurgitation of stomach acid, hypertension, raised

blood lipids, anaemia, peripheral neuropathy (causing numbness and tingling of the limbs), diabetes, blood disorders, and insomnia.
Precautions: etravirine is not recommended for women who are breastfeeding or for people who suffer from acute porphyria. It should be used with caution in people with chronic hepatitis B or C or liver disease and in pregnant women.
Interactions with other drugs: etravirine should not be taken with other NNRTIs or with certain protease inhibitors (e.g. tipranavir), antiepileptic drugs (e.g. phenytoin, carbamazepine) or antimicrobial drugs (e.g. rifabutin).
Proprietary preparation: Intelence.

Etrivex (Galderma) *See* CLOBETASOL PROPIONATE.

etynodiol diacetate <**ethynodiol diacetate**> A synthetic *progestogen used in progestogen-only *oral contraceptives. It is available as tablets on *prescription only.
Side effects, precautions, and interactions with other drugs: *see* PROGESTOGENS.
Proprietary preparation: Femulen.

eucalyptol *See* EUCALYPTUS OIL.

eucalyptus oil An aromatic oil with a cooling effect, distilled from the leaves of various species of eucalyptus tree; its main constituent is **cineole** (or **eucalyptol**). It is used, often in combination with *menthol and/or other volatile substances, in inhalations and other remedies to relieve the congestion associated with colds and catarrh. It is also an ingredient of *rubefacient preparations for the relief of muscular aches and pains. Most preparations containing eucalyptus oil are freely available *over the counter.
Side effects: eucalyptus oil is poisonous in overdose.
Proprietary preparations: *Boots Chillblain Cream (combined with benzyl alcohol); *Boots Mild Vapour Rub 3 Months Plus (combined with levomenthol and racemic camphor); *Boots Vapour Chest Rub (combined with levomenthol and camphor); *Deep Heat Rub (combined with methyl salicylate, menthol, and turpentine oil); *Non-Drowsy Sudafed Inhalant Oil (combined with racemic camphor, menthol, and peppermint oil); *Olbas Oil (combined with menthol, cajuput oil, clove oil, and juniper berry oil); *Olbas Pastilles (combined with menthol, peppermint oil, clove oil, and juniper berry oil); *Vicks Vaporub (combined with turpentine oil, camphor, and menthol).

Eucardic (Roche Products) *See* CARVEDILOL.

Eucerin (Beiersdorf) *See* UREA.

Eucreas (Novartis) A proprietary combination of *metformin hydrochloride and *vildagliptin (oral hypoglycaemic drugs), used for treating type 2 *diabetes mellitus that is not controlled with metformin alone. It is available as tablets on *prescription only.
Side effects and precautions: *see* METFORMIN HYDROCHLORIDE; VILDAGLIPTIN.
Interactions with other drugs: *see* METFORMIN HYDROCHLORIDE.

Eudemine (Goldshield) *See* DIAZOXIDE.

Eumocream (GlaxoSmithKline) *See* GLYCERIN.

Eumovate (GlaxoSmithKline) *See* CLOBETASONE BUTYRATE.

Eurax (Novartis) *See* CROTAMITON.

Eurax-Hydrocortisone (Novartis) A proprietary combination of *crotamiton (a soothing agent) and *hydrocortisone (a corticosteroid), used for the treatment of itching skin conditions. It is available as a cream on *prescription only. **Eurax Hc**, which is packaged in a 15-gram tube, is available from pharmacies without a prescription.
Side effects and precautions: *see* TOPICAL STEROIDS; CROTAMITON.

evening primrose oil An oil pressed from the seeds of the evening primrose plant (*Oenothera biennis*), which is rich in the polyunsaturated fatty acids linoleic acid and gamma linolenic acid. It is used as an *emollient for the treatment of dry skin conditions and is available as a cream without a prescription.
Precautions: the cream should be used with caution by people with epilepsy.
Proprietary preparation: Linola Gamma (Gammaderm).

everolimus An anticancer drug used for the treatment of advanced renal cell carcinoma (a malignant tumour of kidney cells) that has progressed after treatment with other anticancer therapies. It is a *tyrosine kinase inhibitor that reduces levels of *vascular endothelial growth factor (VEGF); thus it inhibits the growth and proliferation of tumour cells. Everolimus is available as tablets on *prescription only.
Side effects: include infections, anaemia, raised blood levels of glucose and lipids, loss of appetite, dehydration, insomnia, abnormal taste, headache, conjunctivitis, hypertension, breathlessness, cough, diarrhoea, vomiting, nausea, dry mouth, abdominal pain, indigestion, rash, dry skin, itching, fatigue, chest pain, fever, and weight loss.
Precautions: everolimus is not recommended for use in children and adolescents, in people with severely impaired liver function, or during pregnancy or breastfeeding. Women capable of bearing children should use contraception. The dose of everolimus should be reduced in people with moderately impaired liver function. The use of live vaccines should be avoided during treatment.
Interactions with other drugs:
Erythromycin: increases the plasma concentration of everolimus.
Ketoconazole: increases the plasma concentration of everolimus.
Rifampicin: decreases the plasma concentration of everolimus.
Verapamil: increases the plasma concentration of everolimus.
Proprietary preparation: Afinitor.

Evista (Daiichi Sankyo UK Ltd) *See* RALOXIFENE.

Evoltra (Genzyme Therapeutics) *See* CLOFARABINE.

Evorel (Janssen-Cilag) *See* ESTRADIOL; HORMONE REPLACEMENT THERAPY.

Evorel Conti (Janssen-Cilag) A proprietary combination of *estradiol and *norethisterone used as continuous combined *hormone replacement therapy for the relief of menopausal symptoms and prevention of osteoporosis in women who have not had a hysterectomy and who have not had a period for a year. It is available as skin patches on *prescription only.
Side effects, precautions, and interactions with other drugs: *see* HORMONE REPLACEMENT THERAPY.

Evorel Sequi (Janssen-Cilag) A proprietary preparation of *estradiol skin patches and combined estradiol/*norethisterone skin patches used as sequential combined *hormone replacement therapy for the relief of menopausal symptoms in women who have not had a hysterectomy. The patches, which are available on *prescription only, must be applied in the prescribed order.
Side effects, precautions, and interactions with other drugs: *see* HORMONE REPLACEMENT THERAPY.

Evra (Janssen-Cilag) A proprietary combination of *ethinylestradiol (an oestrogen) and norelgestromin (a *progestogen), used as a contraceptive in the form of transdermal (skin) patches. It is available on *prescription only.
Side effects and precautions: *see* ETHINYLESTRADIOL, PROGESTOGENS.
Interactions with other drugs: *see* OESTROGENS, PROGESTOGENS.

excipient A substance that is combined with a drug in order to render it suitable for administration; examples are preservatives included in eye drops and skin preparations. Excipients should have no pharmacological action themselves, but some may cause allergic reactions in sensitive individuals (e.g. parabens (preservatives) and lanolin in creams and ointments).

Exelderm (Centrapharm) *See* SULCONAZOLE.

Exelon (Novartis) *See* RIVASTIGMINE.

exemestane An *aromatase inhibitor used for the teatment of early breast cancer in postmenopausal women following 2–3 years of initial *tamoxifen therapy, and for the treatment of advanced breast cancer in postmenopausal women that has progressed following therapy with tamoxifen or other *oestrogen antagonists. It is available as tablets on *prescription only.
Side effects: include loss of appetite, insomnia, depression, headache, dizziness, hot flushes, nausea, abdominal pain, vomiting, constipation, indigestion, diarrhoea, sweating, rash, and hair loss.
Precautions: exemestane should not be taken by women who have not reached menopause or by women who are pregnant or breastfeeding. It should be used with caution in women with liver or kidney disease.
Interactions with other drugs:

Clozapine: increases the risk of agranulocytosis (a blood disorder); the two drugs should therefore not be used together.
Phenytoin: reduces the absorption of exemestane.

Sodium clodronate: may increase the plasma concentration of exemestane.
Proprietary preparation: Aromasin.

exenatide An antidiabetic drug that increases the secretion of *insulin from pancreatic beta cells. It is used in combination with metformin and/or sulphonylureas (*oral hypoglycaemic drugs) for the treatment of type 2 *diabetes mellitus in people whose blood-glucose levels have not been controlled by these oral medicines alone. Exenatide is available as a subcutaneous injection on *prescription only.
Side effects: include low blood-glucose levels, nausea, vomiting, diarrhoea, decreased appetite, headache, dizziness, indigestion, abdominal pain, and abdominal distension.
Precautions: exenatide should not be given to people with type 1 diabetes or ketoacidosis or to people with severe kidney disease, severe gastrointestinal disease, or pancreatitis. It should not be used during pregnancy or breastfeeding.
Interactions with other drugs:
Warfarin: its anticoagulant effect may be increased by exenatide.
Proprietary preparation: Byetta.

Exforge (Novartis) A proprietary combination of *valsartan (an angiotensin II inhibitor) and *amlodipine (a calcium antagonist), used to treat *hypertension. It is available as tablets on *prescription only.
Side effects: *see* ANGIOTENSIN II INHIBITORS; CALCIUM ANTAGONISTS.
Precautions: *see* AMLODIPINE; ANGIOTENSIN II INHIBITORS.
Interactions with other drugs: *see* ACE INHIBITORS; CALCIUM ANTAGONISTS.

Exjade (Novartis) *See* DEFERASIROX.

Ex-Lax Senna (Novartis) *See* SENNA.

Exocin (Allergan) *See* OFLOXACIN.

Exorex (Forrest Laboratories) *See* COAL TAR.

expectorants Drugs that are claimed to decrease the viscosity and increase the volume of mucus in the airways, making it more watery and therefore easier to expel by coughing. Drugs used orally as expectorants irritate the lining of the stomach, which has been said to provide a stimulus for the reflex production of fluid by the glands of the airways. However, there is no evidence that any expectorant works. Expectorants are usually given to relieve chesty productive coughs, but may also be used to increase the secretion of liquid mucus in irritating dry coughs. They include *ammonium chloride, **ammonium acetate**, **ammonium carbonate**, *guaifenesin, **guaiacol**, *ipecacuanha, and *squill, which are incorporated into many proprietary medicines for treating coughs and colds. *Compare* MUCOLYTIC DRUGS.

Extavia (Novartis) *See* INTERFERON BETA.

Exterol (Dermal Laboratories) A proprietary combination of *urea hydrogen

peroxide and *glycerin, used for the softening and removal of earwax. It is available without a prescription, but only from pharmacies.
Side effects: there may be mild effervescence on application and the drops may cause irritation.
Precautions: Exterol should not be used on perforated eardrums.

extrapyramidal reactions A group of reactions caused by a reduction in the activity of the neurotransmitter *dopamine in the brain. This can result from disease (such as Parkinson's disease) or from taking drugs that antagonize the action of dopamine. Drugs having this effect include *antipsychotic drugs and *metoclopramide (an antiemetic). Extrapyramidal reactions consist of tremor, rigidity, and other symptoms of parkinsonism, abnormal face and body movements (such as twisting of the neck, rolling eyes, and writhing movements of the arms), restlessness, and uncontrolled movements of the jaws, tongue, lips, cheeks, and limbs. Drug-induced extrapyramidal reactions are more common in children and young adults and are dose-related. If alternative drugs that do not cause these reactions cannot be used, the reactions can be prevented or treated with *orphenadrine or *procyclidine.

ezetimibe A *lipid-lowering drug that lowers cholesterol levels (*see* HYPERLIPIDAEMIA) by decreasing cholesterol absorption in the intestine. It can be used either alone or in combination with other cholesterol-lowering drugs (usually a *statin). Ezetimibe is available as tablets on *prescription only.
Side effects: include stomach upsets, headache, fatigue, and muscle pain.
Precautions: ezetimibe should not be taken by people with moderate or severe liver disease. It should be used with caution in women who are pregnant or breastfeeding.
Interactions with other drugs:
Ciclosporin: the plasma concentrations of both drugs may increase.
Proprietary preparation: Ezetrol; *Inegy (combined with simvastatin).

Ezetrol (Schering-Plough) *See* EZETIMIBE.

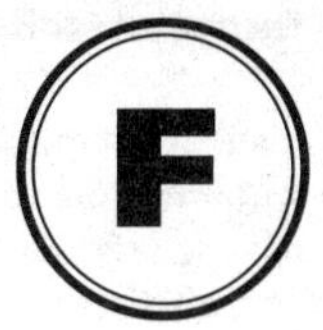

Fabrazyme (Genzyme Therapeutics) *See* AGALSIDASE.

Factor VIIa One of the factors involved in the complex process of blood clotting. Recombinant Factor VIIa, prepared by genetic engineering techniques, is used to control bleeding in people with haemophilia who have developed antibodies to *Factor VIII and *Factor IX. A *prescription only medicine, it is available in a form for injection for use in specialist centres.
Side effects: skin irritation, nausea, fever, malaise, and changes in blood pressure may very rarely occur.
Proprietary preparation: NovoSeven.

Factor VIII (**antihaemophilic factor**) One of the factors involved in the complex process of blood clotting. Freeze-dried Factor VIII fraction, prepared from human plasma, or recombinant human antihaemophilic factor VIII (**octocog alfa** or **moroctocog alfa**), prepared by genetic engineering techniques, is used for the prevention and treatment of bleeding in people with classical haemophilia (haemophilia A; *see* HAEMOSTATIC DRUGS). All preparations are available in a form for injection on *prescription only.
Side effects: include gastrointestinal upsets, alterations in taste, flushing, palpitation, breathlessness, cough, headache, dizziness, and allergic reactions, such as chills and fever.
Proprietary preparations: Alphanate; Fanhdi; Helixate NexGen; Kogenate (octocog alfa); Octanate; ReFacto AF (moroctocog alfa); 8Y; *Haemate P (combined with von Willebrand factor); *Optivate (combined with von Willebrand factor).

Factor IX One of the factors involved in the complex process of blood clotting. Freeze-dried Factor IX fraction, prepared from human plasma, is used for the prevention and treatment of bleeding in people with haemophilia B (*see* HAEMOSTATIC DRUGS). It may also contain other clotting factors. Factor IX preparations are available in a form for injection on *prescription only.
Side effects: there may be gastrointestinal upsets, headache, dizziness, and allergic reactions, such as chills and fever.
Precautions: Factor IX should not be given to people with disseminated intravascular coagulation (DIC), a rare disorder in which there is generalized blood clotting.
Proprietary preparations: AlphaNine; BeneFIX; HT Defix; Mononine; Replenine.

Factor XIII One of the factors involved in the complex process of blood clotting. Freeze-dried Factor XIII is used for the treatment of congenital deficiency of Factor XIII and any bleeding or delayed wound healing that may

result from this deficiency. It is available as a form for intravenous injection on *prescription only.
Side effects: may include allergic reactions and fever.
Precautions: there is a small risk of *anaphylaxis.
Proprietary preparation: Fibrogammin P.

faecal softeners *Laxatives that ease straining and are therefore used by people with painful anal or rectal conditions, such as fissures or haemorrhoids. The most commonly used faecal softener is *arachis oil. *See also* DOCUSATE SODIUM; GLYCERIN; LIQUID PARAFFIN.

famciclovir An *antiviral drug used for the treatment of herpes zoster infections (shingles) and genital herpes. It is converted in the body to *penciclovir and may be used in preference to *aciclovir as it can be given less often. Famciclovir is available as tablets on *prescription only.
Side effects: include nausea, headache, and (less commonly) vomiting, dizziness, and rash.
Precautions: famciclovir should be used with caution in those with impaired liver and kidney function and in women who are pregnant or breastfeeding.
Interactions with other drugs:
Probenecid: increases the plasma concentration of famciclovir.
Proprietary preparation: Famvir.

Famel Linctus (Seton Scholl Healthcare) *See* PHOLCODINE.

Famel Original (Seton Scholl Healthcare) A proprietary combination of *codeine (a cough suppressant) and creosote (an *expectorant), used to relieve the symptoms of dry troublesome coughs. It is available as a syrup without a prescription, but only from pharmacies.
Side effects and interactions with other drugs: *see* CODEINE; OPIOIDS.
Precautions: this medicine is not recommended for children. *See also* OPIOIDS.

Family Meltus Chesty Coughs (SSL International) *See* GUAIFENESIN.

famotidine An *H_2-receptor antagonist used for the treatment of duodenal and gastric ulcers and reflux oesophagitis (*see* ACID-PEPTIC DISEASES). It is available as tablets on *prescription only. Packs containing no more than two weeks' supply of tablets, for the relief of indigestion and heartburn in people over 16 years old, can be obtained from pharmacies without a prescription.
Side effects: include headache, dizziness, dry mouth, constipation, diarrhoea, nausea, rash, weakness, and fatigue. Rarely, famotidine may cause reversible breast enlargement in men.
Precautions: famotidine should be used with caution by people with poor kidney function or stomach cancer and by women who are pregnant or breastfeeding.
Proprietary preparations: Pepcid; *PepcidTwo (combined with calcium carbonate and magnesium sulphate).

Famvir (Novartis) *See* FAMCICLOVIR.

Fanhdi (Grifols) *See* FACTOR VIII.

Fansidar (Roche Products) A proprietary combination of *pyrimethamine (an antimalarial drug) and sulfadoxine (a *sulphonamide), used for the treatment of falciparum *malaria. It is available as tablets on *prescription only.
Side effects, precautions, and interactions with other drugs: *see* PYRIMETHAMINE; CO-TRIMOXAZOLE.

Fareston (Orion Pharma) *See* TOREMIFENE.

Fasigyn (Pfizer) *See* TINIDAZOLE.

Faslodex (AstraZeneca) *See* FULVESTRANT.

Fasturtec (sanofi-aventis) *See* RASBURICASE.

Faverin (Solvay Healthcare) *See* FLUVOXAMINE MALEATE.

Fectrim (DDSA Pharmaceuticals) *See* CO-TRIMOXAZOLE.

Fefol (Intrapharm) A proprietary combination of *ferrous sulphate and *folic acid, used to prevent deficiencies of iron and folic acid during pregnancy. It is available as *modified-release capsules and can be obtained without a prescription, but only from pharmacies. It cannot be prescribed on the NHS.
Side effects, precautions, and interactions with other drugs: *see* IRON.

felbinac An *NSAID that is one of the active agents produced by the metabolism of *fenbufen. Felbinac is applied to the skin to relieve the pain and inflammation of sprains, strains, and similar injuries. It is available as a gel or foam on *prescription only; a gel with a lower concentration of felbinac can be obtained from pharmacies without a prescription.
Side effects and precautions: *see* NSAIDs.
Proprietary preparations: Traxam (gel or foam); Traxam Pain Relief (lower-strength gel).

Feldene, Feldene Gel, Feldene Melt (Pfizer) *See* PIROXICAM.

felodipine A class II *calcium antagonist used for the treatment of all grades of *hypertension and for the prevention of *angina. It is available as *modified-release tablets on *prescription only.
Side effects: *see* CALCIUM ANTAGONISTS.
Precautions: felodipine should not be used to treat unstable angina or to treat patients who have uncontrolled heart failure or who have had a heart attack during the previous month. It should not be taken during pregnancy. *See also* CALCIUM ANTAGONISTS; ANTIHYPERTENSIVE DRUGS.
Interactions with other drugs:

Antiepileptic drugs: the effects of felodipine are reduced by phenytoin, carbamazepine, and primidone.
Antifungal drugs: itraconazole and ketoconazole increase the plasma concentration of felodipine.
Erythromycin: increases the plasma concentration of felodipine.

See also CALCIUM ANTAGONISTS.
Proprietary preparations: Cardioplen XL; Plendil; Vascalpha; *Triapin (combined with ramipril).

Femapak 40 (Solvay Healthcare) A proprietary preparation of *estradiol (40-microgram) patches and *dydrogesterone tablets used as sequential combined *hormone replacement therapy for the relief of menopausal symptoms in women who have not had a hysterectomy. **Femapak 80**, containing 80-microgram estradiol patches, is used in addition for the prevention of postmenopausal osteoporosis. Both preparations are available on *prescription only.

Side effects, precautions, and interactions with other drugs: *see* HORMONE REPLACEMENT THERAPY.

Femara (Novartis) *See* LETROZOLE.

Fematrix (Solvay Healthcare) *See* ESTRADIOL; HORMONE REPLACEMENT THERAPY.

Feminax Period Pain Capsules (Bayer) A proprietary combination of *paracetamol (a non-opioid analgesic) and *codeine (an opioid analgesic), used to treat pains associated with menstruation. It is available as capsules without a prescription, but only from pharmacies.
Side effects and precautions: *see* PARACETAMOL; CODEINE.
Interactions with other drugs: *see* OPIOIDS.

Feminax Ultra (Bayer) *See* NAPROXEN.

Femodene (Bayer) A proprietary combination of *ethinylestradiol and *gestodene, used as an *oral contraceptive. **Femodene ED** contains both active and dummy tablets so that a tablet is taken each day of a 28-day cycle. Both preparations are available as tablets on *prescription only.
Side effects and interactions with other drugs: *see* ORAL CONTRACEPTIVES.
Precautions: these preparations should not be used by women who are at risk of developing thromboembolism, for example because they are very overweight or have varicose veins or a history of thrombosis. They should therefore only be taken by women who cannot tolerate other brands and who are prepared to accept the increased risk. *See also* ORAL CONTRACEPTIVES.

Femodette (Bayer) A proprietary combination of *ethinylestradiol and *gestodene, used as an *oral contraceptive. It is available as tablets on *prescription only.
Side effects, precautions, and interactions with other drugs: *see* ORAL CONTRACEPTIVES.

Femoston 2/10 (Solvay Healthcare) A proprietary preparation of *estradiol (2-milligram tablets) and combined estradiol (2 mg)/*dydrogesterone (10 mg) tablets, used as sequential combined *hormone replacement therapy for the relief of menopausal symptoms and the prevention of osteoporosis in women who have not had a hysterectomy. **Femoston 1/10** (in which the tablets

contain 1 mg estradiol) are used only for the relief of menopausal symptoms. All preparations are available on *prescription only.
Side effects, precautions, and interactions with other drugs: *see* HORMONE REPLACEMENT THERAPY.

Femoston-conti (Solvay Healthcare) A proprietary combination of *estradiol and *dydrogesterone, used as continuous combined *hormone replacement therapy for the relief of menopausal symptoms and the prevention of osteoporosis in women who have not had a hysterectomy. It is available as tablets on *prescription only.
Side effects, precautions, and interactions with other drugs: *see* HORMONE REPLACEMENT THERAPY.

FemSeven (Merck Serono) *See* ESTRADIOL; HORMONE REPLACEMENT THERAPY.

FemSeven Conti (Merck Serono) A proprietary combination of *estradiol and *levonorgestrel, used as continuous combined *hormone replacement therapy for the relief of menopausal symptoms in women who have not had a hysterectomy. It is available as skin patches on *prescription only.
Side effects, precautions, and interactions with other drugs: *see* HORMONE REPLACEMENT THERAPY.

FemSeven Sequi (Merck Serono) A proprietary preparation of estradiol patches and combined estradiol/levonorgestrel patches, used as sequential combined *hormone replacement therapy in women who have not had a hysterectomy. It is available on *prescription only.
Side effects, precautions, and interactions with other drugs: *see* HORMONE REPLACEMENT THERAPY.

Femulen (Pharmacia) *See* ETYNODIOL DIACETATE; ORAL CONTRACEPTIVES.

Fenactol (Discovery Pharmaceuticals) *See* DICLOFENAC SODIUM.

Fenbid Forte Gel, Fenbid Spansule (Goldshield) *See* IBUPROFEN.

fenbufen An *NSAID used for the treatment of pain and inflammation in rheumatoid arthritis and other disorders of the joints or muscles. It is available as tablets or capsules on *prescription only. *See also* FELBINAC.
Side effects: *see* NSAIDs. In addition, fenbufen is more likely than some other NSAIDs to cause rashes, in which case a doctor should be informed as the treatment may need to be discontinued immediately; allergic lung disorders may follow the rash.
Precautions and interactions with other drugs: *see* NSAIDs.
Proprietary preparation: Lederfen.

Fenistil Cold Sore Cream (Novartis) *See* PENCICLOVIR.

Fennings Children's Cooling Powders (Anglian Pharma) *See* PARACETAMOL.

Fennings Little Healers (Anglian Pharma) *See* IPECACUANHA.

fenofibrate A *fibrate used for the treatment of a wide variety of *hyperlipidaemias that have not responded to dietary intervention and other appropriate measures. It is available as capsules or tablets on *prescription only.
Side effects and precautions: *see* FIBRATES.
Interactions with other drugs: *see* BEZAFIBRATE.
Proprietary preparations: Lipantil Micro (in two strengths of capsules); Supralip (tablets).

f

fenoprofen An *NSAID used for the treatment of pain and inflammation in rheumatoid arthritis and other disorders of the joints or muscles. It is also used to relieve mild or moderate pain caused by other conditions. Fenoprofen is available as tablets on *prescription only.
Side effects: *see* NSAIDs. Additional side effects may include infections of the upper airways and cystitis.
Precautions and interactions with other drugs: *see* NSAIDs.
Proprietary preparation: Fenopron.

Fenopron (Typharm) *See* FENOPROFEN.

fenoterol hydrobromide A *sympathomimetic drug that stimulates beta *adrenoceptors. It is used in combination with *ipratropium as a *bronchodilator in the treatment of asthma.
Side effects, precautions, and interactions with other drugs: *see* SALBUTAMOL.
Proprietary preparation: *Duovent (combined with ipratropium).

Fentalis (Sandoz) *See* FENTANYL.

fentanyl A strong *opioid used for the treatment of severe pain, such as that due to cancer. It is also used for pain relief during surgical operations and to depress breathing in patients on ventilators. Fentanyl is a *controlled drug; it is available as *transdermal (skin) patches (for use during surgery or for people on ventilators) and as dispersible tablets, a nasal spray, and an injection.
Side effects and precautions: *see* MORPHINE.
Interactions with other drugs: *see* OPIOIDS.
Proprietary preparations: Abstral (tablets); Actiq (tablets); Durogesic DTrans (skin patches); Effentora (tablets); Fentalis (skin patches); Instanyl (nasal spray); Matrifen (skin patches); Mezolar Matrix Transdermal Patches; Osmanil (skin patches); Sublimaze (injection); Victanyl (skin patches).

Feospan (Intrapharm) *See* FERROUS SULPHATE.

Feprapax (Ashbourne Pharmaceuticals) *See* LOFEPRAMINE.

Ferinject (Syner-Med) *See* FERRIC CARBOXYMALTOSE.

ferric carboxymaltose A complex of iron given by slow intravenous injection or infusion to treat iron deficiency when oral preparations are poorly tolerated or inadequate. It is available on *prescription only.
Side effects: *see* IRON. There may also be rash, headache, and dizziness.

Precautions: *see* IRON. This medicine is not recommended for pregnant women and there is a risk of allergic reactions.
Proprietary preparation: Ferinject.

ferric hydroxide sucrose (iron sucrose) A complex of *iron (in the form of ferric hydroxide) and sucrose, used in the treatment of iron-deficiency anaemia. It is given by slow intravenous injection or infusion and is available on *prescription only.
Side effects: include nausea, vomiting, changes in taste, headache, low blood pressure, and (less commonly) 'pins and needles', abdominal disorders, muscle pain, fever, flushing, and nettle rash.
Precautions: oral iron should not be taken until five days after the last injection. Injections should not be given to pregnant women or to people with liver disease, infection, or a history of asthma or other allergic disorders.
Proprietary preparation: Venofer.

Ferriprox (Swedish Orphan International) *See* DEFERIPRONE.

Ferrograd (Teofarma) *See* FERROUS SULPHATE.

Ferrograd C (Teofarma) A proprietary combination of *ferrous sulphate and ascorbic acid (vitamin C), used for the treatment of iron-deficiency anaemia. It is available as tablets and may be obtained without a prescription, but only from pharmacies.
Side effects, precautions, and interactions with other drugs: *see* IRON.

Ferrograd Folic (Teofarma) A proprietary combination of *ferrous sulphate and *folic acid, used to prevent deficiencies of iron and folic acid during pregnancy. It is available as tablets and can be obtained without a prescription, but only from pharmacies.
Side effects, precautions, and interactions with other drugs: *see* IRON.

ferrous fumarate An *iron supplement used for the treatment of iron-deficiency anaemia. It is available, as tablets, capsules, or a syrup, without a prescription: some preparations are freely available *over the counter; others can be bought only from pharmacies. Ferrous fumarate is also included in many preparations combined with *folic acid.
Side effects, precautions, and interactions with other drugs: *see* IRON.
Proprietary preparations: Fersaday (tablets); Fersamal (tablets and syrup); Galfer (capsules and syrup); *Galfer FA (combined with folic acid); *Pregaday (combined with folic acid).

ferrous gluconate An *iron supplement used for the treatment and prevention of iron-deficiency anaemia. It is available as tablets that can be obtained without a prescription, but only from pharmacies.
Side effects, precautions, and interactions with other drugs: *see* IRON.

ferrous sulphate An *iron supplement used for the treatment of iron-deficiency anaemia. It is available as tablets, oral drops, a solution for

children, and as *modified-release preparations and can be obtained without a prescription, but only from pharmacies.
Side effects, precautions, and interactions with other drugs: *see* IRON.
Proprietary preparations: Feospan (modified-release capsules); Ferrograd (tablets); Ironorm Drops; *Fefol (combined with folic acid); *Ferrograd C (combined with ascorbic acid); *Ferrograd Folic (combined with folic acid).

Fersaday (Goldshield) *See* FERROUS FUMARATE.

Fersamal (Goldshield) *See* FERROUS FUMARATE.

fesoterodine An *antimuscarinic drug used to treat incontinence and abnormal frequency and urgency in passing urine. It is available as tablets on *prescription only.
Side effects: *see* ANTIMUSCARINIC DRUGS. There may also be insomnia.
Precautions: *see* ANTIMUSCARINIC DRUGS. Fesoterodine should not be taken by women who are pregnant or breastfeeding.
Interactions with other drugs: *see* ANTIMUSCARINIC DRUGS.
Proprietary preparation: Toviaz.

fexofenadine hydrochloride One of the newer (non-sedating) *antihistamines, used for the relief of symptoms of such allergic conditions as hay fever and urticaria. It is available as tablets on *prescription only.
Side effects, precautions, and interactions with other drugs: *see* ANTIHISTAMINES.
Proprietary preparations: Telfast 30; Telfast 120; Telfast 180.

fibrates A group of *lipid-lowering drugs that lower plasma *triglycerides and increase the breakdown of LDL-*cholesterol (*see* LIPOPROTEINS), thereby reducing plasma LDL-cholesterol by up to 18%. They also tend to raise plasma HDL-cholesterol (which has a beneficial effect). Fibrates are used to treat a variety of *hyperlipidaemias. *See* BEZAFIBRATE; CIPROFIBRATE; FENOFIBRATE; GEMFIBROZIL.
Side effects: fibrates can cause gastrointestinal upset (nausea and/or vomiting), rash, and muscle pain. Less often itching, impotence, headache, dizziness, drowsiness, and hair loss may occur.
Precautions and interactions with other drugs: Fibrates should not be taken by women who are pregnant or breastfeeding. Fibrates can cause rhabdomyolysis (inflammation and destruction of muscle tissue). Muscle pain, tenderness, or weakness must therefore be reported to a doctor promptly and investigated. Rhabdomyolysis can be a serious condition and is more likely to occur in people who are also taking *statins or *daptomycin; these drugs should therefore preferably be avoided. People with kidney disease or hypothyroidism are at a higher risk of developing rhabdomyolysis.

Ezetimibe: there is an increased risk of gallstones if this drug is taken with fibrates; ezetimibe should be discontinued if symptoms develop.

See also entries for individual drugs.

Fibrazate XL (Sandoz) *See* BEZAFIBRATE.

Fibrelief (Manx) *See* ISPAGHULA HUSK.

fibrinolytic drugs A class of drugs that are used to dissolve blood clots. They act by stimulating production of the body's own enzymes that break down fibrin, the protein that forms the basis of blood clots (thrombi), i.e. they are **thrombolytic drugs**. The common fibrinolytic drugs are *streptokinase, *alteplase, *reteplase, and *tenecteplase. Most of them are used to dissolve blood clots in the coronary arteries (which supply the heart) in people who have had a heart attack; some of them have other uses in addition to or instead of this. Fibrinolytic drugs are available as solutions for injection or infusion on *prescription only.
Side effects: include nausea, vomiting, and bleeding (which is usually limited to the injection site). Back pain and allergic reactions have been reported, and low blood pressure can occur after a heart attack.
Precautions and interactions with other drugs: fibrinolytic drugs should not be given to people who have an active peptic ulcer, a bleeding disorder, active lung disease, severe liver disease, or acute pancreatitis, or to those who have recently had a stroke, haemorrhage, or injury, or who have recently undergone surgery (including tooth extraction). They should be used with caution in pregnant women and in people with high blood pressure. The risk of bleeding is increased if fibrinolytic drugs are used with anticoagulants or antiplatelet drugs.

Fibrogammin P (CSL Behring) *See* FACTOR XIII.

Fibro-Vein (STD Pharmaceutical Products) *See* SODIUM TETRADECYL SULPHATE.

Fiery Jack Cream (J. Pickles & Sons) A proprietary combination of *capsicum oleoresin, *diethylamine salicylate, *glycol salicylate, and *methyl nicotinate, used as a *rubefacient for the relief of muscular aches and pains, including backache, sciatica, lumbago, and strains. It is freely available *over the counter.
Side effects and precautions: *see* RUBEFACIENTS; SALICYLATES.

Fiery Jack Ointment (J. Pickles & Sons) *See* CAPSICUM OLEORESIN.

50:50 Ointment (Boots) A proprietary combination of *liquid paraffin and *white soft paraffin, used as an *emollient for the relief of dry flaky skin. It is available without a prescription, but only from Boots stores.

filgrastim Recombinant human granulocyte-colony stimulating factor, a form of *granulocyte-colony stimulating factor produced by genetic engineering. It is used for the treatment of neutropenia (a decrease in the number of neutrophils, a type of white blood cell) induced by *cytotoxic drug treatment for *cancer or resulting from destruction of the bone marrow prior to bone marrow transplantation. It may be given to cancer patients who are about to undergo blood collection before aggressive treatment; neutrophil production will thus be boosted in this collected blood, which is used to replace the white cells destroyed by the treatment. Filgrastim is also used for

treating some other forms of neutropenia (such as that present at birth) when this causes recurrent serious infections. It is available as a form for injection on *prescription only; its use is restricted to specialist units.
Side effects: include pain in muscles or bones, transient low blood pressure, difficult or painful urination, allergic reactions, headache, diarrhoea, anaemia, nose bleeds, hair loss, osteoporosis, and rash.
Precautions: white blood cell counts should be carefully monitored during treatment. Filgrastim should be used with caution in women who are pregnant or breastfeeding.

Proprietary preparations: Neupogen; Ratiograstim; Zarzio.

Finacea Gel (Meda Pharmaceuticals) *See* AZELAIC ACID.

finasteride An *anti-androgen that acts by inhibiting the enzyme that metabolizes *testosterone to the more active dihydrotestosterone. It is used in the treatment of benign enlargement of the prostate and also to promote hair growth in men in male-pattern baldness. It is available as tablets on *prescription only.
Side effects: include impotence, decreased libido, a reduced volume of semen on ejaculation, breast tenderness and enlargement, and allergic reactions (including lip swelling and rash).
Precautions: finasteride should be used with caution in men with urinary obstruction and prostate cancer. The use of barrier contraception is recommended if the patient's sexual partner is pregnant or capable of becoming pregnant; women who are pregnant or capable of becoming so should avoid handling crushed or broken tablets.
Proprietary preparations: Propecia; Proscar.

Firazyr (Jerini) *See* ICATIBANT.

Firmagon (Ferring Pharmaceuticals) *See* DEGARELIX.

first-line treatment Drug therapy that is the first choice for treating a particular condition; other drugs are only used if first-line therapy has failed.

fish oils *See* OMEGA-3 FATTY ACID COMPOUNDS.

Flagyl (Winthrop Pharmaceuticals) *See* METRONIDAZOLE.

Flamasacard (Abbey) *See* ASPIRIN.

Flamazine (Smith & Nephew Healthcare) *See* SILVER SULFADIAZINE.

flavoxate hydrochloride An *antimuscarinic drug used to treat urinary incontinence, abnormal frequency or urgency in passing urine, and bladder spasms due to the presence of a catheter. It acts in the same way as *oxybutynin but is less effective, although it may be preferred to this drug as its side effects are less severe. Flavoxate is available as tablets on *prescription only.
Side effects: include dry mouth, constipation, blurred vision, nausea, and headache.

Precautions: flavoxate is not recommended for children under 12 years old. *See also* OXYBUTYNIN HYDROCHLORIDE.
Interactions with other drugs: *see* ANTIMUSCARINIC DRUGS.
Proprietary preparation: Urispas 200.

Flebogamma (Grifols) *See* IMMUNOGLOBULINS.

Flebogammadif (Grifols) *See* IMMUNOGLOBULINS.

flecainide acetate A class I *anti-arrhythmic drug used for the treatment of a variety of *arrhythmias. It is available as an injection, tablets, or *modified-release capsules on *prescription only.
Side effects: include dizziness, visual disturbances, and less commonly nausea and vomiting.
Precautions: therapy with flecainide acetate should be initiated under hospital supervision. It should not be taken after a heart attack or in people with heart failure. It should be used with caution in people with liver or kidney disease and in women who are pregnant or breastfeeding. *See also* ANTI-ARRHYTHMIC DRUGS.
Interactions with other drugs:

Other anti-arrhythmic drugs: amiodarone increases the risk of arrhythmias and the dose of flecainide should be reduced; depression of heart function is increased if flecainide is taken with any other anti-arrhythmic.
Antidepressants: tricyclic antidepressants increase the risk of arrhythmias; fluoxetine increases the plasma concentration of flecainide.
Antimalarial drugs: quinine increases the plasma concentration of flecainide; Riamet should not be taken with flecainide.
Beta blockers: depression of heart function is increased if these drugs are taken with flecainide.
Clozapine: increases the risk of arrhythmias.
Diuretics: increase adverse effects on the heart through potassium loss.
Mizolastine: increases the risk of arrhythmias and should not be taken with flecainide.
Ritonavir: increases the plasma concentration of flecainide (and the risk of arrhythmias) and should therefore not be taken with flecainide.
Tolterodine: increases the risk of arrhythmias.
Verapamil: depression of heart function is increased if verapamil is taken with flecainide.

Proprietary preparations: Tambocor; Tambocor XL (modified-release capsules.

Fleet Phospho-soda (Laboratorios Casen Fleet) A proprietary combination of sodium dihydrogen phosphate dihydrate and disodium phosphate dodecahydrate (both *phosphate laxatives), used to evacuate the bowel before investigative procedures or surgery. It is available as an oral solution and can be obtained without a prescription, but only from pharmacies.

Side effects: *see* BOWEL-CLEANSING SOLUTIONS.
Precautions: this solution is not recommended for children. *See also* BOWEL-CLEANSING SOLUTIONS.

Fleet Ready-to-Use Enema (Laboratorios Casen Fleet) A proprietary combination of the osmotic laxatives *sodium acid phosphate and sodium phosphate (*see* PHOSPHATE LAXATIVES), used for the treatment of constipation or to evacuate the bowel before investigative procedures or surgery. It is available from pharmacies without a prescription.
Precautions: this enema is not recommended for children under three years old and should be used with caution in elderly people. *See also* PHOSPHATE LAXATIVES.

Flexotard MR (Pharmacia) *See* DICLOFENAC SODIUM.

Flixonase (Allen & Hanburys) *See* FLUTICASONE PROPIONATE.

Flixotide (Allen & Hanburys) *See* FLUTICASONE PROPIONATE.

Flolan (GlaxoSmithKline) *See* EPOPROSTENOL.

Flomaxtra (Astellas Pharma) *See* TAMSULOSIN HYDROCHLORIDE.

Florinef (E.R. Squibb & Sons) *See* FLUDROCORTISONE ACETATE.

Floxapen (Actavis) *See* FLUCLOXACILLIN.

Flu-Amp (Mylan) *See* CO-FLUAMPICIL.

Fluanxol (Lundbeck) *See* FLUPENTIXOL.

Fluclomix (Ashbourne Pharmaceuticals) *See* FLUCLOXACILLIN.

flucloxacillin A *penicillin that is resistant to beta-lactamase (*see* PENICILLINS). It is used for the treatment of infections due to penicillinase-producing bacteria, including ear infections, pneumonia, impetigo, cellulitis (an infection of the deep layers of the skin), and infections of the lining of the heart cavity or valves. It is available, on *prescription only, as capsules or a syrup for oral use and as an injection.
Side effects: include diarrhoea and allergic reactions (*see* BENZYLPENICILLIN). In addition, hepatitis and jaundice may occur (the jaundice may develop up to several weeks after treatment has stopped).
Precautions: *see* BENZYLPENICILLIN; PENICILLINS.
Interactions with other drugs: *see* BENZYLPENICILLIN.
Proprietary preparations: Floxapen; Fluclomix; Flu-Amp (*see* CO-FLUAMPICIL); Magnapen (*see* CO-FLUAMPICIL).

fluconazole A triazole *antifungal drug used for the treatment of many fungal infections, especially candidiasis (of the mouth, vagina, or throat), athlete's foot, and cryptococcal meningitis (a form of meningitis that can occur as an opportunistic infection in AIDS patients). Available on *prescription, fluconazole can be taken orally, as capsules or a suspension, or it can be given by intravenous infusion. Capsules for treating vaginal

candidiasis (maximum dose 150 mg) can be bought from pharmacies without a prescription.
Side effects: include abdominal discomfort, diarrhoea, and flatulence. Rarely, allergic reactions may occur; if a rash develops, the treatment should be stopped and a doctor consulted.
Precautions: fluconazole should be used with caution by people with impaired kidney function and by women who are pregnant or breastfeeding.
Interactions with other drugs:

Analgesics: the plasma concentrations of celecoxib and parecoxib are increased and their doses therefore need to be reduced; the plasma concentration of alfentanil is increased, which may cause depression of breathing.

Antibiotics: rifampicin reduces the plasma concentration of fluconazole; the plasma concentration of rifabutin is increased by fluconazole.

Anticoagulants: the anticoagulant effects of warfarin and acenocoumarol are enhanced by fluconazole.

Antidiabetic drugs: the plasma concentrations of the sulphonylureas are increased.

Antipsychotic drugs: pimozide and sertindole should not be taken with fluconazole because of the risk of abnormal heart rhythms.

Antiviral drugs: the plasma concentrations of nevirapine, ritonavir, tipranavir, and zidovudine are increased by fluconazole.

Bosentan: its plasma concentration may be increased and it should not be taken with fluconazole.

Ciclosporin: its plasma concentration is increased.

Diuretics: hydrochlorothiazide increases the plasma concentration of fluconazole; the plasma concentration of eplerenone is increased.

Ergotamine: its toxic effects may be increased and it should not be taken with fluconazole.

Midazolam: its plasma concentration (and the risk of prolonged sedation) is increased.

Phenytoin: its effect is enhanced.

Reboxetine: should not be taken with fluconazole.

Theophylline: fluconazole increases the plasma concentration of theophylline, which may increase its side effects in patients receiving high doses of this drug.

Proprietary preparations: Diflucan; Diflucan One (available without a prescription).

flucytosine An *antifungal drug used for the treatment of systemic (generalized) yeast infections, such as candidiasis. It enhances the effects of *amphotericin, and is therefore used with this drug for treating severe or longstanding fungal infections, including cryptococcal meningitis and severe *Candida* infections. Flucytosine is available as a solution for intravenous infusion on *prescription only; tablets may be obtained for named patients.
Side effects: include nausea, vomiting, diarrhoea, rashes, and (more rarely)

confusion, hallucinations, convulsions, headache, sedation, vertigo, and blood disorders (including bone marrow suppression).
Precautions: flucytosine should be used with caution in the elderly, in people with impaired kidney function or blood disorders, and in women who are pregnant or breastfeeding. Regular blood counts and tests for liver and kidney function should be carried out during treatment.
Interactions with other drugs:
Amphotericin: may enhance the adverse effects of flucytosine.
Cytarabine: may reduce the plasma concentration of flucytosine.

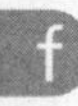

Proprietary preparation: Ancotil.

Fludara (Genzyme Therapeutics) *See* FLUDARABINE.

fludarabine An *antimetabolite that is used for the treatment of chronic lymphocytic leukaemia (*see* CANCER) after treatment with an *alkylating drug has failed. It is available as tablets and as a form for injection or infusion on *prescription only.
Side effects: fludarabine causes *bone marrow suppression and suppression of the immune system; very rarely it may have adverse effects on the nervous system and lungs.
Precautions: fludarabine should not be given to pregnant women or people with severe kidney disease. The dosage may need to be reduced for those with moderate kidney disease. *See also* CYTOTOXIC DRUGS.
Interactions with other drugs:
Clozapine: there is an increased risk of agranulocytosis (a blood disorder) and this drug should not be taken with fludarabine.
Pentostatin: increases the adverse effects of fludarabine on the lungs.
Proprietary preparation: Fludara.

fludrocortisone acetate A mineralocorticoid (*see* CORTICOSTEROIDS) used as replacement therapy in people with a deficiency of the natural hormone (aldosterone), as in Addison's disease or following surgical removal of the adrenal glands. It may also be used to treat a certain kind of low blood pressure (neuropathic orthostatic hypotension), although it does not have a *licence for this. Fludrocortisone is available as tablets on *prescription only.
Side effects: include high blood pressure, sodium and water retention, and potassium loss.
Precautions and interactions with other drugs: *see* CORTICOSTEROIDS.
Proprietary preparation: Florinef.

fludroxycortide <**flurandrenolone**> A moderately potent *topical steroid used for the treatment of a variety of inflammatory skin conditions. It is available, on *prescription only, as a cream, ointment, or impregnated tape.
Side effects and precautions: *see* TOPICAL STEROIDS.
Proprietary preparations: Haelan.

flumazenil A drug that is used to reverse the sedative effects of *benzodiazepines that have been given during anaesthesia, in intensive care,

or in diagnostic procedures. It is available as an injection on *prescription only.
Side effects: include nausea, vomiting, and flushing; agitation, anxiety, and fear can occur if sedation is reversed too rapidly. Patients in intensive care may have a transient increase in heart rate and blood pressure.
Precautions: flumazenil may cause withdrawal symptoms in people who are dependent on benzodiazepines; it should not be used in people who are receiving long-term treatment with benzodiazepines (e.g. for status epilepticus). Flumazenil should be used with caution in people with liver disease or a severe head injury, the elderly, children, and women who are pregnant or breastfeeding.
Proprietary preparation: Anexate.

flumetasone pivalate <**flumethasone pivalate**> A *corticosteroid used in combination with an antibacterial drug for the treatment of inflammation of the outer ear in which eczema is present. It is available as ear drops on *prescription only.
Side effects: flumetasone may cause local allergic reactions. *See* TOPICAL STEROIDS.
Precautions: prolonged use of flumetasone should be avoided. *See* TOPICAL STEROIDS.
Proprietary preparation: *Locorten-Vioform (combined with clioquinol).

flunisolide A *corticosteroid used for the treatment of allergic rhinitis (including hay fever). It is available as a metered-dose nasal spray on *prescription only; a nasal spray specifically for hay fever can be bought from pharmacies without a prescription.
Side effects: include transient local irritation.
Precautions: flunisolide should not be used when infection is present and should be used with caution by pregnant women and by people suffering from ulceration of the nose or who have recently suffered trauma to the nose or undergone nasal surgery.
Proprietary preparations: Syntaris; Syntaris Hayfever Nasal Spray.

fluocinolone acetonide A potent *topical steroid used for the treatment of a variety of skin disorders. It is available, on *prescription only, as a cream or ointment of varying strengths or as a gel.
Side effects and precautions: *see* TOPICAL STEROIDS.
Proprietary preparations: Synalar; Synalar 1 in 4 Dilution, Synalar 1 in 10 Dilution, Synalar Gel; *Synalar C (combined with clioquinol); *Synalar N (combined with neomycin sulphate).

fluocinonide A potent *topical steroid used for the treatment of a variety of severe skin disorders. It is available, on *prescription only, as a cream or ointment.
Side effects and precautions: *see* TOPICAL STEROIDS.
Proprietary preparation: Metosyn.

fluocortolone A moderately potent *topical steroid, consisting of

fluocortolone pivalate and fluocortolone caproate, used for the treatment of a variety of severe skin disorders. These compounds are combined in a cream and an ointment that are available on *prescription only. Fluocortolone combined with a local anaesthetic is used for relieving the symptoms of *haemorrhoids.
Side effects and precautions: *see* TOPICAL STEROIDS.
Proprietary preparations: Ultralanum Plain; *Ultraproct (combined with cinchocaine hydrochloride).

Fluor-a-day (Dental Health Products) *See* FLUORIDE.

fluorescein sodium A dye that is applied to the eye for diagnostic purposes: to highlight damaged areas of the cornea and locate foreign bodies. It is sometimes used in combination with a *local anaesthetic. Fluorescein sodium is available as eye drops or paper strips and can be obtained without a prescription, but only from pharmacies.
Proprietary preparations: Fluorets (paper strips); Minims Fluorescein Sodium (eye drops); *Minims Lidocaine and Fluorescein (combined with lidocaine); *Minims Proxymetacaine and Fluorescein (combined with proxymetacaine).

Fluorets (Bausch & Lomb UK) *See* FLUORESCEIN SODIUM.

fluoride A salt of fluorine, which in solution produces fluoride ions (*see* ELECTROLYTE). The incorporation of fluoride ions into the enamel of developing teeth strengthens the enamel and makes the teeth more resistant to dental caries (tooth decay). An adequate fluoride intake is provided by drinking water with a fluoride content of 1 part per million (ppm). When the natural fluoride content is significantly less than this, fluoride can be added to the public water supplies by the water authorities. In areas where tap water is not fluoridated, **sodium fluoride** supplements may be given to children. Sodium fluoride is available as tablets, drops, mouthwashes, and gels and can be obtained without a prescription, but only from pharmacies.
Monofluorophosphate, which is added to some toothpastes or used in gels, is another source of fluoride; sodium fluoride is also added to some toothpastes.
Side effects: there may be occasional white flecks on the teeth; overdosage may produce yellowish-brown discoloration of the teeth.
Precautions: fluoride supplements should not be used if the fluoride content of drinking water exceeds 0.7 ppm.
Proprietary preparations: Duraphat (mouthwash or toothpaste); En-De-Kay (mouthwash); En-De-Kay Fluotabs (tablets); Fluor-a-day (tablets); FluoriGard (tablets, drops, mouthwash, or gel); *Sensodyne (combined with triclosan).

FluoriGard (Colgate-Palmolive) *See* FLUORIDE.

fluorometholone A *corticosteroid used for the short-term treatment of inflammatory eye conditions that are not infected. It is available as eye drops on *prescription only.

Side effects: include an increase in pressure in the eye after a few weeks' treatment, thinning of the cornea, and fungal infections.
Precautions: fluorometholone should not be used by people with viral, fungal, tuberculous, or weeping infections or by those who wear soft contact lenses; it should be used with caution by people with glaucoma. Prolonged use by pregnant women and infants should be avoided. *See also* TOPICAL STEROIDS.
Proprietary preparation: FML.

fluorouracil (**5-fluorouracil**; **5-FU**) An *antimetabolite used for the treatment of solid tumours (*see* CANCER), especially those of the gastrointestinal tract (such as cancers of the colon and rectum) and breast cancer. It is usually administered intravenously, sometimes in conjunction with *folinic acid, which increases its effectiveness. It is usually given as intensive courses of several days' treatment every 3–4 weeks. Fluorouracil can also be used topically to treat certain malignant skin tumours. A *prescription only medicine, it is available as a solution for injection, capsules, or a cream.
Side effects: injections or capsules may cause *bone marrow suppression, inflammation of the mucous membranes lining the mouth, stomach, and intestine, and nausea and vomiting. *See* CYTOTOXIC DRUGS.
Precautions: *see* CYTOTOXIC DRUGS.
Interactions with other drugs:

Clozapine: there is an increased risk of agranulocytosis (a blood disorder), and the two drugs should not be used together.
Phenytoin: its adverse effects may be increased.
Temoporfin: sensitivity to light is increased if fluorouracil cream is used with it.
Warfarin: its anticoagulant effect is enhanced.

Proprietary preparation: Efudix (cream).

fluoxetine An *antidepressant drug of the *SSRI group. It is used for the treatment of depressive illness, obsessive-compulsive disorder, and bulimia nervosa. Fluoxetine is available as capsules or liquid on *prescription only.
Side effects and precautions: *see* SSRIs.
Interactions with other drugs:

Antiepileptics: the plasma concentrations of carbamazepine and phenytoin are increased by fluoxetine.
Antipsychotics: plasma concentrations of clozapine, haloperidol, risperidone, sertindole, and zotepine are increased by fluoxetine; the risk of ventricular *arrhythmias is increased if droperidol is taken with fluoxetine and the two drugs should not be used together.
Moclobemide: there is an increased risk of adverse effects on the nervous system, and moclobemide should not be started until five weeks after stopping fluoxetine.
Rasagiline: there is an increased risk of adverse effects on the nervous system, and rasagiline should not be started until five weeks after stopping

fluoxetine, which should not be started until two weeks after stopping rasagiline.
Selegiline: there is an increased risk of hypertension and adverse effects on the central nervous system, and selegiline should not be started until five weeks after stopping fluoxetine, which should not be started until two weeks after stopping selegiline.
Sumatriptan: there is an increased risk of adverse effects on the central nervous system.
Tamoxifen: fluoxetine may inhibit its conversion to an active form in the body and it should not be taken with tamoxifen.
For other interactions, *see* SSRIs.

Proprietary preparations: Oxactin; Prozac.

flupentixol <**flupenthixol**> A thioxanthene *antipsychotic drug used for the treatment of schizophrenia and other psychoses, particularly in patients who are apathetic and withdrawn. It is also used for the short-term treatment of depression. Flupentixol is available, on *prescription only, as tablets or as a *depot injection.
Side effects: as for *chlorpromazine hydrochloride, but flupentixol is less sedating and more likely to produce *extrapyramidal reactions.
Precautions: flupentixol should not be used to treat senile confused patients or those who are hyperactive or excitable. *See also* CHLORPROMAZINE HYDROCHLORIDE.
Interactions with other drugs:
Anaesthetics: their effect in lowering blood pressure is enhanced.
Antidepressants: there is an increased risk of antimuscarinic effects and arrhythmias if flupentixol is taken with tricyclic antidepressants.
Antiepileptic drugs: their anticonvulsant effects are antagonized by flupentixol.
Clozapine: should not be used with depot injections of flupentixol.
Ritonavir: may increase the effects of flupentixol.
Sedatives: the sedative effects of flupentixol are increased if it is taken with anxiolytic or hypnotic drugs, or any other drug that causes sedation.
Sibutramine: the risk of adverse effects on the nervous system is increased, and sibutramine should not be taken with flupentixol.
Proprietary preparations: Depixol; Depixol Conc. (depot injection); Depixol Low Volume (depot injection); Fluanxol.

fluphenazine decanoate A phenothiazine *antipsychotic drug used for the treatment of schizophrenia and other psychoses and mania. Fluphenazine is available, on *prescription only, as a *depot injection.
Side effects: as for *chlorpromazine but fluphenazine has more *extrapyramidal reactions, fewer antimuscarinic effects, and is less sedating.
Precautions: fluphenazine should not be used to treat patients who are severely depressed. *See also* CHLORPROMAZINE HYDROCHLORIDE.
Interactions with other drugs: *see* CHLORPROMAZINE HYDROCHLORIDE.
Proprietary preparations: Modecate; Modecate Concentrate.

flurandrenolone *See* FLUDROXYCORTIDE.

flurazepam A long-acting *benzodiazepine used for the short-term treatment of insomnia. It is available as capsules on *prescription only, but cannot be prescribed on the NHS.
Side effects and precautions: *see* BENZODIAZEPINES; DIAZEPAM.
Interactions with other drugs:
Antiviral drugs: fosamprenavir increases the plasma concentration of flurazepam, causing prolonged sedation and depression of breathing; ritonavir increases the plasma concentration of flurazepam, causing profound sedation, and these two drugs should therefore not be taken together.
See also BENZODIAZEPINES.
Proprietary preparation: Dalmane.

flurbiprofen An *NSAID used for the treatment of pain and inflammation in rheumatoid arthritis and other disorders of the muscles or joints. It is also used to treat mild to moderate pain (such as period pains), to relieve postoperative pain, and to relieve sore throats. Flurbiprofen (as the sodium salt) is applied to the eye to prevent constriction of the pupil during eye surgery and to reduce inflammation after surgery or laser treatment. It is available, on *prescription only, as tablets, modified-release capsules, or eye drops; it can be obtained as lozenges without a prescription, but only from *pharmacies.
Side effects: *see* NSAIDs.
Precautions and interactions with other drugs: *see* NSAIDs.
Proprietary preparations: Froben; Froben SR (modified-release capsules); Ocufen (eye drops); Strefen (lozenges) .

flutamide An *anti-androgen used for the treatment of advanced *cancer of the prostate gland. It is available as tablets on *prescription only.
Side effects: include breast enlargement and tenderness (sometimes with milk production), nausea, vomiting, diarrhoea, increased appetite, insomnia, and tiredness.
Precautions: liver function tests will need to be performed regularly during treatment. People with heart disease may suffer from fluid retention.
Interactions with other drugs:
Warfarin: the anticoagulant effect of warfarin is increased.

fluticasone propionate A *corticosteroid most often used as an anti-inflammatory drug for treating skin disorders, such as dermatitis and eczema, and for the prevention of *asthma attacks and the prevention and treatment of allergic rhinitis, including hay fever. When used topically it is classed as a potent steroid. **Fluticasone furoate** is a similar drug used only for the prevention and treatment of allergic rhinitis. Fluticasone is available, on *prescription only, as a cream, an ointment, a metered-dose nasal spray, a metered-dose *inhaler, a breath-activated inhaler, disks of powder to be used

in a breath-activated delivery system, or as single-dose units for use in a *nebulizer.
Side effects: *see* CORTICOSTEROIDS; TOPICAL STEROIDS. The nasal spray may cause irritation, nosebleeds, and disturbances in smell and taste.
Precautions: fluticasone should be used with caution by women who are pregnant or breastfeeding.
Proprietary preparations: Avamys (fluticasone furoate: nasal spray); Cutivate (cream or ointment); Flixonase (nasal spray); Flixotide (inhaler); Flixotide Accuhaler; Flixotide Diskhaler; Flixotide Evohaler; Flixotide Nebules; Nasofan (nasal spray); Seretide (combined with salmeterol.

fluvastatin A *statin used for the treatment of primary hypercholesterolaemia (*see* HYPERLIPIDAEMIA) that has not responded to dietary measures alone. It is available as capsules or *modified-release tablets on *prescription only.
Side effects and precautions: *see* STATINS.
Interactions with other drugs:
Anticoagulants: the effects of warfarin and acenocoumarol are enhanced.
See also STATINS.
Proprietary preparations: Lescol; Lescol XL (modified-release tablets); Luvinsta XL (modified-release tablets).

fluvoxamine maleate An *antidepressant drug of the *SSRI group. It is used for the treatment of depressive illness and obsessive-compulsive disorder. Fluvoxamine is available as tablets on *prescription only.
Side effects and precautions: *see* SSRIs.
Interactions with other drugs:
Antidepressants: there is an increased risk of adverse effects on the central nervous system if duloxetine is taken with fluvoxamine, and the two drugs should not be used together; reboxetine should not be taken with fluvoxamine; the plasma concentration of agomelatine is increased by fluvoxamine.
Antiepileptics: the plasma concentrations of carbamazepine and phenytoin are increased by fluvoxamine.
Antiparkinsonian drugs: there is an increased risk of adverse effects on the nervous system if rasagiline and selegiline are taken with fluvoxamine; the risk of high blood pressure is increased if selegiline is taken with fluvoxamine.
Antipsychotic drugs: the plasma concentration of clozapine may be increased by fluvoxamine; the risk of ventricular *arrhythmias is increased if droperidol is taken with fluvoxamine, and the two drugs should not be used together.
Melatonin: its plasma concentration is increased and it should not be taken with fluvoxamine.
Sumatriptan: there is an increased risk of adverse effects on the central nervous system if sumatriptan is taken with fluvoxamine.
Theophylline and aminophylline: plasma concentrations of these drugs

are increased to toxic values by fluvoxamine, which should therefore not be used in combination with them; if this is unavoidable, the dosage of theophylline or aminophylline must be reduced.

Tizanidine: its plasma concentration is increased and it should not be taken with fluvoxamine.

See also SSRIs.

Proprietary preparation: Faverin.

FML (Allergan) *See* FLUOROMETHOLONE.

folic acid A vitamin of the B group (*see* VITAMIN B COMPLEX) that has an important role in DNA and RNA synthesis. Good dietary sources of folic acid are liver, yeast, and green vegetables. The proper functioning of folic acid depends on that of another B vitamin, B_{12}, and deficiency of one vitamin may lead to deficiency of the other. Deficiency of folic acid causes certain types of *anaemia (including megaloblastic anaemia), in which the cells that give rise to red blood cells do not develop normally. These can be treated with folic acid. A good intake of folic acid is particularly necessary during pregnancy. Folic acid supplements taken before and during pregnancy help to prevent spina bifida and other neural-tube defects (in which the spinal cord or brain fail to develop normally) in the fetus. It is recommended that women should take 400 micrograms of folic acid daily while trying to conceive and for the first three months of pregnancy. This dosage should be increased to 400–500 milligrams for women who have previously given birth to a baby with a neural-tube defect. Folic acid is also combined with *iron supplements in preparations used to prevent deficiencies of folic acid and iron during pregnancy. Folic acid is available as tablets, a syrup, or a solution and can be obtained from pharmacies without a prescription, but preparations in which the daily dose exceeds 500 micrograms are *prescription only medicines.

Side effects: there may be mottling of the teeth.

Proprietary preparations: Folicare (solution); Lexpec (syrup); *Fefol (combined with ferrous fumarate); *Ferrograd Folic (combined with ferrous sulphate); *Galfer FA (combined with ferrous fumarate); *Pregaday (combined with ferrous fumarate).

Folicare (Rosemont Pharmaceuticals) *See* FOLIC ACID.

folinic acid An agent that counteracts the side effects of *methotrexate and is given as 'rescue' treatment, usually 24 hours after administration of methotrexate, when inflammation of the lining of the mouth and other mucous membranes or *bone marrow suppression are causing problems. It also enhances the activity of *fluorouracil and is used as part of the combination treatment for cancers of the colon and rectum. Folinic acid is given in the form of **calcium folinate** (or **calcium leucovorin**), available as tablets or a solution for injection, or **calcium levofolinate** (**levofolinic acid**), (**calcium levoleucovorin**), **disodium folinate**, or **disodium levofolinate**, which are available as injections. All these drugs are *prescription only medicines.

Side effects: include allergic reaction; fever occasionally occurs after injection.
Proprietary preparations: Isovorin (calcium levofolinate); Refolinon (calcium folinate); Sodiofolin (disodium folinate).

follitropin A synthetic preparation of follicle-stimulating hormone (a *gonadotrophin) used for the treatment of infertility in men and women that is due to underactivity of the pituitary gland (resulting in insufficient production of gonadotrophins). It is also used to induce superovulation (production of a large number of eggs) in women undergoing fertility treatment, such as *in vitro* fertilization. Follitropin is given by subcutaneous or intramuscular injection and is available on *prescription only.
Side effects: include ovarian hyperstimulation (the uncontrolled production of large numbers of follicles in the ovaries) and multiple pregnancy; allergic reactions may occur in both sexes.
Precautions: follitropin should be used with caution in women with ovarian cysts and in people with thyroid or adrenal disorders or pituitary tumours.
Proprietary preparations: Gonal-F (follitropin alpha); Puregon (follitropin beta); *Pergoveris (combined with lutropin alpha).

fondaparinux sodium An *anticoagulant used for the prevention of venous thromboembolism (VTE; *see* THROMBOSIS) in patients after major orthopaedic surgery of the legs or abdominal surgery and in patients who are judged to be at high risk for VTE and are immobilized due to acute illness. It is available as a subcutaneous injection on *prescription only.
Side effects: include bleeding, anaemia, and purpura (a rash resulting from bleeding).
Precautions: fondaparinux should not be given to patients with active bleeding, acute bacterial endocarditis (inflammation of the heart lining), or severe kidney disease. Fondaparinux should not be prescribed to pregnant women unless clearly necessary. Breastfeeding is not recommended during treatment.
Proprietary preparation: Arixtra.

Foradil (Novartis) *See* FORMOTEROL FUMARATE.

Foraven XL (Forum Health Products) *See* VENLAFAXINE.

Forceval (Alliance) A proprietary combination of *vitamin A, vitamins of the B group (*see* VITAMIN B COMPLEX), ascorbic acid (*see* VITAMIN C), vitamin D_2 (*see* ERGOCALCIFEROL), *vitamin E, and various minerals and trace elements, used as a multivitamin and mineral supplement for treating vitamin and mineral deficiency and for people on special diets that lack these substances. It is available as capsules or junior capsules (which also contain *vitamin K) and can be obtained without a prescription, but only from pharmacies.

formaldehyde A caustic liquid that is used to remove verrucas and warts (*see* KERATOLYTICS). It is available as a lotion or gel that can be obtained without a prescription, but only from pharmacies.
Side effects: formaldehyde may cause irritation of the treated skin.

Precautions: formaldehyde should not be used on facial or genital warts or on warts around the anus. It should not be applied to healthy skin around the wart or to broken skin.
Proprietary preparation: Veracur.

formoterol fumarate <**eformoterol fumarate**> A *sympathomimetic drug that stimulates beta *adrenoceptors in the airways. It is used as a *bronchodilator mainly to prevent asthma attacks during the night and exercise-induced asthma in people who are taking long-term prophylactic anti-inflammatory drugs (such as corticosteroids). It is not suitable for the treatment of acute attacks of asthma. Formoterol may also be used for the treatment of severe chronic obstructive pulmonary disease (COPD). It is available, on *prescription only, as a powder or aerosol for use in a breath-activated *inhaler.
Side effects: *see* SALBUTAMOL. In addition, there may be irritation of the mouth, throat, and eyes, altered taste, rash, insomnia, nausea, and itching.
Precautions: formoterol should not be taken by women who are pregnant or breastfeeding.
Interactions with other drugs: *see* SALBUTAMOL.
Proprietary preparations: Atimos Modulite (aerosol inhaler); Foradil (powder inhaler); Oxis Turbohaler (powder inhaler); *Fostair (combined with beclometasone dipropionate); *Symbicort (combined with budesonide).

formulation The form in which a drug is presented. Tablets, a syrup, and an injection are examples.

Forsteo (Eli Lilly & Co) *See* TERIPARATIDE.

Fortipine LA 40 (Goldshield) *See* NIFEDIPINE.

Fortral (Winthrop Pharmaceuticals) *See* PENTAZOCINE.

Fortum (GlaxoSmithKline) *See* CEFTAZIDIME.

Fosamax, Fosamax Once Weekly (Merck Sharp & Dohme) *See* ALENDRONIC ACID.

fosamprenavir A protease inhibitor (*see* ANTIVIRAL DRUGS) used, in combination with *ritonavir, for the treatment of *HIV infection. It is available as tablets or an oral suspension on *prescription only.
Side effects: include heachache, dizziness, diarrhoea, nausea, vomiting, fatigue, and rash. If the rash is severe, treatment should be stopped.
Precautions: fosamprenavir should not be taken by women who are breastfeeding and should be used with caution in people with diabetes, haemophilia, or liver disease and in pregnant women.
Interactions with other drugs: fosamprenavir inhibits an enzyme system in the liver that is involved in metabolizing drugs and therefore has the potential to interact with many drugs. A doctor should be consulted before taking fosamprenavir with any other drug.
Proprietary preparation: Telzir.

fosaprepitant A drug that is metabolized in the liver to produce the antiemetic *aprepitant. It is used as an *adjunct to *dexamethasone and *ondansetron (or a similarly acting drug) to prevent nausea and vomiting in patients receiving chemotherapy and is available as a form for intravenous infusion on *prescription only.
Side effects, precautions, and interactions with other drugs: *see* APREPITANT.
Proprietary preparation: Ivemend.

Fosavance (Merck Sharp & Dohme) A proprietary combination of *colecalciferol (vitamin D_3) and *alendronic acid (a bisphosphonate), used for the treatment of osteoporosis in postmenopausal women who are risk of developing vitamin D deficiency. It is available as tablets on *prescription only.
Side effects, precautions, and interactions with other drugs: *see* ALENDRONIC ACID; VITAMIN D.

Foscan *See* TEMOPORFIN.

foscarnet An *antiviral drug used for the treatment of cytomegalovirus retinitis, a serious eye infection, occurring mainly in AIDS patients, that can lead to blindness. It is also used for treating herpes simplex infections, such as cold sores and genital herpes, in people whose immune systems are compromised and who have not responded to *aciclovir. However, it does not deplete white blood cells to the same extent as ganciclovir. Foscarnet is available as an intravenous infusion on *prescription only.
Side effects: include nausea, vomiting, diarrhoea, abdominal pains, headache, fatigue, impairment of kidney function, reduced concentrations of calcium and haemoglobin in the blood, rash, fever, and genital irritation or ulcers.
Precautions: foscarnet should be used with caution in people with kidney disease and it should not be given to women who are pregnant or breastfeeding. Plenty of fluids should be taken during treatment.
Proprietary preparation: Foscavir.

Foscavir (AstraZeneca) *See* FOSCARNET.

fosinopril An *ACE inhibitor used alone for the treatment of *hypertension and as an adjunct to *diuretics for the treatment of *heart failure. It is available as tablets on *prescription only.
Side effects, precautions, and interactions with other drugs: *see* ACE INHIBITORS.
Proprietary preparation: Staril.

fosphenytoin *See* PHENYTOIN.

Fosrenol (Shire Pharmaceuticals) *See* LANTHANUM.

Fostair (Chiesi) A proprietary combination of *beclometasone dipropionate (a corticosteroid) and *formoterol fumarate (a bronchodilator), used for the treatment and prevention of asthma. It is available as a metered-dose aerosol inhaler on *prescription only.

Side effects and precautions: *see* BECLOMETASONE; FORMOTEROL.
Interactions with other drugs: *see* CORTICOSTEROIDS; SALBUTAMOL.

Fostimon (Pharmasure) *See* UROFOLLITROPIN.

Frador (Fenton) A proprietary combination of *chlorobutanol (an antiseptic), *menthol, *styrax, and balsamic benzoin (an antiseptic and astringent) in the form of a *tincture, used to relieve the pain of mouth ulcers. It is freely available *over the counter.

Fragmin (Pharmacia) *See* DALTEPARIN SODIUM.

f

framycetin sulphate An *aminoglycoside antibiotic used, in combination with a corticosteroid, for the treatment of bacterial infections of the eyes (such as conjunctivitis) or the outer ear. It is available as eye or ear drops on *prescription only.
Side effects: there is a small risk of ear damage, especially if the eardrum is perforated; local allergic reactions may occur.
Precautions: ear drops containing framycetin should not be used in people with a perforated eardrum. Contact lenses should not be worn by people taking eye drops containing framycetin.
Proprietary preparations: *Sofradex (combined with dexamethasone and gramicidin).

frangula *See* NORMACOL PLUS.

Freederm (Diomed Developments) *See* NICOTINAMIDE.

friars' balsam *See* BENZOIN TINCTURE COMPOUND.

Frisium (sanofi-aventis) *See* CLOBAZAM.

Froben, Froben SR (Abbott) *See* FLURBIPROFEN.

Froop (Ashbourne Pharmaceuticals) *See* FUROSEMIDE.

frovatriptan A *5HT$_1$ agonist used for the treatment of headache in acute migraine attacks. It is available as tablets on *prescription only.
Side effects: include dizziness, fatigue, headache, flushing, sensations of tingling, heat, heaviness, pressure, or tightness; if tightness in the chest or throat is severe, treatment should be discontinued.
Precautions: frovatriptan should not be taken by people with certain heart diseases, uncontrolled hypertension, or disease of the peripheral blood vessels or by those who have previously had a heart attack or stroke. It should be used with caution by women who are pregnant or breastfeeding and by people with liver disease.
Interactions with other drugs:

Antidepressants: there is an increased risk of adverse effects on the nervous system if MAO inhibitors, SSRIs, or St John's wort are taken with frovatriptan; St John's and frovatriptan should not be taken together.
Other antimigraine drugs: the risk of spasm of the blood vessels is increased if ergotamine or methysergide are taken with frovatriptan; these

drugs should not be started for 24 hours after stopping frovatriptan, and frovatriptan should not be started for 24 hours after stopping ergotamine or methysergide.
Proprietary preparation: Migard.

Frumil, Frumil LS (sanofi-aventis) *See* CO-AMILOFRUSE.

frusemide *See* FUROSEMIDE.

Frusene (Orion Pharma) A proprietary combination of *furosemide (a loop diuretic) and *triamterene (a potassium-sparing diuretic), used for the treatment of *oedema associated with congestive heart failure, liver disease, or kidney disease. It is available as tablets on *prescription only.
Side effects, precautions, and interactions with other drugs: *see* LOOP DIURETICS; POTASSIUM-SPARING DIURETICS.
See also DIURETICS.

Frusol (Rosemont Pharmaceuticals) *See* FUROSEMIDE.

5-FU *See* FLUOROURACIL.

Fucibet (Leo Pharmaceuticals) A proprietary combination of *fusidic acid (an antibiotic) and *betamethasone (a potent steroid), used for the treatment of eczema occurring with bacterial infection. It is available as a cream on *prescription only.
Side effects, precautions, and interactions with other drugs: *see* CORTICOSTEROIDS.

Fucidin (Leo Pharmaceuticals) *See* FUSIDIC ACID.

Fucidin H (Leo Pharmaceuticals) A proprietary combination of *fusidic acid (an antibiotic) and *hydrocortisone (a moderately potent steroid), used for the treatment of eczema and dermatitis occurring with bacterial infection. It is available, on *prescription only, as a cream.
Side effects, precautions, and interactions with other drugs: *see* CORTICOSTEROIDS.

Fucithalmic (Leo Pharmaceuticals) *See* FUSIDIC ACID.

fulvestrant An *oestrogen antagonist used to treat breast cancer in postmenopausal women in which oestrogen stimulates growth of the tumour. It is used when other hormonal treatments have been unsuccessful. Fulvestrant is given by deep intramuscular injection and is available on *prescription only.
Side effects: include flushing, nausea, vomiting, loss of appetite, rash, and urinary-tract infections.
Precautions: fulvestrant it is not recommended for people with severely impaired liver function or for pregnant or breastfeeding women.
Proprietary preparation: Faslodex.

Fungilin (E.R. Squibb & Sons) *See* AMPHOTERICIN.

Fungizone (E.R. Squibb & Sons) *See* AMPHOTERICIN.

Furadantin (Goldshield) *See* NITROFURANTOIN.

furosemide <**frusemide**> A *loop diuretic used for the treatment of *oedema associated with heart failure, liver disease with ascites (accumulation of fluid in the abdominal cavity), or kidney disease. It is also used to treat hypertension that has not responded to antihypertensive drugs. Furosemide is available, on *prescription only, as tablets, a suspension, or a solution for intravenous injection. *See also* CO-AMILOFRUSE.
Side effects, precautions, and interactions with other drugs: *see* LOOP DIURETICS.
Proprietary preparations: Froop; Frusol; Lasix; Rusyde; *Diumide-K Continus (combined with potassium chloride); Frumil (*see* CO-AMILOFRUSE); *Frusene (combined with triamterene); *Lasilactone (combined with spironolactone).
See also DIURETICS.

fusidic acid A narrow-spectrum *antibiotic used, often in the form of its salt, **sodium fusidate**, for the treatment of infections caused by penicillin-resistant staphylococci, especially bone and skin infections and abscesses. It is available, on *prescription only, as a cream or ointment for topical use, as eye drops, as tablets or a solution for oral use, or as an *intravenous infusion.
Side effects: the tablets or injection may cause nausea, vomiting, rashes, and reversible jaundice, especially after high doses.
Precautions: regular monitoring of liver function during treatment with the tablets or injection is desirable.
Interactions with other drugs:
Ritonavir: its plasma concentration is increased and it increases the plasma concentration of fusidic acid and therefore should not be used with it.
Statins: the risk of muscle damage is increased if simvastatin and possibly atorvastatin are taken with fusidic acid.
Proprietary preparations: Fucidin; Fucithalmic (eye drops); *Fucibet (combined with betamethasone); *Fucidin H (combined with hydrocortisone).

Fuzeon (Roche Products) *See* ENFUVIRTIDE.

Fybogel (Forum Health Products) *See* ISPAGHULA HUSK.

Fybogel Mebeverine (Forum Health Products) A proprietary combination of *mebeverine hydrochloride (an antispasmodic) and *ispaghula husk (a bulking agent), used for the treatment of irritable bowel syndrome. It is available as effervescent granules on *prescription only.
Precautions: Fybogel Mebeverine should not be taken by people with intestinal obstruction. This medicine should be taken with a full glass of water and should not be taken immediately before going to bed.

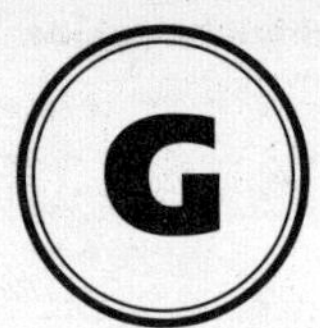

gabapentin An *anticonvulsant drug used alone or as an *adjunct in the treatment of partial epilepsy and alone for the relief of pain associated with nerve damage (including pain due to shingles). It is available as capsules and tablets on *prescription only.
Side effects: include somnolence, dizziness, shaky movements, fatigue, headache, nausea and vomiting, rhinitis, weight gain, and nervousness.
Precautions: dosages should be reduced gradually when stopping medication. The dosage may need to be reduced in the elderly. Women who are planning to become pregnant, or who are already pregnant, should seek specialist advice. Gabapentin is not recommended for women who are breastfeeding.
Interactions with other drugs:
Anatacids: reduce the absorption of gabapentin.
Antidepressants: may reduce the anticonvulsant effect of gabapentin; St John's wort should not be taken with gabapentin.
Antimalarial drugs: mefloquine reduces the anticonvulsant effect of gabapentin; chloroquine and hydroxychloroquine may increase the risk of convulsions.
Proprietary preparation: Neurontin.

Gabitril (Cephalon) *See* TIAGABINE.

galantamine An *acetylcholinesterase inhibitor used for the treatment of mild to moderate Alzheimer's disease. It is available as tablets, *modified-release capsules, and an oral solution on *prescription only.
Side effects: include diarrhoea, nausea, vomiting, abdominal pain, dizziness, headache, and fatigue.
Precautions: galantamine should not be taken by people with kidney disease or by breastfeeding women. It should be used with caution in people with heart disease, asthma, chronic obstructive lung disease, or liver disease.
Interactions with other drugs:
Erythromycin: increases the plasma concentration of galantamine.
Proprietary preparations: Reminyl; Reminyl XL (modified-release capsules).

Galcodine, Galcodine Paediatric (Thornton & Ross) *See* CODEINE.

Galenamox (Allphar Services) *See* AMOXICILLIN.

Galenphol, Galenphol Paediatric, Galenphol Strong (Thornton & Ross) *See* PHOLCODINE.

Galfer (Thornton & Ross) *See* FERROUS FUMARATE.

Galfer FA (Thornton & Ross) A proprietary combination of *ferrous fumarate and *folic acid, used to prevent deficiencies of iron and folic acid during pregnancy. It is available as tablets and can be obtained without a prescription, but only from pharmacies.
Side effects, precautions, and interactions with other drugs: *see* IRON.

Galpseud (Thornton & Ross) *See* PSEUDOEPHEDRINE.

galsulfase An enzyme produced by genetic engineering that is used for the treatment of Maroteau-Lamy syndrome, a rare genetic disorder caused by a deficiency of this enzyme. It is given by intravenous infusion under expert supervision and is available on *prescription only.
Side effects: include breathing difficulties, chest pain, headache, fever, and abdominal pain.
Precautions: reactions relating to the infusion often occur, and these can be minimized by giving an antihistamine and an antipyretic before treatment. Galsulfase should not be given to people with acute fever or respiratory illness or to breastfeeding women. It should be used with caution during pregnancy.
Proprietary preparation: Naglazyme.

Galvus (Novartis) *See* VILDAGLIPTIN.

Gammaderm *See* EVENING PRIMROSE OIL.

Gammaplex (Bio Products Laboratory) *See* IMMUNOGLOBULINS.

ganciclovir An *antiviral drug used for the treatment of cytomegalovirus (CMV) infections. These occur mainly in AIDS patients and in the recipients of transplants. The most serious CMV infection in AIDS patients is retinitis (which may lead to blindness); in transplant patients it is CMV pneumonia. Ganciclovir is available, on *prescription only, as an intravenous infusion or eye gel.
Side effects: the most serious side effect is *bone marrow suppression, resulting in susceptibility to infection and bleeding; other side effects include anaemia, fever, and rash may occur. Less frequently, chills, fever, malaise, nausea, vomiting, abdominal pain, mouth ulcers, diarrhoea, loss of appetite, headache, and itching may occur.
Precautions: ganciclovir should not be given to women who are pregnant or breastfeeding; pregnancy during treatment should be avoided by using adequate contraceptive measures. Blood counts must be monitored during treatment.
Interactions with other drugs:

Imipenem: ganciclovir increases the side effects of this antibiotic.
Zidovudine: causes profound reduction of white-blood-cell production by the bone marrow and should not be used with ganciclovir.

Proprietary preparations: Cymevene (infusion); Virgan (eye gel).

Ganfort (Allergan) A proprietary combination of *timolol maleate (a beta blocker) and *bimatoprost (a prostaglandin analogue), used to reduce pressure inside the eye in people with glaucoma or high blood pressure in the

eye. It is taken when treatment with beta blockers or prostaglandin analogues alone has failed to reduce the pressure. Ganfort is available as eye drops on *prescription only.
Side effects and precautions: *see* BETA BLOCKERS; LATANOPROST.
Interactions with other drugs: *see* BETA BLOCKERS.

ganirelix A drug that inhibits the secretion of *gonadotrophin-releasing hormone. It is used in the treatment of women undergoing assisted reproduction techniques to prevent the premature release of luteinizing hormone, thus allowing time for egg-producing follicles in the ovary to develop. It is given by subcutaneous injection, together with follicle-stimulating hormone, until sufficient follicles are present. Ganirelix is available on *prescription only.
Side effects: include local irritation, headache, and nausea.
Precautions: ganirelix should not be given to women who have impaired liver of kidney function or to women who are pregnant or breastfeeding.
Proprietary preparation: Orgalutran.

Gastrocote (Actavis) A proprietary combination of *alginic acid, *aluminium hydroxide, *magnesium trisilicate, and *sodium bicarbonate, used as an *antacid in the treatment of indigestion, oesophagitis, and heartburn due to reflux (*see* ACID-PEPTIC DISEASES). It is freely available *over the counter as chewable tablets or a sugar-free liquid.
Side effects and interactions with other drugs: *see* ANTACIDS.
Precautions: the tablets are not recommended for children under six years old and should be used with caution by people with diabetes, since they have a high sugar content.

gastro-oesophageal reflux *See* ACID-PEPTIC DISEASES.

Gaviscon Advance (Reckitt Benckiser) A proprietary combination of sodium alginate (*see* ALGINIC ACID) and *potassium bicarbonate, used for the treatment of heartburn, oesophagitis, and indigestion due to reflux (*see* ACID-PEPTIC DISEASES). It is available as a sugar-free suspension and chewable tablets (**Gaviscon Advance Tablets**) and can be obtained without a prescription, but only from pharmacies.
Precautions: Gaviscon Advance has a high sodium content and should therefore be avoided by people following salt-restricted diets and by those who have heart failure or impaired liver or kidney function.

Gaviscon Double Action (Reckitt Benckiser) A proprietary combination of sodium alginate (*see* ALGINIC ACID), *calcium carbonate, and *sodium bicarbonate, used as an *antacid to relieve heartburn and indigestion. It is freely available *over the counter in the form of tablets.
Side effects, precautions, and interactions with other drugs: *see* ANTACIDS.

Gaviscon Infant (Reckitt Benckiser) *See* ALGINIC ACID.

Gaviscon Liquid (Reckitt Benckiser) A proprietary combination of sodium alginate (*see* ALGINIC ACID), *sodium bicarbonate, and *calcium carbonate,

used as an *antacid for the treatment of heartburn, oesophagitis, and indigestion due to reflux (*see* ACID-PEPTIC DISEASES). It can be obtained without a prescription, but only from pharmacies.
Side effects and interactions with other drugs: *see* ANTACIDS.
Precautions: Gaviscon Liquid has a high sodium content and should therefore be avoided by people following salt-restricted diets and by those who have heart failure or impaired liver or kidney function.

Gaviscon Tablets (Reckitt Benckiser) A proprietary combination of *alginic acid, *aluminium hydroxide, *magnesium trisilicate, and *sodium bicarbonate, used as an *antacid for the treatment of heartburn, oesophagitis, and indigestion due to reflux (*see* ACID-PEPTIC DISEASES). It can be obtained without a prescription, but only from pharmacies. **Gaviscon 500** is a similar formulation; **Gaviscon 250** (half-strength tablets) cannot be prescribed on the NHS.
Side effects and interactions with other drugs: *see* ANTACIDS.
Precautions: Gaviscon Tablets have a high sodium content and should therefore be avoided by people following salt-restricted diets and by those who have heart failure or impaired liver or kidney function.

Gee's Linctus (Boots) A proprietary combination of opium tincture (a weak *opioid) and *squill vinegar, used to provide relief from chesty coughs. It is available without a prescription, but only from pharmacies.
Precautions: the linctus may cause drowsiness, and people taking it should not drive or operate machinery. It should not be taken by children under 12 years old.

gefitinib A *tyrosine kinase inhibitor that prevents epidermal growth factor receptor (EGFR), a protein present in increased amounts in tumour cells, from binding to epidermal growth factor, which causes growth and proliferation of these cells. It is used to treat a type of advanced lung cancer and is available as tablets on *prescription only.
Side effects: include rash, acne, nausea, diarrhoea, loss of appetite, and conjunctivitis.
Precautions: gefitinib is not recommended for pregnant or breastfeeding women.
Interactions with other drugs:
Antifungal drugs: itraconazole and ketoconazole increase plasma concentrations of gefitinib.
H_2-receptor antagonists: may reduce plasma concentrations of gefitinib and therefore its efficacy.
Phenytoin: decreases plasma concentrations of gefitinib.
Rifampicin: decreases plasma concentrations of gefitinib.
Warfarin: its anticoagulant effect may be increased by gefitinib.
Proprietary preparation: Iressa.

gel A jelly-like substance consisting of a colloid in which a liquid is dispersed in a solid. Some drugs are formulated as gels for *topical application. The bases may be soluble or insoluble in water.

GelTears (Bausch & Lomb UK) *See* CARBOMER.

gemcitabine An *antimetabolite used intravenously for the treatment of some forms of advanced lung *cancer and of advanced pancreatic cancer (*see* CYTOTOXIC DRUGS) and, in combination with other medicines, for the treatment of advanced bladder, ovarian, and breast cancer. It is available as an injection on *prescription only.
Side effects: include mild nausea and vomiting and rashes; influenza-like symptoms and kidney impairment may also occur. *See* CYTOTOXIC DRUGS.
Precautions: gemcitabine should not be given with radiotherapy or to pregnant or breastfeeding women. *See* CYTOTOXIC DRUGS.
Proprietary preparation: Gemzar.

gemeprost A *prostaglandin that is used to soften and dilate the cervix (neck of the uterus) to induce abortion (*see also* MIFEPRISTONE) or to cause expulsion of a fetus that has died in the uterus. Gemeprost is available, on *prescription only, as pessaries to be inserted into the vagina.
Side effects: include vaginal bleeding, pain in the uterus, nausea, vomiting, diarrhoea, headache, muscle weakness, dizziness, flushing, chills, backache, breathlessness, chest pain, bouts of palpitation, and mild fever.
Precautions: gemeprost should be used with caution in women with obstructive airways disease (e.g. asthma), certain heart conditions, glaucoma, or inflammation of the cervix or vagina.

gemfibrozil A *fibrate used for the treatment of a wide variety of *hyperlipidaemias and to prevent coronary heart disease in men who have not responded to dietary modification and other appropriate measures. It is available as capsules or tablets on *prescription only.
Side effects and precautions: *see* FIBRATES. Gemfibrozil can also cause blurred vision, jaundice, atrial fibrillation (*see* ARRHYTHMIA), and painful extremities. It should not be taken by people with alcoholism, liver disease, or gallstones.
Interactions with other drugs:

Bexarotene: its plasma concentration is increased and it should not be taken with gemfibrozil.
Repaglinide: the risk of severely lowered blood glucose levels is increased and repaglinide should not be taken with gemfibrozil.
Rosiglitazone: its plasma concentration is increased by gemfibrozil.
See also FIBRATES.

Proprietary preparation: Lopid.

Gemzar (Eli Lilly & Co) *See* GEMCITABINE.

generic name The nonproprietary name of a drug or chemical, which is not protected by a trademark. *Compare* PROPRIETARY NAME.

Genotropin (Pharmacia) *See* SOMATROPIN.

gentamicin The most important of the *aminoglycoside antibiotics. It is widely used for the treatment of serious infections, when it may be given with a *penicillin and/or *metronidazole. It is used for the treatment of septicaemia, septicaemia in the newborn, meningitis and other infections of the central nervous system, infections of the bile ducts, kidney infections, infections of the prostate, infections of the membranes or valves of the heart, and pneumonia. It is also used to treat ear and eye infections. Gentamicin is available on *prescription only. For *systemic infections it is given by injection; for ear and eye infections as drops.
Side effects: damage to the ears and kidneys may occur if concentrations in the blood become high.
Precautions: gentamicin should not be taken by pregnant women or by people with myasthenia gravis. It should be used with caution in those with kidney disease, in children, and in the elderly, and should not be used for prolonged periods. Blood and urine tests are required to monitor concentrations of gentamicin and kidney function.
Interactions with other drugs (with injections only):
Amphotericin: increases the risk of kidney toxicity.
Antibacterials: there is an increased risk of ear and kidney toxicity with cephalosporins, colistin, capreomycin, teicoplanin, and vancomycin.
Ciclosporin: increases the risk of kidney toxicity.
Cisplatin: increases the risk of kidney toxicity.
Loop diuretics: increase the risk of ear toxicity.
Muscle relaxants: the effects of some muscle relaxants used during surgery is increased.
Neostigmine and pyridostigmine: the effects of these drugs are antagonized.
Tacrolimus: increases the risk of kidney toxicity.
Proprietary preparations: Cidomycin (injection); Genticin (injection, ear and eye drops); Isotonic Gentamicin Injection; *Gentisone HC (combined with hydrocortisone).

gentian violet *See* CRYSTAL VIOLET.

Genticin (Amdipharm) *See* GENTAMICIN.

Gentisone HC (Amdipharm) A proprietary combination of *gentamicin (an antibiotic) and *hydrocortisone (a corticosteroid), used for the treatment of infections of the outer ear. It is available as ear drops on *prescription only.
Side effects, precautions, and interactions with other drugs: *see* GENTAMICIN; TOPICAL STEROIDS.

Germolene Antiseptic Cream (Bayer) A proprietary combination of the antiseptics *chlorhexidine and *phenol, used for the treatment of minor cuts and grazes, minor burns, scalds, blisters, insect bites, stings, and spots. It is freely available *over the counter.

Germolene Antiseptic Ointment (Bayer) A proprietary combination of *zinc oxide, *methyl salicylate, *phenol, and *octafonium chloride, used as an emollient antiseptic treatment for minor cuts and grazes, burns, scalds, blisters, sore or rough skin, sunburn, muscular pain, and stiffness. It is freely available *over the counter.

Germoloids (Bayer) A proprietary combination of *zinc oxide (an astringent) and *lidocaine (a local anaesthetic), used to relieve the pain and discomfort of *haemorrhoids and anal itching. It is freely available *over the counter in the form of a cream, ointment, or suppositories.

gestodene A synthetic *progestogen used as an ingredient in combined *oral contraceptives. There is a higher risk of thromboembolism with this progestogen than with certain others. Gestodene is available on *prescription only.
Side effects and interactions with other drugs: *see* ORAL CONTRACEPTIVES.
Precautions: gestodene should not be used by women who are at risk of developing thromboembolism, for example because they are very overweight or have varicose veins or a history of thrombosis. It should therefore only be taken by women who cannot tolerate other oral contraceptives and who are prepared to accept the increased risk. *See also* ORAL CONTRACEPTIVES.
Proprietary preparations: *Femodene and Femodene ED (combined with ethinylestradiol); *Femodette (combined with ethinylestradiol). *Sunya 20/75 (combined with ethinylestradiol). *Triadene (combined with ethinylestradiol).

Gestone (Nordic Pharma) *See* PROGESTERONE.

GHRH Ferring (Ferring Pharmaceuticals) *See* SOMATORELIN ACETATE.

ginger tincture An extract from the root of the ginger plant (*Zingiber officinale*). It is used as a flavouring agent and is included as an ingredient in preparations to relieve flatulence and wind pain.

Glandosane (Fresenius) A proprietary combination of carboxymethylcellulose (a protective agent; *see* CARMELLOSE), salts of potassium, sodium, magnesium, and calcium (*see* ELECTROLYTE), and sorbitol (a sugar), used as an artificial saliva to relieve dry mouth, which occurs, for example, after radiotherapy. It is freely available *over the counter in the form of an aerosol spray.

glatiramer acetate A drug that modifies the body's immune response and is used for the treatment of people who have developed the first symptoms of multiple sclerosis and to reduce the frequency of relapses in people with relapsing-remitting multiple sclerosis. It is available as a subcutaneous injection on *prescription only.
Side effects: include reactions at the injection site, anxiety, depression, headache, flushing, breathlessness, nausea, rash, back pain, and chest pain.
Precautions: glatiramer should not be given to pregnant women. In patients with kidney disease, renal function should be monitored during treatment. Glatiramer should be used with caution in people with heart disease.
Proprietary preparation: Copaxone.

glaucoma A condition in which loss of vision occurs because of damage to the optic nerve, which in most cases is caused by an abnormally high pressure in the eye. This is known as **primary glaucoma** and there are two distinct types. In **acute** (or **closed-angle**) **glaucoma**, there is an abrupt rise in pressure due to sudden closure of the angle between the cornea and iris where aqueous fluid usually drains from the eye. This is accompanied by pain and marked blurring of vision. In the more common **chronic simple** (or **open-angle**) **glaucoma**, the pressure increases gradually, usually without producing pain, and the visual loss is insidious. The same type of visual loss may rarely occur in eyes with a normal pressure: this is called **low-tension glaucoma.** Primary glaucoma occurs increasingly with age and is an important cause of blindness. **Secondary glaucoma** may occur when some other eye disease impairs the normal circulation of the aqueous fluid and causes the pressure inside the eye to rise.

In all types of glaucoma treatment is focused on reducing the pressure inside the eye. Drops are instilled into the eye at regular intervals to improve the outflow of aqueous fluid from the eye and/or to reduce the production of aqueous fluid. Drugs used include some *beta blockers (*see* BETAXOLOL HYDROCHLORIDE; CARTEOLOL HYDROCHLORIDE; LEVOBUNOLOL HYDROCHLORIDE; METIPRANOLOL; TIMOLOL MALEATE); *miotics, such as *pilocarpine; *adrenaline and drugs with similar effects to adrenaline (*see* DIPIVEFRINE); the sympathomimetic drugs *apraclonidine and *brimonidine; and the prostaglandin analogues *bimatoprost, *latanoprost, and *travoprost. Carbonic anhydrase inhibitors, in the form of tablets or eye drops, are also used (*see* ACETAZOLAMIDE; BRINZOLAMIDE; DORZOLAMIDE).

Gliadel (Link Pharmaceuticals) *See* CARMUSTINE.

glibenclamide A long-acting *sulphonylurea used for the treatment of type II (noninsulin-dependent) *diabetes mellitus. It is available as tablets on *prescription only.
Side effects: *see* SULPHONYLUREAS.
Precautions: glibenclamide should not be used in the elderly. *See also* SULPHONYLUREAS.
Interactions with other drugs:

Bosentan: the risk of liver damage is increased and therefore bosentan should not be given with glibenclamide.
See also SULPHONYLUREAS.

Glibenese (Pfizer) *See* GLIPIZIDE.

gliclazide A *sulphonylurea used for the treatment of type II (noninsulin-dependent) *diabetes mellitus. It is available as tablets and *modified-release tablets on *prescription only.
Side effects and precautions: *see* SULPHONYLUREAS.
Interactions with other drugs:

Miconazole: enhances the effects of gliclazide and should not be taken with it.

See also SULPHONYLUREAS.
Proprietary preparations: Diamicron, Diamicron MR (modified-release tablets).

glimepiride A *sulphonylurea used for the treatment of type II (noninsulin-dependent) *diabetes mellitus. It is available as tablets on *prescription only.
Side effects and interactions with other drugs: *see* SULPHONYLUREAS.
Precautions: blood tests and monitoring of liver function should be carried out regularly during treatment. Glimepiride should not be taken by those with severely impaired liver or kidney function or by pregnant women (*see also* SULPHONYLUREAS).
Interactions with other drugs: *see* SULPHONYLUREAS.
Proprietary preparation: Amaryl.

glipizide A *sulphonylurea used for the treatment of type II (noninsulin-dependent) *diabetes mellitus. It is available as tablets on *prescription only.
Side effects and precautions: *see* SULPHONYLUREAS.
Interactions with other drugs:
Miconazole: enhances the effects of glipizide and should not be taken with it.
See also SULPHONYLUREAS.
Proprietary preparations: Glibenese; Minodiab.

Glivec (Novartis) *See* IMATINIB.

GlucaGen (Novo Nordisk) *See* GLUCAGON.

glucagon A protein hormone secreted by the alpha cells of the islets of Langerhans in the pancreas. It acts in opposition to *insulin and increases blood glucose by stimulating the breakdown of glycogen to glucose in the liver. Glucagon is used to counteract *hypoglycaemia resulting from insulin overdosage in the treatment of *diabetes mellitus. It is given by intramuscular, subcutaneous, or intravenous injection and is available on *prescription only.
Side effects: include nausea, vomiting, diarrhoea, and low concentrations of *potassium in the blood; rarely, allergic reactions may occur.
Precautions: glucagon must not be given to people with tumours of the insulin- or glucagon-producing cells of the islets of Langerhans in the pancreas or to those with phaeochromocytoma (a tumour of the adrenal gland).
Proprietary preparation: GlucaGen.

Glucobay (Bayer) *See* ACARBOSE.

glucocorticoids *See* CORTICOSTEROIDS.

gluconolactone A compound that can bind free calcium and is included in solutions for washing out catheters.
Proprietary preparation: *Uriflex R (combined with disodium edetate, citric acid, and magnesium carbonate).

Glucophage, Glucophage SR (Merck Serono) *See* METFORMIN HYDROCHLORIDE.

glucosamine A drug used to relieve the symptoms associated with mild to moderate osteoarthritis of the knee. It is available as tablets on *prescription only.
Side effects: include nausea, abdominal pain, indigestion, diarrhoea, constipation; headache, and fatigue.
Precautions: glucosamine should not be taken by people with shellfish allergy or by pregnant or breastfeeding women. People with impaired glucose tolerance should have their blood glucose monitored before and during treatment. People at high risk of developing cardiovascular disease should have their plasma cholesterol levels monitored during treatment.
Interactions with other drugs:
Warfarin: glucosamine enhances its anticoagulant effect, therefore simultaneous use of these medicines should be avoided where possible.
Proprietary preparation: Alateris.

glutaraldehyde A caustic liquid that is used to destroy warts and verrucas (*see* KERATOLYTICS). The process is slow and the wart may need to be pared down and repainted several times. Glutaraldehyde is available as a liquid and can be obtained without a prescription, but only from pharmacies.
Side effects: glutaraldehyde stains the skin brown and may cause local irritation.
Precautions: glutaraldehyde should not be used on facial or genital warts or on warts around the anus. It should not be applied to healthy skin around the wart or to broken skin or come into contact with the eyes, mouth, or other mucous membranes.
Proprietary preparation: Glutarol.

Glutarol (Dermal Laboratories) *See* GLUTARALDEHYDE.

glycerin (**glycerol**) A clear viscous liquid obtained by hydrolysis of fats and mixed oils. It is used as an *emollient in many skin preparations, as an earwax softener, as a *stimulant laxative and faecal softener (particularly in the form of suppositories and enemas), as a *demulcent and sweetening agent in linctuses and pastilles, and in combination with *thymol in a mouthwash.
Proprietary preparations: Boots Constipation Relief Suppositories; Boots Cough Syrup 3 Months Plus; Boots Glycerin and Blackcurrant Soothing Cough Syrup; Boots Nirolex Dry Cough Relief Linctus; Calcough Tickly; Eumocream; Neutrogena Norwegian Formula Dermatological Cream; Tixylix Baby Syrup, Tixylix Toddler Syrup; *Earex Plus Ear Drops (combined with choline salicylate); *Exterol (combined with urea hydrogen peroxide); *Lemsip Cough Dry (combined with honey); *Micolette Micro-enema (combined with sodium lauryl sulphoacetate and sodium citrate); *Optive (combined with carmellose).

glycerol *See* GLYCERIN.

glyceryl trinitrate A *nitrate drug used in treatment of *angina, to prevent or shorten attacks. It is short acting and rapidly absorbed across the lining of the mouth. Therefore to abort attacks it is usually taken as tablets to be dissolved in the mouth – often under the tongue (sublingual) or between the upper lip and the gum (buccal) – or as a sublingual spray. Relief of pain is

Proprietary preparations of glyceryl trinitrate

Preparation	Formulation	Availability
Coro-Nitro Pump Spray	metered-dose sublingual aerosol spray	*P
Deponit	24-hour skin patches	P
Glytrin Spray	metered-dose sublingual aerosol spray	P
GTN 300 mcg	sublingual tablets	P
Minitran	24-skin patches	P
Nitrocine	injection	†POM
Nitro-Dur	24-hour skin patches	P
Nitrolingual Pumpspray	metered-dose sublingual aerosol spray	P
Nitromin	metered-dose sublingual aerosol spray	P
Nitronal	injection	POM
Percutol	ointment	P
Rectogesic	rectal ointment	P
Suscard	modified-release buccal tablets	P
Sustac	modified-release tablets	P
Transiderm-Nitro	24-hour skin patches	P
Trintek	24-hour skin patches	P

* P = pharmacy medicine
† POM = prescription only medicine

rapid. Glyceryl trinitrate can be taken before exercise to prevent an angina attack. Prevention of symptoms is achieved by means of *modified-release tablets or by ointment or skin patches applied to the chest. Glyceryl trinitrate is also available for injection. Some preparations are *prescription only medicines; others can be obtained from pharmacies without a prescription. Glyceryl trinitrate tablets are unstable; they must be stored in light-proof, containers, without cotton wool wadding, and discarded after eight weeks. Glyceryl trinitrate spray can be stored for a long time.
Side effects, precautions, and interactions with other drugs: *see* NITRATES.
Proprietary preparations: see table.

glycol monosalicylate *See* GLYCOL SALICYLATE.

glycol salicylate (**glycol monosalicylate**) A *salicylate that is an ingredient of many *rubefacient creams and sprays for the relief of aches, pains, and stiffness in muscles, joints, and tendons. It is also included in preparations for soothing *haemorrhoids. These preparations are freely available *over the counter.
Side effects and precautions: *see* SALICYLATES.
Proprietary preparations: *Deep Heat Spray (combined with methyl salicylate, methyl nicotinate, and ethyl salicylate); *Dubam Spray (combined with ethyl salicylate, methyl salicylate, and methyl nicotinate); *Fiery Jack Cream (combined with capsicum oleoresin, diethylamine salicylate, and

methyl nicotinate); *Pain Relief Balm (combined with ethyl nicotinate and nonylic acid vanillylamide); *Ralgex Cream (combined with capsicum oleoresin and methyl nicotinate); *Ralgex Freeze Spray (combined with methoxymethane and isopentane); *Ralgex Heat Spray (combined with methyl nicotinate).

glycopyrronium bromide An *antimuscarinic drug that is used before surgery to reduce the secretion of saliva and of mucus in the airways (which are increased when a tube is inserted into the air passage and anaesthetics are inhaled). It is also used as a powerful antiperspirant for the treatment of excessive sweating of the palms and soles. Glycopyrronium is available as an injection or as a powder for preparing a topical solution on *prescription only.
Side effects, precautions, and interactions with other drugs: *see* ANTIMUSCARINIC DRUGS.
Proprietary preparation: Robinul (powder).

g

Glypressin (Ferring Pharmaceuticals) *See* TERLIPRESSIN.

Glytrin Spray (sanofi-aventis) *See* GLYCERYL TRINITRATE.

Goddard's Muscle Lotion (Actavis) A proprietary combination of dilute *acetic acid, *turpentine oil, and dilute *ammonia solution, used as a *rubefacient for the relief of pain and stiffness in muscles, joints, and tendons, including backache, sciatica, lumbago, and fibrositis. It is available without a prescription, but only from pharmacies.
Side effects and precautions: *see* RUBEFACIENTS.

goitre *See* IODINE; THYROID HORMONES.

Golden Eye, Golden Eye Ointment (Typharm) *See* PROPAMIDINE ISETHIONATE.

gold salts *See* SODIUM AUROTHIOMALATE.

gonadorelin *Gonadotrophin-releasing hormone, which is used to assess the functioning of the pitutary gland. Normally, it increases the concentrations of pituitary *gonadotrophins in the blood. Gonadorelin is given by intravenous injection and is available on *prescription only.

*Analogues of gonadorelin are more powerful than the natural hormone, initially increasing the secretion of gonadotrophins by the pituitary gland (and hence of oestrogen by the ovaries or testosterone by the testes). However, continued use acts to inhibit the further release of gonadotrophins, resulting in decreased secretion of oestrogen or testosterone. Gonadorelin analogues are used to treat *endometriosis, infertility, breast cancer, and prostate cancer. *See* BUSERELIN; GOSERELIN; LEUPRORELIN; NAFARELIN; TRIPTORELIN.
Side effects: include nausea, headache, abdominal pain, and increased menstrual bleeding; there may be local reactions at the site of injection.
Proprietary preparation: HRF.

gonadotrophin-releasing hormone (GnRH) A hormone that is produced by the hypothalamus and acts on the pituitary gland to promote the release of *gonadotrophins; since it stimulates the production of luteinizing hormone (LH) and follicle-stimulating hormone (FSH), it is also called **LH-RH** or **LH-FSH-RH**. *See* GONADORELIN.

gonadotrophins Hormones produced by the pituitary gland that act on the ovaries in women and on the testes in men to promote the production of sex hormones and either ova (eggs) or sperm. In pregnancy another gonadotrophin, *human chorionic gonadotrophin (HCG), is produced by the placenta. Its presence in the urine is the basis of pregnancy tests. Gonadotrophins are used mainly in the treatment of female infertility that is caused by underactivity of the pituitary gland, which results in poor ovulation. They are also used to induce superovulation (the production of large numbers of eggs) in women undergoing assisted conception (such as *in vitro* fertilization). The gonadotrophins for therapeutic use are natural and synthetic forms of follicle-stimulating hormone (FSH), which stimulates the growth of the egg-producing follicles in the ovaries (*see* UROFOLLITROPIN; FOLLITROPIN), and luteinizing hormone (LH), which stimulates the release of the egg from the ovary (*see* LUTROPIN ALFA). These hormones are available in combination as *human menopausal gonadotrophin (HMG or menotrophin).

Gonal-F (Merck Serono) *See* FOLLITROPIN.

Gonapeptyl Depot (Ferring Pharmaceuticals) *See* TRIPTORELIN.

Gopten (Abbott) *See* TRANDOLAPRIL.

goserelin An analogue of *gonadorelin that is used to treat *endometriosis and to reduce the thickness of the endometrium (lining of the uterus) before a surgical 'scrape' to treat excessively heavy periods. It is also used to suppress the release of gonadotrophins by the pituitary gland before stimulating ovulation in women undergoing fertility treatment, such as *in vitro* fertilization. Goserelin initially causes increased secretion of gonadotrophins by the pituitary gland, which stimulates secretion of oestrogen by the ovaries, but this acts on the pituitary gland to suppress further release of gonadotrophins and therefore production of oestrogen. In men goserelin is used to treat prostate cancer, having an action similar to that of *leuprorelin; in women it is used to treat breast cancer. It is available as a solution for *depot subcutaneous injection on *prescription only.
Side effects: in women these include hot flushes, changes in libido, vaginal dryness, mood changes and other symptoms similar to those of the menopause. There may be weight gain, reduction in bone density (which can exacerbate osteoporosis), and (rarely) nausea, headache, and abdominal pain. Side effects in men include hot flushes, decreased libido, impotence, a temporary increase in bone pain from secondary tumours in the bones, allergic reactions at the injection site, and a temporary increase in blood pressure. Rarely there may be enlargement of the breasts, nausea, vomiting, and dizziness.

Precautions: goserelin should not be taken by women with undiagnosed vaginal bleeding or by those who are pregnant or breastfeeding; a nonhormonal method of contraception should be used during treatment. The drug should be used with caution by women at risk of developing osteoporosis. Treatment should not be continued to longer than six months. In men there is a risk of compression of the spinal cord and of kidney stones blocking the ureters leading from the kidneys; patients should be monitored carefully during the first month of treatment.
Proprietary preparations: Novgos; Zoladex.

gramicidin An *antibiotic that is only used topically, to treat eye and ear infections, since it is too toxic to be given systemically (i.e. by mouth or injection). It is combined with other antimicrobial agents, such as *neomycin and *polymyxin B, or with a *corticosteroid. Preparations containing gramicidin are available on *prescription only.
Side effects: gramicidin may cause allergic reactions (rash or itching).
Proprietary preparations: *Neosporin (combined with neomycin and polymyxin B); *Sofradex (combined with dexamethasone and framycetin sulphate).

granisetron An *antiemetic used for the prevention or treatment of nausea and vomiting associated with *cytotoxic chemotherapy or radiotherapy or occurring after surgery. It acts by opposing the action of the neurotransmitter 5-hydroxytryptamine (*serotonin) at receptors in the central nervous system and in the gut. It is available, on *prescription only, as tablets or an intravenous injection.
Side effects: include headache, constipation, and rash.
Precautions: granisetron should be used with caution in women who are pregnant or breastfeeding.
Proprietary preparation: Kytril.

Granocyte (Chugai Pharma) *See* LENOGRASTIM.

granulocyte-colony stimulating factor (G-CSF) A protein that stimulates the cells of the bone marrow that produce granulocytes (a type of white blood cell with granular cytoplasm), including neutrophils, which have an important role in the body's defence against infection by destroying bacteria. **Recombinant human granulocyte-colony stimulating factor** is manufactured in the laboratory by genetic engineering techniques. It is used to boost neutrophil production in people whose natural production is poor or in those who have received drugs, especially *cytotoxic drugs, that suppress their natural white cell production (*see* FILGRASTIM; LENOGRASTIM; PEGFILGRASTIM).

Graves' disease *See* THYROID HORMONES.

Grazax (ALK) A proprietary preparation consisting of an extract of grass pollen, used to treat allergic rhinitis and conjunctivitis caused by grass pollen. It is available as dispersible *sublingual tablets on *prescription only.

Precautions: Grazax is not recommended for children under 5 years old or adults over 65 years old and should not be taken by children with asthma or upper airways infections.

Grepid (Beacon Pharmaceuticals) *See* CLOPIDOGREL.

griseofulvin An *antifungal drug that is used for treating fungal infections of the skin, scalp, hair, and nails. Treatment may need to be continued for weeks or even months, but side effects are uncommon. Griseofulvin is available as a spray or tablets on *prescription only.
Side effects: include headache, nausea, vomiting, and less commonly rashes, dizziness, fatigue, and sensitivity to light; blood disorders have also been reported.
Precautions: griseofulvin should not be taken by people with liver failure, lupus erythematosus, or porphyria or by pregnant or breastfeeding women. Women should avoid becoming pregnant for one month after treatment has ceased, and men should not father a child within six months of treatment. Griseofulvin enhances the effects of alcohol and may impair the ability to drive and operate machinery.
Interactions with other drugs:

Anticoagulants: the effects of warfarin and acenocoumarol are reduced.
Oral contraceptives: their effects are reduced by griseofulvin; additional contraceptive measures should be taken during treatment and for one month after treatment has ceased.
Phenobarbital: reduces the effect of griseofulvin.

Proprietary preparations: Grisol AF (spray).

Grisol AF (Transdermal) *See* GRISEOFULVIN.

growth hormone A hormone, secreted by the pituitary gland, that promotes growth of the long bones in the limbs and increases protein synthesis. Its release is controlled by the opposing actions of two hormones: **growth hormone releasing hormone** (or **somatorelin**), which stimulates its release, and **somatostatin**, which inhibits this. Excessive production of growth hormone results in gigantism before puberty and acromegaly in adults. Lack of growth hormone in children causes dwarfism. Acromegaly can be treated by injections of somatostatin analogues (*see* OCTREOTIDE; LANREOTIDE); dwarfism is treated with a genetically engineered form of human growth hormone (*see* SOMATROPIN).

GSL (general sales list) *See* OVER THE COUNTER.

GTN 300-mcg (Martindale Pharmaceuticals) *See* GLYCERYL TRINITRATE.

guaifenesin <**guaiphenesin**> A drug that is reported to reduce the viscosity of sputum and is included as an *expectorant in many cough preparations. However, there is no good evidence that it is effective. Guaifenesin is available without a prescription, but preparations containing other ingredients can usually only be bought from pharmacies.

Side effects: gastrointestinal discomfort has occasionally been reported; very large doses cause nausea and vomiting.
Precautions: guaifenesin should not be taken by people with porphyria.
Proprietary preparations: Beechams Veno's Expectorant; Benylin Children's Chesty Coughs; Boots Nirolex Chesty Cough Relief Linctus; Calcough Six Plus; Family Meltus Chesty Coughs; Hill's Balsam Chesty Cough Syrup; Jackson's All Fours; Lemsip Cough Chesty; Robitussin Chesty Cough; Tixylix Chesty Cough; Vicks Cough Syrup for Chesty Coughs; *Adult Meltus Chesty Coughs with Congestion (combined with pseudoephedrine and menthol); *Beechams All-in-One (combined with paracetamol and phenylephrine); *Benylin Chesty Coughs Non Drowsy (combined with menthol); *Benylin Mucus Cough (combined with levomenthol); *Benylin Mucus Cough Night (combined with diphenhydramin and levomenthol); *Boots Bronchial Cough Mixture (combined with ammonium carbonate and ammonium chloride); *Boots Cough and Decongestant Syrup 2 Years Plus (combined with pseudoephedrine); *Boots Nirolex Chesty Cough & Congestion Relief Linctus (combined with pseudoephedrine hydrochloride); *Junior Meltus Chesty Coughs with Catarrh (combined with cetylpyridinium chloride); *Multi-Action Actifed Chesty Coughs (combined with pseudoephedrine and triprolidine); *Non-Drowsy Sudafed Expectorant (combined with pseudoephedrine); *Robitussin Chesty Cough with Congestion (combined with pseudoephedrine).

guaiphenesin *See* GUAIFENESIN.

guanethidine A drug that prevents the release of noradrenaline from nerve endings in the *sympathetic nervous system and may be used, in combination with other antihypertensive drugs, in the treatment of resistant *hypertension. It is given by intramuscular injection and is available on *prescription only.
Side effects: include low blood pressure, and therefore dizziness, on standing up (orthostatic hypotension), fluid retention, slow heart rate, failure of ejaculation, and diarrhoea.
Precautions: guanethidine should not be taken by people with phaeochromocytoma (a tumour of the adrenal gland), kidney disease, or heart failure.
Interactions with other drugs:
Anaesthetics: their effect in lowering blood pressure is increased.
Sympathomimetic drugs: methylphenidate, dexamfetamine, and some drugs used in cough and cold remedies (e.g. ephedrine) antagonize the effect of guanethidine in lowering blood pressure.
Proprietary preparations: Ismelin.

Gygel (Marlborough) *See* NONOXINOL-9.

Gynest (Marlborough) *See* ESTRIOL.

Gyno-Daktarin (Janssen-Cilag) *See* MICONAZOLE.

Gyno-Pevaryl 1 (Janssen-Cilag) *See* ECONAZOLE NITRATE.

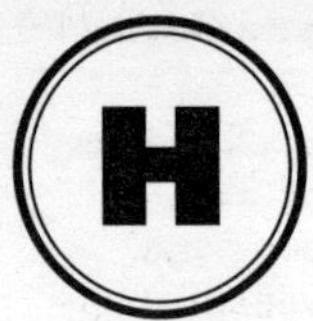

Haelan (Typharm) *See* FLUDROXYCORTIDE.

Haemate P (CSL Behring) A proprietary combination of *Factor VIII and *von Willebrand factor (both blood-clotting factors), used for the prevention and treatment of bleeding in people with haemophilia A and von Willebrand disease (*see* HAEMOSTATIC DRUGS), which are due to a deficiency of these clotting factors. It is available as a form for injection on prescription only. ***Side effects:*** *see* FACTOR VIII.

haemophilia *See* HAEMOSTATIC DRUGS.

Haemorrhoid Relief Ointment (Boots) A proprietary combination of *zinc oxide (an astringent) and *lidocaine (a local anaesthetic), used to relieve the pain of *haemorrhoids. It is freely available *over the counter, but only from Boots stores.

haemorrhoids (piles) Swelling of the spongy blood-filled cushions in the wall of the anus, usually a consequence of prolonged constipation or, occasionally, diarrhoea. Haemorrhoids may protrude beyond the anus. They bleed and may cause pain after defaecation due to an **anal fissure** (a break in the skin lining the anal canal). Soothing preparations available for relief of the symptoms of haemorrhoids contain *local anaesthetics (such as *lidocaine or *pramocaine hydrochloride), mild astringents (such as *zinc oxide, *bismuth subgallate, or *hamamelis), and often lubricants, mild antiseptics, and *vasoconstrictor drugs. Some preparations also contain *corticosteroids to relieve inflammation. If bleeding persists, an irritant fluid (such as *phenol) may be injected around the haemorrhoids to make them shrivel up (*see* SCLEROTHERAPY).

Soothing preparations containing local anaesthetics and/or corticosteroids can be absorbed and may cause *systemic effects; local anaesthetics may irritate the skin around the anus. For these reasons such preparations should not be used for prolonged periods; treatment should be directed towards avoiding precipitating factors for haemorrhoids, such as constipation.

haemostatic drugs Drugs that are used to stop or prevent haemorrhage (excessive bleeding). **Antifibrinolytic drugs** inhibit or prevent the activation of enzymes that digest blood clots in the circulation; they include *tranexamic acid. *Etamsylate acts by encouraging platelets (specialized blood cells) to stick together, which is part of the blood-clotting process. **Haemophilia** is an inherited bleeding disorder in which blood does not clot naturally, or does so only very slowly. The clotting process is a complex reaction involving several clotting factors, some of which are missing in haemophiliacs. The most important of these are *Factor VIII, lack of which results in classical haemophilia (haemophilia A) and von Willebrand's disease; and *Factor IX, lack of which causes Christmas disease (haemophilia B). Blood products containing these factors are used in the treatment of these disorders. *See also* PHYTOMENADIONE; VITAMIN K.

Haldol, Haldol Decanoate (Janssen-Cilag) *See* HALOPERIDOL.

Half-Inderal LA (AstraZeneca) *See* PROPRANOLOL HYDROCHLORIDE.

Half Securon SR (Abbott) *See* VERAPAMIL HYDROCHLORIDE.

Half Sinemet CR (Bristol-Myers Squibb) *See* CO-CARELDOPA.

halibut-liver oil A combination of *vitamin A and *vitamin D used as a vitamin supplement. It is freely available *over the counter in the form of capsules.
Side effects, precautions, and interactions with other drugs: *see* VITAMIN A.

haloperidol A butyrophenone *antipsychotic drug used for the treatment of schizophrenia and other psychoses and mania. In the short term it is used to calm severely agitated or violent patients and to relieve severe anxiety. Haloperidol is also used to treat intractable hiccups, tics, and severe nausea. It is available, on *prescription only, as tablets, capsules, an oral solution, an injection, and a *depot injection.
Side effects: as for *chlorpromazine, but haloperidol has more pronounced *extrapyramidal reactions, fewer antimuscarinic effects, and is less sedating.
Precautions: *see* CHLORPROMAZINE HYDROCHLORIDE.
Interactions with other drugs:

Amiodarone: should not be taken with haloperidol as this combination increases the risk of abnormal heart rhythms.
Anaesthetics: their effect in lowering blood pressure is enhanced.
Antibiotics: there is an increased risk of arrhythmias if moxifloxacin is taken with haloperidol, and these two drugs should not be used together; rifampicin reduces the effects of haloperidol.
Antidepressants: there is an increased risk of antimuscarinic effects and arrhythmias if haloperidol is taken with tricyclic antidepressants; fluoxetine increases the plasma concentration of haloperidol.
Antiepileptic drugs: their anticonvulsant effects are antagonized by haloperidol; carbamazepine reduces the effects of haloperidol.
Antipsychotics: there is an increased risk of arrhythmias if haloperidol is taken with droperidol or sulpride, and droperidol should not be used with haloperidol; clozapine should not be given with depot injections of haloperidol.
Ritonavir: may increase the effects of haloperidol.
Sedatives: the sedative effects of haloperidol are increased if it is taken with anxiolytic or hypnotic drugs, or any other drug that causes sedation.
Sibutramine: should not be taken with haloperidol as this combination increases the risk of adverse effects on the central nervous system.

Proprietary preparations: Dozic; Haldol; Haldol Decanoate (depot injection); Serenace.

hamamelis (witch hazel) An extract of the shrub *Hamamelis virginiana*, which has mild *astringent properties. It is used in lotions to soothe and cool bruises, sprains, or tired sore eyes. It is also included in preparations for soothing *haemorrhoids.
Proprietary preparation: Optrex (eye drops and eye lotion).

Happinose Nasal Decongestant Balm (Diomed Developments) *See* MENTHOL.

Harmogen (Pharmacia) *See* ESTROPIPATE.

h

Hay-Crom (Norton Healthcare) *See* SODIUM CROMOGLICATE.

Haymine (Chemidex Pharma) A proprietary combination of *chlorphenamine maleate (an antihistamine) and *ephedrine (a decongestant), used for the treatment of hay fever, urticaria, and other allergic conditions. It is available as sustained-release tablets and may be bought from pharmacies without a prescription.
Side effects and interactions with other drugs: *see* ANTIHISTAMINES; EPHEDRINE HYDROCHLORIDE.
Precautions: Haymine should not be taken by people who have suffered from coronary thrombosis, high blood pressure, or thyroid problems. *See also* ANTIHISTAMINES; EPHEDRINE HYDROCHLORIDE.

Hc45 (Crookes Healthcare) *See* HYDROCORTISONE.

HDL (high-density lipoproteins) *See* LIPOPROTEINS.

Health Salt (Boots) A proprietary combination of *sodium bicarbonate and *magnesium sulphate, used as an *antacid to relieve indigestion and for its laxative effect. It is available as a powder to be dissolved in water and can be obtained without prescription.
Side effects: *see* MAGNESIUM SALTS.
Precautions: *see* SODIUM BICARBONATE; MAGNESIUM SALTS. This medicine is not recommended for children under 12 years old.
Interactions with other drugs: *see* ANTACIDS.

Healthy Start Children's Vitamin Drops A combination of vitamins A, C, and D, used as a vitamin supplement for children. It is available as oral drops without a prescription and is free of charge to children under four years of age through the Healthy Start Scheme.

heart block *See* ARRHYTHMIA.

heartburn *See* ACID-PEPTIC DISEASES.

heart failure (congestive heart failure) A condition caused by inadequate output of blood from the heart. Because the tissues of the body do not receive enough blood, and therefore enough oxygen, the body takes actions to compensate for this deficiency, which include: constricting the peripheral blood vessels (so that the overall volume of the blood vessels is smaller), retaining sodium and thus water (so that blood volume increases), and making the heart pump faster. These effects occur because a hormonal system called the **renin-angiotensin** system is stimulated. The symptoms of heart failure are *oedema, fatigue, breathlessness, reduced ability to exercise, and attacks of shortness of breath on exercise or during the night. Heart failure is treated with a variety of drugs, including *ACE inhibitors (which prevent the activation of the renin-angiotensin system), *cardiac glycosides (which improve the force of contraction and therefore the output of the heart), *nitrates, *beta blockers, and *diuretics.

Hedex Caplets, Hedex Tablets (GlaxoSmithKline) *See* PARACETAMOL.

Hedex Extra (GlaxoSmithKline) A proprietary combination of *paracetamol (an analgesic) and *caffeine (a stimulant), used to relieve headache (including migraine), toothache, neuralgia, rheumatic pains, and period pains. It is freely available *over the counter in the form of tablets.
Precautions: Hedex Extra should not be given to children, except on medical advice. *See also* PARACETAMOL; CAFFEINE.

Hedex Ibuprofen (GlaxoSmithKline) *See* IBUPROFEN.

Hedrin (Thornton & Ross) *See* DIMETICONE.

Helicobacter *See* ACID-PEPTIC DISEASES.

Helixate NexGen (CSL Behring) *See* FACTOR VIII.

Hemabate (Pharmacia) *See* CARBOPROST.

Heminevrin (AstraZeneca) *See* CLOMETHIAZOLE.

Hemocane (Eastern Pharmaceuticals) A proprietary combination of *lidocaine (a local anaesthetic), *benzoic acid and cinnamic acid (which have antiseptic properties), and *zinc oxide and *bismuth oxide (astringents), used to relieve the pain and itching of *haemorrhoids. It is freely available *over the counter in the form of a cream.

heparin A naturally occurring *anticoagulant that consists of several molecules of different sizes. Heparin is used to treat deep-vein *thrombosis and pulmonary embolism, and is given before and after surgery to prevent these conditions. People undergoing kidney dialysis may be given heparin to prevent clots forming. Heparin may also be given to people who have had a heart attack if there is a risk of further blood clots. Solutions of heparin are used to wash out cannulas (tubes inserted into veins for *infusion of substances) to stop blood clots forming. A *prescription only medicine, heparin (in the form of heparin calcium or heparin sodium) is available as a solution for intravenous or subcutaneous injection. *See also* LOW MOLECULAR WEIGHT HEPARINS; DANAPAROID SODIUM.
Side effects: excessive bleeding is the most serious side effect (*see*

ANTICOAGULANTS); if this occurs, treatment should be stopped and *protamine sulphate may need to be given. Other side effects include destruction of the skin surrounding the injection site and thrombocytopenia (loss of platelets, blood cells that are involved in the clotting process, resulting in bruising and prolonged bleeding after injury). Long-term use of heparin can cause osteoporosis.
Precautions: the anticoagulant effect of heparin should be monitored with regular blood tests, particularly if it is given intravenously. Heparins should be used with caution in people with haemophilia or other bleeding disorders, active peptic ulcer disease, recent cerebral haemorrhage, severe *hypertension, severe liver disease, or kidney failure, or after major trauma or recent surgery.
Interactions with other drugs:

Aspirin: increases the anticoagulant effect of heparin and the risk of excessive bleeding.
Dipyridamole: increases the anticoagulant effect of heparin and the risk of excessive bleeding.
Drotrecogin alfa: should not be used with high doses of heparin.
Glyceryl trinitrate: infusion of glyceryl trinitrate reduces the anticoagulant effect of heparin.
NSAIDs: there is an increased risk of gastric bleeding with diclofenac and ketorolac, which should therefore not be used with heparin.

Proprietary preparations: Canusal; Hepsal; Multiparin.

heparinoids Derivatives of *heparin that have the anticoagulant properties of heparin. They are used in creams, ointments, and gels to improve the circulation in such conditions as bruising, superficial thrombophlebitis (inflammation of a vein with the formation of small blood clots), chilblains, varicose veins, and haemorrhoids. They are not thought to be very effective. Heparinoids can be obtained without a prescription, but only from pharmacies. *Danaparoid sodium is a heparinoid that is injected before and after surgery to prevent deep vein thrombosis and pulmonary embolism.
Proprietary preparations: Hirudoid (cream or ointment); *Anacal (combined with lauromacrogols); *Movelat (combined with salicyclic acid).

Hepsal (Wockhardt UK) *See* HEPARIN.

Hepsera (Gilead Sciences) *See* ADEFOVIR DIPIVOXIL.

Herceptin (Roche Products) *See* TRASTUZUMAB.

heroin hydrochloride *See* DIAMORPHINE HYDROCHLORIDE.

Herpid (Astellas Pharma) *See* IDOXURIDINE.

Hewletts Cream (Kestrel) A proprietary combination of *zinc oxide and *white soft paraffin, used as an *emollient to soothe the dry skin. It is freely available *over the counter.

hexachlorophene <hexachlorophane> An *antiseptic that is active against a wide range of bacteria. It is used for disinfecting the hands before performing surgery and disinfecting the skin, especially pre-operatively. Hexachlorophene can be obtained without a prescription but only from pharmacies.

hexamine hippurate *See* METHENAMINE HIPPURATE.

hexetidine An *antiseptic with activity against bacteria and fungi that is used in mouthwashes or gargles for minor mouth and throat conditions, such as oral thrush, gingivitis (inflammation of the gums), sore throat, recurrent mouth ulcers, and halitosis. It is also used before and after dental surgery. Hexetidine, in the form of a solution, is freely available *over the counter.
Side effects: hexetidine may cause local irritation; alterations in taste and smell have occasionally been reported.
Proprietary preparation: Oraldene.

Hexopal (Genus Pharmaceuticals) *See* INOSITOL NICOTINATE.

hexyl nicotinate A *rubefacient similar to *methyl nicotinate. It is an ingredient of a cream that is freely available *over the counter.
Side effects and precautions: *see* RUBEFACIENTS.
Proprietary preparation: *Transvasin Heat Rub (combined with ethyl nicotinate and tetrahydrofurfuryl salicylate).

hexylresorcinol An *antiseptic used in solutions for cleansing wounds and in mouthwashes and throat lozenges for the relief of minor infections of the mouth and throat. Preparations containing hexylresorcinol are freely available *over the counter.
Proprietary preparations: Boots Sore Throat Relief Dual Action Lozenges; Buttercup Max Strength Sore Throat Lozenges; Lemsip Sore Throat Triple Action Lozenges; Strepsils Extra; TCP Sore Throat Lozenges; *Beechams Throat-Plus Sugar Free Lozenges (combined with benzalkonium chloride).

hiatus hernia *See* ACID-PEPTIC DISEASES.

HiBi Liquid Hand Rub (Molnlycke Health Care) *See* CHLORHEXIDINE.

Hibiscrub (Molnlycke Health Care) *See* CHLORHEXIDINE.

Hibitane (Molnlycke Health Care) *See* CHLORHEXIDINE.

Hill's Balsam Chesty Cough for Children Syrup (Boehringer Ingelheim) *See* IPECACUANHA.

Hill's Balsam Chesty Cough Pastilles (Boehringer Ingelheim) A proprietary combination of *ipecacuanha (an expectorant), *benzoin tincture compound, *menthol, and *peppermint oil, used for the relief of coughs, colds, and catarrh. **Hill's Balsam Extra Strong '2 in 1' Pastilles** contains a higher concentration of menthol. Both preparations are freely available *over the counter.
Side effects: *see* IPECACUANHA.
Precautions: this medicine is not recommended for children. *See also* IPECACUANHA.

Hill's Balsam Chesty Cough Syrup (Boehringer Ingelheim) *See* GUAIFENESIN.

Hill's Balsam Dry Cough Syrup (Boehringer Ingelheim) *See* PHOLCODINE.

Hill's Balsam Nasal Congestion Pastilles (Boehringer Ingelheim) *See* MENTHOL.

Hiprex (Meda Pharmaceuticals) *See* METHENAMINE HIPPURATE.

Hirudoid (Genus Pharmaceuticals) *See* HEPARINOIDS.

Histalix (Wallace) A proprietary combination of *ammonium chloride (an expectorant), *diphenhydramine (a sedative antihistamine), and *menthol, used to relieve the symptoms of coughs and colds. It is available as a syrup without a prescription, but only from pharmacies. It cannot be prescribed on the NHS.
Side effects and interactions with other drugs: *see* ANTIHISTAMINES.
Precautions: this medicine should not be given to children under one year old. *See also* ANTIHISTAMINES.

histamine A compound found in nearly all tissues of the body, with high concentrations in the skin, lungs, and intestines. Histamine causes dilatation of blood vessels and contraction of smooth muscle (for example in the airways) and regulates the secretion of gastric (stomach) acid. It plays an important role in inflammation and is released in large amounts after skin damage (such as that due to animal venoms). It is also released in anaphylactic reactions (*see* ANAPHYLAXIS) and allergic conditions, giving rise to some of the symptoms of these conditions. Histamine acts at specific sites (receptors) in the tissues, of which there are two main types, H_1 receptors and H_2 receptors. *Antihistamines (H_1-receptor antagonists) block H_1 receptors in the skin, nose, and airways and are used for treating such allergic reactions as urticaria (nettle rash) and hay fever. *H_2-receptor antagonists block H_2 receptors, which are found mainly in the stomach; they are used for treating peptic ulcers and other types of *acid-peptic diseases.

histrelin acetate An analogue of *gonadorelin used to reduce levels of testosterone in the treatment of advanced prostate cancer that requires testosterone for growth (*see* LEUPRORELIN). It is available as a subcutaneous *implant on *prescription only.
Side effects: include headache, hot flushes, constipation, joint pain, and weight gain.
Proprietary preparation: Vantas.

HIV The human immunodeficiency virus, which destroys a subgroup of white blood cells (the helper T-cells, or CD4 lymphocytes), resulting in suppression of the body's immune response. HIV infection is predominantly sexually transmitted; the two other main routes of spread are via infected blood or blood products and from an infected woman to her fetus (it may also be acquired from maternal blood during childbirth or be transmitted in breast milk). Acute infection following exposure to the virus results in the production of antibodies, their presence indicating that infection has taken place. Some people who are HIV-positive progress to chronic infection. This can include the **AIDS-related complex** – persistent generalized involvement of the lymph nodes marked by intermittent fever, weight loss, diarrhoea, fatigue, and night sweats – and **AIDS** itself, in which the individual is susceptible to opportunistic infections – especially pneumonia caused by the protozoan *Pneumocystis jirovecii* (*carinii*), cytomegalovirus (CMV) infections, generalized candidiasis or other fungal infections, and tuberculosis – and/or tumours, such as **Kaposi's sarcoma**.

Although there is currently no cure for HIV infection, a combination of antiretroviral drugs (*see* ANTIVIRAL DRUGS) has been shown to be effective in delaying the progress of the disease.

homatropine hydrobromide An *antimuscarinic drug that is very similar to *atropine sulphate. Like atropine, it is used to dilate the pupils and paralyse the ciliary muscle during examination of the interior of the eye. Homatropine hydrobromide is available as eye drops on *prescription only.
Side effects, precautions, and interactions with other drugs: *see* ATROPINE SULPHATE; ANTIMUSCARINIC DRUGS.

hormone replacement therapy (**HRT**) The use of female hormones to relieve the symptoms that occur when the ovaries cease to function, either naturally (the menopause) or following surgical removal of the ovaries ('surgical menopause'). HRT controls such symptoms as hot flushes and vaginal dryness, and there is often an improvement in psychological wellbeing. It also has beneficial effects on bone density, preventing osteoporosis, and on plasma lipids (fats), which may decrease the incidence of coronary heart disease. HRT may, however, increase the incidence of endometrial cancer and possibly of breast cancer.

Replacement is usually with natural *oestrogens (*see* ESTRADIOL; ESTRIOL; ESTRONE) or conjugated oestrogens (a mixture of natural oestrogens obtained from the urine of pregnant mares). In women who have had a hysterectomy oestrogens alone may be given, in the form of tablets, skin patches, a gel for topical application, or a vaginal cream, ring, or tablets. For women who still have a uterus a *progestogen must also be taken to protect against overgrowth of the endometrium (lining of the uterus), which is stimulated by oestrogens and may give rise to cancer. In **sequential combined therapy** a progestogen is added for 10–14 days at the end of each monthly (or for some preparations three-monthly) cycle. The combination of an oestrogen and a progestogen on a cyclical basis may give episodes of monthly or three-monthly bleeding. In **continuous combined therapy** an oestrogen and a progestogen are given every day. With this therapy, which is suitable for women who have not had a natural period for at least a year, most women stop having episodes of bleeding after an initial 2–3 month period of adjustment. Sequential and continuous combined preparations are available as tablets and/or skin patches; in sequential therapy these must be taken (or applied) in the

Hormone replacement therapy

Proprietary preparation	Oestrogen	Progestogen (alone or combined with an oestrogen)
Sequential combined therapy		
Climagest	estradiol tablets	norethisterone tablets
Cyclo-Progynova	estradiol tablets	levonorgestrel/estradiol tablets
Elleste Duet	estradiol tablets	norethisterone tablets
Evorel Sequi	estradiol patches	norethisterone/estradiol patches
Femapak	estradiol patches	dydrogesterone tablets
Femoston	estradiol tablets	dydrogesterone/estradiol tablets
FemSeven Sequi	estradiol patches	levonorgestrel/estradiol patches
Novofem	estradiol tablets	estradiol/norethisterone tablets
Premique Cycle	conjugated oestrogen tablets	medroxyprogesterone tablets
Prempak-C	conjugated oestrogen tablets	norgestrel tablets
Tridestra	estradiol tablets	medroxyprogesterone/ estradiol tablets
Trisequens	estradiol/estriol tablets	norethisterone/estradiol/ estriol tablets

Proprietary preparation	Oestrogen	Progestogen	Formulation
Continuous combined therapy			
Angeliq	estradiol	drospirenone	tablets
Climesse	estradiol	norethisterone	tablets
Clinorette	estradiol	norethisterone	tablets
Elleste Duet Conti	estradiol	norethisterone	tablets
Evorel Conti	estradiol	norethisterone	patches
FemSeven Conti	estradiol	levonorgestrel	patches
Femoston-conti	estradiol	dydrogesterone	tablets
Indivina	estradiol	medroxyprogesterone	tablets
Kliofem	estradiol	norethisterone	tablets
Kliovance	estradiol	norethisterone	tablets
Nuvelle Continuous	estradiol	norethisterone	tablets
Premique	conjugated oestrogens	medroxyprogesterone	tablets
Oestrogen-only therapy			
Bedol	estradiol		tablets
Climaval	estradiol		tablets

Proprietary preparation	Oestrogen	Progestogen	Formulation
Elleste Solo	estradiol		tablets
Elleste Solo MX	estradiol		patches
Estraderm TTS	estradiol		patches
Estraderm MX	estradiol		patches
Estradiol Implants	estradiol		implants
Estradot	estradiol		patches
Estring	estradiol		vaginal ring
Evorel	estradiol		patches
Fematrix	estradiol		patches
FemSeven	estradiol		patches
Gynest	estriol		vaginal cream
Harmogen	estropipate		tablets
Hormonin	estriol/ estradiol/estrone		tablets
Oestrogel	estradiol		gel
Ortho-Gynest	estriol		pessary or vaginal cream
Ovestin	estriol		vaginal cream
Premarin	conjugated oestrogens		tablets or vaginal cream
Progynova	estradiol		tablets
Progynova TS	estradiol		patches
Sandrena	estradiol		gel
Vagifem	estradiol		vaginal tablets
Zumenon	estradiol		tablets
Adjunctive progestogen therapy			
Utrogestan		progesterone	capsules

prescribed order as the dosage of oestrogens may vary or the progestogen may be added on specific days. Progestogens may alternatively be taken in the form of capsules as an *adjunct to oestrogen-only therapy. Synthetic and semisynthetic oestrogens are also used in HRT (*see* ESTROPIPATE; TIBOLONE). All HRT preparations are *prescription only medicines.
Side effects: include nausea, vomiting, weight gain, breast tenderness and enlargement, breakthrough bleeding, headache, dizziness, migraine, and increased blood pressure. The occurrence of migraine-type headaches for the first time, frequent severe headaches, or acute visual disturbances should be reported to a doctor immediately.
Precautions: HRT should not be used by women who have cancer of the breast, uterus, or genital tract, thrombosis, or severe heart, liver, or kidney disease or by those who are pregnant or breastfeeding. It should be used with caution by women who have had thrombosis or thromboembolism, migraine, diabetes, epilepsy, porphyria, fibroids, or tetanus. If pregnancy occurs HRT

should be stopped immediately. HRT may need to be discontinued before surgery.
Interactions with other drugs: as for *oestrogen, but interactions are much less likely to occur as the doses of oestrogen are relatively low.
Proprietary preparations: see table.

Hormonin (Amdipharm) A proprietary combination of *estriol, *estrone, and *estradiol used as *hormone replacement therapy to relieve menopausal symptoms and to prevent postmenopausal osteoporosis. Women who have not had a hysterectomy may also need to take *progestogen supplements. Hormonin is available as tablets on *prescription only.
Side effects, precautions, and interactions with other drugs: *see* HORMONE REPLACEMENT THERAPY.

h

H_2-receptor antagonists (**histamine H_2-receptor antagonists**) A class of drugs that block a type of *histamine receptor in the stomach (called H_2 receptors) and thereby reduce the secretion of gastric (stomach) acid. They reduce both the volume and the acidity of gastric juice and are used in the treatment of gastric and duodenal ulcers, gastro-oesophageal reflux, and indigestion (*see* ACID-PEPTIC DISEASES). *See* CIMETIDINE; FAMOTIDINE; NIZATIDINE; RANITIDINE.
Side effects: side effects are generally rare and minor. Dizziness, drowsiness or fatigue, and rash have been reported with all H_2-receptor antagonists; more rarely headache, changes in liver function, blood disorders, and enlargement of the breasts in men may occur. More information is provided in the entries for individual H_2-receptor antagonists.
Precautions and interactions with other drugs: see entries for individual H_2-receptor antagonists.

HRF (Monmouth Pharmaceuticals) *See* GONADORELIN.

HRT *See* HORMONE REPLACEMENT THERAPY.

$5HT_1$ agonists (**triptans**) Drugs that stimulate receptors for the neurotransmitter *serotonin (5-hydrotryptamine; 5HT) and are used in the treatment of *migraine. They have effects similar to serotonin, rapidly reversing the dilatation of the blood vessels in the brain that is thought to cause a migraine attack. $5HT_1$ agonists are used to treat acute attacks of migraine; they should not be taken with other drugs used for this purpose. *See* ALMOTRIPTAN; ELETRIPTAN; FROVATRIPTAN; NARATRIPTAN; RIZATRIPTAN; SUMATRIPTAN; ZOLMITRIPTAN.
Side effects, precautions, and interactions with other drugs: see entries for individual $5HT_1$ agonists.

HT Defix (Scottish National Blood Transfusion Service) *See* FACTOR IX.

Humalog (Eli Lilly & Co) *See* INSULIN.

Humalog Mix25, Humalog Mix50 (Eli Lilly & Co) *See* INSULIN.

human chorionic gonadotrophin (**HCG**) A *gonadotrophin produced

during pregnancy by the placenta. Therapeutically, it is used in males for the treatment of undescended testicles, delayed puberty, and poor sperm production. In women it is used for the treatment of infertility due to failure of the ovary to release mature eggs. It is used in conjunction with *human menopausal gonadotrophin to promote superovulation (the production of large numbers of eggs) in women undergoing fertility treatment. It is given by subcutaneous or intramuscular *injection and is available on *prescription only.
Side effects: include oedema (fluid retention; particularly in men), headache, tiredness, mood changes, and allergic reactions; high doses result in increased sexuality.
Precautions: HCG should be used with caution by people with asthma, epilepsy, migraine, or disorders of the heart or kidneys.
Proprietary preparations: Choragon; Ovitrelle; Pregnyl.

human menopausal gonadotrophin (**menotrophin**) A combination of follicle-stimulating hormone and luteinizing hormone (*see* GONADOTROPHINS), extracted from the urine of postmenopausal women. It is used for the treatment of infertility in women and men caused by underactivity of the pituitary gland (resulting in insufficient production of gonadotrophins). It is also used to stimulate the ovaries in women undergoing fertility treatment. Human menopausal gonadotrophin is given by subcutaneous or intramuscular injection and is available on *prescription only.
Side effects: include ovarian hyperstimulation (the uncontrolled production of large numbers of follicles in the ovaries) and multiple pregnancy; in both sexes there may be allergic reactions.
Precautions: the drug should not be given to women with ovarian cysts or tumours of the breast, uterus or ovaries, to men with tumours of the testes or prostate gland, or to people with pituitary or hypothalamic tumours.
Proprietary preparations: Merional; Menopur.

Humatrope (Eli Lilly & Co) *See* SOMATROPIN.

humectants *See* EMOLLIENTS.

Humira (Abbott) *See* ADALIMUMAB.

Humulin I (Eli Lilly & Co) *See* INSULIN.

Humulin M3 (Eli Lilly & Co) *See* INSULIN.

Humulin S (Eli Lilly & Co) *See* INSULIN.

Hyalase (Wockhardt UK) *See* HYALURONIDASE.

hyaluronidase An enzyme that increases the permeability of connective tissue and is given in conjunction with injections of other drugs (such as local anaesthetics) to enhance the penetration of the drug into the tissues. It is available, on *prescription only, as a form for injection. Hyaluronidase is also used to encourage the resorption of blood and other fluids in inflamed tissues.

Side effects: hyaluronidase may cause oedema (fluid retention) and occasionally a severe allergic reaction.
Precautions: hyaluronidase should not be used to reduce the swelling of bites or stings and must not be given intravenously. It should not be applied to the eyes or to infected or cancerous tissues.
Proprietary preparation: Hyalase.

Hycamtin (GlaxoSmithKline) *See* TOPOTECAN.

hydralazine hydrochloride A *vasodilator drug used as an adjunct to a *nitrate for the treatment of moderate to severe *heart failure and, in conjunction with beta blockers, moderate to severe *hypertension. Its use is declining, especially for treatment of hypertension, due to its side effects. It is available, on *prescription only, as tablets or as a solution for injection.
Side effects: include a rapid heart rate, dizziness, headache, nausea, vomiting, fluid retention, and (less commonly) diarrhoea, constipation, rashes, and numbness or tingling in the hands or feet.
Precautions: hydralazine should not be taken by people with systemic lupus erythematosus or some types of heart disease. It should be used with caution in people with liver or kidney disease or a history of stroke and in women who are pregnant or breastfeeding. *See also* ANTIHYPERTENSIVE DRUGS.
Interactions with other drugs: the effects of hydralazine in lowering blood pressure are enhanced by many other drugs.
Proprietary preparation: Apresoline.

Hydrea (E.R. Squibb & Sons) *See* HYDROXYCARBAMIDE.

Hydrex (Ecolab) *See* CHLORHEXIDINE.

hydrochlorothiazide A *thiazide diuretic used, in combination with other antihypertensive drugs, for the treatment of *hypertension and *oedema associated with *heart failure, liver disease, or kidney disease. *See also* CO-AMILOZIDE.
Side effects, precautions, and interactions with other drugs: *see* THIAZIDE DIURETICS; ANTIHYPERTENSIVE DRUGS.
Proprietary preparations: *Accuretic (combined with quinapril); *Capozide (combined with captopril); *Carace Plus (combined with lisinopril); *CoAprovel (combined with irbesartan); *Co-Diovan (combined with valsartan); *Cozaar-Comp (combined with losartan); *Dyazide (combined with triamterene); *Innozide (combined with enalapril); *Micardis Plus (combined with telmisartan); Moduret 25 (*see* CO-AMILOZIDE); *Olmetec Plus (combined with olmesartan); *Triam-Co (combined with triamterene); *Zestoretic (combined with lisinopril).
See also DIURETICS.

hydrocortisone (**cortisol**; **17-hydroxycorticosterone**) A moderately potent *corticosteroid with both mineralocorticoid and glucocorticoid activity, used for the treatment of poorly functioning adrenal glands, anaphylactic shock (*see* ANAPHYLAXIS), inflammatory bowel disease, *haemorrhoids, rheumatic

disease, and inflammatory conditions of the eyes, ears, or skin. It is available as tablets, a solution for injection, eye drops or ointment, ear drops, a cream or ointment for skin conditions, and a rectal foam, usually on *prescription only. A few preparations, containing low doses of hydrocortisone, are available without a prescription.
Side effects: *see* CORTICOSTEROIDS; TOPICAL STEROIDS. In addition, perineal or scrotal warmth, irritation, and pain can occur if intravenous injections are given too rapidly.
Precautions and interactions with other drugs: *see* CORTICOSTEROIDS; TOPICAL STEROIDS.
Proprietary preparations: Boots Bite & Sting Hydrocortisone Cream; Colifoam (rectal foam); Corlan (lozenges); Dermacort (cream); Dioderm (cream); Efcortesol (injection); Hc45 (cream); Hydrocortistab (injection); Mildison Lipocream; Solu-Cortef (injection); *Alphaderm (combined with urea); *Alphosyl HC (combined with coal tar and allantoin); *Anugesic-HC (combined with pramocaine hydrochloride, zinc oxide, Peru balsam, benzyl benzoate, and bismuth oxide); *Anugesic-HC Suppositories (combined with zinc oxide, bismuth oxide, bismuth subgallate, pramocaine hydrochloride, and Peru balsam); *Anusol-HC (combined with benzyl benzoate, bismuth subgallate, Peru balsam, and zinc oxide); *Calmurid HC (combined with lactic acid); *Canesten HC (combined with clotrimazole); *Daktacort (combined with miconazole nitrate); *Eurax-Hydrocortisone (combined with crotamiton); *Fucidin H (combined with fusidic acid); *Gentisone HC (combined with gentamicin); *Nystaform-HC (combined with nystatin and chlorhexidine); *Otosporin (combined with polymyxin B sulphate and neomycin sulphate); *Perinal (combined with lidocaine hydrochloride); *Proctofoam HC (combined with pramocaine hydrochloride); *Proctosedyl (combined both cinchocaine hydrochloride); *Timodine (combined with nystatin, benzalkonium chloride, and dimeticone); *Uniroid-HC (combined with cinchocaine hydrochloride); *Xyloproct (combined with zinc oxide, lidocaine, and aluminium acetate).

hydrocortisone butyrate A potent *topical steroid used for the treatment of eczema, psoriasis, and other inflammatory skin diseases. It is available, on *prescription only, as a cream, ointment, emulsion, or scalp lotion.
Side effects and precautions: *see* TOPICAL STEROIDS.
Proprietary preparations: Locoid; Locoid Crelo; Locoid Lipocream; Locoid Scalp Lotion.

Hydrocortistab (Sovereign Medical) *See* HYDROCORTISONE.

hydroflumethiazide A *thiazide diuretic used for the treatment of *hypertension or *oedema associated with heart failure, liver disease, or kidney disease. It is available, in combination with spironolactone, as tablets on *prescription only (*see* CO-FLUMACTONE).
Side effects, precautions, and interactions with other drugs: *see* THIAZIDE DIURETICS; ANTIHYPERTENSIVE DRUGS.

Proprietary preparations: Aldactide 25; Aldactide 50 (*see* CO-FLUMACTONE).
See also DIURETICS.

hydrogen peroxide An oxidizing agent that has *antiseptic, disinfectant, and deodorizing properties. It is a weak antibacterial agent. Diluted hydrogen peroxide is used in preparations for cleansing, disinfecting, and removing dead tissue from wounds, ulcers, and pressure sores and to release dressings compacted with dried blood, but it may cause more harm than good. A solution is used for disinfecting contact lenses. Hydrogen peroxide is available as a solution, mouthwash, or cream and may be bought without a *prescription, but only from pharmacies.
Precautions: preparations should not be allowed to come into contact with the eyes. Stronger solutions can be irritating and bleaching.

Proprietary preparations: Crystacide (cream); Peroxyl (mouthwash).
See also UREA HYDROGEN PEROXIDE.

Hydromol Cream (Alliance) A proprietary combination of *arachis oil and *liquid paraffin (both emollients), *isopropyl myristate, sodium lactate, and *sodium pyrrolidone carboxylate (a humectant), used for the relief of dry skin conditions. It is freely available *over the counter.

Hydromol Emollient (Alliance) A proprietary combination of light *liquid paraffin (an emollient) and an *isopropyl myristate, used to relieve dry skin conditions. It is available as an emulsion to be added to the bath and can be obtained without a prescription, but only from pharmacies.

hydromorphone hydrochloride An *opioid analgesic that is a derivative of *morphine. It is used for the treatment of severe pain in people terminally ill with cancer. Hydromorphone is available as capsules or *modified-release capsules; it is a *controlled drug.
Side effects and precautions: *see* MORPHINE; OPIOIDS.
Interactions with other drugs: *see* OPIOIDS.
Proprietary preparations: Palladone; Palladone SR (modified-release capsules).

hydrotalcite A compound preparation of aluminium magnesium carbonate hydroxide hydrate, used as an *antacid for the treatment of indigestion. It is available as a suspension and can be obtained without a prescription, but only from pharmacies.
Side effects, precautions, and interactions with other drugs: *see* ANTACIDS.
Proprietary preparation: *Altacite Plus (combined with dimeticone).

hydroxocobalamin A form of vitamin B_{12} (*see* VITAMIN B COMPLEX) used to treat pernicious *anaemia, which is caused by lack of intrinsic factor, a substance that is produced in the intestines and allows vitamin B_{12} to be absorbed. Hydroxocobalamin has replaced *cyanocobalamin for treating this condition since it remains in the body for a longer period; it is available as an intramuscular injection on *prescription only.

Side effects: include itching, rash, fever, chills, hot flushes, nausea, and dizziness.
Proprietary preparations: Cobalin-H; Neo-Cytamen.

hydroxycarbamide <**hydroxyurea**> A *cytotoxic drug used to treat chronic myeloid leukaemia (*see* CANCER) and, combined with radiotherapy, cervical cancer. It may occasionally be used to treat the blood disease polycythaemia. It is also used to prevent sickle-cell crises, in which patients with sickle-cell disease experience episodes of severe pain due to blockage of small blood vessels. Hydroxycarbamide is available as capsules or tablets on *prescription only, and is likely to be used only in specialist units.
Side effects: include nausea (and possibly vomiting), *bone marrow suppression, and skin reactions (*see* CYTOTOXIC DRUGS).
Precautions: *see* CYTOTOXIC DRUGS.
Interactions with other drugs:
Antiviral drugs: there is an increased risk of adverse effects if didanosine and stavudine are taken with hydroxycarbamide and these drugs should therefore not be used together.
Clozapine: should not be taken with hydroxycarbamide as this combination increases the risk of agranulocytosis (a blood disorder).
Proprietary preparations: Hydrea (capsules); Siklos (tablets).

hydroxychloroquine sulphate A drug similar to *chloroquine, used for the treatment of rheumatoid arthritis, juvenile arthritis, and lupus erythematosus (a chronic inflammatory condition of connective tissue). It is also used to treat skin conditions that are aggravated by sunlight. Available as tablets on *prescription only, it should be administered under specialist supervision.
Side effects, precautions, and interactions with other drugs: *see* CHLOROQUINE.
Proprietary preparation: Plaquenil.

17-hydroxycorticosterone *See* HYDROCORTISONE.

hydroxyethylcellulose An agent used in the treatment of dry eyes due to deficient production of natural tears. It is available as single-dose eye drops and can be obtained without a prescription, but only from pharmacies.
Proprietary preparation: *Minims Artificial Tears (combined with sodium chloride).

2-hydroxyethyl salicylate A *salicylate that is included in *rubefacients for the relief of muscular and rheumatic aches and pains. It is an ingredient of preparations that are freely available *over the counter.
Side effects and precautions: *see* SALICYLATES.
Proprietary preparation: *Transvasin Heat Spray (combined with diethylamine salicylate and methyl nicotinate).

5-hydroxytryptamine *See* SEROTONIN.

hydroxyurea *See* HYDROXYCARBAMIDE.

hydroxyzine hydrochloride One of the original (sedating) *antihistamines, used to relieve the symptoms of such allergic conditions as hay fever and urticaria. It is also used for the short-term treatment of anxiety. Hydroxyzine is available as tablets or a syrup on *prescription only.
Side effects, precautions, and interactions with other drugs: *see* ANTIHISTAMINES.
Proprietary preparations: Atarax; Ucerax.

Hygroton (Alliance) *See* CHLORTALIDONE.

Hylo-Forte (Scope Ophthalmics) *See* SODIUM HYALURONATE.

Hylo-Tear (Scope Ophthalmics) *See* SODIUM HYALURONATE.

h

hyoscine butylbromide An *antimuscarinic drug (known as **scopolamine** in the USA) that is used for the relief of gut spasms; for example, those associated with irritable bowel syndrome (*see* ANTISPASMODICS). It is available as tablets or an injection on *prescription only, but packs containing limited quantities of tablets can be obtained from pharmacies without a prescription.
Side effects and precautions: *see* ANTIMUSCARINIC DRUGS.
Proprietary preparation: Buscopan.

hyoscine hydrobromide An *antimuscarinic drug (known as **scopolamine** in the USA) that is used to prevent or treat motion sickness and is given before surgery to reduce secretions and prevent vomiting. Hyoscine is available as tablets (for motion sickness) that can be obtained from pharmacies without a prescription, and as skin patches (for motion sickness) and an injection, which are available on *prescription only.
Side effects: include drowsiness and dizziness. *See also* ANTIMUSCARINIC DRUGS.
Precautions: drowsiness may affect driving and the performance of other skilled tasks and is enhanced by alcohol. *See also* ANTIMUSCARINIC DRUGS.
Proprietary preparations: Boots Travel Calm Tablets; Joy Rides; Kwells; Scopoderm TTS (patches).

hypercholesterolaemia The presence of high concentrations of *cholesterol in the blood. *See* HYPERLIPIDAEMIA.

hyperlipidaemia (**hyperlipoproteinaemia**) A condition in which the plasma concentration of *lipoproteins carrying *cholesterol and/or *triglycerides is increased. There are different classes of hyperlipidaemia, depending on which lipids are present in excess and the underlying cause of the condition. In **primary** and **familial hypercholesterolaemia** the main lipid to be elevated is cholesterol; in **hypertriglyceridaemia** triglycerides are present in excess. **Mixed** (or **combined**) **hyperlipidaemias** are conditions in which both cholesterol and triglycerides are increased. Different *lipid-lowering drugs can be used to treat the various types of hyperlipidaemia.

hypertension High blood pressure, i.e. an elevation of arterial blood pressure above the normal range expected for a person of a particular age and sex. It may result from a variety of disorders, such as kidney or endocrine (glandular) disease. However, more often the cause is not known; in these cases it is called **essential hypertension**. Hypertension is initially symptomless, although severely raised blood pressure may cause headaches and palpitations. It usually requires long-term drug treatment to prevent such complications as damage to arteries (*atherosclerosis), heart attack, *heart failure, stroke, and kidney failure. Certain individuals are more at risk of hypertension, including people with *diabetes mellitus, smokers, and those whose blood lipids (fats) are high (*see* HYPERLIPIDAEMIA). Weight loss, a low salt diet, avoidance of excess alcohol and smoking, and regular exercise are important measures to reduce high blood pressure, but for more severe cases drug therapy may be necessary. Drugs used in the treatment of hypertension are known as *antihypertensive drugs, of which there are several groups (*see* ACE INHIBITORS; ALPHA BLOCKERS; BETA BLOCKERS; CALCIUM ANTAGONISTS; DIURETICS; VASODILATORS).

hyperthyroidism *See* THYROID HORMONES.

hypertriglyceridaemia The presence of high concentrations of *triglycerides in the blood. *See* HYPERLIPIDAEMIA.

hypnotic drugs Drugs that produce sleep by depressing brain function. They are used to treat insomnia, but should only be taken for short periods – no more than three weeks and preferably only one week. Hypnotics should be avoided in elderly people, who are at risk of becoming unsteady on their feet and confused, and therefore likely to fall and injure themselves. They should not be given to children unless there are exceptional reasons for doing so (such as night terrors). Hypnotics may impair judgment and increase reaction time, affecting the ability to drive or operate machinery. They increase the effects of alcohol, and the hangover effects of a dose may impair driving the following day. The commonly used hypnotics are the *benzodiazepines and some sedative *antihistamines; *zopiclone, *zolpidem tartrate, *zalepon, and *melatonin are newer hypnotics. *Barbiturates were formerly used as hypnotics but can now only be prescribed for patients who are already taking them. *See also* CHLORAL HYDRATE; CLOMETHIAZOLE; TRICLOFOS SODIUM.

Hypnovel (Roche Products) *See* MIDAZOLAM.

hypoglycaemia A deficiency of glucose in the bloodstream, which can cause muscular weakness and incoordination, mental confusion, and sweating. If severe it can lead to convulsions, unconsciousness, and coma. Low blood sugar most commonly occurs with overdosage of *insulin or *sulphonylureas in the treatment of *diabetes mellitus. Mild hypoglycaemia can be treated by giving glucose or sugar, usually in a readily absorbable form, such as dextrose tablets, sweet tea, fruit juice, or jam, but if the individual is unconscious an injection of *glucagon or glucose (50%) is necessary. Chronic hypoglycaemia due to excessive secretion of insulin by a tumour is rare but can be treated with surgery and *diazoxide.

hypoglycaemic drugs *See* ORAL HYPOGLYCAEMIC DRUGS.

Hypolar Retard (Sandoz) *See* NIFEDIPINE.

hypolipidaemic drugs *See* LIPID-LOWERING DRUGS.

hypothyroidism *See* THYROID HORMONES.

Hypovase (Pfizer) *See* PRAZOSIN.

hypromellose A drug used for the treatment of dry eyes when the watery component of natural tears is absent or reduced. It is available as eye drops and can be obtained from pharmacies without a prescription.
Precautions: hypromellose should not be used with soft contact lenses.
Proprietary preparations: Artelac; Isopto Alkaline; Isopto Plain; *Ilube (combined with acetylcysteine); *Maxitrol (combined with dexamethasone, neomycin sulphate, and polymyxin B sulphate); *Tears Naturale (combined with dextran).

Hypurin Bovine Isophane (Wockhardt UK) *See* INSULIN.

Hypurin Bovine Lente (Wockhardt UK) *See* INSULIN.

Hypurin Bovine Neutral (Wockhardt UK) *See* INSULIN.

Hypurin Bovine Protamine Zinc (Wockhardt UK) *See* INSULIN.

Hypurin Porcine 30/70 Mix (Wockhardt UK) *See* INSULIN.

Hypurin Porcine Isophane (Wockhardt UK) *See* INSULIN.

Hypurin Porcine Neutral (Wockhardt UK) *See* INSULIN.

Hytrin (Amdipharm) *See* TERAZOSIN.

ibandronic acid A *bisphosphonate used mainly to prevent bone damage and fractures in women with breast cancer that has spread to the bones and to reduce high plasma calcium levels in people with cancer. It is available as tablets or forms for intravenous injection or infusion on *prescription only.
Side effects: include low plasma calcium levels, bone pain, fever, flu-like illness, infection, headache, dizziness, pharyngitis, diarrhoea, vomiting, and gastrointestinal pain.
Precautions: ibandronic acid should not be given to children or to pregnant or breastfeeding women.
Interactions with other drugs:
Aminoglycosides: in combination with ibandronic acid, they may cause abnormally low concentrations of calcium in the plasma.
Proprietary preparations: Bondronat; Bonviva.

ibritumonab tiuxetan A *monoclonal antibody labelled with radioactive yttrium, used for the treatment of certain forms of lymphoma (*see* CANCER) of the B cells (a type of white blood cell). It is given by intravenous infusion, after infusion of *rituximab, and attaches to the cancerous B cells, which are killed by the radiation. Ibritumonab is a *prescription only medicine.
Side effects: the most common are weakness, fever, chills, fatigue, nausea, infection, low counts of platelets and white blood cells, and anaemia.
Precautions: ibritumonab should not be given to women who are pregnant or breastfeeding. Blood cell and platelet counts should be monitored during treatment.
Proprietary preparation: Zevalin.

Ibuderm (Diomed Developments) *See* IBUPROFEN.

Ibufem (GalPharm International) *See* IBUPROFEN.

Ibugel (Dermal Laboratories) *See* IBUPROFEN.

Ibuleve (Diomed Developments) *See* IBUPROFEN.

Ibumousse (Dermal Laboratories) *See* IBUPROFEN.

ibuprofen An *NSAID used for the treatment of pain and inflammation in rheumatoid arthritis (including arthritis in children) and other disorders of the muscles or joints. It is also used to treat period pains, pain after surgery, and fever and pain in children. Ibuprofen is applied to the skin to relieve the pain of sprains, strains, bruises, and rheumatic and muscular pain. Ibuprofen has the lowest incidence of gastrointestinal side effects of all the NSAIDs, but its anti-inflammatory effects are weaker. It is available as tablets, effervescent

granules, *modified-release tablets and capsules, a syrup, a gel for topical application, and a solution for injection. Some preparations are *prescription only medicines. Some non-prescription preparations are freely available *over the counter, but higher dosages and large pack sizes must be bought from pharmacies.
Side effects, precautions, and interactions with other drugs: *see* NSAIDs.
Proprietary preparations: Anadin Ibuprofen; Anadin Ultra; Arthrofen; Boots Fever and Pain Relief 6 Months Plus Ibuprofen; Boots Ibuprofen Pain Relief 6 Months Plus; Brufen; Brufen Retard (modified-release tablets); Calprofen; Cuprofen; Cuprofen Gel; Cuprofen Maximum Strength; Ebufac; Fenbid Forte Gel; Fenbid Spansule (modified-release capsules); Hedex Ibuprofen; Ibrufhalal; Ibuderm; Ibufem; Ibugel (gel); Ibuleve (gel and spray); Ibumousse (foam); Ibuspray; Motrin; Nurofen; Nurofen for Children (suspension); Pedea (solution for injection); Proflex (tablets and cream); Radian B Ibuprofen Gel; Relcofen; Rimafen; *Deep Relief (combined with menthol); *Lemsip Flu 12 Hr (combined with pseudoephedrine); *Non-Drowsy Sudafed Dual Relief Max (combined with pseudoephedrine); *Nurofen Plus (combined with codeine); *Solpadeine Migraine Ibuprofen & Codeine (combined with codeine).

Ibuspray (Dermal Laboratories) *See* IBUPROFEN.

icatibant A drug used for treatment of acute attacks of hereditary angioedema, a severe allergic reaction that involves swelling of the lips, eyes, and tongue and is due to *C1-esterase inhibitor deficiency. It is available as a form for subcutaneous injection on *prescription only.
Side effects: include skin pain, nausea, abdominal pain, dizziness, and headache.
Precautions: icatibant is not recommended for pregnant women, and breastfeeding should be avoided for 12 hours after the injection is given. This medicine should be used with caution in people who have had a stroke or have heart disease.
Proprietary preparation: Firazyr.

ichthammol A *keratolytic that is milder than *coal tar; it is used for the treatment of chronic *eczema in which the skin has become thick and hard. It is available as an ointment and – combined with *zinc oxide – as a cream or medicated bandage that can be obtained without a prescription, but only from pharmacies.
Side effects: ichthammol may cause local irritation of the skin.
Proprietary preparations: *Icthaband (combined with zinc oxide); *Icthopaste (combined with zinc oxide).

Icthaband (Molnlycke Health Care) A proprietary preparation consisting of a bandage impregnated with a paste containing *zinc oxide (an astringent protective agent) and *ichthammol (a mild keratolytic). It is used in the treatment of chronic *eczema in which the skin has become lichenified (thick and hard). Icthaband can be obtained from pharmacies without a prescription.

Icthopaste (Smith & Nephew Healthcare) A proprietary preparation consisting of a bandage impregnated with a paste containing *zinc oxide (an astringent protective agent) and *ichthammol (a mild keratolytic). It is used in the treatment of chronic *eczema in which the skin has become thick and hard. Icthopaste can be obtained from pharmacies without a prescription.

idarubicin A *cytotoxic antibiotic used for the treatment of advanced breast cancer that has not responded to other chemotherapy. It is also used to treat acute leukaemias, myeloma (cancer of the plasma cells of the bone marrow), and non-Hodgkin's lymphoma (*see* CANCER). Idarubicin is available as capsules or an injection on *prescription only.
Side effects: *see* DOXORUBICIN; CYTOTOXIC DRUGS.
Precautions: idarubicin should not be given to people who have arrhythmias (abnormal heart rhythms) or who have recently had a heart attack or to pregnant women and should be used with caution in people with liver or kidney disease. *See also* DOXORUBICIN; CYTOTOXIC DRUGS.
Proprietary preparation: Zavedos.

idoxuridine A nucleoside analogue (*see* ANTIVIRAL DRUGS) used for the treatment of herpes zoster (shingles) and herpes simplex infections (such as cold sores and genital herpes). A *prescription only medicine, it is available as a solution for topical application with *dimethyl sulfoxide to aid its absorption.
Side effects: include skin irritation and allergic reactions; there may be a strange taste when applied near the mouth.
Precautions: idoxuridine should not be used by women who are pregnant or breastfeeding. It may damage or stain clothing.
Proprietary preparation: Herpid (combined with dimethyl sulfoxide).

Idrolax (UCB Pharma) *See* POLYETHYLENE GLYCOLS.

idursulfase A genetically engineered form of the enzyme iduronate-2-sulfatase, used to treat the genetic disorder Hunter's syndrome, which is due to a deficiency of this enzyme. It is available as a form for intravenous infusion on *prescription only and is used under specialist supervision.
Side effects: include headache, hypertension, indigestion, wheezing, urticaria (nettle rash), itching, and swelling at the infusion site.
Precautions: reactions relating to the infusion often occur, and these can be minimized by giving an antihistamine and an antipyretic before treatment. Idursulfase should not be given to women who are capable of having children. It should be used with caution in people with breathing problems and in breastfeeding women.
Proprietary preparation: Elaprase.

ifosfamide An *alkylating drug, similar to *cyclophosphamide, that is used for the treatment of a wide variety of *cancers. Like cyclophosphamide, it releases acrolein in the body, which can cause irritation and bleeding in the bladder. It is therefore given with *mesna to prevent this effect. Ifosfamide is available as an injection on *prescription only.

Side effects: include nausea and vomiting, blood in the urine, *bone marrow suppression, lack of periods in women, and decreased fertility in men. In high doses ifosfamide can cause drowsiness, confusion, and fits. *See also* CYTOTOXIC DRUGS.
Precautions: ifosfamide should not be given to people who are already passing blood in their urine, those who have a urinary-tract infection or liver disease, or to women who are pregnant or breastfeeding. *See also* CYTOTOXIC DRUGS.
Interactions with other drugs:
Clozapine: should not be given with ifosfamide as this combination increases the risk of agranulocytosis (a blood disorder).
Warfarin: ifosfamide enhances the anticoagulant effect of warfarin.
Proprietary preparation: Mitoxana.

i

Iglu Gel (Diomed Developments) A proprietary combination of *lidocaine (a local anaesthetic) and *aminoacridine hydrochloride (an antiseptic), used to relieve pain from mouth ulcers, sore gums, and ill-fitting dentures. It is available without a prescription, but only from pharmacies.

Ikorel (sanofi-aventis) *See* NICORANDIL.

iloprost A *prostaglandin analogue used for the treatment of pulmonary arterial hypertension (raised blood pressure in the vessels supplying the lungs). It is available as a solution for use in a *nebulizer on *prescription only.
Side effects: include low blood pressure, fainting, cough, headache, and throat or jaw pain.
Precautions: iloprost should not be used within six months of a heart attack or within three months of a stroke, or by people with unstable angina, severe arrhythmias, heart-valve defects, or conditions that increase the risk of bleeding, or by women who are pregnant or breastfeeding. It should be used with caution in people with lung disease or infection, severe asthma, or liver disease.
Proprietary preparation: Ventavis.

Ilube (Alcon Laboratories) A proprietary combination of *acetylcysteine (a mucolytic drug) and *hypromellose (a lubricant), used for the treatment of dry eyes associated with excessive production of mucus in the eyes. It is available as eye drops on *prescription only.
Precautions: Ilube should not be used with soft contact lenses.

imatinib A *tyrosine kinase inhibitor used for the treatment of several forms of leukaemia (*see* CANCER), gastrointestinal stromal tumours (a form of stomach cancer), and some other cancers. It is available as tablets on *prescription only.
Side effects: *see* CYTOTOXIC DRUGS. There may also be weight gain, headache, indigestion, abdominal pain, rash, muscle cramps, muscle, joint, and bone pain, fluid retention, and fatigue.
Precautions: *see* CYTOTOXIC DRUGS. Imatinib is not recommended for

breastfeeding women and should be used with caution in people with liver, kidney, or heart disease.
Interactions with other drugs:

Antiepileptic drugs: the plasma concentration of imatinib is reduced by carbamazepine, oxcarbazepine, and phenytoin, and these drugs should not be used with it.

Clozapine: this drug increases the risk of agranulocytosis (a blood disorder) and should not be used with imatinib.

Rifampicin: reduces the plasma concentration of imatinib and should not be used with it.

Proprietary preparation: Glivec.

Imdur Durules (AstraZeneca) *See* ISOSORBIDE MONONITRATE.

imidapril hydrochloride An *ACE inhibitor used for the treatment of essential *hypertension. It is available as tablets on *prescription only.
Side effects: *see* ACE INHIBITORS. There may also be dry mouth.
Precautions and interactions with other drugs: *see* ACE INHIBITORS.
Proprietary preparation: Tanatril.

imidazoles A group of chemically related drugs that are active against fungi and are also effective against a wide range of bacteria. The group includes the *antifungal drugs *econazole nitrate, *clotrimazole, *ketoconazole, *miconazole *sulconazole, and *tioconazole. Some imidazoles, such as *mebendazole, have marked activity against parasitic worms and are used chiefly as (*anthelmintics).

imiglucerase An enzyme preparation produced by genetic engineering techniques that is used to replace an enzyme whose deficiency results in Gaucher's disease, an inherited disorder in which lipids accumulate in the bone marrow, liver, spleen, lymph nodes, and other tissues. Imiglucerase is available, on *prescription only, as a form for intravenous infusion; its use is restricted to specialists.
Side effects: include itching, pain or swelling at the injection site, and allergic reactions; nausea, vomiting, and diarrhoea have also been reported.
Precautions: imiglucerase should be used with caution in women who are pregnant or breastfeeding.
Proprietary preparation: Cerezyme.

Imigran, Imigran RADIS (GlaxoSmithKline) *See* SUMATRIPTAN.

imipenem A broad-spectrum beta-lactam *antibiotic, structurally similar to the *penicillins, that is used for the treatment of intra-abdominal, genitourinary, and gynaecological infections and for infections of the lower respiratory tract, bones, joints, skin, and soft tissues. It is also used to treat septicaemia and to prevent infections after surgery. Imipenem is given in combination with **cilastatin**, an agent that inhibits its breakdown in the kidneys and therefore prolongs its action. It is administered by intravenous infusion and is available on *prescription only.

Side effects: include nausea, vomiting, diarrhoea, taste disturbances, blood disorders, allergic reactions, convulsions, confusion, and mental disturbances.
Precautions: imipenem should not be given to women who are breastfeeding. It should be used with caution in patients allergic to other beta-lactam antibiotics, in those with kidney disease or any disease of the central nervous system (such as epilepsy), and in pregnant women.
Interactions with other drugs:
Ganciclovir: the adverse effects of imipenem are increased if it is administered with this drug.
Proprietary preparation: Primaxin (combined with cilastatin).

imipramine hydrochloride A *tricyclic antidepressant drug used for the treatment of depressive illness and also bedwetting in children; it is less sedative than *amitriptyline. It is available as tablets on *prescription only.
Side effects, precautions, and interactions with other drugs: see AMITRIPTYLINE HYDROCHLORIDE; TRICYCLIC ANTIDEPRESSANTS.

imiquimod A drug that modifies the body's immune response. It is used for the treatment of genital and anal warts, small superficial basal cell carcinomas (a type of skin cancer), and actinic keratoses (horny overgrowths of the skin) on the face or scalp. It is available as a cream on *prescription only.
Side effects: include pain, itching, burning, irritation, and redness at the application site, headache, flu-like symptoms, and muscle pain.
Precautions: the cream should be used with caution by pregnant women, by people with autoimmune conditions, and by people who have received an organ transplant. Treatment is not recommended until the skin has healed after any previous drug or surgical treatment.
Proprietary preparation: Aldara.

Immukin (Boehringer Ingelheim) *See* INTERFERON GAMMA.

immunoglobulins A group of proteins that act as antibodies as part of the immune response to help the body fight infection. They belong to a class of proteins called **gammaglobulins** and are produced by certain white blood cells in response to the presence of antigens, substances that the body regards as foreign or potentially dangerous, which occur, for example, on the surface of bacteria or viruses.

Normal immunoglobulin, which is prepared from human plasma and contains antibodies to a number of viruses, is used to treat immunoglobulin deficiency that occurs in congenital agammaglobulinaemia and hypogammaglobulinaemia, conditions that are present at birth and result in extreme susceptibility to infections. It is also used to prevent damage to the coronary arteries in Kawasaki syndrome, in which inflammation of the blood vessels is associated with fever and rash, and in the treatment of idiopathic thrombocytopenic purpura, in which platelets (blood cells involved in blood clotting) are destroyed by the body's own antibodies. In addition, normal immunoglobulin is given to prevent infections developing in patients who

have received a bone marrow transplant, which is preceded by treatment to destroy the patient's own bone marrow (*see* BONE MARROW SUPPRESSION). For all these purposes immunoglobulin is given by intravenous injection; for immunoglobulin deficiency states it may also be given by subcutaneous injection. Intramuscular or subcutaneous injections of normal immunoglobulin may be used to provide temporary immunity against hepatitis A, hepatitis B, chickenpox in adults, measles, and rubella in people at risk. Normal immunoglobulin is available as a solution for injection on *prescription only.
Side effects: include malaise, chills, and fever.
Precautions: normal immunoglobulin should not be given within three weeks of vaccination as it may interfere with the immune response to vaccines that contain live viruses.
Proprietary preparations: Flebogamma; Flebogammadif; Gammaplex; Kiovig; Octagam; Privigen; Sandoglobulin; Subcuvia; Subgam; Vigam; Vivaglobin.

Immunoprin (Ashbourne Pharmaceuticals) *See* AZATHIOPRINE.

immunosuppressants Drugs that suppress the activity of the immune system. They are given after organ transplantation to prevent the body's immune system causing tissue rejection. Some are also used in the treatment of autoimmune diseases (in which the body's immune system attacks the body's own tissues), including rheumatoid arthritis and myasthenia gravis. The immunosuppressants used to prevent transplant rejection include *azathioprine, *ciclosporin, *mycophenolate mofetil, *corticosteroids (such as prednisolone), *sirolimus, *tacrolimus, and *basiliximab.

Because immunity is lowered during treatment with immunosuppressants, there is an increased susceptibility to infection (*see* BONE MARROW SUPPRESSION), and regular blood counts may need to be carried out. Some drugs, especially the *cytotoxic drugs used to treat cancer, cause immunosuppression as a side effect.

Imodium (McNeil Ltd) *See* LOPERAMIDE HYDROCHLORIDE.

Imodium Plus (McNeil Ltd) A proprietary combination of *loperamide hydrochloride (an antidiarrhoeal drug) and simeticone (an antifoaming agent; *see* DIMETICONE), used to treat acute diarrhoea with colic. It is available as tablets without a prescription, but only from pharmacies.
Side effects and precautions: *see* LOPERAMIDE HYDROCHLORIDE.

Implanon (Organon Laboratories) *See* ETONOGESTREL.

implant A medicinal preparation that is inserted into the patient's tissues, usually beneath the skin. This enables slow and steady release of the active ingredient over a period of weeks or months. Some hormonal contraceptives can be administered in this way.

Imuderm (Goldshield) A proprietary combination of *almond oil and *liquid paraffin (both emollients), which is added to the bath or applied directly to the skin for the treatment of *eczema, *psoriasis, and other skin conditions associated with dry, itching, scaly, or cracked skin. It is freely available *over the counter in the form of an oil.

Imunovir (Ardern Healthcare) *See* INOSINE PRANOBEX.

Imuran (GlaxoSmithKline) *See* AZATHIOPRINE.

Increlex (Ipsen) *See* MECASERMIN.

indapamide A thiazide-like diuretic (*see* THIAZIDE DIURETICS) used for the treatment of *hypertension. It is available as tablets or *modified-release tablets on *prescription only.
Side effects: include headache, dizziness, fatigue, and muscle cramps due to loss of potassium.
Precautions: indapamide should be discontinued if there are signs of deteriorating kidney function, and it should not be taken by people who have low concentrations of sodium or potassium in the blood, Addison's disease, or by those with severe liver disease.
Interactions with other drugs: *see* THIAZIDE DIURETICS.
Proprietary preparations: Ethibide XL (modified-release tablets); Indipam; Natrilix; Natrilex SR (modified-release tablets); *Coversyl Arginine Plus (combined with perindopril).

Inderal, Inderal LA (AstraZeneca) *See* PROPRANOLOL HYDROCHLORIDE.

indigestion *See* ACID-PEPTIC DISEASES.

indinavir A protease inhibitor (*see* ANTIVIRAL DRUGS) that is used in combination with other antiretroviral drugs (nucleoside reverse transcriptase inhibitors) for the treatment of *HIV infection. Indinavir is available as capsules on *prescription only.
Side effects: include stomach and bowel upsets, headache, fatigue, dizziness, insomnia, dry mouth, disturbances of taste, blood disorders, rash, tingling in the extremities, and aching muscles.
Precautions: indinavir should not be taken by women who are breastfeeding. It should be used with caution in people with diabetes, haemophilia, or liver or kidney disease and in pregnant women.
Interactions with other drugs:

Anti-arrhythmic drugs: indinavir increases plasma concentrations of amiodarone and flecainide and should not be taken with them.

Antibiotics: indinavir increases the plasma concentration of rifabutin and decreases that of rifampicin and should not be taken with them.

Antifungal drugs: itraconazole and ketoconazole increase the plasma concentration of indinavir and should not be taken with it.

Antipsychotics: indinavir increases the plasma concentrations of pimozide and sertindole and should not be taken with them.

Antiviral drugs: atazanavir should not be taken with indinavir; etravirine may reduce the plasma concentration of indinavir and should not be taken with it; indinavir increases the plasma concentration of maraviroc.

Ciclosporin: its plasma concentration is increased.
Cilostazol: its plasma concentration may be increased and it should not be taken with indinavir.
Eletriptan: its adverse effects are increased and it should not be taken with indinavir.
Ergotamine: its adverse effects are increased and it should not be taken with indinavir.
Sedatives: the risk of prolonged sedation is increased if alprazolam or midazolam are taken with indinavir, which should therefore not be taken with them.
Sildenafil: its plasma concentration is increased and therefore its dosage may need to be reduced.
Statins: the risk of muscle damage is increased if rosuvastatin or simvastatin are taken with indinavir, which should therefore not be used with them.
St John's wort: reduces the plasma concentration of indinavir and should not be taken with it.
Vardenafil: its plasma concentration is increased and it should not be taken with indinavir.

Proprietary preparation: Crixivan.

Indipam (Actavis) *See* INDAPAMIDE.

Indivina 1 mg/2.5 mg (Orion Pharma) A proprietary combination of *estradiol (1 milligram) and *medroxyprogesterone (2.5 mg), used as continuous combined *hormone replacement therapy for the relief of menopausal symptoms and prevention of osteoporosis in women who have not had a hysterecomy. **Indivina 1 mg/5 mg** (containing 5 mg medroxyprogesterone) or **Indivina 2 mg/5 mg** (containing 2 mg estradiol and 5 mg medroxyprogesterone) may be given if breakthrough bleeding occurs. All these preparations are available as tablets on *prescription only.

Side effects and interactions with other drugs: *see* HORMONE REPLACEMENT THERAPY.

Precautions: *see* HORMONE REPLACEMENT THERAPY. Indivina is less suitable for women whose last menstrual period occurred during the preceeding three years.

Indolar SR (Sandoz) *See* INDOMETACIN.

indometacin <**indomethacin**> An *NSAID used for the treatment of the pain and inflammation in rheumatoid arthritis and other disorders of muscles or joints. It is also used to relieve the pain of acute gout and period pains. Indometacin is available, on *prescription only, as capsules, *modified-release capsules, and suppositories.

Side effects: indometacin commonly causes indigestion, nausea, vomiting, and diarrhoea, gastrointestinal ulceration and bleeding, dizziness, headache, and light-headedness. It may rarely cause drowsiness, confusion, insomnia,

psychiatric disturbances, blood disorders, and blurred vision. Suppositories can cause local irritation and occasionally bleeding.
Precautions: *see* NSAIDs. In addition, indometacin should be used with caution in people with epilepsy, parkinsonism, or psychiatric illness; suppositories should not be used in people with haemorrhoids. Eye and blood tests are advisable for those taking indometacin on a long-term basis.
Interactions with other drugs:

Triamterene: should not be taken with indometacin as this combination may decrease kidney function.
See also NSAIDs.

Proprietary preparations: Indolar SR (modified-release capsules); Pardelprin (modified-release capsules); Rimacid; Slo-Indo (modified-release capsules).

indoramin hydrochloride An *alpha blocker used to treat all grades of *hypertension and to relieve the obstruction of urine flow that can occur in men with an enlarged prostate gland. It is available as tablets on *prescription only.
Side effects and interactions with other drugs: *see* ALPHA BLOCKERS.
Precautions: people with heart failure should be treated appropriately before taking indoramin. Indoramin should be used with caution in people with liver or kidney disease, epilepsy, Parkinson's disease, or depression. Alcohol should be avoided by people taking indoramin. *See also* ANTIHYPERTENSIVE DRUGS.
Proprietary preparations: Baratol; Doralese.
See also VASODILATORS.

Inegy (Merck Sharp & Dohne) A proprietary combination of *simvastatin (a statin) and *ezetimibe (another lipid-lowering drug), used for the treatment of hypercholesteroleamia and mixed *hyperlipidaemia in people whose lipid levels are not adequately controlled with either drug alone. It is available as tablets on *prescription only.
Side effects, precautions, and interactions with other drugs: *see* EZETIMIBE; SIMVASTATIN.

Infacol (Forest Laboratories) *See* DIMETICONE.

Infaderm Therapeutic Body Oil (Goldshield) A proprietary combination of *almond oil and *liquid paraffin (both emollients), which is added to the bath or applied directly to the skin for the treatment of *eczema, *psoriasis, and other skin conditions associated with dry, itching, scaly, or cracked skin. It is freely available *over the counter.

infliximab A *monoclonal antibody that inhibits tumour necrosis factor alpha (*see* DISEASE-MODIFYING ANTIRHEUMATIC DRUGS). It is used to treat rheumatoid arthritis, ankylosing spondylitis (inflammation of the joints of the backbone), psoriatic arthritis, Crohn's disease, ulcerative colitis, and *psoriasis. Infliximab is given by intravenous infusion under specialist supervision and is available on *prescription only.
Side effects: include airways and other infections, nausea, indigestion, diarrhoea, abdominal pain, headache, flushing, and sweating.

Precautions: infliximab may cause allergic reactions (including fever, chest pain, breathlessness, itching, and rash); antipyretics, antihistamines, or hydrocortisone may be given to prevent these. Infliximab should not be given to people with severe infections or to women who are pregnant or breastfeeding. It should be used with caution in patients with tuberculosis or heart failure.

Interactions with other drugs:

Anakinra: should not be used with infliximab.

Vaccines: should not be given with infliximab.

Proprietary preparation: Remicade.

infusion The slow injection of a substance, usually into a vein (**intravenous infusion**; *see* INTRAVENOUS INJECTION), enabling large volumes to be administered over a period of minutes, hours, or even days. This is a common method for replacing water, electrolytes, and blood products and is also used for the continuous administration of drugs (e.g. antibiotics, painkillers) or *parenteral nutrition. The infused substance flows under gravity from a suspended bottle through a tube ending in a hollow needle inserted into the patient's vein. Many infusions are controlled by electronically regulated infusion pumps to ensure an accurate rate of flow.

inhaler A device for breathing in a drug in order to deliver it to the airways or lungs. Inhalers are most commonly used for administering bronchodilators or corticosteroids in the treatment of *asthma. They enable the drug to be delivered rapidly directly to the lungs and a much lower dosage can be used than if the drug was given in tablet or intravenous form. **Aerosol** (or **metered-dose**) **inhalers** deliver a measured dose of the drug in the form of a suspension of extremely small liquid or solid particles, which is dispensed from the inhaler by a propellant under pressure. Such inhalers are placed into the mouth and depressed (activated) to release drug as the individual takes a breath. This requires a certain amount of coordination and may therefore be unsuitable for children. **Spacers** (or **spacing devices**), which are available for use with some aerosol inhalers, extend the space between the inhaler and the mouth. This reduces the speed at which the aerosol travels to the back of the mouth, allowing more time for the propellant to evaporate and therefore reducing the impact of the propellant on the back of the mouth (which can cause irritation) and enabling a higher proportion of the particles of the drug to be inhaled. There is also less need to coordinate breathing in with activation of the inhaler. **Breath-activated** (or **breath-actuated**) **inhalers** deliver the drug, in the form of an aerosol or a dry powder, only when the user places his (or her) mouth over the outlet and breathes in. This obviates the need to coordinate breathing in with depressing the dispenser. The dose of drug will still be measured (metered) and is not dependent on the size of breath taken. **Dry-powder inhalers** are loaded with capsules of the drug in powder form; as the inhaler is activated (by taking a breath), the capsule is punctured and a type of fan mechanism disperses the powder so that it can be inhaled (these inhalers are called 'Spinhalers' or 'Rotahalers'). 'Turbohalers' are fitted with canisters that deliver measured doses of the drug in powder form. *See also* NEBULIZER.

injection The introduction into the body of drugs in liquid form by means of a syringe, usually drugs that would be destroyed by the digestive processes if taken by mouth. Common routes for injection are below the skin (*subcutaneous), e.g. for insulin; into a muscle (*intramuscular), for drugs that are slowly absorbed; and into a vein (*intravenous), for drugs to be rapidly absorbed. *Enemas are also regarded as injections.

Innohep (Leo Pharmaceuticals) *See* TINZAPARIN SODIUM.

Innovace (Merck Sharp & Dohme) *See* ENALAPRIL MALEATE.

Innozide (Merck Sharp & Dohme) A proprietary preparation consisting of *enalapril (an ACE inhibitor) and *hydrochlorothiazide (a thiazide diuretic), used in the treatment of mild to moderate *hypertension. It is available as tablets on *prescription only.
Side effects, precautions, and interactions with other drugs: *see* ACE INHIBITORS; THIAZIDE DIURETICS.
See also ANTIHYPERTENSIVE DRUGS; DIURETICS.

inosine pranobex An *antiviral drug used for the treatment of herpes simplex infections in mucous membranes and adjacent skin, such as cold sores and genital herpes, and genital warts. It is available as tablets on *prescription only.
Side effects: there may be reversible increases in the concentrations of uric acid in the blood and urine.
Precautions: inosine pranobex should be not be taken by pregnant women and should be used with caution in people with kidney disease, gout, or raised plasma concentrations of uric acid.
Proprietary preparation: Imunovir.

inositol *See* VITAMIN B COMPLEX.

inositol nicotinate A *nicotinic acid derivative used for the treatment of Raynaud's syndrome (poor circulation of hands and feet) or intermittent claudication (cramping pain in the legs on walking due to insufficient blood to the muscles). It is available as tablets on *prescription.
Side effects: as for *nicotinic acid, but side effects are less severe and occur less frequently.
Precautions: inositol nicotinate should not be taken by people who have recently had a heart attack or by those with a stroke or during pregnancy.
Proprietary preparation: Hexopal.

Inovelon (Eisai) *See* RUFINAMIDE.

Inspra (Pfizer) *See* EPLERENONE.

Instanyl (Nycomed UK) *See* FENTANYL.

Instillagel (CliniMed) A proprietary combination of *lidocaine hydrochloride (a local anaesthetic) and *chlorhexidine gluconate (an antiseptic), used for the disinfection, lubrication, and local anaesthesia of the urethra preparatory to passing a catheter or a cystoscope (a fibre-optic viewing device) through the urethra to the bladder. It is instilled into the urethra before the procedure and is available as a gel in a disposable syringe without a prescription.

instillation The application of liquid medication drop by drop, as into the eye or the bladder.

Insulatard (Novo Nordisk) *See* INSULIN.

insulin A protein hormone, secreted by the beta cells of the islets of Langerhans in the pancreas, that controls the concentration of glucose in the blood. It is secreted in response to a rise in blood glucose, which occurs after a meal; its secretion is inhibited by low blood glucose and its action is opposed by some other hormones, mainly *glucagon and *adrenaline. Insulin's actions are to promote the uptake of glucose from the blood by the body's cells, mainly in muscles, where it is used as energy, and in the liver, where it is converted to glycogen for storage. It also stops fat stores being broken down in the body to provide energy and increases protein synthesis. A lack of insulin causes *diabetes mellitus. People with type I (insulin-dependent) diabetes usually require injections of insulin once or twice a day; those with type II (noninsulin-dependent) diabetes may require insulin rather than *oral hypoglycaemic drugs. Insulin cannot be taken orally (it is broken down in the gut) and must therefore always be injected; after instruction, patients can inject themselves subcutaneously (beneath the skin) in the thigh, buttocks, upper arm, or abdomen. In emergencies soluble insulin can be injected intramuscularly or intravenously; this should only be done in hospital.

Preparations of insulin for therapeutic use are derived from animal sources; they are **highly purified insulins**, which have been treated to remove impurities that would cause allergic reactions. Pork (or porcine) insulin (from pigs) is closer chemically to human insulin and causes fewer local reactions than beef (or bovine) insulin (from cows), but most preparations are synthetic **human insulins**. These are manufactured by altering the structure of pork insulin, either by enzymatic modification or by genetic engineering (to produce recombinant insulin), using bacteria or yeasts. They are labelled according to their method of manufacture: **emp** (enzyme-modified pork), **prb** (pork recombinant, using bacteria), or **pyr** (pork recombinant, using yeasts).

Insulin is available in formulations that are short-acting, intermediate-acting, or long-acting. **Short-acting insulins** are solutions of highly purified soluble insulin that, when given subcutaneously, act rapidly (within 30–60 minutes) and are effective for up to eight hours; blood concentrations have a peak between two and four hours. Administration of short-acting insulins should usually be followed by a meal within 15–30 minutes. They are used for diabetic emergencies since they can be injected intravenously as well as subcutaneously or intramuscularly. The effect of intravenous insulin disappears within 30 minutes. **Insulin lispro**, **insulin aspart**, and **insulin**

Proprietary preparations of insulin

Proprietary preparation	Type of insulin (highly purified)	Packaged as
Short-acting		
Actrapid	human neutral insulin (pyr)	vials, prefilled pens, cartridges for reusable pens
Apidra	insulin glulisine	prefilled pens
Humalog	insulin lispro	vials or cartridges for reusable pens
Humulin S	human neutral insulin (prb)	vials, prefilled pens, cartridges for reusable pens
Hypurin Bovine Neutral	beef neutral insulin	vials, cartridges for reusable pens
Hypurin Porcine Neutral	pork neutral insulin	vials, cartridges for reusable pens
Insuman Rapid	human neutral insulin	cartridges for reusable pens, prefilled pens
NovoRapid	insulin aspart	vials or cartridges for reusable pens, prefilled pens
Intermediate-acting		
Humulin I	human isophane insulin (prb)	vials, prefilled pens, cartridges for reusable pens
Hypurin Bovine Isophane	beef isophane insulin	vials, cartridges for reusable pens
Hypurin Porcine Isophane	pork isophane insulin	vials, cartridges for reusable pens
Insulatard	human isophane insulin (pyr)	vials, prefilled pens, cartridges for reusable pens
Long-acting		
Hypurin Bovine Lente	long-acting beef insulin	vials
Hypurin Bovine Protamine Zinc	beef protamine zinc insulin	vials
Lantus	insulin glargine	cartridges for reusable pens, prefilled pens
Levemir	insulin detemir	cartridges for reusable pens, prefilled pens

Biphasic

Humalog Mix25	25% insulin lispro + 75% insulin lispro protamine	prefilled pens, cartridges for reusable pens
Humalog Mix50	50% insulin lispro + 50% insulin lispro protamine	prefilled pens, cartridges for reusable pens
Humulin M3	30% human neutral insulin (prb) + 70% human isophane insulin (prb)	vials, prefilled pens, cartridges for reusable pens
Hypurin Porcine 30/70 Mix	30% pork neutral insulin + 70% pork isophane insulin	vials, prefilled pens, cartridges for reusable pens
Insuman Combi 15	15% human neutral insulin + 85% human isophane insulin	prefilled pens
Insuman Combi 25	25% human neutral insulin + 75% human isophane insulin	prefilled pens
Insuman Combi 50	50% human neutral insulin + 50% human isophane insulin	prefilled pens
Mixtard 30	30% human neutral insulin + 70% human isophane insulin	vials, cartridges for reusable pens, prefilled pens
NovoMix 30	30% insulin aspart + 70% insulin aspart protamine	cartridges for reusable pens, prefilled pens

glulisine are *analogues of human insulin that act very rapidly (15 minutes after injection) and have a short duration of action (2–3 hours), which allows doses to be timed more accurately to coincide with meals. The duration of action of soluble insulin can be prolonged by the addition of zinc, producing **insulin zinc suspensions** (**IZS**), or by zinc and protamine (a protein), producing **protamine zinc insulin** (**PZI**). Zinc and protamine combine with insulin to delay its release in the body. **Intermediate-acting insulins** include **amorphous IZS** and **isophane insulin** (neutral protamine Hagedorn, or NPH insulin). When injected subcutaneously, they start to act at around 1 hour after injection, with maximum effects at 2–8 hours; activity lasts 18–20 hours. Some intermediate-acting insulins are given twice daily in conjunction with short-acting insulin; others are given once a day. **Long-acting insulins** include amorphous IZS and **crystalline IZS** (**ultralente**), or a mixture of these (**lente**), and protamine zinc insulin. They start to act 2–3 hours after subcutaneous injection, with peak activity at 4–16 hours, and can have a duration of action up to 36 hours. The analogues **insulin detemir** and **insulin glargine** have a duration of action of 24 hours. Often combinations of short-, intermediate-, and long-acting insulins are prescribed. **Biphasic insulins** are stable mixtures of a short-acting and an intermediate-acting insulin in fixed proportions, which give a two-stage action. The speed of onset of action will vary with the proportion of short-acting insulin (the higher the proportion, the more rapid the onset). Generally, peak activity is at 1–9 hours and duration of action is around 18–20 hours.

Insulin is supplied either as a solution in vials to be drawn up into a syringe for injection or in dispensing **insulin pens** designed to inject measured doses. These pens are available as prefilled disposable devices or as reusable devices that can be fitted with cartridges of insulin and disposable needles. When taking insulin it is usually necessary to measure glucose concentrations in the blood or urine to ensure that the dose is correct. Most diabetic people can make these measurements themselves at home. Short-acting insulins may also be given by continuous subcutaneous infusion via a pump worn under the clothing when blood glucose concentrations are difficult to control. Insulin is available from pharmacies without a prescription, but the preparations listed in the table are *prescription only medicines and several formulations of insulin, reusable pens, and needles cannot be prescribed on the NHS.

Side effects: the most common side effect is *hypoglycaemia (low blood sugar), which occurs when the patient receives too much insulin or misses a meal and can cause loss of consciousness if untreated (e.g. by taking a glucose sweet). However, most individuals learn to recognize the warning signs of a 'hypo' attack, which include sweating, irritability, muscular weakness, and confusion. Local reactions (e.g. irritation, rash) may occur at the injection site. Hyperglycaemia (high blood sugar; *see* DIABETES MELLITUS) can result when the patient takes too little insulin for the food consumed; changes to the dosing regime are necessary to avoid this problem.

Precautions: expert counselling, training, and dosage adjustment are needed when an individual first starts taking insulin. People using insulin should drive or operate machinery only if they are aware of the nature and risks of hypoglycaemia; alcohol enhances the effect of insulin in lowering blood sugar. Insulin requirements usually fall during the first three months of pregnancy and rise during the last six months; close monitoring of insulin requirements is necessary during pregnancy. Any diabetic woman should consult a doctor if she suspects that she is pregnant.

Interactions with other drugs:

ACE inhibitors: possibly enhance the effect of insulin in lowering blood glucose.

Anabolic steroids: possibly enhance the effect of insulin in lowering blood glucose.

Beta blockers: enhance the effect of insulin in lowering blood glucose and mask many of the symptoms of hypoglycaemia.

Corticosteroids: reduce the effect of insulin in lowering blood glucose.

Diuretics: loop and thiazide diuretics reduce the effect of insulin in lowering blood glucose.

MAOIs: enhance the effect of insulin in lowering blood glucose.

Oral contraceptives: reduce the effect of insulin in lowering blood glucose.

Proprietary preparations: see table.

insulin aspart *See* INSULIN.

insulin detemir *See* INSULIN.

insulin glargine *See* INSULIN.

insulin glulisine *See* INSULIN.

insulin lispro *See* INSULIN.

Insuman Comb 15 (Sanofi-aventis) *See* INSULIN.

Insuman Comb 25 (Sanofi-aventis) *See* INSULIN.

Insuman Comb 50 (Sanofi-aventis) *See* INSULIN.

Insuman Rapid (Sanofi-aventis) *See* INSULIN.

Intal CFC-free Inhaler (Sanofi-aventis) *See* SODIUM CROMOGLICATE.

Integrilin (GlaxoSmithKline) *See* EPTIFIBATIDE.

Intelence (Janssen-Cilag) *See* ETRAVIRINE.

interferon alfa A type of *interferon used for the treatment of certain cancers: it has some activity against lymphomas, leukaemias, and Kaposi's sarcoma (a skin cancer prevalent in AIDS patients) and is capable of reducing the size of certain solid tumours (*see* CANCER). Its use is usually restricted to specialist cancer centres since it has many side effects. Interferon alfa is also used in the treatment of genital warts, genital herpes, hepatitis B, and hepatitis C. It is available, on *prescription only, as forms for injection.
Side effects: include influenza-like symptoms (chills, fever, fatigue, aching muscles and joints), loss of appetite, weight loss, and (less commonly) dizziness, vertigo, forgetfulness, depression, drowsiness, confusion, nervousness, sleep disturbance, and depressed production of blood cells by the bone marrow. Changes in blood pressure, abnormal heart rhythms, and allergic reactions have also been reported.
Precautions: interferon alfa should not be given to people with severe kidney or liver disease, epilepsy or other neurological disorders, or severe heart disease. It should only be given by a specialist and should be used with caution in people who have diabetes. It may impair the ability to drive and operate machinery.
Interactions with other drugs:
Telbivudine: the risk of peripheral neuropathy (causing numbness and tingling of the limbs) is increased if this drug is given with interferon alfa.
Theophylline: its effects are enhanced by interferon alfa.
Proprietary preparations: IntronA; Roferon-A.

interferon beta A type of *interferon used for reducing the frequency and degree of severity of relapses in patients with relapsing remitting multiple sclerosis. It is usually given only to those individuals who have had at least two attacks in the last 2–3 years and in whom the disease has not progressed between relapses, but may be given during an attack; it is not usually given to

those who are wheelchair bound. Interferon beta is available as an injection on *prescription only.
Side effects: include reactions at the injection site, influenza-like symptoms, menstrual disturbances, depression, allergic reactions, insomnia, mood swings, anxiety, confusion, sometimes nausea and vomiting, and rarely hair loss.
Precautions: interferon beta should not be given to women who are pregnant or breastfeeding or to people with liver disease, severe depression, or suicidal tendencies. It should be used with caution in people with uncontrolled epilepsy or kidney disease.
Proprietary preparations: Avonex; Betaferon; Extavia; Rebif.

interferon gamma A type of *interferon used to reduce the frequency of severe infections in people with chronic granulomatous disease (which causes a variety of infections) or severe malignant osteopetrosis (a bone disease). It is available as a form for subcutaneous injection on *prescription only.
Side effects: include headache, nausea, vomiting, diarrhoea, abdominal pain, rash, fever, and muscle and joint pain.
Precautions: interferon gamma can cause exacerbations of heart disease, and it should be used with caution in patients with impaired liver or kidney function. Blood tests and liver and kidney function tests should be carried out before and during treatment. Interferon gamma is not recommended for pregnant or breastfeeding women.
Proprietary preparation: Immukin.

interferons Proteins that are produced by cells infected with a virus and have the ability to enhance the resistance of other cells to attack by other viruses. Interferons are active against many different viruses, but particular interferons are effective only in the species that produces them. There are three types of human interferon: alpha (from white blood cells), beta (from fibroblasts), and gamma (from lymphocytes). Human interferon can now be produced by genetic engineering for clinical use in treating hepatitis B and C, hairy-cell leukaemia, Kaposi's sarcoma, and certain other forms of *cancer, and multiple sclerosis. Side effects, including influenza-like symptoms, lethargy, and depression, may be severe. *See* INTERFERON ALFA; INTERFERON BETA; INTERFERON GAMMA; PEGINTERFERON ALFA.

interleukins A family of proteins that control some aspects of the immune response by conveying signals between white blood cells. Different interleukins are designated by numbers. For example, **interleukin-2** (IL-2) stimulates activity in certain T-lymphocytes that results in the destruction of virus-infected cells. A genetically engineered form of IL-2 is used in the treatment of certain cancers (*see* ALDESLEUKIN).

intramuscular injection The *injection of a drug into the body of a muscle. Usually a larger volume of liquid is injected than for *subcutaneous injections (more than 2 mL) and a slightly wider needle is used. Common sites for intramuscular injections are the deltoid muscle on the outer side of the shoulder and the gluteal muscles of the buttocks.

intravenous injection *Injection of a drug directly into a vein. A small or large volume can be injected; large volumes can be injected over a long period: this is known as intravenous *infusion. Because the drug mixes rapidly with the bloodstream, intravenous injection is the fastest way of introducing a drug into the body.

Intrinsa (Procter & Gamble) *See* TESTOSTERONE.

IntronA (Schering-Plough) *See* INTERFERON ALFA.

Invanz (Merck Sharp & Dohme) *See* ERTAPENEM SODIUM.

Invega (Janssen-Cilag) *See* PALIPERIDONE.

Invirase (Roche Products) *See* SAQUINAVIR.

Iocare (CIBA Vision Ophthalmics) *See* BALANCED SALT SOLUTION.

iodine An element required in small amounts for healthy growth and development. Iodine accumulates in the thyroid gland, where it is required for the production of *thyroid hormones. A deficiency of iodine leads to **goitre** (swelling of the neck due to enlargement of the thyroid gland). Aqueous iodine oral solution (**Lugol's solution**) is given to patients with thyrotoxicosis (overproduction of thyroid hormones) in order to reduce the size of the thyroid gland before surgery. It acts as a signal to turn off production of thyroid hormones by the gland. This solution is available from pharmacies without a prescription.

Iodine is also an *antiseptic and is used to disinfect the skin (*see* POVIDONE–IODINE).

Side effects: Lugol's solution can cause allergic reactions, headache, tear production, conjunctivitis, pain in the salivary glands, laryngitis, bronchitis, and rashes. Prolonged use results in depression, insomnia, and impotence.

Precautions: Lugol's solution should not be used for long-term treatment. It should not be taken by women who are breastfeeding and should be used with caution in pregnant women and in children.

Iodoflex (Smith & Nephew Healthcare) *See* CADEXOMER IODINE.

Iodosorb (Smith & Nephew Healthcare) *See* CADEXOMER IODINE.

Iopidine (Alcon Laboratories) *See* APRACLONIDINE.

ipecacuanha (**ipecac**) A plant extract that contains two alkaloids, emetine and cephaeline, that irritate the lining of the stomach and intestines and act as *emetics. Ipecacuanha was formerly used to induce vomiting in people (especially children) who had swallowed a non-corrosive poison. In very small doses it can act as an *expectorant, being available as syrups and tablets and included in many cough medicines. Ipecacuanha is freely available *over the counter.

Side effects: large doses produce excessive vomiting, bleeding from the stomach and intestines, and damage to the heart.
Precautions: overdosage can be fatal in children.
Proprietary preparations: Fennings Little Healers (tablets); Hill's Balsam Chesty Cough for Children Syrup; *Hill's Balsam Chesty Cough Pastilles (combined with benzoin tincture, menthol, and peppermint oil).

Ipocol (Sandoz) *See* MESALAZINE.

ipratropium bromide An *antimuscarinic drug used as a *bronchodilator to relieve the wheezing and breathlessness associated with chronic obstructive pulmonary disease (chronic bronchitis or emphysema), especially in people who fail to respond to beta-adrenoceptor stimulants (such as salbutamol or terbutaline). It is also used to treat perennial allergic rhinitis. Ipratropium has its maximum effect 30–60 minutes after use; its duration of action is 3–6 hours. It is available, on *prescription only, as an aerosol or powder for inhalation, a nasal spray, and a solution for use in a *nebulizer.
Side effects: these are rare – a dry mouth and dryness and irritation of the nose may occur; difficulties in urinating and constipation are less likely.
Precautions: ipratropium should be used with caution by people with glaucoma, men with an enlarged prostate, and pregnant women.
Proprietary preparations: Atrovent (metered-dose aerosol inhaler); Atrovent Aerocaps (powder for inhalation); Atrovent UDV (solution for use in a nebulizer); Ipratropium Steri-Neb (solution for use in a nebulizer); Respontin (solution for use in a nebulizer); Rinatec (nasal spray); *Combivent (combined with salbutamol); *Duovent (combined with fenoterol hydrobromide).

Ipratropium Steri-Neb (IVAX) *See* IPRATROPIUM BROMIDE.

irbesartan An *angiotensin II inhibitor used in the treatment of *hypertension, including that in diabetics with kidney disease. It is available as tablets on *prescription only.
Side effects: include headache, dizziness, and muscle and bone pain.
Precautions: irbesartan should not be taken by women who are pregnant or breastfeeding. It should be used with caution by people with kidney disease, severe liver disease, heart failure, and some types of heart disease.
Interactions with other drugs: *see* ACE INHIBITORS.
Proprietary preparations: Aprovel; *CoAprovel (combined with hydrochlorothiazide).

Iressa (AstraZeneca) *See* GEFITINIB.

irinotecan A *topoisomerase inhibitor used for the treatment of *cancers of the colon and rectum that have failed to respond to treatment with *fluorouracil. It is available as a solution for intravenous infusion on *prescription only.
Side effects: include diarrhoea occurring more than 24 hours after treatment (which should be reported to a doctor immediately), early diarrhoea (i.e. less than 24 hours after treatment), nausea, vomiting (which can be severe), loss of

appetite, *bone marrow suppression, hair loss, weakness, fatigue, breathlessness, cramps, and tingling in fingers or toes. *See also* CYTOTOXIC DRUGS.

Precautions: irinotecan should not be given to people with chronic inflammatory bowel disease, bowel obstruction, liver or kidney disease, or bone marrow suppression or to women who are pregnant or breastfeeding. *See also* CYTOTOXIC DRUGS.

Interactions with other drugs:

Atazanavir: the risk of it causing adverse effects is increased.

Clozapine: should not be taken with irinotecan because of an increased risk of this combination causing agranulocytosis (a blood disorder).

Ketoconazole: increases the plasma concentration of the active form of irinotecan and should therefore not be given with it.

St John's wort: reduces the plasma concentration of irinotecan and should therefore not be taken with it.

Proprietary preparation: Campto.

iron A metallic element essential to life: most importantly, it is a constituent of haemoglobin, the oxygen-carrying pigment of red blood cells. The main dietary sources of iron are meat and liver. Iron deficiency, which results in iron-deficiency *anaemia, can be caused by blood loss (for example due to heavy menstrual periods or a bleeding peptic ulcer or occurring after childbirth), pregnancy, low dietary intake, or illnesses in which absorption of iron from the gut is affected. It can also occur in premature babies, babies born by Caesarean section, and in patients after surgical removal of the stomach.

Iron supplements are used for the treatment and prevention of iron-deficiency anaemia. They contain soluble iron in the form of iron salts (*see* FERROUS SULPHATE; FERROUS FUMARATE; FERROUS GLUCONATE; POLYSACCHARIDE–IRON COMPLEX; SODIUM FEREDETATE). Iron salts are sometimes combined with *folic acid; this combination is used mainly during pregnancy to prevent deficiencies of iron and folic acid. Preparations for use during pregnancy often contain other supplemental vitamins and minerals. Some preparations include *vitamin C (ascorbic acid) to help absorption. Iron is best absorbed on an empty stomach, but this can result in gastrointestinal upsets. These can be largely avoided by using *modified-release preparations (although iron from these is sometimes poorly absorbed), by gradually increasing the dose, or by taking the supplements after meals. Iron supplements are usually taken orally – as tablets, modified-release capsules, or syrup; they may occasionally need to be given by injection (*see* FERRIC CARBOXYMALTOSE; FERRIC HYDROXIDE SUCROSE; IRON DEXTRAN). Most iron supplements are available without a prescription.

Side effects: include nausea, stomach pain, diarrhoea and constipation (which may cause problems in the elderly). Iron salts colour the stools black.

Precautions: iron supplements should be used with caution by people with gastrointestinal obstruction (since they may worsen constipation) or inflammatory bowel disease (because the iron may not be absorbed).

Interactions with other drugs (oral iron):

Antacids: reduce the absorption of iron.
Antibiotics: the absorption of both tetracyclines and iron is reduced; iron reduces the absorption of quinolones.
Antiparkinsonian drugs: the absorption of entacapone and levodopa is reduced by iron.
Dimercaprol: should not be taken with iron.
Penicillamine: its absorption is reduced by iron.
Vitamin C: enhances the absorption of iron.
Zinc salts: the absorption of both zinc and iron salts is reduced.

iron dextran A complex of *iron (in the form of ferric hydroxide) and dextran, given by deep intramuscular injection for the treatment of iron-deficiency anaemia when oral iron preparations cannot be tolerated or are unsuccessful. It is available on *prescription only.

Side effects: include nausea, vomiting, abdominal pain, flushing, breathlessness, numbness, cramps, blurred vision, itching, and rash.
Precautions: iron dextran should not be given to people with a history of asthma or other allergic disorders, active rheumatoid arthritis, severely impaired liver function, or acute kidney failure. Oral iron supplements should not be given until at least five days after injection of iron dextran. This medicine should be used with caution in pregnant women. Because of a risk of *anaphylaxis, a test dose of iron dextran should be given before each injection and the patient monitored for signs of the reaction.
Proprietary preparation: CosmoFer.

Ironorm Drops (Wallace MFG) *See* FERROUS SULPHATE.

iron sucrose *See* FERRIC HYDROXIDE SUCROSE.

Irriclens (ConvaTec) *See* SODIUM CHLORIDE.

irrigation The process of washing out a wound or a hollow organ (such as the bladder) with a continuous flow of water or medicated solution. For example, an infected bladder may be irrigated with an antibiotic or antiseptic solution.

Irripod (CD Medical) *See* SODIUM CHLORIDE.

Isentress (Merck Sharp & Dohme) *See* RALTEGRAVIR.

Isib 60XL (Ranbaxy) *See* ISOSORBIDE MONONITRATE.

Ismelin (Amdipharm) *See* GUANETHIDINE.

Ismo, Ismo Retard (Riemser) *See* ISOSORBIDE MONONITRATE.

isocarboxazid A *monoamine oxidase inhibitor used for the treatment of depressive illness. It is available as tablets on *prescription only.
Side effects, precautions, and interactions with other drugs: *see* MONOAMINE OXIDASE INHIBITORS.

Isodur (Galen) *See* ISOSORBIDE MONONITRATE.

Isogel (Potters) *See* ISPAGHULA HUSK.

Isoket, Isoket Retard (UCB Pharma) *See* ISOSORBIDE DINITRATE.

isometheptene mucate A *sympathomimetic drug that acts as a *vasoconstrictor; it is used in combination with *paracetamol (an analgesic) for the relief of *migraine attacks. Isometheptene is available as capsules with or without a prescription (depending on the dosage).
Side effects: include dizziness and (more rarely) disorders of blood circulation and rashes.
Precautions: isometheptene should not be taken by people with glaucoma, severe heart disease or hypertension, severe liver or kidney disease, or by women who are pregnant or breastfeeding. It should be used with caution in people with diabetes or an overactive thyroid gland.
Interactions with other drugs:
Antidepressants: a severe rise in blood pressure can occur if MAOIs or moclobemide are taken with isometheptene.
Antiparkinsonian drugs: there is an increased risk of adverse effects if isometheptene is taken with bromocriptine; rasagiline should not be taken with isometheptene.
Guanethidine: its effect in lowering blood pressure is reduced.
Proprietary preparation: *Midrid (combined with paracetamol).

isoniazid A bactericidal *antibiotic used for the treatment of *tuberculosis; it is usually given in combination with other antituberculosis agents, such as *rifampicin and *pyrazinamide. A *prescription only medicine, it is available as tablets, an elixir, or as a solution for injection.
Side effects: include nausea, vomiting, insomnia, and restlessness. Nerve damage, producing weakness, numbness, and 'pins and needles', may occur; this can be prevented by taking isoniazid with *pyridoxine (vitamin B_6). More serious (but rare) are psychiatric disturbances and hepatitis.
Precautions: isoniazid should be used with caution in patients with liver or kidney disease or a history of psychosis or alcoholism and in women who are pregnant or breastfeeding.
Interactions with other drugs:
Antacids: reduce the absorption of isoniazid.
Antiepileptics: the effects of carbamazepine, ethosuximide, and phenytoin are enhanced.
Cycloserine: the toxic effects of this drug may be increased.
Diazepam: the effects of this drug are enhanced.
Proprietary preparations: *Rifater (combined with rifampicin and pyrazinamide); *Rifinah (combined with rifampicin).

isopropyl myristate An oily liquid that is readily absorbed by the skin and is used as a base for relatively nongreasy creams and ointments. It also acts as a solvent for many medications that need to be applied to the skin. Isopropyl

myristate is an ingredient or base of several *emollient skin preparations used for treating dry skin conditions.
Proprietary preparations: *Dermol (combined with liquid paraffin); *Diprobath (combined with light liquid paraffin); *Doublebase Emollient Shower Gel (combined with liquid paraffin); *Emulsiderm (combined with benzalkonium chloride); *Hydromol Emollient (combined with light liquid paraffin).

Isopto Alkaline (Alcon Laboratories) *See* HYPROMELLOSE.

Isopto Plain (Alcon Laboratories) *See* HYPROMELLOSE.

isosorbide dinitrate A *nitrate drug used in treatment of *angina and also as an adjunct to *cardiac glycosides and *diuretics in the treatment of congestive *heart failure. Isosorbide dinitrate is converted in the body to *isosorbide mononitrate, which is the active form of the drug. It is available as *modified-release tablets, a sublingual spray, and an intravenous injection. The injection is a *prescription only medicine; the others can be obtained from pharmacies without a prescription. Oral preparations (unlike those of *glyceryl trinitrate) are stable and can be stored for a long time.
Side effects, precautions, and interactions with other drugs: *see* NITRATES.
Proprietary preparations: Angitak (sublingual spray); Isoket (injection); Isoket Retard (modified-release tablets).

isosorbide mononitrate A *nitrate drug used in the treatment of *angina and also as an adjunct to *cardiac glycosides and *diuretics in the treatment of congestive *heart failure. It is available as tablets or capsules, in either short-acting or *modified-release formulations. Some preparations are *prescription only medicines; others can be obtained from pharmacies without a prescription. Unlike some oral preparations of *glyceryl trinitrate, isosorbide mononitrate is stable and can be stored for a long time.
Side effects, precautions, and interactions with other drugs: *see* NITRATES.
Proprietary preparations: see table.

Isotard (ProStrakan) *See* ISOSORBIDE MONONITRATE.

Isotonic Gentamicin Injection (Baxter Healthcare) *See* GENTAMICIN.

isotretinoin A *retinoid used topically for the treatment of *acne. It may also be given by mouth, under the supervision of a hospital specialist, for severe cases of acne that are unresponsive to antibiotics. Isotretinoin is available, on *prescription only, as a gel or capsules.
Side effects: the gel may cause redness, local irritation, and peeling of the skin at the start of treatment, but this should not last; it may cause changes in skin pigmentation and make the skin more sensitive to light. The capsules commonly cause dryness, flaking, and thinning of the skin, dryness of the nose (with nosebleeds), throat, and eyes, and pain in the joints and muscles. Other side effects may include visual impairment (which should be reported to a doctor immediately), hair loss, nausea, headache, drowsiness, sweating, mood changes, and menstrual irregularities.

Proprietary preparations of isosorbide mononitrate

Preparation	Formulation	Availability
Angeze	tablets	*P
Angeze SR	modified-release tablets	P
Chemydur 60XL	modified-release tablets	P
Dynamin	tablets	P
Elantan 10	tablets (10 mg)	P
Elantan 20	tablets (20 mg)	†POM
Elantan 40	tablets (40 mg)	POM
Elantan LA 25 or LA 50	modified-release capsules (25 or 50 mg)	P
Imdur Durules	modified-release tablets	POM
Isib 60XL	modified-release tablets	P
Ismo 10 or 20	tablets (10 or 20 mg)	P
Ismo Retard	modified-release tablets	P
Isodur 25XL or 50XL	modified-release capsules (25 or 50 mg)	P
Isotard 25XL, 40XL, 50XL, or 60XL	modified-release tablets (25, 40, 50, or 60 mg)	P
Modisal LA25 or LA50	modified-release capsules (25 or 50 mg)	P
Modisal XL	modified-release tablets	P
Monomax SR	modified-release capsules	P
Monomax XL	modified-release tablets	P
Monomil XL	modified-release tablets	P
Monosorb XL 60	modified-release tablets	P
Tragena XL	modified-release tablets	P
Xismox 60XL	modified-release tablets	P
Zemon 40XL or 60XL	modified-release tablets (40 or 60 mg)	P

* P = pharmacy medicine
† POM = prescription only medicine

Precautions: the gel should not be used on damaged or sunburnt skin, by people with eczema or a personal or family history of skin cancer, or by pregnant women. It should not come into contact with the eyes, nostrils, or mouth, and exposure of treated skin to ultraviolet light (including excessive sunlight) should be avoided. The gel should not be used with other topical preparations (e.g. *keratolytics) that may irritate the skin. The capsules should not be taken by women who are pregnant or breastfeeding, and contraception must be used for one month before and during treatment and for at least one month after treatment (*see* RETINOIDS). They should not be taken by people with liver disease or *hyperlipidaemia. Tests to monitor liver function and to measure concentrations of fats in the blood should be performed before and during treatment. Donation of blood should be avoided during treatment and for at least one month after stopping treatment.

Interactions with other drugs:

Tetracyclines: should not be taken with isotretinoin capsules as this increases the risk of raised blood pressure in the brain.

Vitamin A: the risk of vitamin A poisoning is increased if supplements are taken with isotretinoin capsules.

Proprietary preparations: Isotrex (gel); Roaccutane (capsules); *Isotrexin (combined with erythromycin).

Isotrex (GlaxoSmithKline) *See* ISOTRETINOIN.

Isotrexin (GlaxoSmithKline) A proprietary combination of *isotretinoin (a retinoid) and *erythromycin (an antibiotic), used for the treatment of mild to moderate acne. A *prescription only medicine, it is available as a gel to be applied to the skin.
Side effects, precautions, and interactions with other drugs: *see* ISOTRETINOIN.

Isovorin (Pfizer) *See* FOLINIC ACID.

Ispagel Orange (LPC) *See* ISPAGHULA HUSK.

ispaghula husk A natural fibre used as a *bulk-forming laxative. Ispaghula is available as powder or granules and can be obtained without a prescription, but only from pharmacies.
Side effects: include flatulence and abdominal distension.
Precautions: ispaghula should not be taken by people who have difficulty in swallowing, intestinal obstruction, impacted faeces, or colonic atony (a poorly functioning large bowel). Preparations containing ispaghula should always be taken with plenty of fluid and should not be taken immediately before going to bed.
Proprietary preparations: Fybogel; Fibrelief; Isogel; Ispagel Orange; Regulan; *Fybogel Mebeverine (combined with mebeverine hydrochloride).

isradipine A class II *calcium antagonist used for the treatment of *hypertension. It is available as tablets on *prescription only.
Side effects and precautions: *see* CALCIUM ANTAGONISTS; ANTIHYPERTENSIVE DRUGS.

Interactions with other drugs:

Antiepileptic drugs: the effects of isradipine are reduced by phenytoin, carbamazepine, phenobarbital, and primidone.

See also CALCIUM ANTAGONISTS.

Proprietary preparation: Prescal.

Istin (Pfizer) *See* AMLODIPINE.

itraconazole A triazole *antifungal drug that is used to treat a wide variety of fungal infections, including tinea (ringworm) of the skin, scalp, and nails, and candidiasis (thrush), and to prevent fungal infections in people whose immune systems are functioning poorly, such as AIDS patients and the recipients of transplants. Itraconazole is taken by mouth, as capsules or a liquid, or given by intravenous infusion and is available on *prescription only.

Side effects: include nausea, abdominal pain, indigestion, constipation (people taking the liquid may have diarrhoea), itching, headache, dizziness, menstrual disorders, and allergic reactions.
Precautions: itraconazole should not be taken by people with liver disease or porphyria or by women who are breastfeeding. It should be used with caution during pregnancy.
Interactions with other drugs:

Antacids: reduce the absorption of itraconazole.

Antibiotics: rifabutin and rifampicin reduce the plasma concentration of itraconazole, which should not be taken with rifabutin.

Anticoagulants: the effects of warfarin and acenocoumarol are enhanced; rivaroxaban should not be taken with itraconazole.

Antipsychotics: pimozide and sertindole should not be taken with itraconazole because of the risk of irregular heart rhythms.

Antiviral drugs: efavirenz reduces the plasma concentration of itraconazole; itraconazole increases the plasma concentration of indinavir, whose dosage may therefore need to be reduced; the plasma concentrations of both drugs may be increased if itraconazole is taken with ritonavir.

Ciclosporin: its plasma concentrations (and therefore side effects) are increased by itraconazole.

Cytotoxic drugs: lapatinib and nilotinib should not be taken with itraconazole; the risk of nerve damage is increased if vincristine is given with itraconazole.

Digoxin: its plasma concentrations (and therefore side effects) are increased by itraconazole.

Eletriptan: its plasma concentration is increased and it should not be taken with itraconazole.

Eplerenone: its plasma concentration is increased and it should not be taken with itraconazole.

Ergotamine: its adverse effects are increased and it should not be taken with itraconazole.

Ivabradine: its plasma concentration is increased and it should not be taken with itraconazole.

Midazolam: its plasma concentrations (and therefore side effects) are increased by itraconazole.

Mizolastine: its plasma concentration is increased and it should not be taken with itraconazole.

Phenytoin: reduces the plasma concentration of itraconazole.

Ranolazine: its plasma concentration is increased and it should not be taken with itraconazole.

Reboxetine: should not be taken with itraconazole.

Sirolimus: its plasma concentration is increased and it should not be taken with itraconazole.

Statins: there is an increased risk of myopathy (muscle disease) with atorvastatin and simvastatin and therefore these drugs should not be used with itraconazole.

Tacrolimus: its plasma concentration is increased.
Ulcer-healing drugs: H_2-receptor antagonists and proton pump inhibitors reduce the absorption of itraconazole.
Vardenafil: its plasma concentration is increased and it should not be taken with itraconazole.
Proprietary preparations: Sporanox; Sporanox Capsules; Sporanox Pulse.

ivabradine A drug used to relieve the symptoms of *angina: ivabradine works by slowing the heart's pacemaker current and thus reducing the heart rate. It is used when *beta blockers cannot be taken and is available as tablets on *prescription only.
Side effects: include slowing of the heart rate, headache, dizziness, and visual disturbance (including blurred vision; treatment should be stopped if vision deteriorates).
Precautions: ivabradine should not be taken by people with various heart diseases or severe liver disease, by people who have just had a stroke, or by women who are pregnant or breastfeeding.
Interactions with other drugs: ivabradine is metabolized by several enzyme systems in the liver, and drugs that inhibit these systems will alter plasma ivabradine concentrations and should therefore be used with caution or not taken with them. These drugs include some antibiotics, antifungal drugs, antiviral drugs, and calcium antagonists. A doctor should be consulted before taking ivabradine with any other drug.
Proprietary preparation: Procoralan.

Ivemend (Merck Sharp & Dohme) *See* FOSAPREPITANT.

i

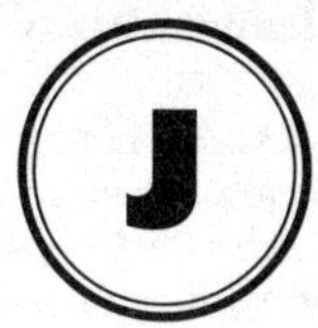

Jaap's Health Salts (Roche Products) A proprietary combination of *sodium bicarbonate, sodium potassium tartrate, and *tartaric acid, used as an *antacid for the relief of indigestion and heartburn and as a mild *laxative. It is freely available *over the counter as a powder to be dissolved to make an effervescent drink.
Precautions and interactions with other drugs: *see* ANTACIDS.

Jackson's All Fours (Anglian Pharma) *See* GUAIFENESIN.

Januvia (Merck Sharp & Dohme) *See* SITAGLIPTIN.

J Collis Browne's Mixture (Thornton & Ross) A proprietary combination of *morphine (which reduces gut motility) and *peppermint oil (an antispasmodic), used to treat diarrhoea and stomach upsets (*see* ANTIDIARRHOEAL DRUGS). It can be obtained from pharmacies without a prescription.
Side effects and interactions with other drugs: *see* MORPHINE; OPIOIDS.
Precautions: the mixture should not be given to children under six years old.
See also MORPHINE.

J Collis Browne's Tablets (Thornton & Ross) A proprietary combination of *calcium carbonate (an antacid), *kaolin (an adsorbent), and *morphine (which reduces gut motility), used for the treatment of diarrhoea and stomach upsets (*see* ANTIDIARRHOEAL DRUGS). It can be obtained without a prescription, but only from pharmacies.
Side effects and interactions with other drugs: *see* MORPHINE.
Precautions: these tablets should not be taken by children under six years old.
See KAOLIN; MORPHINE.

Joy Rides (GlaxoSmithKline) *See* HYOSCINE HYDROBROMIDE.

Junior Meltus Chesty Coughs with Catarrh (SLL International) A proprietary combination of *guaifenesin (an expectorant) and *cetylpyridinium chloride (an antiseptic), used to relieve coughs and catarrh associated with influenza, colds, and mild throat infections. It is available without a prescription, but only from pharmacies.
Precautions: large doses can cause nausea and vomiting. This medicine is not suitable for children under six years of age.

Junior Meltus Dry Coughs with Congestion (SSL International) A proprietary combination of *dextromethorphan (a cough suppressant) and *pseudoephedrine (a decongestant), used for the relief of dry coughs

accompanied by congestion of the upper airways. It is available as a liquid without a prescription, but only from pharmacies.
Side effects, and interactions with other drugs: *see* DEXTROMETHORPHAN; OPIOIDS; EPHEDRINE HYDROCHLORIDE; DECONGESTANTS.
Precautions: this medicine should not be taken by children under two years old. *See also* OPIOIDS; EPHEDRINE HYDROCHLORIDE; DECONGESTANTS.

juniper berry oil An oil extracted from juniper berries. It relieves flatulence, has a *diuretic action, and has antiseptic and anti-inflammatory properties. Juniper berry oil is an ingredient of remedies for treating infections of the urinary tract and of topical preparations for the relief of muscle and joint pain. Combined with other aromatic oils, it is included in inhalations and pastilles to relieve congestion due to colds and catarrh.
Side effects and precautions: prolonged use can irritate the stomach and high doses can damage the kidneys.
Proprietary preparations: *Olbas Oil (combined with eucalyptus oil, menthol, cajuput oil, and clove oil); *Olbas Pastilles (combined with eucalyptus oil, menthol, peppermint oil, and clove oil).

juniper tar *See* CADE OIL.

Kaletra (Abbott) A proprietary combination of lopinavir and *ritonavir (both protease inhibitors), used, in combination with other antiretroviral drugs (*see* ANTIVIRAL DRUGS), in the treatment of *HIV infection. It is available as tablets on *prescription only.
Side effects: include diarrhoea, nausea and vomiting, abdominal pain, appetite changes, blood disorders, raised blood lipids, disturbed sleep, pancreatitis (treatment should be stopped if signs of this develop), headache, dizziness, and 'pins and needles'.
Precautions: Kaletra should not be taken by women who are breastfeeding or by people with porphyria. It should be used with caution in people with diabetes, haemophilia, or impaired liver or kidney function, in those who are also taking drugs that may cause arrhythmias, and in pregnant women.
Interactions with other drugs:
Ranolazine: its plasma concentration may be increased by Kaletra and the two medicines should not be taken together.
See also RITONAVIR.

Kalspare (DHP Healthcare) A proprietary combination of *chlortalidone (a thiazide-like diuretic) and *triamterene (a potassium-sparing diuretic), used for the treatment of *hypertension or *oedema associated with heart failure, liver disease, or kidney disease. It is available as tablets on *prescription only.
Side effects, precautions, and interactions with other drugs: *see* THIAZIDE DIURETICS; POTASSIUM-SPARING DIURETICS.
See also ANTIHYPERTENSIVE DRUGS; DIURETICS.

Kamillosan (Norgine) A proprietary preparation consisting of extracts of chamomile (camomile) in a base containing purified *lanolin and *yellow soft paraffin, used as an *emollient for the relief of sore nipples, napkin rash, and chapped hands. It is freely available *over the counter in the form of an ointment.

Kao-C (Torbet Laboratories) A proprietary combination of *calcium carbonate (an antacid) and *kaolin (an adsorbent), used for the treatment of diarrhoea in children (*see* ANTIDIARRHOEAL DRUGS). It is freely available *over the counter in the form of a sugar-free suspension.
Precautions: Kao-C is not recommended for treating acute diarrhoea and should not be given to children under one year old. *See also* KAOLIN.

kaolin A purified and powdered adsorbent white clay. It adsorbs fluid and irritants from the gut and is used in the treatment of diarrhoea, but is not recommended for acute diarrhoea. It is used alone (as an oral suspension) or in combination with other ingredients, including morphine, in a variety of

*antidiarrhoeal preparations. Kaolin is also used in dusting powders to adsorb moisture and as an ingredient in poultices. It is available as a suspension or an ingredient in tablets, pastes, and powders, and can be obtained without a prescription.
Precautions: kaolin should not be taken by people with gastrointestinal obstruction.
Proprietary preparations: *J Collis Browne's Tablets (combined with calcium carbonate and morphine); *Kao-C (combined with calcium carbonate).

Kapake (Galen) *See* CO-CODAMOL.

Kaplon (APS-Berk) *See* CAPTOPRIL.

Karvol (Crookes Healthcare) A proprietary combination of levomenthol (*see* MENTHOL), *chlorobutanol (an antiseptic), *terpineol, *thymol, *pumilio pine oil, and pine oil sylvestris in the form of capsules or drops, used for the relief of nasal congestion. The contents of the capsules or the drops are placed on a handkerchief or added to hot water, and the vapour is inhaled. Karvol preparations are freely available *over the counter.

Kay-Cee-L (Geistlich Pharma) *See* POTASSIUM CHLORIDE.

Kefadim (Flynn Pharma) *See* CEFTAZIDIME.

Keflex (Flynn Pharma) *See* CEFALEXIN.

Kemadrin (GlaxoSmithKline) *See* PROCYCLIDINE.

Kemicetine (Pharmacia) *See* CHLORAMPHENICOL.

Kenalog Intra-articular/Intramuscular (E.R. Squibb & Sons) *See* TRIAMCINOLONE ACETONIDE.

Kentera (Recordati Pharmaceuticals) *See* OXYBUTYNIN HYDROCHLORIDE.

Kepivance (Amgen) *See* PALIFERMIN.

Keppra (UCB Pharma) *See* LEVETIRACETAM.

Keral (A. Menarini Pharma U.K. S.R.L.) *See* DEXKETOPROFEN.

keratolytics Drugs that cause softening and swelling of the cells at the surface of the skin, so that the outer layer of the skin peels off or can easily be removed. Keratolytics are used to remove thickened and horny patches of skin or scaly areas produced by *eczema or *psoriasis. They are also used in the treatment of acne, warts, and corns. Keratolytics include *salicylic acid, *benzoic acid, *benzoyl peroxide, *coal tar, *tar, and *sulphur. **Caustics** are drugs that are applied to the skin to destroy tissue. Used for treating warts and corns, they include *silver nitrate, *podophyllum, *podophyllotoxin, *formaldehyde, and *glutaraldehyde.

Ketek (Sanofi-aventis) *See* TELITHROMYCIN.

Ketocid (Chiesi) *See* KETOPROFEN.

ketoconazole A powerful imidazole *antifungal drug used for the treatment of fungal infections and to prevent fungal infections in those whose immune systems are functioning poorly (such as AIDS patients and the recipients of transplants). Ketoconazole is particularly useful for treating resistant candidiasis (thrush), gastrointestinal infections, and infections of the skin, nails, and scalp. It is available on *prescription only as tablets for oral use and as a cream or shampoo for topical application; shampoos for the prevention and treatment of dandruff can be bought without a prescription.
Side effects: when taken by mouth, side effects include nausea, vomiting, abdominal pain, headache, rashes, itching, and (more rarely) tingling sensations, dizziness, hair loss, breast enlargement in men, and liver damage. When applied topically it can irritate the skin.
Precautions: ketoconazole tablets should not be taken by people with liver disease or by women who are pregnant or breastfeeding. Liver function should be monitored before and during treatment.
Interactions with other drugs:

Antacids: reduce the absorption of ketoconazole.

Anticoagulants: the effects of warfarin and acenocoumarol are enhanced; the plasma concentration of rivaroxaban is increased and it should not be given with ketoconazole.

Antimuscarinics: reduce the absorption of ketoconazole.

Antipsychotics: pimozide and sertindole should not be taken with ketoconazole because of the risk of irregular heart rhythms; the plasma concentration of aripiprazole is increased and its dosage may therefore need to be reduced.

Antiviral drugs: nevirapine reduces the plasma concentration of ketoconazole and should not be taken with it; the doseage of indinavir and maraviroc may need to be reduced; the plasma concentrations of both drugs may be increased if ritonavir is taken with ketoconazole.

Buprenorphine: its plasma concentration is increased and its dosage may therefore need to be reduced.

Ciclosporin: its plasma concentration is increased.

Cilostazol: its plasma concentration is increased and it should not be taken with ketoconazole.

Cytotoxic drugs: the plasma concentration of lapatinib, nilotinib, and temsirolimus are increased and these drugs should not be taken with ketoconazole.

Disopyramide: should not be taken with ketoconazole because of the risk of irregular heart rhythms.

Domperidone: may increase the risk of irregular heart rhythms.

Eletriptan: its plasma concentrations (and risk of adverse effects) are increased and it should not be taken with ketoconazole.

Eplerenone: its plasma concentration is increased and it should not be taken with ketoconazole.

Ergotamine: its adverse effects may be increased and it should not be taken with ketoconazole.

Felodipine: its plasma concentration is increased.
Ivabradine: its plasma concentration is increased and it should not be given with ketoconazole.
Midazolam: its sedative effect is increased.
Mizolastine: its plasma concentration may be increased and it should not be taken with ketoconazole.
Oral contraceptives: their effect may be reduced.
Phenytoin: reduces the plasma concentration of ketoconazole.
Ranolazine: its plasma concentration is increased and it should not be taken with ketoconazole.
Rifampicin: the plasma concentrations of both drugs are reduced.
Simvastatin: the risk of muscle damage is increased and this drug should not be taken with ketoconazole.
Sirolimus: its plasma concentration is increased and it should not be taken with ketoconazole.
Tacrolimus: its plasma concentration is increased.
Theophylline: its plasma concentration may be increased.
Vardenafil: its plasma concentration is increased and it should not be taken with ketoconazole.

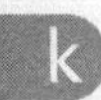

Proprietary preparations: Boots Anti-Dandruff Ketoconazole Shampoo; Daktarin Gold; Nizoral; Nizoral Dandruff Shampoo; Nizoral Shampoo.

ketoprofen An *NSAID used for the treatment of pain and mild inflammation in rheumatoid arthritis and other disorders of muscles or joints. It is also used to relieve period pains, acute gout, sciatica, and pain occurring after orthopaedic surgery. It is available, on *prescription only, as capsules, *modified-release capsules, suppositories, an injection, and a gel for topical application (some gel formulations are also available without a prescription).
Side effects: *see* NSAIDs. Suppositories may cause local irritation; there may be pain at the site of the injection.
Precautions and interactions with other drugs: *see* NSAIDs.
Proprietary preparations: Boots Muscular Pain Relief Gel; Ketocid (modified-release capsules); Ketoprofen CR (modified-release capsules); Ketovail (modified-release capsules); Orudis (capsules); Orudis Suppositories; Oruvail (modified-release capsules, gel, and injection); Powergel (gel).

Ketoprofen CR (Du Pont Pharmaceuticals) *See* KETOPROFEN.

ketorolac trometamol An *NSAID used for the treatment of moderate to severe postoperative pain. It is applied to the eye to prevent or reduce inflammation following eye surgery. Ketorolac is available, on *prescription only, as tablets, an injection, or eye drops.
Side effects: include altered taste, dry mouth, flushing, palpitations, breathlessness, and muscle pain. *See also* NSAIDs.
Precautions: *see* NSAIDs.
Interactions with other drugs: *see* NSAIDs. In addition:
Analgesics: ketorolac should not be taken with other NSAIDs as this increases their adverse effects.

Anticoagulants: should not be used with injections of ketorolac as the risk of bleeding is increased.
Lithium: should not be used with ketorolac tablets or injection, which reduce its excretion and therefore increase the risk of it having adverse effects.
Pentoxifylline: should not be used with ketorolac tablets or injection since it increases the risk of ketorolac causing bleeding.
Probenecid: delays the excretion of ketorolac tablets or injection, which increases the risk of it having adverse effects; therefore the two drugs should not be taken together.

Proprietary preparations: Acular (eye drops); Toradol (tablets and injection).

ketotifen A drug that is thought to prevent the release of *histamine, an important mediator of allergic responses (*see* ANTIHISTAMINES). It is used for the treatment of hay fever and allergic conjunctivitis. Ketotifen is available, on *prescription only, as eye drops, tablets, or an elixir.
Side effects: include drowsiness, impaired reactions, dry mouth, and occasionally excitement and weight gain.
Precautions: alcohol enhances its sedative effect. Ketotifen should not be taken by women who are pregnant or breastfeeding. Dosage should be reduced gradually over 2–4 weeks at the end of treatment.
Interactions with other drugs:
Metformin: there is a risk of blood disorders.
Proprietary preparation: Zaditen.

k

Ketovail (sanofi-aventis) *See* KETOPROFEN.

Ketovite (Paines & Byrne) A proprietary combination of vitamins used to prevent vitamin deficiency in people with metabolic disorders. It is available as tablets or a liquid; these can be taken together as a vitamin supplement by people on special diets that lack vitamins. The tablets, which are available on *prescription only, contain ascorbic acid (*see* VITAMIN C), members of the *vitamin B complex (including inositol, riboflavin, and thiamine), and alpha tocopheryl acetate (*see* VITAMIN E). The liquid contains *vitamin A, *ergocalciferol (vitamin D_2), and the B vitamins choline chloride and cyanocobalamin; it can be obtained from pharmacies without a prescription.

Kineret (Amgen) *See* ANAKINRA.

Kiovig (Baxter) *See* IMMUNOGLOBULINS.

Kivexa (GlaxoSmithKline) A proprietary combination of *abacavir and *lamivudine (nucleoside reverse transcriptase inhibitors; *see* ANTIVIRAL DRUGS), used in the treatment of *HIV infection. It is available as tablets on *prescription only.
Side effects, precautions, and interactions with other drugs *see* ABACAVIR; LAMIVUDINE.

Klaricid, Klaricid XL (Abbott) *See* CLARITHROMYCIN.

Klean-Prep (Norgine) A proprietary combination of macrogol '3350' (*see* POLYETHYLENE GLYCOLS), anhydrous *sodium sulphate, *sodium bicarbonate, *sodium chloride, and *potassium chloride, used to evacuate the bowel before investigative procedures or surgery. It is available as an oral powder to be mixed with water and can be obtained without a prescription, but only from pharmacies.
Side effects and precautions: *see* BOWEL-CLEANSING SOLUTIONS; POLYETHYLENE GLYCOLS.

Kliofem (Novo Nordisk) A proprietary combination of *estradiol and *norethisterone, used as continuous combined *hormone replacement therapy for the relief of menopausal symptoms and prevention of osteoporosis in women who have not had a hysterectomy and who have not had a period for a year. It is available as tablets on *prescription only.
Side effects, precautions, and interactions with other drugs: *see* HORMONE REPLACEMENT THERAPY.

Kliovance (Novo Nordisk) A proprietary combination of *estradiol and *norethisterone, used as continuous combined *hormone replacement therapy for the relief of menopausal symptoms in women who have not had a hysterectomy and who have not had a period for a year. It is available as tablets on *prescription only.
Side effects, precautions, and interactions with other drugs: *see* HORMONE REPLACEMENT THERAPY.

Kogenate (Bayer) *See* FACTOR VIII.

Kolanticon Gel (Peckforton Pharmaceuticals) A proprietary combination of *dicycloverine hydrochloride (an antispasmodic), *aluminium hydroxide and light *magnesium oxide (antacids), and activated *dimeticone (an antifoaming agent), used for the treatment of gut spasm, excess stomach acid, flatulence, and peptic ulceration. It is available as a sugar-free gel and can be obtained without a prescription, but only from pharmacies.
Side effects: *see* ANTIMUSCARINIC DRUGS.
Precautions: Kolanticon should not be taken by people with gastrointestinal obstruction, severe ulcerative colitis, or myasthenia gravis. It should be used with caution by people with glaucoma or an enlarged prostate gland.

Konakion MM (Roche Products) *See* PHYTOMENADIONE.

Kuvan (Merck Serono) *See* SAPROPTERIN.

Kwells (Bayer) *See* HYOSCINE HYDROBROMIDE.

Kytril (Roche Products) *See* GRANISETRON.

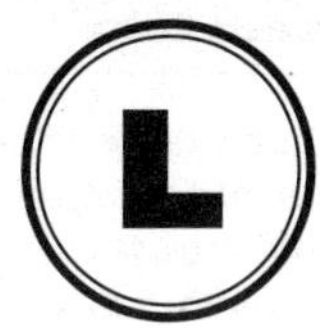

labetalol hydrochloride A combined *alpha and *beta blocker used in the treatment of *hypertension, including hypertension during pregnancy. It is available on *prescription only as tablets or as a solution for intravenous injection or infusion.
Side effects: include low blood pressure on standing, tiredness, weakness, headache, rash, tingling of the scalp, difficulty in passing urine, stomach pain, nausea, vomiting, and liver damage (in which case treatment may need to be stopped).
Precautions: labetalol should not be given to people with certain liver disorders as it has the potential for causing liver damage. *See also* ANTIHYPERTENSIVE DRUGS; BETA BLOCKERS.
Interactions with other drugs: *see* BETA BLOCKERS.
Proprietary preparation: Trandate.

lacidipine A class II *calcium antagonist used in the treatment of *hypertension. It is available as tablets on *prescription only.
Side effects and interactions with other drugs: *see* CALCIUM ANTAGONISTS.
Precautions: lacidipine should not be taken by people who have had a heart attack within the previous month or who have unstable *angina or by women who are pregnant or breastfeeding. *See also* CALCIUM ANTAGONISTS; ANTIHYPERTENSIVE DRUGS.
Proprietary preparation: Motens.

lacosamide A drug used as an *adjunct in the treatment of partial epileptic seizures (*see* ANTICONVULSANT DRUGS) and pain due to nerve damage in people with diabetes. It is available, on *prescription only, as tablets, a syrup, or a form for intravenous infusion.
Side effects: include dizziness, headache, double vision, nausea, vomiting, constipation, depression, and somnolence.
Precautions: lacosamide should be used with caution in people with heart disease or impaired liver or kidney function, in women who are pregnant or breastfeeding, and in people who are prone to falls (as dizziness is a common side effect).
Interactions with other drugs: drugs that may cause arrhythmias should be used with caution; these include anti-arrhythmic drugs, carbamazepine, and lamotrigine.

Antidepressants: increase the risk of convulsions; St John's wort should not be taken with lacosamide.

Mefloquine: increases the risk of convulsions and should not be taken with lacosamide.

Proprietary preparation: Vimpat.

Lacri-Lube (Allergan) A proprietary combination of *white soft paraffin, *liquid paraffin, and wool fat (anhydrous *lanolin), used for the lubrication of dry eyes. It is available as an eye ointment and can be obtained without a prescription, but only from pharmacies.

lactic acid A weak acid that has mild *antibiotic properties and is also a *keratolytic. It is used, usually in combination with *salicylic acid, for the removal of warts. It is also included as an ingredient in preparations for the treatment of skin conditions.
Proprietary preparations: *Bazuka Gel (combined with salicylic acid); *Calmurid (combined with urea); *Calmurid HC (combined with hydrocortisone and urea); *Cuplex (combined with salicylic acid); *Duofilm (combined with salicylic acid); *Salactol (combined with salicylic acid); *Salatac (combined with salicylic acid).

Lactugal (Intrapharm) *See* LACTULOSE.

lactulose An *osmotic laxative used for the treatment of constipation. Lactulose is a semisynthetic derivative of sugar that is not absorbed from the gut; it may take up to 48 hours to work. It is available as a solution and can be obtained without a prescription, but only from pharmacies. Some preparations cannot be prescribed on the NHS.
Side effects: lactulose may cause flatulence, cramps, and abdominal discomfort.
Precautions: lactulose should not be taken by people with intestinal obstruction or galactosaemia (a congenital inability to metabolize certain sugars).
Proprietary preparations: Duphalac; Lactugal; Regulose.

Lamictal (GlaxoSmithKline) *See* LAMOTRIGINE.

Lamisil (Novartis) *See* TERBINAFINE.

lamivudine An *antiviral drug that prevents retrovirus replication: it is a reverse transcriptase inhibitor. Lamivudine is used, in combination with other antiretroviral drugs, to delay the progression of disease in *HIV-infected patients; it is also used to treat chronic hepatitis B infection. Lamivudine is available, on *prescription only, as tablets or a solution.
Side effects: include nausea, vomiting, diarrhoea, abdominal pain, cough, headache, insomnia, malaise, muscle and joint pain, fatigue, peripheral neuropathy (causing numbness and tingling of the limbs), muscle disorders, and (rarely) pancreatitis.
Precautions: lamivudine should be used with caution in people with impaired kidney function (the dosage is usually reduced). It should not be taken by women who are breastfeeding and is generally not recommended in the first three months of pregnancy.
Interactions with other drugs:

Trimethoprim: increases the plasma concentration (and therefore side effects) of lamivudine.

Proprietary preparations: Epivir; Zeffix; *Combivir (combined with zidovudine); *Kivexa (combined with abacavir); Trizivir (combined with zidovudine and abacavir).

lamotrigine An *anticonvulsant drug used for the treatment of partial seizures and generalized tonic-clonic seizures. It is available, on *prescription only, as tablets or dispersible tablets.
Side effects: include rashes, fever, malaise, influenza-like symptoms, drowsiness, and (rarely) liver disorders.
Precautions: people taking lamotrigine should be closely monitored initially: liver, kidney, and blood-clotting functions should be assessed. If rashes, influenza-like symptoms, or drowsiness occur, or if the drug becomes less effective in controlling seizures, treatment may need to be stopped. When stopping medication, lamotrigine should be withdrawn gradually over a two-week period.
Interactions with other drugs: taking two or more anticonvulsants together may enhance their toxicity.
Antidepressants: increase the risk of convulsions; St John's wort should not be taken with lamotrigine.
Antimalarial drugs: chloroquine, hydroxychloroquine, and mefloquine increase the risk of convulsions.
Oral contraceptives: reduce the plasma concentration of lamotrigine.
Rifampicin: reduces the plasma concentration of lamotrigine.
Proprietary preparation: Lamictal.

lanolin (**hydrous wool fat**) A mixture of **wool fat** (obtained from the wool of sheep) and 25–30% water. Wool fat itself is also called **anhydrous lanolin**. Lanolin and wool fat are used as a base for creams and as *emollients: when mixed with vegetable oil or soft paraffin (*see* YELLOW SOFT PARAFFIN) they form creams that are readily absorbed.
Side effects: lanolin and wool fat may cause allergic reactions. Highly purified lanolin causes fewer allergic reactions.

Lanoxin, Lanoxin-PG (GlaxoSmithKline) *See* DIGOXIN.

lanreotide A long-acting *analogue of **somatostatin**, a hormone that is produced in the brain, gastrointestinal tract, and pancreas and inhibits the release of *growth hormone. It is used for the short-term treatment of patients awaiting surgery for acromegaly (a condition due to excessive secretion of growth hormone by a tumour of the pituitary gland) and for the long-term treatment of acromegaly that does not respond to surgery, *dopamine receptor antagonists, or radiotherapy. It can also be used as an interim treatment until radiotherapy has been effective in reducing concentrations of growth hormone. Lanreotide is also used to inhibit the secretions (and thus relieve the symptoms) of hormone-secreting tumours of the gastrointestinal tract and for the treatment of thyroid tumours. It is available as an injection on *prescription only.
Side effects: include pain, stinging, and swelling at the injection site, loss of

appetite, nausea, vomiting, and abdominal pain; gallstones may develop with long-term treatment.
Precautions: lanreotide should be used with caution in women who are pregnant or breastfeeding. Diabetic patients may need to reduce their dosage of insulin or oral antidiabetic drugs. Gall-bladder function should be monitored. Lanreotide should be withdrawn gradually at the end of treatment.
Interactions with other drugs:
Antidiabetic drugs: doses of these may need to be reduced (see Precautions).
Ciclosporin: lanreotide reduces the absorption of ciclosporin.
Proprietary preparations: Somatuline LA; Somatuline Autogel.

lansoprazole A *proton pump inhibitor used for the treatment of reflux oesophagitis, gastric and duodenal ulcers (including those associated with *Helicobacter pylori* infection and the use of *NSAIDs), Zollinger-Ellison syndrome, and other kinds of *acid-peptic disease. It is available as capsules or dispersible tablets on *prescription only.
Side effects: include headache, dizziness, fatigue, malaise, diarrhoea, constipation, sore throat, rashes, and muscle aches.
Precautions: *see* PROTON PUMP INHIBITORS.
Interactions with other drugs:
Antiplatelet drugs: the effects of clopidogrel and prasugrel may be reduced and these drugs should not be taken with lansoprazole.
Antifungal drugs: the absorption of ketoconazole and itraconazole may be reduced by lansoprazole.
Atazanavir: its plasma concentration is reduced.
Cilostazol: its plasma concentration may be reduced and it should not be taken with lansoprazole.
Proprietary preparation: Zoton FasTab.

lanthanum A *phosphate-binding agent used to reduce high levels of phosphate in the blood in people with chronic kidney failure who are undergoing dialysis treatment. It is available as tablets on *prescription only.
Side effects: include abdominal pain, constipation, diarrhoea, indigestion, flatulence, nausea, vomiting, and low blood-calcium levels.
Precautions: lanthanum is not recommended for pregnant or breastfeeding women. It should be used with caution in people with peptic ulcers, inflammatory bowel disease, or impaired liver function.
Proprietary preparation: Fosrenol.

Lantus (sanofi-aventis) *See* INSULIN.

Lanvis (GlaxoSmithKline) *See* TIOGUANINE.

lapatinib A *tyrosine kinase inhibitor used for the treatment of advanced breast cancer in which the tumour cells are covered with excess amounts of a protein, human epidermal growth factor 2 (HER2), that stimulates tumour growth. It works by blocking the action of HER2. Lapatinib is used in

combination with *capecitabine. It is available as tablets on *prescription only.
Side effects: *see* CYTOTOXIC DRUGS. There may also be loss of appetite, diarrhoea, fatigue, rash, and liver damage.
Precautions: lapatinib should not be taken by women who are breastfeeding and should be used with caution in people with liver disease (liver function should be monitored before and during treatment) or kidney disease and in pregnant women. *See also* CYTOTOXIC DRUGS.
Interactions with other drugs: the following drugs should not be used with lapatinib: carbamazepine, clozapine, itraconazole, ketoconazole, phenytoin, pimozide, posaconazole, repaglinide, rifampicin, ritonavir, saquinavir, St John's wort, and telithromycin.
Proprietary preparation: Tyverb.

Largactil (sanofi-aventis) *See* CHLORPROMAZINE HYDROCHLORIDE.

Lariam (Roche Products) *See* MEFLOQUINE.

laronidase An enzyme produced by genetic engineering and used for treating people with Hurler's disease, a rare inherited disorder due to deficiency of this enzyme. It is available as an intravenous infusion on *prescription only.
Side effects: include headache, nausea, abdominal pain, rash, joint pain, pain at the extremities, flushing, fever, reactions at the infusion site, increased blood pressure, a fast heart rate, and chills.
Precautions: reactions to the infusion often occur, and these can be minimized by giving an antihistamine and an antipyretic before treatment.
Proprietary preparation: Aldurazyme.

laropiprant *See* TREDAPTIVE.

Laryngojet (UCB Pharma) *See* LIDOCAINE.

Lasilactone (sanofi-aventis) A proprietary combination of *furosemide (a loop diuretic) and *spironolactone (a potassium-sparing diuretic), used for the treatment of *oedema associated with congestive *heart failure, liver disease, or kidney disease. It is available as capsules on *prescription only.
Side effects, precautions, and interactions with other drugs: *see* LOOP DIURETICS; POTASSIUM-SPARING DIURETICS.

See also DIURETICS.

Lasix (sanofi-aventis) *See* FUROSEMIDE.

Lassar's paste A preparation consisting of *salicylic acid (a keratolytic) and *zinc oxide (an astringent), used to treat conditions characterized by thick or hard skin. Combined with *dithranol, it is used for the treatment of psoriasis.

latanoprost A *prostaglandin analogue that is used to reduce the pressure inside the eye in the treatment of open-angle (chronic) *glaucoma and raised blood pressure in the eye. It acts by increasing the outflow of aqueous fluid from the eye. Latanoprost is used for treating people who have not responded

to or cannot tolerate other drugs. It is available as eye drops on *prescription only.
Side effects: latanoprost may increase the brown pigment in the iris, and people should be warned to notice any changes in eye colour. The eyes may become irritated or bloodshot, and the eyelashes may become darker, longer, and thicker.
Precautions: latanoprost should be used with caution by people with asthma and is not recommended for women who are pregnant or breastfeeding.
Proprietary preparations: Xalatan; *Xalacom (combined with timolol maleate).

lauromacrogols A group of compounds that are used as *surfactants. They also have some local *antipruritic activity and are included in preparations to treat dry skin conditions or haemorrhoids.
Side effects: lauromacrogols occasionally cause allergic skin reactions.
Proprietary preparations: *Anacal (combined with heparinoid); *Balneum Plus Cream (combined with urea); *Balneum Plus Oil (combined with soya oil); *E45 Itch Relief Cream (combined with urea).

laxatives Drugs that stimulate, or increase the frequency of, bowel evacuation (these laxatives are also called **cathartics** or **purgatives**) or that encourage the passage of a softer or bulkier stool. Laxatives should not be used for prolonged periods. Excessive use can lead to low plasma concentrations of *potassium and colonic atony (a nonfunctioning large bowel). A balanced diet with adequate fibre and fluid intake and the development of a regular bowel habit should obviate the need for laxatives in most people. However, laxatives are required when drugs are causing constipation or if bowel evacuation is necessary, for example before childbirth or surgery (*see also* BOWEL-CLEANSING SOLUTIONS). The main types of laxatives are *bulk-forming laxatives, *faecal softeners, *osmotic laxatives, and *stimulant laxatives.

Laxido Orange (Galen Ltd) A proprietary combination of macrogol '350' (*see* POLYETHYLENE GLYCOLS), *sodium chloride, *sodium bicarbonate, and *potassium chloride, used as an *osmotic laxative for the treatment of chronic constipation and impacted faeces. It is available as an oral powder to be dissolved in water and can be obtained without a prescription, but only from pharmacies.
Side effects and precautions: *see* POLYETHYLENE GLYCOLS; STIMULANT LAXATIVES.

LDL (low-density lipoproteins) *See* LIPOPROTEINS; CHOLESTEROL.

Ledclair (Durbin) *See* SODIUM CALCIUM EDETATE.

Ledermycin (Pfizer) *See* DEMECLOCYCLINE HYDROCHLORIDE.

leflunomide A *disease-modifying antirheumatic drug (DMARD) used in the treatment of rheumatoid arthritis and psoriatic arthritis under specialist supervision. It is available as tablets on *prescription only.
Side effects: include raised blood pressure, 'pins and needles', headache,

dizziness, diarrhoea, nausea, vomiting, mouth ulcers, abdominal pain, hair loss, rash, itching, dry skin, loss of appetite, weight loss, and mild allergic reactions.
Precautions: leflunomide should not be taken by pregnant women because of a risk of abnormalities in the fetus. Women should use effective contraception during and for at least two years after treatment. Leflunomide should not be taken by people with liver disease, severe immunodeficiency states (e.g. AIDS), impaired bone marrow function, serious infections, or kidney disease or by breastfeeding women. Because leflunomide may cause severe liver damage, liver function tests should be carried out during treatment, which should be stopped or the dosage reduced if there are any signs of abnormality. Other drugs affecting liver function should not be taken with leflunomide as this increases the risk of liver damage.
Interactions with other drugs:
Colestyramine: decreases the effect of leflunomide.
Methotrexate: increases the risk of adverse effects.
Vaccines: should not be given with leflunomide.
Proprietary preparation: Arava.

Lemsip Cold & Flu Capsules (Reckitt Benckiser) A proprietary combination of *paracetamol (an analgesic and antipyretic), *caffeine (a stimulant), and *phenylephrine (a decongestant), used to relieve the symptoms of colds and influenza, including aches and pains, nasal congestion, and fever. **Lemsip Max Cold & Flu Capsules** contains higher doses of the active ingredients. Both preparations are freely available *over the counter.
Side effects and interactions with other drugs: *see* PHENYLEPHRINE.
Precautions: this medicine should not be given to children, except on medical advice. *See also* PARACETAMOL; CAFFEINE; PHENYLEPHRINE.

Lemsip Cold & Flu Lemon (Reckitt Benckiser) A proprietary combination of *paracetamol (an analgesic and antipyretic), *phenylephrine (a decongestant), and *vitamin C, used to relieve the symptoms of colds and influenza, including aches, pains, fevers, and nasal congestion. Similar preparations are **Lemsip Cold & Flu Breathe Easy** and **Lemsip Cold & Flu Blackcurrant**; **Lemsip Max Cold & Flu Sachets** contain higher doses of the active ingredients. All these preparations are freely available *over the counter in the form of powders.
Side effects and interactions with other drugs: *see* PHENYLEPHRINE.
Precautions: these medicines should not be given to children except on medical advice. *See also* PARACETAMOL; PHENYLEPHRINE.

Lemsip Cough Chesty (Reckitt Benckiser) *See* GUAIFENESIN.

Lemsip Cough Dry (Reckitt Benckiser) A proprietary combination of honey and *glycerin, used as a *demulcent for the relief of dry irritating coughs. It is freely available *over the counter in the form of a liquid.

Lemsip Flu 12 Hr (Reckitt Benckiser) A proprietary combination of

*ibuprofen (an NSAID) and *pseudoephedrine (a decongestant), used to relieve the symptoms of colds and influenza, including nasal congestion, aches and pains, headaches, sore throat, and fever. It is available as *modified-release capsules and can be obtained without a prescription, but only from pharmacies.
Side effects and interactions with other drugs: *see* NSAIDS; DECONGESTANTS; EPHEDRINE HYDROCHLORIDE.
Precautions: these preparations should not be taken by children. *See also* NSAIDS; DECONGESTANTS.

Lemsip Max Flu Lemon (Reckitt Benckiser) A proprietary combination of *paracetamol (an analgesic and antipyretic) and *pseudoephedrine (a decongestant), used to relieve the symptoms of colds and influenza, including nasal congestion, fever, and aches and pains. It is available in the form of powders and can be obtained without a prescription, but only from pharmacies.
Side effects and interactions with other drugs: *see* EPHEDRINE HYDROCHLORIDE; DECONGESTANTS.
Precautions: this medicine should not be given to children, except on medical advice. *See also* PARACETAMOL; DECONGESTANTS; EPHEDRINE HYDROCHLORIDE.

Lemsip Sore Throat Triple Action Lozenges (Reckitt Benckiser) *See* HEXYLRESORCINOL.

lenalidomide A drug that modifies or regulates the immune system. Lenalidomide is used, in combination with *dexamethasone, to treat multiple myeloma (cancer of antibody-forming cells in the bone marrow). It is available as capsules on *prescription only.
Side effects: include deep vein *thrombosis, neutropenia (a deficiency of neutrophils, a type of white blood cell), low blood pressure, breathlessness, fatigue, and loss of strength.
Precautions: lenalidomide can cause abnormalities in the fetus. Therefore women should use effective contraception for at least one month before, during, and for at least one month after treatment; men should use condoms during and for a least one week after treatment. Blood counts should be carried out before and during treatment, and signs of neutropenia (e.g. fever, sore throat) should be reported to a doctor. Signs of thrombosis (e.g. chest pain, limb swelling) should also be reported. Lenalidomide should not be taken by women who are breastfeeding.
Proprietary preparation: Revlimid.

lenograstim Recombinant human granulocyte-colony stimulating factor, a form of *granulocyte-colony stimulating factor produced by genetic engineering. It is used for the treatment of neutropenia (a decrease in the number of neutrophils, a type of white blood cell) induced by *cytotoxic drug treatment for *cancer or resulting from destruction of the bone marrow prior to bone marrow transplantation. It may be given to cancer patients who are about to undergo blood collection before aggressive treatment; neutrophil

production will thus be boosted in this collected blood, which is used to replace the white cells destroyed by the treatment. Lenograstim is available as a form for subcutaneous injection or intravenous infusion on *prescription only; its use is restricted to specialist units.
Side effects and precautions: *see* FILGRASTIM.
Proprietary preparation: Granocyte.

lepirudin An *anticoagulant used for the prevention and treatment of *thrombosis and thromboembolism in people who have developed thrombocytopenia with *heparin therapy. It is available in a form for intravenous injection or infusion on *prescription only.
Side effects: include bleeding (*see* ANTICOAGULANTS), anaemia, fever, and allergic reactions (such as rashes).
Precautions and interactions with other drugs: lepirudin should not be given to women who are pregnant or breastfeeding and should be used with caution in people with liver or kidney disease and in people who have recently undergone major surgery. The risk of bleeding is increased if lepirudin is used with other anticoagulants, antiplatelet drugs, or fibrinolytic drugs.
Proprietary preparation: Refludan.

lercanidipine A class II *calcium antagonist used for the treatment of mild to moderate *hypertension. It is available as tablets on *prescription only.
Side effects: *see* CALCIUM ANTAGONISTS.
Precautions: lercanidipine should not be taken by people with unstable angina or uncontrolled heart failure, by those who have had a heart attack within the previous month, or by those with severe kidney disaese or by women who are pregnant or breastfeeding. *See also* CALCIUM ANTAGONISTS.
Interactions with other drugs:

Ciclosporin: the plasma concentrations of either or both drugs may be increased, and lercanidipine should not be taken with ciclosporin.

See also CALCIUM ANTAGONISTS.

Proprietary preparation: Zanidip.

Lescol, Lescol XL (Novartis) *See* FLUVASTATIN.

letrozole An *aromatase inhibitor used for the treatment of breast *cancer in postmenopausal women. It is available as tablets on *prescription only.
Side effects: include pain in muscles or bones, headache, fatigue, indigestion, nausea and vomiting, constipation, diarrhoea, and hot flushes.
Precautions: letrozole should not be taken by women who have not reached the menopause, who are pregnant or breastfeeding, or who have severe liver disease. It should be used with caution in those with kidney disease.
Proprietary preparation: Femara.

leukaemia *See* CANCER.

Leukeran (GlaxoSmithKline) *See* CHLORAMBUCIL.

leukotriene receptor antagonists A class of drugs that block leukotriene receptors in the body. Leukotrienes are a group of compounds that are released from cells and cause actions that result in inflammation. They are responsible for the swelling, redness, and warmth of inflamed tissue and constriction of the airways in people with *asthma and severe hay fever. Leukotriene receptor antagonists thus prevent the inflammatory response produced by leukotrienes; the drugs of this class in current use are *montelukast and *zafirlukast, which are used for the prevention of asthma.

leuprorelin An analogue of *gonadorelin that is used for the treatment of *endometriosis. It is also used to treat advanced prostate cancer that depends on the male sex hormone testosterone for growth. Here leuprorelin acts by causing an initial rise in plasma concentrations of testosterone, followed by a reduction to the same low concentrations achieved by castration. It is given by intramuscular or subcutaneous injection and is available on *prescription only.
Side effects: in women, *see* GOSERELIN. In men side effects include impotence, decreased libido, and (rarely) fatigue, nausea, and irritation at the injection site; there may be bone pain and difficulty in passing urine at the start of treatment, when testosterone concentrations are high.
Precautions: *see* GOSERELIN. In men an *anti-androgen may need to be given at the start of treatment, when high concentrations of testosterone may cause adverse effects.
Proprietary preparations: Prostap SR; Prostap 3.

l

Leustat (Janssen-Cilag) *See* CLADRIBINE.

Levemir (Novo Nordisk) *See* INSULIN.

levetiracetam An antiepileptic drug (*see* ANTICONVULSANT DRUGS) that is used alone or as an *adjunct to treat partial seizures and as an adjunct to treat tonic-clonic seizures and myoclonic seizures (in which sudden muscle spasms occur between seizures). It is available, on *prescription only, as tablets, an oral solution, and a form for intravenous infusion.
Side effects: include dizziness, sleepiness, liver or kidney disease, headache, nausea, vomiting, and indigestion.
Precautions: levetiracetam is not recommended for pregnant or breastfeeding women.
Interactions with other drugs:

Antidepressants and antimalarial drugs: there may be an increased risk of convulsions if some of these drugs are taken with levetiracetam.

Proprietary preparation: Keppra.

Levitra (Bayer) *See* VARDENAFIL.

levobunolol hydrochloride A *beta blocker used for the treatment of chronic (open-angle) *glaucoma. It is available, on *prescription only, as eye drops – either as a solution or in single-dose preservative-free units.
Side effects: include irritation of the eyes, headache, and dizziness. The drops can trickle into the back of the nose and be swallowed, causing *systemic effects and possibly interactions with other drugs (*see* BETA BLOCKERS).

Precautions: levobunolol should not be used by people with asthma, breathing problems, or heart failure. *See also* BETA BLOCKERS.
Proprietary preparations: Betagan; Betagan Unit Dose.

levobupivacaine *See* LOCAL ANAESTHETICS.

levocetirizine A nonsedating *antihistamine used for the treatment of hay fever and urticaria (nettle rash). It is available as tablets or an oral solution on *prescription only.
Side effects and interactions with other drugs: *see* ANTIHISTAMINES.
Precautions: levocetirizine should not be taken by people with severe kidney disease. *See also* ANTIHISTAMINES.
Proprietary preparation: Xyzal.

levodopa An *antiparkinsonian drug used to increase concentrations of *dopamine in the brain in people with idiopathic parkinsonism (i.e. parkinsonism of unknown origin). Levodopa is converted to dopamine in the body, but to be effective it must cross into the brain before conversion. However, a large proportion of levodopa is transformed to dopamine in peripheral tissues (those outside the brain), which can cause the side effects of vomiting and low blood pressure. To prevent this effect levodopa is given in combination with *carbidopa or *benserazide. After several years of levodopa therapy patients may deteriorate, as the effectiveness of the treatment wanes, and unpredictable fluctuations in mobility can occur (the 'on-off' effect). Symptoms can usually be improved by increasing the dosage or dividing the existing daily dose into smaller and more frequent quantities. Alternatively, *modified-release preparations may be of benefit. In some cases a low protein diet may increase the absorption of levodopa. (*See also* APOMORPHINE HYDROCHLORIDE.)
Side effects: include nausea and vomiting, loss of appetite, involuntary abnormal movements of the limbs and face, insomnia, agitation, postural hypotension (a sudden drop in blood pressure on standing), dizziness, fast heart rate, and a reddish discoloration of the urine (which is harmless). Rarely, allergic reactions may occur.
Precautions: levodopa should be used with caution in people with lung disease, peptic ulcers, diabetes, psychiatric illness, cardiovascular disease, glaucoma, or a history of convulsions. Those who do benefit from therapy should resume normal activities slowly. Dosage should be reduced gradually at the end of treatment. Levodopa should not be taken by women who are breastfeeding.
Interactions with other drugs:

Anaesthetics: there is a risk of abnormal heart thythms if levodopa is given with general anaesthetics that are inhaled.

MAOIs: a dangerous rise in blood pressure can occur; levodopa should be avoided for at least two weeks after stopping MAOIs.

Proprietary preparations: Caramet CR (*see* CO-CARELDOPA); Duodopa (*see* CO-CARELDOPA); Madopar and Madopar CR (*see* CO-BENELDOPA); Sinemet (*see* CO-CARELDOPA); Stalevo (*see* CO-CARELDOPA);.

levofloxacin A *quinolone antibiotic used for the treatment of pneumonia, acute sinusitis, chronic bronchitis, infections of the urinary tract, skin and soft tissue infections, and eye infections. It is available, on *prescription only, as tablets, a solution for intravenous infusion, or eye drops.
Side effects: *see* QUINOLONES.
Precautions: levofloxacin eye drops should not be used in children under one year old and should be used with caution by women who are pregnant or breastfeeding. The eye drops may cause local irritation, sensitivity to light, and headache. *See also* QUINOLONES.
Interactions with other drugs: *see* QUINOLONES.
Proprietary preparations: Oftaquix (eye drops); Tavanic.

levofolinic acid *See* FOLINIC ACID.

levomenthol *See* MENTHOL.

levomepromazine <**methotrimeprazine**> A phenothiazine *antipsychotic drug used for the treatment of schizophrenia and manic-depressive psychosis, especially when sedation is desirable. It is also given to terminally ill patients to relieve nausea and vomiting, restlessness, or distress. Levomepromazine is available as tablets or an injection on *prescription only.
Side effects: as for *chlorpromazine hydrochloride, but levomepromazine is more sedating.
Precautions and interactions with other drugs: *see* CHLORPROMAZINE HYDROCHLORIDE.
Proprietary preparation: Nozinan.

Levonelle 1500, Levonelle One Step (Bayer) *See* LEVONORGESTREL.

levonorgestrel A synthetic *progestogen used mainly in *oral contraceptives, either in combination with an *oestrogen or as a progestogen-only preparation. As the latter, it may be used for emergency contraception, taken as a single dose within 72 hours of unprotected sexual intercourse. It is also used in *depot contraceptives in the form of an intrauterine system. This consists of an intrauterine contraceptive device (IUCD) that releases levonorgestrel for up to three years; it can be removed at any time within this period. This formulation is a more effective contraceptive than an IUCD alone and is associated with a lower incidence of pelvic inflammatory disease, a potential risk for IUCD users. Levonorgestrel is also used in *hormone replacement therapy (HRT). It is available on *prescription only, but a preparation for emergency contraception can be obtained from pharmacies without a prescription.
Side effects: *see* ORAL CONTRACEPTIVES; PROGESTOGENS. The IUCD and the emergency contraceptive may cause pain in the lower abdomen; the emergency contraceptive may also cause menstrual irregularities, nausea, fatigue, headache, and dizziness.
Precautions (with oral contraceptives and HRT): *see* ORAL CONTRACEPTIVES; PROGESTOGENS. The IUCD should not be used during pregnancy or by women with undiagnosed vaginal bleeding, severe anaemia, genital cancers, or pelvic

inflammatory disease; it should be used with caution by women with heart disease or diabetes, who are on long-term steroid therapy, or who have had an ectopic pregnancy. Women who take the emergency contraceptive should use barrier contraception until the next period.
Interactions with other drugs: *see* PROGESTOGENS.
Proprietary preparations: Levonelle 1500, Levonelle One Step (emergency contraceptive); Mirena (IUCD); Norgeston (contraceptive pill); *Cyclo-Progynova (combined with estradiol); *Logynon and Logynon ED (combined with ethinylestradiol); *Microgynon 30 and Microgynon 30 ED (combined with ethinylestradiol); *Ovranette (combined with estradiol); *Prempak-C (combined with conjugated oestrogens).

Levophed (Hospira) *See* NORADRENALINE.

levothyroxine sodium <**thyroxine sodium**> A preparation of the *thyroid hormone thyroxine that is given to replace a lack of the natural hormone. It is also used for the treatment of goitre and thyroid cancer. Levothyroxine sodium is available as tablets or an oral solution on *prescription only.
Side effects: these are usually the result of overdosage at the start of treatment and diminish as the dosage is adjusted according to the level of thyroid hormones measured in the blood. They include irregular heart rhythms, anginal pain, muscle cramps, headache, restlessness, excitability, insomnia, flushing, sweating, diarrhoea, excessive weight loss, and muscular weakness.
Precautions: levothyroxine sodium should be used with caution by people with poorly functioning adrenal glands, cardiovascular disorders, diabetes mellitus, or diabetes insipidus and by women who are pregnant or breastfeeding.
Interactions with other drugs:
Antiepileptic drugs: carbamazepine, phenobarbital, phenytoin, and primidone increase the requirement for levothyroxine sodium.
Colestyramine: reduces the absorption of levothyroxine sodium.
Oral anticoagulants: their anticoagulant effects are enhanced.
Propranolol: reduces the effect of levothyroxine sodium.
Rifampicin: increases the requirement for levothyroxine sodium.
Sucralfate: reduces the absorption of levothyroxine sodium.
Proprietary preparation: Eltroxin (tablets).

Lexpec (Rosemont Pharmaceuticals) *See* FOLIC ACID.

Librium (Meda Pharmaceuticals) *See* CHLORDIAZEPOXIDE.

lice Small wingless insects that live as parasites on the skin. Lice infestations cause intense itching; scratching to relieve this may result in secondary infection. Head lice are common in schoolchildren and do not indicate poor hygiene. They can be treated with *malathion, *permethrin, or *dimeticone, which kill the lice (i.e. they are **pediculicides**); some health authorities suggest that malathion should be alternated with carbaryl to prevent the development of resistance. Crab (or pubic) lice adhere to body hair (in the pubic region and armpits); they may also infest the eyelashes. Carbaryl and malathion provide effective treatment.

licence A document given to a pharmaceutical company that allows that company to market a particular drug. The company must apply for a licence to the regulatory body that issues them: in the UK this is the Medicines and Healthcare products Regulatory Agency (MHRA); in the USA it is the Food and Drug Administration (FDA). The regulatory body issues the licence only for defined uses (called indications), which should be adhered to by the doctor prescribing the drug. However, some drugs may be given for an 'unlicensed indication'; in these circumstances the doctor not adhering to the licence may be vulnerable to litigation if anything untoward occurs due to use of the drug.

lidocaine <**lignocaine**> A *local anaesthetic that is applied to parts of the body where pain relief is required or given by local injection for infiltration anaesthesia. It is a component of preparations used to treat *haemorrhoids and other causes of anal pain and itching. It is used for relieving sore throats, teething discomfort in babies, and mouth discomfort due to ulcers in adults, to numb areas of skin before injections, and to numb regions of the body before such procedures as insertion of urinary catheters, vaginal examinations, and ophthalmic procedures. It is combined with a *corticosteroid for local use in inflammatory or rheumatic conditions. Lidocaine is also a class I *anti-arrhythmic drug administered by intravenous injection for the treatment of ventricular *arrhythmias, especially after a heart attack. It is available as solutions for injection (for local anaesthesia lidocaine may be combined with *adrenaline) and is included in a variety of ointments, gels, creams, and other preparations for topical application. Solutions for injection are *prescription only medicines; topical preparations are usually available without a prescription.

Side effects: injections of lidocaine may cause dizziness, 'pins and needles', or drowsiness. Less often confusion and hypotension (low blood pressure) may occur.

Precautions: lidocaine injections should not be given to patients with heart block or certain other heart conditions and should be used with caution in people with liver or kidney disease, breathing difficulties, or epilepsy and in pregnant women.

Interactions with other drugs:

Antipsychotics: the risk of arrhythmias is increased if lidocaine is given with some antipsychotics.

Antiviral drugs: atazanavir, darunavir, and fosamprenavir increase the plasma concentration of lidocaine, which should not be given with darunavir or fosamprenavir.

Beta blockers: increase depression of heart function.

Cimetidine: increases the plasma concentration (and adverse effects) of lidocaine.

Diuretics: acetazolamide, loop diuretics, and thiazide diuretics reduce the action of lidocaine.

Synercid: should not be given with lidocaine as this combination increases the risk of arrhythmias.
Proprietary preparations: Boots Pharmacy Anaesthetic Throat Spray; Laryngojet (jet spray); LMX 4 (cream); Vagisil Medicated Creme; Versatis (medicated plaster); Xylocaine (injection (with or without adrenaline) or spray); *Boots Teething Gel 3 Months + (combined with cetylpyridinium chloride); *Calgel (combined with cetylpyridinium); *Dentinox Teething Gel (combined with cetylpyridinium); *Depo-Medrone with Lidocaine (combined with methylprednisolone); *Emla (combined with prilocaine); *Germoloids (combined with zinc oxide); *Haemorrhoid Relief Ointment (combined with zinc oxide); *Instillagel (combined with chlorhexidine); *Medijel (combined with aminoacridine); *Minims Lidocaine and Fluorescein (combined with fluorescein); *Perinal (combined with hydrocortisone); *Rapydan (combined with tetracaine); *Xyloproct (combined with aluminium acetate, zinc oxide, and hydrocortisone).

lignocaine *See* LIDOCAINE.

Li-Liquid (Rosemont Pharmaceuticals) *See* LITHIUM CITRATE.

linctus A syrupy liquid medicine, particularly one used in the treatment of irritating coughs.

linezolid An *antibiotic used to treat severe infections that are resistant to other antibacterials, including streptococcal infections, *vancomycin-resistant infections, and meticillin-resistant *Staphylococcus aureus* (MRSA). It is available, on *prescription only, as tablets, an oral suspension, or a solution for intravenous infusion.
Side effects: include headache, diarrhoea, nausea, vomiting, and blood disorders.
Precautions and interactions with other drugs: linezolid should not be given to people with uncontrolled *hypertension, phaeochromocytoma (a tumour of the adrenal gland), carcinoid (an intestinal tumour), an overactive thyroid gland, bipolar disorder, schizophrenia, or liver disease or to women who are breastfeeding. Since it inhibits monoamine oxidase enzymes, it should not be taken by people who are also receiving *monoamine oxidase inhibitors, SSRIs, $5HT_1$ agonists, tricyclic antidepressants, sympathomimetic drugs, or dopamine receptor agonists. Blood counts should be monitored throughout treatment.
Proprietary preparation: Zyvox.

liniment A medicinal preparation that is rubbed onto the skin or applied on a surgical dressing. Liniments often contain camphor.

Linola Gamma (Linderma) *See* EVENING PRIMROSE OIL.

Lioresal (Novartis) *See* BACLOFEN.

liothyronine sodium (L-triiodothyronine) A preparation of the *thyroid hormone triiodothyronine that is given to replace a lack of natural thyroid

hormone and is also used for the treatment of goitre, thyroid cancer, and coma induced by a severe lack of thyroid hormone. Liothyronine has a more rapid onset and shorter duration of action than *levothyroxine sodium. It is available as tablets and an intravenous injection on *prescription only.
Side effects, precautions, and interactions with other drugs: *see* LEVOTHYROXINE SODIUM.
Proprietary preparation: Triiodothyronine (injection).

Lipantil Micro (Solvay Healthcare) *See* FENOFIBRATE.

lipid-lowering drugs (**hypolipidaemic drugs**) Drugs that lower the concentrations of *lipoproteins, the agents that transport *cholesterol and *triglycerides, in blood. It is advised that these drugs are given when other risk factors for coronary heart disease have been controlled or eliminated. The most important risk factors are smoking, alcohol consumption, *obesity, *diabetes, *hypertension, and inactivity. Dietary intervention is the first-line treatment of raised lipid concentrations, and adherence to a low-fat/high-fibre diet should accompany the use of lipid-lowering drugs, along with maintenance of near-ideal body weight, reduction of blood pressure, and cessation of smoking. The lipid-lowering drugs include *statins, *fibrates, *bile-acid sequestrants, *nicotinic acid, *acipimox, *ezetimibe, *omega-3 fatty acid compounds, and *ispaghula husk.

Lipitor (Pfizer) *See* ATORVASTATIN.

Lipobase (Astellas Pharma) A proprietary combination of cetostearyl alcohol, cetomacrogol, *liquid paraffin, and *white soft paraffin, used as an *emollient for the relief of dry and itching skin conditions. It is freely available *over the counter.

lipoproteins Complex molecules that transport lipids, especially *cholesterol and *triglycerides, in the blood. Lipids do not mix with water (the blood is largely water), and in order to circulate and be taken up by tissues these fatty compounds need to be 'tucked' inside larger molecules, the lipoproteins, which do mix with blood. Lipoproteins are classified according to their density; the most important lipoproteins in terms of heart disease are the **high-density lipoproteins** (**HDL**) and **low-density lipoproteins** (**LDL**). High concentrations of LDL-cholesterol in the blood increase the risk for coronary heart disease; HDL-cholesterol has a protective effect. *See* LIPID-LOWERING DRUGS.

Liposic (Bausch & Lomb UK) *See* CARBOMER.

Lipostat (E.R. Squibb & Sons) *See* PRAVASTATIN.

liquid paraffin A mineral oil used as an *emollient and as an ingredient in lubricants to treat dry eyes. It was formerly widely used as a *faecal softener to lubricate the passage of faeces in the treatment of constipation, but is no longer recommended for this purpose. It can be obtained without a

prescription, but some preparations containing liquid paraffin are available only from pharmacies.
Side effects: when used as a faecal softener, anal seepage of paraffin and anal irritation occur after long-term use, absorption of fat-soluble vitamins may be affected, and life-threatening pneumonia can develop if it is accidentally taken into the lungs.
Proprietary preparations: Cetraben Emollient Bath Additive; Doublebase Emollient Bath Additive; Oilatum Emollient and Oilatum Junior Emollient (bath additive); *Cetraben Emollient Cream (combined with white soft paraffin); *Dermamist (combined with white soft paraffin); *Dermol (combined with benzalkonium chloride, isopropyl myristate, and chlorhexidine hydrochloride); *Diprobase (combined with white soft paraffin); *Doublebase Emollient Shower Gel (combined with isopropyl myristate); *E45 Bath Oil (combined with dimeticone); *E45 Cream (combined with lanolin and white soft paraffin); *E45 Wash Cream (combined with zinc oxide); *Emollin (combined with white soft paraffin); *Emulsiderm (combined with benzalkonium chloride and isopropyl myristate); *Epaderm (combined with yellow soft paraffin and wax); *50:50 Ointment (combined with white soft paraffin); *Hydromol Cream (combined with isopropyl myristate, arachis oil, sodium lactate, and sodium pyrrolidone carboxylate); *Hydromol Emollient (combined with isopropyl myristate); *Imuderm (combined with almond oil); *Infaderm Therapeutic Body Oil (combined with almond oil); *Lacri-Lube (combined with white soft paraffin and wool fat); *Lipobase (combined with white soft paraffin); *Lubri-Tears (combined with white soft paraffin and wool fat); *Milpar (combined with magnesium hydroxide); *Oilatum Plus (combined with benzalkonium chloride and triclosan); *Ultrabase (combined with white soft paraffin); *Unguentum M (combined with white soft paraffin and other emollients).

Liquifilm Tears (Allergan) *See* POLYVINYL ALCOHOL.

Liquivisc (Allergan) *See* CARBOMER.

liraglutide A *glucagon-like protein produced by genetic engineering, used, in combination with *metformin and/or a *sulphonylurea, to control blood glucose levels in type 2 *diabetes mellitus and to promote weight loss. It works by suppressing glucagon secretion and increasing *insulin secretion when blood glucose levels are high; it also intensifies feelings of satiety and delays stomach emptying. Liraglutide is given by subcutaneous injection and is available on *prescription only.
Side effects: include headache, decreased appetite, diarrhoea, nausea, vomiting, indigestion, and low blood glucose levels.
Precautions: liraglutide should not be given to women who are pregnant or breastfeeding and is not recommended for people with liver disease or severe kidney disease.
Proprietary preparation: Victoza.

lisinopril An *ACE inhibitor used as an adjunct to *diuretics for the

treatment of *heart failure. It is also taken after myocardial infarction (heart attack) to reduce recurrence and is used to treat all grades of *hypertension. Available as tablets on *prescription only, it is usually taken once a day.
Side effects, precautions, and interactions with other drugs: *see* ACE INHIBITORS.
Proprietary preparations: Zestril; *Carace Plus (combined with hydrochlorothiazide); *Zestoretic (combined with hydrochlorothiazide).
See also ANTIHYPERTENSIVE DRUGS.

Liskonum (GlaxoSmithKline) *See* LITHIUM CARBONATE.

LITAK (Lipomed) *See* CLADRIBINE.

lithium A drug used in the form of its salts for the prevention and treatment of mania and in the prevention of bipolar disorder and recurrent depression (unipolar depression). Its mechanism of action is unclear, but it inhibits the action of an important enzyme involved in the transmission of signals in the brain. Lithium may be added to *tricyclic antidepressants to increase their effectiveness. The concentrations of lithium in the blood that are therapeutically effective may be close to those that produce toxic effects. Plasma concentrations of lithium should therefore be monitored carefully and the dosage adjusted as necessary. Overdosage can be fatal. Lithium is available as *lithium carbonate and *lithium citrate. Different products have different absorption characteristics, therefore it is not advisable to change brands of medication unless specifically instructed to do so.
Side effects: these are dose-related and develop as concentrations of lithium in the blood increase. They include nausea, vomiting, and diarrhoea, fine tremor, increased urine production, weight gain, and oedema. Signs of lithium intoxication include blurred vision, increasing gastrointestinal disturbances, drowsiness and lethargy, giddiness, coarse tremor, and lack of coordination. Treatment may need to be stopped.
Precautions: lithium salts should not be used to treat children, people with kidney or heart disease, or those with *sodium imbalance (lithium toxicity is exacerbated by sodium depletion). They should be used with caution in elderly people and in women who are pregnant or breastfeeding.
Interactions with other drugs: lithium interacts with a wide variety of drugs, including:
ACE inhibitors: increase concentrations of lithium in the blood.
Amiodarone: should not be given with lithium as this combination increases the risk of ventricular *arrhythmias.
Angiotensin II inhibitors: increase concentrations of lithium in the blood.
Anticonvulsants: carbamazepine and phenytoin may increase lithium toxicity without increasing plasma concentrations of lithium.
Calcium antagonists: diltiazem and verapamil may increase lithium toxicity without increasing plasma concentrations of lithium.
Diuretics: increase concentrations of lithium in the blood. As lithium toxicity is exacerbated by sodium depletion, the use of diuretics, especially thiazides, with lithium is hazardous and should be avoided.

Methyldopa: may increase toxicity of lithium without increasing plasma lithium concentrations.
Metronidazole: increases concentrations of lithium in the blood.
NSAIDs: increase concentrations of lithium in the blood; the use of ketorolac with lithium should be avoided.
Sertindole: should not be given with lithium as this combination increases the risk of ventricular arrhythmias.
SSRIs: increase concentrations of lithium in the blood.
Theophylline: may reduce concentrations of lithium in the blood.

lithium carbonate A *lithium salt used for the treatment and prevention of mania, bipolar disorder, and recurrent depression. It is also used to treat aggressive and self-mutilating behaviour. It is available as tablets and *modified-release tablets on *prescription only.
Side effects, precautions, and interactions with other drugs: *see* LITHIUM.
Proprietary preparations: Camcolit; Liskonum; Priadel.

lithium citrate A *lithium salt used for the treatment and prevention of mania, bipolar disorder, and recurrent depression. It is also used to treat aggressive and self-mutilating behaviour. It is available as *modified-release tablets or a liquid on *prescription only.
Side effects, precautions, and interactions with other drugs: *see* LITHIUM.
Proprietary preparations: Li-Liquid; Priadel Liquid.

l

Livial (Organon Laboratories) *See* TIBOLONE.

LMX 4 (Ferndale) *See* LIDOCAINE.

local anaesthetics Drugs that inhibit the conduction of impulses in sensory nerves in the region where they are applied and therefore reduce or abolish sensations in that area of the body. Local anaesthetics are used for local pain relief, including that required before painful procedures, such as venepuncture (taking a blood sample) or injections. They are usually applied topically, to the skin or mucous membranes, for **surface anaesthesia**, but some (e.g. **bupivacaine**, **levobupivacaine**, *lidocaine, and *prilocaine) can be injected for **infiltration** (or **local**) **anaesthesia**. Although local anaesthetics are used for their local analgesic effects, most of them also cause dilatation of blood vessels, so that they are quickly absorbed into the bloodstream and removed from their intended site of action. For this reason they are often administered with a *vasoconstrictor drug, such as *adrenaline or *phenylephrine. Local anaesthetics absorbed into the bloodstream can cause unwanted *systemic effects (see side effects below).

Local anaesthetics that are ingredients of creams, sprays, or gels for the skin, to relieve the pain of stings or minor cuts, abrasions, and burns, include *tetracaine, *benzocaine, and lidocaine. These anaesthetics are also included in sprays and lozenges for painful conditions of the mouth, gums, and throat, and lidocaine is used in teething gels. Local anaesthetics applied in eye drops include tetracaine, **oxybuprocaine**, **proxymetacaine**, and lidocaine. Soothing preparations for the relief of haemorrhoids often contain local anaesthetics,

such as lidocaine, benzocaine, *pramocaine hydrochloride, or *cinchocaine hydrochloride.
Side effects: rapid and extensive absorption of local anaesthetics causes light-headedness followed by sedation. Some local anaesthetics cause allergic reactions. For specific side effects, see entries for individual drugs.

Loceryl, Loceryl Lacquer (Galderma) *See* AMOROLFINE.

Locoid, Locoid Crelo, Locoid Lipocream, Locoid Scalp Lotion (Astellas Pharma) *See* HYDROCORTISONE BUTYRATE.

Locorten-Vioform (Amdipharm) A proprietary combination of *clioquinol (an antibiotic) and *flumetasone pivalate (a topical steroid), used for the treatment of inflammatory conditions of the outer ear in which secondary infection is suspected. It is available as ear drops on *prescription only.
Side effects: this preparation may irritate the skin and discolour the hair.
Precautions: this medicine should not be used on perforated eardrums or for treating primary infections of the outer ear. It should be used with caution by women who are pregnant or breastfeeding. It is not recommended for children under two years old.

Lodine, Lodine SR (Almirall) *See* ETODOLAC.

lodoxamide A drug used for the treatment of allergic conjunctivitis. It is available as eye drops on *prescription only.
Side effects: include mild transient stinging, burning, itching, and tear production.
Precautions: lodoxamide should not be used by wearers of soft contact lenses, and should be used with caution by women who are pregnant or breastfeeding.
Proprietary preparation: Alomide.

Loestrin 20 (Galen) A proprietary combination of *ethinylestradiol (20 micrograms) and *norethisterone acetate used as an *oral contraceptive. **Loestrin 30** contains 30 micrograms of ethinylestradiol. Both preparations are available as tablets on *prescription only.
Side effects, precautions, and interactions with other drugs: *see* ORAL CONTRACEPTIVES.

lofepramine A *tricyclic antidepressant drug used for the treatment of depressive illness; it is less sedating than *amitriptyline hydrochloride. Lofepramine is available as tablets or an oral suspension on *prescription only.
Side effects: similar to those of amitriptyline hydrochloride, but lofepramine has fewer antimuscarinic effects (e.g. dry mouth, blurred vision, difficulty in urinating) than amitriptyline; it can have adverse effects on the liver.
Precautions and interactions with other drugs: *see* TRICYCLIC ANTIDEPRESSANTS.
Proprietary preparations: Feprapax (tablets); Lomont (suspension).

lofexidine hydrochloride A drug used to relieve the symptoms in people who are undergoing withdrawal from physical *dependence on opioids, such as heroin (*diamorphine). It acts on alpha-adrenoceptors in the brain to reduce impulses in the *sympathetic nervous system. Lofexidine is available as tablets on *prescription only.
Side effects: include drowsiness, dry mouth, throat, and nose, low blood pressure, and slowing of the heart rate. Overdosage can cause sedation and coma.
Precautions: lofexidine should be used with caution in people who have certain heart conditions, slow heart rate, or kidney disease and in women who are pregnant or breastfeeding. Treatment with lofexidine should be stopped gradually (over several days) to prevent a sudden increase in blood pressure.
Interactions with other drugs:
Anxiolytic and hypnotic drugs: lofexidine increases their sedative effects.
Proprietary preparation: BritLofex.

Logynon (Bayer) A proprietary combination of *ethinylestradiol and *levonorgestrel used as an *oral contraceptive of the triphasic type. These tablets are packaged in three phases, which differ in the amounts of the active ingredients they contain. **Logynon ED** contains both active and dummy tablets, so that a tablet is taken each day of a 28-day cycle. Both preparations are available on *prescription only.
Side effects, precautions, and interactions with other drugs: *see* ORAL CONTRACEPTIVES.

Lomont (Rosemont Pharmaceuticals) *See* LOFEPRAMINE.

lomustine An *alkylating drug used for the treatment of Hodgkin's disease, melanoma (skin cancer), and certain solid tumours (*see* CANCER). It is available as capsules on *prescription only.
Side effects: include nausea and vomiting, which may be moderately severe. *See also* CYTOTOXIC DRUGS.
Precautions: *see* CYTOTOXIC DRUGS.
Interactions with other drugs:
Clozapine: increases the risk of agranulocytosis (a blood disorder) and therefore should not be taken with lomustine.
Proprietary preparation: CCNU.

Loniten (Pharmacia) *See* MINOXIDIL.

loop diuretics The most powerful class of *diuretics. Loop diuretics act rapidly, causing large volumes of urine to be excreted, but have a short duration of action. The name comes from the fact that they inhibit salt reabsorption in the loop of Henle, part of the tubular structure of the kidney. They are used for the treatment of *heart failure, nephrotic syndrome (a condition in which there is a large loss of protein in the urine, causing low blood protein and *oedema), and pulmonary oedema (fluid in the spaces of the lungs). Loop diuretics cause a marked loss of potassium, which may be corrected by the use of *potassium supplements or the addition of a *potassium-sparing diuretic. They start to act rapidly within one hour, and diuresis is complete within six hours. *See* BUMETANIDE; FUROSEMIDE; TORASEMIDE.

Side effects: these diuretics can sometimes have too powerful an action, causing depletion of potassium, sodium, and water; these effects in turn can cause weakness, lethargy, cramps, and dizziness. The dizziness often occurs as a result of low blood pressure on standing up from a lying or sitting posture (postural hypotension). Other side effects include a loss of calcium. Loop diuretics may worsen diabetic control because they reduce insulin secretion and therefore increase blood sugar concentration. There is a risk of gout with loop diuretics due to their effect of reducing uric acid excretion. Large doses of furosemide intravenously can disturb hearing transiently. Rashes, pancreatitis, and thrombocytopenia (decreased number of platelets in the blood, causing easy bruising) are rare side effects of loop diuretics.

Precautions: potassium supplements will often be required. Loop diuretics should not be taken by people with advanced cirrhosis of the liver. They are not usually given to pregnant women and should be used with caution in men with an enlarged prostate gland and in people with diabetes or gout. Loop diuretics can increase the likelihood of dehydration and hangovers after drinking.

Interactions with other drugs:

ACE inhibitors: the blood-pressure-lowering effect of ACE inhibitors is enhanced; since ACE inhibitors cause potassium retention, the loss of potassium is not so great when these drugs are taken together.

Aminoglycoside antibiotics: increase the risk of hearing problems.

Anti-arrhythmic drugs: if potassium loss occurs, amiodarone, disopyramide, and flecainide are more likely to have adverse effects on the heart and the action of lidocaine is antagonized.

Antihypertensive drugs: their effects in lowering blood pressure are increased.

Antipsychotics: if potassium loss occurs, amisulpride, pimozide, and sertindole are more likely to cause ventricular *arrhythmias, and pimozide should not be taken with loop diuretics.

Atomoxetine: if potassium loss occurs, this drug is more likely to cause ventricular arrhythmias.

Corticosteroids: may further increase the loss of potassium.

Digitalis drugs: the adverse effects of these drugs are increased if potassium loss occurs.

Lithium: concentrations of lithium in the blood may be increased, causing adverse effects.

NSAIDs: may reduce the diuretic effect of loop diuretics.

Sotalol: if potassium loss occurs, sotalol is more likely to cause ventricular arrhythmias.

loperamide hydrochloride An *opioid that slows down movements of the gut and is used in the treatment of acute diarrhoea in adults and children over four years old and chronic diarrhoea in adults only (*see* ANTIDIARRHOEAL

DRUGS). Loperamide is available as capsules, tablets, or a syrup on *prescription, but capsules or tablets for treating acute diarrhoea can be obtained from pharmacies without a prescription.
Side effects: abdominal cramps, bloating, and rashes may occur.
Precautions: loperamide should not be taken by people with acute ulcerative colitis, antibiotic-associated colitis, paralysis of the small intestine, or abdominal distension.
Proprietary preparations: Boots Diareze; Diocalm Ultra; Imodium (capsules or syrup); Norimode; *Boots Dual Action Diarrhoea Relief (tablets: packaged with sodium chloride, potassium chloride, sodium citrate, and citric acid); *Imodium Plus (combined with simeticone).

Lopid (Pfizer) *See* GEMFIBROZIL.

lopinavir *See* KALETRA.

loprazolam A short-acting *benzodiazepine used for the short-term treatment of insomnia. It is available as tablets on *prescription only.
Side effects and precautions: *see* BENZODIAZEPINES; DIAZEPAM.
Interactions with other drugs: *see* BENZODIAZEPINES.

Lopresor, Lopresor SR (Novartis) *See* METOPROLOL TARTRATE.

Loramyc (Laboratoires BioAlliance) *See* MICONAZOLE.

loratadine One of the newer (non-sedating) *antihistamines, used to relieve the symptoms of such allergic conditions as hay fever and urticaria. It is available as tablets or a syrup from pharmacies without a prescription.
Side effects and interactions with other drugs: *see* ANTIHISTAMINES.
Precautions: loratadine should not be taken by women who are pregnant or breastfeeding. *See also* ANTIHISTAMINES.

lorazepam A short-acting *benzodiazepine used for the short-term treatment of anxiety and insomnia and to relax patients before operations. It is also given by injection in the treatment of status epilepticus (repeated epileptic seizures). Lorazepam is available as tablets and an injection on *prescription only.
Side effects and precautions: *see* DIAZEPAM; BENZODIAZEPINES.
Interactions with other drugs: *see* BENZODIAZEPINES.
Proprietary preparation: Ativan.

lormetazepam A short-acting *benzodiazepine used for the short-term treatment of insomnia. It is available as tablets on *prescription only.
Side effects and precautions: *see* BENZODIAZEPINES; DIAZEPAM.
Interactions with other drugs: *see* BENZODIAZEPINES.

Loron 520 (Roche Products) *See* SODIUM CLODRONATE.

losartan potassium An *angiotensin II inhibitor used in the treatment of *hypertension and of chronic heart failure when ACE inhibitors cannot be used. It is available as tablets or an oral suspension on *prescription only.

Side effects and precautions: *see* ANGIOTENSIN II INHIBITORS.
Interactions with other drugs: *see* ACE INHIBITORS.
Proprietary preparations: Cozaar; *Cozaar-Comp (combined with hydrochlorothiazide).

Losec, Losec MUPS (AstraZeneca) *See* OMEPRAZOLE.

Lotemax (Bausch & Lomb UK) *See* LOTEPREDNOL ETABONATE.

loteprednol etabonate A *corticosteroid used for the short-term treatment of inflammation following eye surgery. It is available as eye drops on *prescription only.
Side effects: include an increase in pressure in the eye after a few weeks' treatment and thinning of the cornea and sclera.
Precautions: loteprednol should not be used by people with viral, fungal, tuberculous, or weeping infections or by those who wear soft contact lenses; it should be used with caution by people with glaucoma. Prolonged use by pregnant women and infants should be avoided. *See also* TOPICAL STEROIDS.
Proprietary preparation: Lotemax.

lotion A medicinal solution for washing or bathing the external parts of the body. Lotions usually have a cooling, soothing, or antiseptic action.

Lotriderm (Teva UK) A proprietary combination of *betamethasone dipropionate (a potent steroid) and *clotrimazole (an antifungal agent), used for the treatment of short-term fungal infections of the skin. It is available as a cream on *prescription only.
Side effects: there may be local mild burning, irritation, and allergic reactions. *See also* TOPICAL STEROIDS.
Precautions: *see* TOPICAL STEROIDS.

low molecular weight heparins Forms of *heparin that consist of smaller molecules than standard heparin. They have a longer duration of action than standard heparin and are used for the prevention and treatment of deep-vein *thrombosis and in the treatment of pulmonary embolism and unstable *angina. They are also used in patients undergoing kidney dialysis, in order to prevent the formation of blood clots. The low molecular weight heparins include *bemiparin sodium, *dalteparin sodium, *enoxaparin, and *tinzaparin sodium; they are administered by injection (usually subcutaneous) and are available on *prescription only. *See also* DANAPAROID SODIUM.
Side effects, precautions, and interactions with other drugs: *see* HEPARIN.

lozenge A medicinal tablet containing sugar. Lozenges are usually solid and rigid (compared to a *pastille, which is soft) and should be sucked, so that the medication is applied to the mouth and throat.

Luborant (Goldshield) *See* CARMELLOSE.

Lubri-Tears (Alcon Laboratories) A proprietary combination of *white soft paraffin, *liquid paraffin, and wool fat (anhydrous *lanolin), used for the lubrication of dry eyes. It is available as an eye ointment and can be obtained without a prescription, but only from pharmacies.

Lucentis (Novartis) *See* RANIBIZUMAB.

Lugol's solution *See* IODINE.

lumefantrine *See* RIAMET.

Lumigan (Allergan) *See* BIMATOPROST.

Lustral (Pfizer) *See* SERTRALINE.

lutropin alfa A genetically engineered form of human luteinizing hormone, used in the treatment of infertility to stimulate development of egg follicles in the ovary in women with deficiencies of luteinizing hormone and follicle-stimulating hormone (*see* GONADOTROPHINS). It is given by subcutaneous injection, with *follitropin. Treatment should be supervised in a specialist infertility clinic in order to monitor follicle development and to guide correct dosage and the timing of coitus. Lutropin alfa is available on *prescription only.
Side effects: include nausea, vomiting, abdominal pain, headache, sleepiness, reactions at the injection site, breast pain, and ovarian hyperstimuation (the uncontrolled production of large number of follicles).
Precautions: lutropin alfa should not be given to women with ovarian cysts, vaginal bleeding, tumours of the pituitary or hypothalamus, or cancer of the ovaries, uterus, or breast.
Proprietary preparations: Luveris; *Pergoveris (combined with follitropin alfa).

Luveris (Merck Serono) *See* LUTROPIN ALFA.

Luvinsta XL (Actavis) *See* FLUVASTATIN.

Lyclear Creme Rinse, Lyclear Dermal Cream (Chefaro UK) *See* PERMETHRIN.

Lyflex (Chemidex Pharma) *See* BACLOFEN.

lymecycline A tetracycline antibiotic used for the treatment of chronic bronchitis, brucellosis, chlamydial infections, and infections caused by mycoplasmas and rickettsias (*see* TETRACYCLINES). It is also used to treat mouth ulcers and acne. It is available on *prescription only as capsules.
Side effects, precautions, and interactions with other drugs: *see* TETRACYCLINES.
Proprietary preparation: Tetralysal 300.

lymphoma *See* CANCER.

Lypsyl Cold Sore Gel (Novartis) A proprietary combination of *lidocaine (a local anaesthetic), *cetrimide (an antiseptic), and *zinc sulphate (an astringent), used for the relief of cold sores. It reduces pain, discharge, and secondary infection, but is unlikely to have any effect on the duration of symptoms. The gel is available from pharmacies without a prescription.

Lyrica (Pfizer) *See* PREGABALIN.

Lyrinel XL (Janssen-Cilag) *See* OXYBUTYNIN HYDROCHLORIDE.

Lysodren (HRA Pharma) *See* MITOTANE.

Lysovir (Alliance) *See* AMANTADINE HYDROCHLORIDE.

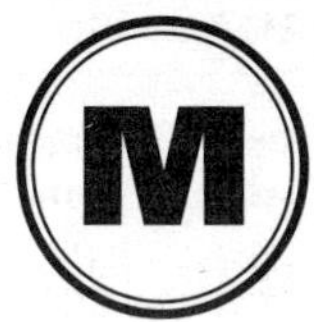

Maalox (sanofi-aventis) *See* CO-MAGALDROX.

Maalox Plus (sanofi-aventis) A proprietary combination of *aluminium hydroxide and *magnesium hydroxide (antacids) and activated *dimeticone (an antifoaming agent), used for the relief of indigestion (*see* ACID-PEPTIC DISEASES). It is freely available *over the counter in the form of a suspension or tablets; the tablets cannot be prescribed on the NHS.
Side effects, precautions, and interactions with other drugs: *see* ANTACIDS.

MabCampeth (Genzyme Therapeutics) *See* ALEMTUZUMAB.

Mabron (Morningside) *See* TRAMADOL HYDROCHLORIDE.

MabThera (Roche Products) *See* RITUXIMAB.

Mackenzies Smelling Salts (Actavis) A proprietary combination of strong *ammonia solution and *eucalyptus oil, used as an aromatic inhalation for the relief of nasal congestion associated with catarrh and head colds. It is freely available *over the counter.
Precautions: Mackenzies Smelling Salts should not be used in babies under three months old.

Macrobid (Goldshield) *See* NITROFURANTOIN.

Macrodantin (Goldshield) *See* NITROFURANTOIN.

macrogols *See* POLYETHYLENE GLYCOLS.

macrolide antibiotics A group of antibiotics that are bacteriostatic, i.e. they prevent bacteria from multiplying, but do not kill them. They have a similar spectrum of activity to the *penicillins and are therefore useful for treating infections in patients who are allergic to penicillin. The original, and probably best known, macrolide is *erythromycin. Its major drawback is that it can have gastrointestinal side effects; this effect is not so marked with the other macrolide antibiotics, *azithromycin and *clarithromycin.

Macugen (Pfizer) *See* PEGAPTANIB SODIUM.

Madopar, Madopar CR (Roche Products) *See* CO-BENELDOPA.

Magnapen (Wockhardt UK) *See* CO-FLUAMPICIL.

magnesia, cream of *See* MAGNESIUM HYDROXIDE.

magnesium alginate *See* ALGINIC ACID.

magnesium carbonate A salt of magnesium that is used as an *antacid for

the relief of indigestion (*see* ACID-PEPTIC DISEASES). It is available in the form of a mixture and is also included as an ingredient in a variety of compound antacid preparations. Most preparations containing magnesium carbonate are freely available *over the counter.
Side effects and precautions: *see* MAGNESIUM SALTS.
Interactions with other drugs: *see* ANTACIDS.
Proprietary preparations: *Actonorm Powder (combined with other antacids and atropine sulphate); *Andrews Antacid (combined with calcium carbonate); *Bisodol Antacid Powder (combined with sodium bicarbonate); *Bisodol Antacid Tablets (combined with sodium bicarbonate and calcium carbonate); *Bisodol Extra Tablets (combined with sodium bicarbonate, calcium carbonate, and dimeticone); *Osvaren (combined with calcium acetate); *Rennie (combined with calcium carbonate); *Rennie Deflatine (combined with calcium carbonate and dimeticone); *Topal (combined with aluminium hydroxide and alginic acid); *Uriflex R (combined with citric acid, gluconolactone, and disodium edetate).

magnesium citrate An *osmotic laxative used for total evacuation of the bowel before X-ray examination or surgery of the bowel. It is available without a prescription in the form of an effervescent powder to be dissolved in water.
Side effects and precautions: *see* BOWEL-CLEANSING SOLUTIONS.
Proprietary preparations: Citramag; *CitraFleet (combined with sodium picosulfate); *Picolax (combined with sodium picosulfate).

m

magnesium hydroxide A salt of magnesium that is included as an ingredient in a variety of *antacid preparations for the relief of indigestion (*see* ACID-PEPTIC DISEASES). Magnesium hydroxide, in the form of a mixture (**cream of magnesia**), is also used as an *osmotic laxative. Most preparations containing magnesium hydroxide are freely available *over the counter. *See also* CO-MAGALDROX.
Side effects and precautions: *see* MAGNESIUM SALTS.
Interactions with other drugs: *see* ANTACIDS.
Proprietary preparations: Phillips' Milk of Magnesia (laxative); *Boots Wind Relief Tablets (combined with aluminium hydroxide and simeticone); *Carbellon (combined with charcoal and peppermint oil); Maalox (*see* CO-MAGALDROX); *Maalox Plus (combined with aluminium hydroxide and dimeticone); *Milpar (combined with liquid paraffin); Mucogel (*see* CO-MAGALDROX).

magnesium oxide A salt of magnesium that has laxative properties and is therefore included as an ingredient in aluminium-containing *antacids, such as aluminium hydroxide, to reduce their constipating effect. Antacid preparations containing magnesium oxide are freely available *over the counter.
Side effects and precautions: *see* MAGNESIUM SALTS.
Interactions with other drugs: *see* ANTACIDS.
Proprietary preparations: *Asilone Suspension (combined with aluminium

hydroxide and dimeticone); *Kolanticon Gel (combined with aluminium hydroxide, dimeticone, and dicycloverine hydrochloride).

magnesium salts A group of magnesium-containing compounds. Magnesium salts used as *antacids include *magnesium carbonate, *magnesium trisilicate, and *magnesium hydroxide. The latter is also an *osmotic laxative, as are *magnesium sulphate and *magnesium citrate; they are used to treat constipation or as *bowel-cleansing solutions.
Side effects: magnesium salts in antacid preparations can cause diarrhoea; in laxatives they can cause colic. *See also* ANTACIDS.
Precautions: magnesium salts should not be taken by people with kidney disease as this can cause dangerously high plasma concentrations of magnesium.
Interactions with other drugs: *see* ANTACIDS.

magnesium sulphate A salt of magnesium used as an *osmotic laxative; it produces rapid evacuation of the bowel. Magnesium sulphate given by intravenous infusion or intramuscular injection is used to treat magnesium deficiency. Intravenous injections of magnesium sulphate are used for the emergency treatment of serious *arrhythmias. Intravenous magnesium sulphate is also used to prevent the recurrence of seizures in eclampsia, a serious condition that can affect pregnant women. Magnesium sulphate paste can be used to treat boils. Laxatives (which include **Epsom salts**) and pastes containing magnesium sulphate are available without a prescription; injections are *prescription only medicines.
Side effects: colic and diarrhoea can occur when magnesium sulphate is taken by mouth. Injections of magnesium sulphate may cause nausea, vomiting, thirst, flushing, low blood pressure, and drowsiness.
Precautions: *see* MAGNESIUM SALTS.
Interactions with other drugs:
Nifedipine: may cause severe lowering of blood pressure if given with magnesium sulphate injections for treating eclampsia.
See also ANTACIDS.
Proprietary preparations: *Health Salt (combined with sodium bicarbonate); *Original Andrews Salts (combined with sodium bicarbonate and citric acid); *PepcidTwo (combined with calcium carbonate and famotidine).

magnesium trisilicate A salt of magnesium that is used as an *antacid for the relief of indigestion (*see* ACID-PEPTIC DISEASES). It is available in the form of tablets or a mixture and is also an ingredient of a variety of compound antacid preparations. Preparations containing magnesium silicate can be obtained without a prescription.
Side effects and precautions: *see* MAGNESIUM SALTS.
Interactions with other drugs: *see* ANTACIDS.
Proprietary preparations: Peppermint Indigestion Tablets; *Asilone Heartburn (combined with alginic acid, aluminium hydroxide, and sodium bicarbonate); *Gastrocote (combined with alginic acid, aluminium hydroxide,

m

and sodium bicarbonate); *Gaviscon Tablets (combined with aluminium hydroxide, alginic acid, and sodium bicarbonate).

malaria An infectious disease due to the presence of parasitic protozoa of the genus *Plasmodium* within the red blood cells. *P. falciparum* causes **falciparum** (or **malignant**) **malaria** (the most serious kind); *P. vivax* (or less commonly *P. malariae* or *P. ovale*) cause **benign malarias**. Malaria is transmitted by the *Anopheles* mosquito and is confined mainly to tropical and subtropical areas.

When the mosquito bites an individual, parasites are injected into the bloodstream and migrate to the liver and other organs, where they multiply. After an incubation period varying from 12 days (*P. falciparum*) to 10 months (some varieties of *P. vivax*), parasites return to the bloodstream and invade the red blood cells. Rapid multiplication of the parasites results in destruction of the red cells and the release of more parasites capable of infecting other red cells. This causes a short bout of shivering, fever, and sweating, and the loss of healthy red cells results in *anaemia. When the next batch of parasites is released symptoms reappear. The interval between fever attacks varies in different types of malaria: two or three days in benign malarias, and from a few hours to two days in falciparum malaria.

Drugs used to treat falciparum malaria include *quinine, *Malarone (a combination of *proguanil hydrochloride and atovaquone), and *Riamet (a combination of artemether and lumefantrine, two drugs derived from a species of wormwood) (*see also* FANSIDAR; PALUDRINE/AVLOCLOR). For benign malarias, *chloroquine is the treatment of choice. Drugs used to prevent travellers from contracting malaria include chloroquine, *mefloquine, and proguanil hydrochloride.

Malarone (GlaxoSmithKline) A proprietary combination of *proguanil hydrochloride and *atovaquone, used for the treatment of falciparum *malaria that is thought to be resistant to other antimalarial drugs. **Malarone Paediatric** is a lower-strength formulation for children. Both preparations are available as tablets on *prescription only.
Side effects: include nausea, vomiting, and diarrhoea (which can reduce its absorption), abdominal pain, loss of appetite, headache, and cough.
Precautions: Malarone should be used with caution in people with acute kidney failure and in pregnant women. It should not be taken by women who are breastfeeding.
Interactions with other drugs: *see* PROGUANIL HYDROCHLORIDE; ATOVAQUONE.

malathion A pesticide that is used clinically to treat infestations of *lice and *scabies. It is available as a liquid or shampoo; liquids are preferable since contact time is longer (12 hours or overnight is recommended). Some liquids contain alcohol; these are not recommended for treating scabies or crab lice (see also Precautions below). Hair treated with malathion preparations should be allowed to dry naturally. Malathion can be obtained without a prescription, but only from pharmacies.
Side effects: malathion may irritate the skin.

Precautions: malathion should not be applied near the eyes or on broken skin; treatment of infants under six months old should be supervised by a doctor. Lotions containing alcohol should not be used to treat scabies or crab lice; they should also not be used for treating head lice in young children or people with asthma (since inhalation of the fumes can be dangerous). Continuous or prolonged use of alcoholic lotions should be avoided.
Proprietary preparation: Derbac-M.

malic acid An acid present in apples, pears, and many other fruits. It is used as an ingredient in skin preparations (combined with *benzoic acid and *salicylic acid) for the removal of dead skin from ulcers, burns, and wounds. As it can cause increased salivation when taken by mouth, malic acid is also an ingredient in artifical saliva preparations.
Proprietary preparation: *Salivix (combined with acacia).

Manerix (Roche Products) *See* MOCLOBEMIDE.

Manevac (Galen) A proprietary combination of *senna (a stimulant laxative) and *ispaghula husk (a bulk-forming laxative), used for the treatment of constipation. It is available as granules and can be obtained without a prescription, but only from pharmacies.
Side effects: there may be flatulence, abdominal distention, and diarrhoea.
Precautions: *see* ISPAGHULA HUSK.

MAOIs *See* MONOAMINE OXIDASE INHIBITORS.

maraviroc An antiretroviral drug (*see* ANTIVIRAL DRUGS) used, in combination with other antiretrovirals, in the treatment of HIV infection in people who have previously been treated with antiretrovirals. It acts by preventing the virus from entering cells. Maraviroc is available as tablets on *prescription only.
Side effects: include diarrhoea, nausea, headache, dizziness, 'pins and needles', somnolence, cough, rash, itching, back pain, muscle spasms, and insomnia.
Precautions: maraviroc should not be taken by women who are breastfeeding. It should be used with caution in the elderly, pregnant women, and people with liver or kidney disease or hepatitis B or C.
Interactions with other drugs:
Antivirals: the plasma concentration of maraviroc may be increased by most protease inhibitors and reduced by efavirenz.
Ketoconazole: increases the plasma concentration of maraviroc.
Macrolide antibiotics: may increase the plasma concentration of maraviroc.
St John's wort: may reduce the plasma concentration of maraviroc and should not be taken with it.
Proprietary preparation: Celsentri.

Marevan (Goldshield) *See* WARFARIN SODIUM.

Marvelon (Organon Laboratories) A proprietary combination of

*ethinylestradiol and *desogestrel used as an *oral contraceptive. It is available as tablets on *prescription only.
Side effects and interactions with other drugs: *see* ORAL CONTRACEPTIVES.
Precautions: Marvelon should not be used by women who are at risk of developing thromboembolism, for example because they are very overweight or have varicose veins or a history of thrombosis. It should therefore only be taken by women who cannot tolerate other brands and who are prepared to accept the increased risk. *See also* ORAL CONTRACEPTIVES.

Matrifen (Nycomed UK) *See* FENTANYL.

Maxalt, Maxalt Melt (Merck Sharp & Dohme) *See* RIZATRIPTAN.

Maxepa (Seven Seas) *See* OMEGA-3 FATTY ACID COMPOUNDS.

Maxidex (Alcon Laboratories) *See* DEXAMETHASONE.

Maxitrol (Alcon Laboratories) A proprietary combination of *dexamethasone (a corticosteroid), *neomycin sulphate and *polymyxin B sulphate (antibiotics), and *hypromellose (a lubricant), used for the treatment of local inflammation of the eye. It is available as drops or an ointment on *prescription only.
Side effects: include increased pressure in the eye, thinning of the cornea, cataracts, and fungal infections.
Precautions: Maxitrol should not be used when viral or fungal infections are present, during pregnancy, or by children, people with glaucoma or a perforated eardrum, or by wearers of soft contact lenses.

Maxolon (Shire Pharmaceuticals) *See* METOCLOPRAMIDE.

Maxtrex (Pharmacia) *See* METHOTREXATE.

mebendazole An *anthelmintic that immobilizes and kills parasitic worms in the intestine; it is active against roundworms, threadworms, whipworms, and hookworms. Mebendazole is available on *prescription as tablets or a suspension, but packs of tablets containing no more than 800 mg mebendazole can be obtained from pharmacies without a prescription.
Side effects: there may be diarrhoea and abdominal pain; otherwise side effects are rare as the drug is poorly absorbed from the intestine.
Precautions: mebendazole should not be used during pregnancy.
Interactions with other drugs:

Cimetidine: may increase the plasma concentration (and therefore side effects) of mebendazole.

Proprietary preparations: Ovex; Vermox.

mebeverine hydrochloride An *antispasmodic drug used in the treatment of irritable bowel syndrome (IBS) and other conditions marked by gut spasms. It is available as tablets, *modified-release capsules, or a liquid on *prescription only, but limited quantities of tablets can be obtained from pharmacies without a prescription.
Precautions: mebeverine should be used with caution by people with

intestinal obstruction due to loss of intestinal movement and by women who are pregnant or breastfeeding.
Proprietary preparations: Boots IBS Relief; Colofac; Colofac 100; Colofac IBS; Colofac MR (modified-release capsules); *Fybogel Mebeverine (combined with ispaghula).

mecasermin A genetically engineered form of somatomedin (or insulin-like growth factor), a hormone that stimulates growth. It is used for the treatment of growth failure in children and adolescents who have a deficiency of this hormone. Mecasermin is available as a form for subcutaneous injection on *prescription only.
Side effects: include low blood-glucose levels, enlarged tonsils, headache, snoring, and hearing loss.
Precautions: mecasermin should not be given to people with tumours or during pregnancy or breastfeeding.
Proprietary preparation: Increlex.

meclozine hydrochloride An *antihistamine, similar to *cyclizine, that is used for the treatment of motion sickness. It is available as tablets that can be obtained without a prescription, but only from pharmacies.
Side effects, precautions, and interactions with other drugs: *see* ANTIHISTAMINES.
Proprietary preparation: Sea-Legs.

m

Medijel (DDD) A proprietary combination of *aminoacridine hydrochloride (an antiseptic) and *lidocaine hydrochloride (a local anaesthetic), used to relieve the pain of mouth ulcers, sore gums, and ill-fitting dentures. It is available as a gel or pastilles. The pastilles are available without a prescription, but only from pharmacies; the gel is freely available *over the counter.

Medikinet XL (Flynn Pharma) *See* METHYLPHENIDATE HYDROCHLORIDE.

Medinol (SSL International) *See* PARACETAMOL.

Medised (SSL International) A proprietary combination of *paracetamol (an analgesic and antipyretic) and *promethazine (a sedative antihistamine), formulated for young children. It is used to relieve mild to moderate pain (including headache and toothache) and the symptoms of influenza, colds, and chickenpox. It is available as a liquid (standard or sugar-free) and can be obtained without a prescription, but only from pharmacies.
Side effects: *see* ANTIHISTAMINES.
Precautions: Medised should not be given to children under one year old. *See also* PARACETAMOL; ANTIHISTAMINES.
Interactions with other drugs: *see* ANTIHISTAMINES.

Medrone (Pharmacia) *See* METHYLPREDNISOLONE.

medroxyprogesterone A synthetic *progestogen used to treat menstrual disorders (including irregular bleeding and absence of periods), *endometriosis, cancer of the endometrium (lining of the uterus), and (rarely)

breast cancer in postmenopausal women and cancers of the kidney and prostate gland. Deep intramuscular injections of medroxyprogesterone are used as a *depot contraceptive, providing contraception for periods of up to three months. Medroxyprogesterone is also used with oestrogens in *hormone replacement therapy. It is available as tablets or injections on *prescription only.
Side effects: include weight gain, fluid retention, and breast tenderness. Depot injections may also cause irregular, prolonged, or heavy vaginal bleeding during the first 2–3 cycles, headache, abdominal pain, dizziness, and weakness, and there may be temporary infertility when the treatment stops.
Precautions: medroxyprogesterone should not be used during pregnancy or by women with hormone-dependent cancer (some kinds of breast or genital cancer), undiagnosed vaginal bleeding, or liver disease. It should be used with caution in women with asthma, diabetes, epilepsy, migraine, a history of depression, heart disease, or clotting problems.
Interactions with other drugs: *see* PROGESTOGENS.
Proprietary preparations: Climanor (tablets); Depo-Provera (depot injection); Provera (tablets); *Premique Cycle (packaged with conjugated oestrogens); *Indivina 1 mg/2.5 mg (combined with estradiol); *Premique (combined with conjugated oestrogens); *Tridestra (combined with estradiol).

m

mefenamic acid An *NSAID used for the treatment of mild to moderate pain in rheumatoid arthritis (including arthritis in children), osteoarthritis, period pains, and heavy periods; it is also used to relieve postoperative pain. Mefenamic acid is available, on prescription only, as capsules, tablets, and a suspension for children.
Side effects: *see* NSAIDs. Additional side effects may include a rash or diarrhoea (in which case a doctor should be informed as treatment may need to be discontinued) and drowsiness.
Precautions: *see* NSAIDs. In addition, mefenamic acid should not be taken by people with inflammatory bowel disease.
Interactions with other drugs: *see* NSAIDs.
Proprietary preparations: Ponstan; Ponstan Forte; Ponstan Paediatric Suspension.

mefloquine A drug used for the prevention of *malaria, especially in areas where chloroquine-resistant malaria parasites are common. It may rarely also be used to treat falciparum malaria in people who have not used it previously for prevention. Mefloquine is available as tablets on *prescription only.
Side effects: mefloquine has a range of side effects, which should be reported to a doctor if they occur. These include nausea, vomiting, diarrhoea, abdominal pain, dizziness, loss of balance, headache, sleep disorders, tremor, shaking with unsteady gait, anxiety, depression, panic attacks, agitation, and hallucinations. Other possible side effects are tinnitus, visual disturbances, circulatory disorders, slowing or increasing of the heart rate, muscle weakness, muscle or joint pain, itching, hair loss, malaise, fever, fatigue, loss

of appetite, and blood disorders. If any of these side effects occur, medical advice should be obtained before the next dose.
Precautions: this drug should not be used for prevention of malaria in people who have liver disease or epilepsy. It should not be taken during pregnancy, and contraception should be used for three months after treatment has been stopped. It should not be taken by women who are breastfeeding or by people with a history of depression or other psychiatric disorders. Mefloquine should be used with caution in people with certain heart disorders. Dizziness or a disturbed sense of balance may impair the performance of such skilled tasks as driving.
Interactions with other drugs:

Amiodarone: there is an increased risk of *arrhythmias and amiodarone should not be taken with mefloquine.
Antibiotics: there is an increased risk of arrhythmias if mefloquine is taken with moxifloxacin, which should therefore not be used with it; rifampicin reduces plasma concentrations of mefloquine and should not be used with it.
Antiepileptic drugs: their anticonvulsant effects are antagonized by mefloquine.
Atomoxetine: there is an increased risk of arrhythmias.
Antimalarial drugs: there is an increased risk of convulsions if chloroquine or quinine are taken with mefloquine; Riamet should not be taken with mefloquine.
Ivabradine: there is a danger of abnormal heart rhythms.
Pimozide: there is an increased risk of arrhythmias and pimozide should not be taken with mefloquine.

Proprietary preparation: Lariam.

Megace (Bristol-Myers Squibb) *See* MEGESTROL ACETATE.

megestrol acetate A synthetic *progestogen used to treat *cancer of the endometrium (lining of the womb) and (more rarely) breast cancer and a type of kidney cancer. It is available as tablets on *prescription only.
Side effects and precautions: *see* MEDROXYPROGESTERONE.
Interactions with other drugs: *see* PROGESTOGENS.
Proprietary preparation: Megace.

melatonin A naturally occurring hormone produced by the pineal gland and structurally related to *serotonin. Melatonin is associated with the control of circadian (daily) rhythms and an increased propensity for sleep. It is used as a *hypnotic drug for the short-term treatment of insomnia characterized by poor quality of sleep in people who are aged 55 or over. Melatonin is available as tablets on *prescription only.
Side effects: include pharyngitis, back pain, headache, and weakness.
Precautions: melatonin is not recommended for people with impaired liver function or autoimmune disease or for pregnant or breastfeeding women. It should be used with caution in people with kidney disease. Melatonin may cause drowsiness and therefore should be used with caution if the effects of

drowsiness are likely to be associated with a risk to safety. Alcohol should not be taken during treatment, as it reduces the effectiveness of melatonin in inducing sleep.
Interactions with other drugs:
Carbamazepine: may reduce the efficacy of melatonin.
Fluvoxamine: may increase the plasma concentration of melatonin.
Quinolones: may increase the plasma concentration of melatonin.
Rifampicin: may reduce the efficacy of melatonin.
Proprietary preparation: Circadin.

meloxicam An *NSAID used for the short-term treatment of acute osteoarthritis and for the long-term treatment of rheumatoid arthritis and ankylosing spondylitis (a type of arthritis of the spine). It is available as tablets or suppositories on *prescription only.
Side effects and interactions with other drugs: *see* NSAIDs.
Precautions: *see* NSAIDs. The suppositories should not be used in people with haemorrhoids.
Proprietary preparation: Mobic.

melphalan An *alkylating drug used for the treatment of myeloma (cancer of the plasma cells of the bone marrow), solid tumours (ovarian and breast cancer), and polycythaemia vera (in which the number of red cells in the blood is greatly increased). It is available, on *prescription only, as a solution for injection or infusion or as tablets.
Side effects: these are rare, but *bone marrow suppression can occur. *See also* CYTOTOXIC DRUGS.
Precautions: *see* CYTOTOXIC DRUGS.
Interactions with other drugs:
Ciclosporin: the risk of this drug having adverse effects on the kidneys is increased.
Clozapine: there is a risk of agranulocytosis (a blood disorder) and this drug should not be taken with melphalan.
Proprietary preparation: Alkeran.

Meltus Decongestant (SSL International) *See* PSEUDOEPHEDRINE.

Meltus Dry Cough (SSL International) A proprietary combination of *dextromethorphan (a cough suppressant) and *pseudoephedrine (a decongestant), used for the relief of dry coughs and congestion associated with colds. It is available as a liquid without a prescription, but only from pharmacies. It cannot be prescribed on the NHS.
Side effects, precautions, and interactions with other drugs: *see* DEXTROMETHORPHAN; OPIOIDS; EPHEDRINE HYDROCHLORIDE; DECONGESTANTS.

memantine A drug used to treat moderate to severe Alzheimer's disease. It acts by blocking the release of glutamate, a neurotransmitter that is produced in increased amounts in the disease and causes further damage to the brain. Memantine is available as tablets or oral drops on *prescription only.

Side effects: include sleepiness, dizziness, hypertension, headache, and constipation.
Precautions: memantine should not be taken by breastfeeding women. It should be used with caution in people with a history of epilepsy or a predisposition to convulsions.
Interactions with other drugs:
Amantadine: should not be taken with memantine.
Dextromethorphan: should not be taken with memantine.
Proprietary preparation: Ebixa.

menadiol sodium phosphate A synthetic form of *vitamin K that is given to correct vitamin K deficiency and to reverse the effects of *warfarin sodium if too large a dose has been used. It is available as tablets that can be obtained without a prescription, but only from pharmacies.
Precautions: menadiol should not be taken by newborn babies and infants or by women in the late stages of pregnancy. This vitamin should be used with caution by people with glucose-6-phosphate dehydrogenase (G6PD) deficiency and vitamin E deficiency.
Interactions with other drugs:
Oral anticoagulants: their effects may be reduced by menadiol sodium phosphate.

Menopur (Ferring Pharmaceuticals) *See* HUMAN MENOPAUSAL GONADOTROPHIN.

m

menotrophin *See* HUMAN MENOPAUSAL GONADOTROPHIN.

menthol (**levomenthol**) An aromatic substance with a minty taste, extracted from peppermint oil. It is commonly used, with or without *eucalyptus oil, *camphor, and *turpentine oil, in vapour inhalations, vapour rubs, and cough remedies to relieve nasal or catarrhal congestion associated with colds, influenza, rhinitis, or sinusitis and it is also included, together with more active ingredients, in many other proprietary cough medicines. Menthol is used as a counterirritant (*see* RUBEFACIENTS) in preparations that are rubbed into the skin to relieve muscle or joint pain, and is included in oral preparations to treat gallstones or kidney stones.
Proprietary preparations: Deep Freeze Cold Gel; Happinose Nasal Decongestant Balm; Hill's Balsam Nasal Congestion Pastilles; Vicks Cough Syrup with Honey for Dry and Irritating Coughs; *Boots Dual Action Cold Sore Lotion (combined with dichlorobenzyl alcohol, benzyl alcohol, and camphor); *Boots Mild Vapour Rub 3 Months Plus (combined with eucalyptus oil and camphor); *Non-Drowsy Sudafed Inhalant Oil (combined with camphor, eucalyptus oil, and peppermint oil); *Vicks Inhaler (combined with camphor); *Vicks Vaporub (combined with turpentine oil, camphor, and eucalyptus oil); plus many other proprietary medicines (see individual entries).

Mepradec (Discovery Pharmaceuticals) *See* OMEPRAZOLE.

meprobamate An *anxiolytic drug used for the short-term treatment of anxiety. It is not recommended, since it is less effective than the *benzodiazepines, has a higher incidence of side effects, and is more dangerous in overdosage. Combined with analgesics, it is used for the treatment of muscle pain. Meprobamate is available as tablets; it is a *controlled drug.
Side effects: include drowsiness (the most common effect), light-headedness, confusion, shaky movements, unsteadiness, amnesia, paradoxical overexcitedness, headache, blurred vision, nausea, vomiting, diarrhoea, low blood pressure, 'pins and needles', and weakness. *Dependence can develop.
Precautions: meprobamate should not be taken by people with respiratory depression or severe breathing problems, or by women who are breastfeeding; it is not recommended for children. Meprobamate should be used with caution in pregnant women, elderly or debilitated people, and in people with lung disease, muscle weakness, epilepsy, liver or kidney disease, a history of drug or alcohol abuse, or a marked personality disorder. Drowsiness can affect driving and the performance of other skilled tasks and is increased by alcohol. Treatment should be stopped gradually; sudden withdrawal can lead to convulsions.
Interactions with other drugs: the sedative effect of meprobamate is increased by a number of drugs, including anaesthetics, opioid analgesics, antidepressants, antihistamines, and antipsychotic drugs.

meptazinol An *opioid analgesic used for the treatment of moderate to severe pain, including postoperative pain and pain in childbirth. It is available as tablets or an injection on *prescription only.
Side effects and precautions: *see* MORPHINE.
Interactions with other drugs: *see* OPIOIDS.
Proprietary preparation: Meptid.

Meptid (Almirall) *See* MEPTAZINOL.

mepyramine An *antihistamine that is used topically to relieve the irritation and itching caused by insect bites or stings and allergic skin conditions, such as urticaria (nettle rash). It is available in the form of creams and sprays that can be obtained from pharmacies without a prescription.
Side effects: mepyramine may occasionally cause allergic reactions.
Precautions: preparations containing mepyramine should not be used for longer than three days and should not be applied to broken skin.
Proprietary preparations: Anthisan (cream); Boots Bite and Sting Antihistamine Cream; *Wasp-Eze Spray (combined with benzocaine).

Merbentyl, Merbentyl 20 (sanofi-aventis) *See* DICYCLOVERINE HYDROCHLORIDE.

mercaptopurine An *antimetabolite used to prevent the recurrence of the acute leukaemias and to treat chronic myeloid leukaemia (*see* CANCER). It is available as tablets on *prescription only.

Side effects: include *bone marrow suppression, loss of appetite, nausea and vomiting, and liver damage. *See also* CYTOTOXIC DRUGS.
Precautions: mercaptopurine should not be taken by breastfeeding or pregnant women or by people with severe kidney or liver disease. *See also* CYTOTOXIC DRUGS.
Interactions with other drugs:
Allopurinol: the dosage of mercaptopurine should be reduced if it is taken with allopurinol since this drug increases the adverse effects of mercaptopurine.
Clozapine: there is an increased risk of agranulocytosis (a blood disorder), and therefore this drug should not be taken with mercaptopurine.
Co-trimoxazole: increases the risk of blood disorders.
Proprietary preparation: Puri-Nethol.

Mercilon (Organon Laboratories) A proprietary combination of *ethinylestradiol and *desogestrel used as an *oral contraceptive. It is available as tablets on *prescription only.
Side effects and interactions with other drugs: *see* ORAL CONTRACEPTIVES.
Precautions: Mercilon should not be used by women who are at risk of developing thromboembolism, for example because they are very overweight or have varicose veins or a personal or family history of thrombosis. It should therefore only be taken by women who cannot tolerate other brands and who are prepared to accept the increased risk. *See also* ORAL CONTRACEPTIVES.

Merional (Pharmasure) *See* HUMAN MENOPAUSAL GONADOTROPHIN.

Merocaine (sanofi-aventis) A proprietary combination of *benzocaine (a local anaesthetic) and *cetylpyridinium chloride (an antiseptic), used for the treatment of mouth and throat infections and as an *adjunct for tonsillitis, pharyngitis, and dental procedures. It is available as lozenges and can be obtained without a prescription, but only from pharmacies.
Precautions: Merocaine is not recommended for children under 12 years old.

Merocet, Merocets (sanofi-aventis) *See* CETYLPYRIDINIUM CHLORIDE.

Meronem (AstraZeneca) *See* MEROPENEM.

meropenem A beta-lactam antibiotic, similar to *penicillins, that is used for the treatment of pneumonia, urinary-tract, intra-abdominal, and skin and soft-tissue infections, septicaemia, and fevers associated with a low white blood cell count. It is also used to treat chronic lower respiratory-tract infections in those with cystic fibrosis. It is available as an injection on *prescription only.
Side effects: include nausea, vomiting, diarrhoea, abdominal pain, blood disorders, headache, 'pins and needles', rash, itching, urticaria (nettle rash), and pain at the injection site.
Precautions: meropenem should not be given to people who are allergic to it and should be used with caution in anyone allergic to other beta-lactam

antibiotics. It should also be used with caution in patients who have liver or kidney disease and in women who are pregnant or breastfeeding.
Proprietary preparation: Meronem.

mesalazine An *aminosalicylate used for the treatment of mild to moderate attacks of ulcerative colitis and to maintain remission in ulcerative colitis and colitis due to Crohn's disease. It is available, on *prescription only, as tablets, *modified-release tablets and granules, suppositories, an enema, or a rectal foam.
Side effects: include nausea, diarrhoea, headache, abdominal pain, blood disorders (see Precautions below), and kidney damage.
Precautions: mesalazine should not be taken by people with severe liver disease or a blood-clotting disorder; any unexplained bleeding, bruising, sore throat, or malaise should be reported immediately to a doctor, as this may indicate a blood disorder. *See* AMINOSALICYLATES.
Proprietary preparations: Asacol; Asacol MR (modified-release tablets); Ipocol; Mezavant XL (modified-release tablets); Pentasa; Salofalk.

mesna A drug that is given in conjunction with *cyclophosphamide or *ifosfamide to prevent the adverse effects of these cytotoxic drugs on the bladder. It is available, on *prescription only, as a solution for injection or as tablets.
Proprietary preparation: Uromitexan.

mesterolone A drug used for the treatment of *androgen deficiency and male infertility. It is available as tablets on *prescription only.
Side effects: include excessive frequency and duration of penile erection, fluid retention and weight gain, and liver disorders.
Precautions and interactions with other drugs: *see* TESTOSTERONE.
Proprietary preparation: Pro-Viron.

Mestinon (Valeant) *See* PYRIDOSTIGMINE.

mestranol A synthetic *oestrogen that is used in combination with *norethisterone (a progestogen) in *oral contraceptives. It is available as tablets on *prescription only.
Side effects, precautions, and interactions with other drugs: *see* OESTROGENS; ORAL CONTRACEPTIVES.
Proprietary preparation: *Norinyl-1.

Metalyse (Boehringer Ingelheim) *See* TENECTEPLASE.

Metanium (Ransom) A proprietary combination of *titanium dioxide, titanium peroxide, and titanium salicylate in a cream base that includes *dimeticone, light *liquid paraffin, and *white soft paraffin. It is used as a *barrier preparation for the prevention and treatment of napkin rash and is freely available *over the counter in the form of an ointment.

metaraminol A *sympathomimetic drug that causes blood vessels to constrict and therefore raises blood pressure. It is used to restore or maintain

blood pressure in patients undergoing surgery, especially those who have low blood pressure due to spinal anaesthesia. It is available as a solution for intravenous injection or infusion on *prescription only.
Side effects, precautions, and interactions with other drugs: *see* NORADRENALINE.

metastases *See* CANCER.

Meted (Alliance) A proprietary combination of *sulphur and *salicylic acid (both keratolytics), used for the treatment of scaly disorders of the scalp, such as seborrhoeic *eczema, *psoriasis, and dandruff. It is available as a shampoo and can be obtained without a prescription, but only from pharmacies.
Side effects: Meted may cause local irritation.

Metenix 5 (sanofi-aventis) *See* METOLAZONE.

metered-dose inhaler *See* INHALER.

metformin hydrochloride An *oral hypoglycaemic drug that lowers blood-glucose concentrations by increasing the uptake of glucose into the body's tissues and reducing its release from the liver. It belongs to a group of drugs called **biguanides** and is the only drug of this group that is currently available. Metformin is used for the treatment of type II (noninsulin-dependent) *diabetes mellitus and is of particular value in obese people. It is available as tablets, *modified-release tablets, and an oral solution on *prescription only.
Side effects: include loss of appetite, nausea, vomiting, and diarrhoea (usually transient). Uptake of vitamin B_{12} is reduced, and prolonged treatment may cause anaemia. Occasionally metformin causes lactic acidosis (resulting in coma); this risk is increased in people with kidney or liver disease and in certain other vulnerable groups, in whom metformin should be avoided (see below).
Precautions: metformin should not be taken by people with liver or kidney disease, heart failure, or severe infections, after surgery or injury, by those who are dehydrated, or by those who have recently had a heart attack. Alcohol should be avoided, as it increases the risk of *hypoglycaemia and may cause lactic acidosis.
Interactions with other drugs:
Cimetidine: increases the plasma concentration of metformin and therefore the risk of hypoglycaemia (low blood-glucose levels).
Proprietary preparations: Bolamyn SR (modified-release tablets); Glucophage; Glucophage SR (modified-release tablets); *Avandamet (combined with rosiglitazone); *Competact (combined with pioglitazone); *Eucreas (combined with vildagliptin).

methadone hydrochloride An *opioid analgesic used in the treatment of people who are physically dependent on diamorphine (heroin) or other opioids, in whom it prevents the occurrence of withdrawal symptoms (*see* DEPENDENCE). It is also sometimes used to treat severe pain in people who

cannot tolerate morphine and occasionally to control coughing in terminally ill patients. Methadone is a *controlled drug; it is available as tablets, an oral solution, or an injection.
Side effects and precautions: *see* MORPHINE.
Interactions with other drugs:

Amisulpride: increases the risk of ventricular *arrhythmias and should not be taken with methadone.
Atomoxetine: increases the risk of ventricular arrhythmias.
Carbamazepine: reduces the effects of methadone.
Phenytoin: reduces the effects of methadone and may cause withdrawal symptoms.
Sodium oxybate: its effects are enhanced and it should not be used with methadone.
Zidovudine: its plasma concentration may be increased by methadone.
See also OPIOIDS.

Proprietary preparations: Methadose; Metharose; Physeptone.

Methadose (Rosemont Pharmaceuticals) *See* METHADONE HYDROCHLORIDE.

Metharose (Rosemont Pharmaceuticals) *See* METHADONE HYDROCHLORIDE.

methenamine hippurate <**hexamine hippurate**> An *antiseptic used for the treatment of recurrent infections of the urinary tract; it acts by being transformed to *formaldehyde. It is available as tablets without a *prescription, but only from pharmacies.
Side effects: include gastrointestinal disturbances, bladder irritation, and rash.
Precautions: hexamine should not be taken by people who are severely dehydrated or by those with severe kidney disease.
Proprietary preparation: Hiprex.

methionine An amino acid used for the treatment of paracetamol overdose when *acetylcysteine is not available or not tolerated. It is available as tablets on *prescription only.
Side effects: include nausea, vomiting, drowsiness, and irritability.
Precautions: methionine should be used with caution in people with liver disease.
Proprietary preparation: *Paradote (combined with paracetamol).

methocarbamol A *muscle relaxant that is used for the short-term relief of muscle spasms. It is available as tablets on *prescription only.
Side effects: include lassitude, light-headedness, drowsiness, dizziness, restlessness, anxiety, confusion, nausea, and an allergic rash.
Precautions: methocarbamol should not be given to anyone who is in a coma or who has brain damage, epilepsy, or myasthenia gravis. It should be used with caution in people with impaired liver or kidney function and in women who are pregnant or breastfeeding. Drowsiness may affect driving or the ability to operate machinery, and methocarbamol can enhance the sedative effects of alcohol.
Proprietary preparation: Robaxin.

methotrexate An *antimetabolite that is used for the treatment of acute lymphoblastic leukaemia in children and adults and of choriocarcinoma (a form of cancer occurring in the uterus during or after pregnancy), non-Hodgkin's lymphoma, and a number of solid tumours in adults (*see* CANCER). Methotrexate is also used as an *immunosuppressant to treat severe *psoriasis and rheumatoid arthritis that have not responded to other treatments. It may be taken orally, injected into a vein, an artery, a muscle, or around the spinal cord, or infused into a vein, and *folinic acid is often given afterwards to prevent side effects. It is available as tablets or solutions for injection on *prescription only.
Side effects: include *bone marrow suppression, inflammation and ulceration of the mucous membranes, especially the mouth, and rarely inflammation of the lungs. It can also cause liver damage. *See* CYTOTOXIC DRUGS.
Precautions: methotrexate should not be given to people with severe kidney or liver disease or to pregnant women. *See also* CYTOTOXIC DRUGS.
Interactions with other drugs:

Acitretin: increases the plasma concentrations of methotrexate and the risk of adverse effects on the liver; it should not be used with methotrexate.
Aspirin: increases the risk of adverse effects of methotrexate.
Ciclosporin: the adverse effects of both methotrexate and ciclosporin are increased.
Cisplatin: increases the risk of adverse effects on the lungs.
Clozapine: there is an increased risk of agranulocytosis (a blood disorder), and therefore this drug should not be given with methotrexate.
Corticosteroids: increase the risk of adverse effects on the blood.
Co-trimoxazole: increases the risk of adverse effects on the blood.
Leflunomide: increases the risk of adverse effects of methotrexate.
NSAIDs: increase the risk of adverse effects of methotrexate; azapropazone should not be taken with methotrexate.
Probenecid: increases the risk of adverse effects of methotrexate.
Pyrimethamine: increases the risk of adverse effects of methotrexate.

Proprietary preparations: Maxtrex (tablets); Metoject (injection).

methotrimeprazine *See* LEVOMEPROMAZINE.

methyl aminolevulinate A drug that makes the skin more sensitive to light. It is used for the treatment of actinic keratoses on the face or scalp (scaly red spots due to overexposure to sunlight) and, less commonly, for types of skin cancer not considered suitable for surgery. The drug is applied as a cream to the skin, which is then illuminated by red light. This causes activation of the compound leading to death of the affected cells. Methyl aminolevulinate is available on *prescription only.
Side effects: the most common side effects are pain, a burning sensation, and reddening of the skin, with the formation of scars.
Precautions: methyl aminolevulinate should not be used in people with porphyria and is not recommended for women who are pregnant or

breastfeeding. Exposure to sunlight should be avoided for two days after treatment.
Proprietary preparation: Metvix.

methylcellulose A synthetic *bulk-forming laxative used for treating constipation and for managing chronic diarrhoea in bowel disease. It is also used in the treatment of *obesity to reduce food intake, since its bulk-forming properties are supposed to induce feelings of fullness. Methylcellulose is freely available *over the counter in the form of tablets.
Side effects and precautions: *see* ISPAGHULA HUSK.
Proprietary preparation: Celevac.

methylcysteine hydrochloride A *mucolytic drug that reduces the viscosity of bronchial secretions by liquefying mucus. It is used to relieve congestion of the airways, for example in bronchitis. Methylcysteine is available as tablets without a prescription, but only from pharmacies. It cannot be prescribed on the NHS.
Side effects: stomach and bowel upsets may occur.
Proprietary preparation: Visclair.

methyldopa An alpha stimulant (*see* SYMPATHOMIMETIC DRUGS) that acts centrally (on receptors in the brain). It is used in the treatment of all grades of *hypertension, including hypertension during pregnancy. It is available as tablets on *prescription only.
Side effects: include sedation, headache, depression, nasal congestion, dry mouth, and gastrointestinal upsets; rarely it can cause anaemia.
Precautions: methyldopa should not be taken by people with depression or liver disease. Blood counts and liver function should be monitored before and during treatment.
Interactions with other drugs:
MAOIs: these drugs should not be used with methyldopa.
Proprietary preparation: Aldomet.
See also ANTIHYPERTENSIVE DRUGS.

methylnaltrexone bromide A drug that opposes the action of *opioids, used as an *adjunct for the treatment of constipation induced by opioid analgesics in people with terminal illness when response to standard laxatives has failed. It is given by subcutaneous injection and is available on *prescription only.
Side effects: include nausea, abdominal pain, diarrhoea, and flatulence.
Precautions: methylnaltrexone should not be given to people with an obstructed intestine or severe liver disease. It should be used with caution in people with impacted faeces, a colostomy, or kidney disease and in women who are pregnant or breastfeeding.
Proprietary preparation: Relistor.

methyl nicotinate A drug that is used as a *rubefacient for the relief of aches and pains in muscles, tendons, and joints. It is an ingredient of creams, ointments, and sprays most of which are freely available *over the counter.

Side effects and precautions: *see* RUBEFACIENTS.
Proprietary preparations: *Deep Heat Spray (combined with ethyl salicylate, methyl salicylate, and glycol salicylate); *Dubam Spray (combined with ethyl salicylate, methyl salicylate, and glycol salicylate); *Fiery Jack Cream (combined with capsicum oleoresin, diethylamine salicylate, and glycol salicylate); *Ralgex Cream (combined with capsicum oleoresin and glycol monosalicylate); *Ralgex Heat Spray (combined with glycol salicylate); *Transvasin Heat Spray (combined with diethylamine salicylate and 2-hydroxyethyl salicylate).

methylphenidate hydrochloride A *stimulant of the central nervous system, similar to *dexamfetamine sulphate, that is used for the treatment of attention deficit hyperactivity disorder in children under specialist supervision. A *controlled drug, it is available as tablets and *modified-release tablets or capsules.
Side effects: *see* DEXAMFETAMINE SULPHATE. In addition, rashes, urticaria, fever, muscle aches, hair loss, and dermatitis can occur.
Precautions: *see* DEXAMFETAMINE SULPHATE. In addition, methylphenidate should not be taken by people with anxiety, severe depression, or suicidal thoughts.
Interactions with other drugs:
Anaesthetics: there is an increased risk of high blood pressure if inhaled general anaesthetics are given with methylphenidate.
Antidepressants: there is a risk of a dangerous rise in blood pressure if MAOIs or moclobemide are given with methylphenidate.
Clonidine: may cause serious adverse effects.
Guanethidine: its effect in lowering blood pressure is reduced.
Warfarin: its anticoagulant effect may be enhanced.
Proprietary preparations: Concerta XL (modified-release tablets); Equasym; Equasym XL (prolonged release tablets); Ritalin (tablets); Medikinet XL (modified-release capsules).

methylprednisolone A *corticosteroid used for treatment of inflammatory disorders (including rheumatic and bowel disease), and cerebral oedema (swelling of the brain). It is available, on *prescription only, as tablets or a solution for injection.
Side effects, precautions, and interactions with other drugs: *see* CORTICOSTEROIDS.
Proprietary preparations: Depo-Medrone (*depot injection into a muscle or a joint); Medrone (tablets); Solu-Medrone (injection); *Depo-Medrone with Lidocaine (combined with lidocaine hydrochloride).

methyl salicylate A *salicylate that is an ingredient of many *rubefacient creams and sprays for the relief of aches, pains, and stiffness in muscles, tendons, and joints. It is also used in preparations for treating fungal skin infections, relieving congestion due to colds and catarrh, and soothing *haemorrhoids. Preparations containing methyl salicylate are available without a prescription, but some can only be obtained from pharmacies.

Side effects and precautions: *see* SALICYLATES.
Proprietary preparations: *Balmosa (combined with camphor, capsicum oleoresin, and menthol); *Boots Pain Relief Warming Spray (combined with camphor and ethyl nicotinate); *Deep Heat Massage Liniment (combined with menthol); *Deep Heat Rub (combined with eucalyptus oil, menthol, and turpentine oil); *Deep Heat Spray (combined with ethyl salicylate, glycol salicylate, and methyl nicotinate); *Dubam Cream (combined with menthol and cineole); *Dubam Spray (combined with ethyl salicylate, glycol salicylate, and methyl nicotinate); *Germolene Antiseptic Ointment (combined with zinc oxide, octafonium chloride, and phenol); *Olbas Oil (combined with eucalyptus oil, menthol, cajuput oil, clove oil, and juniper berry oil); *Olbas Pastilles (combined with eucalyptus oil, menthol, peppermint oil, clove oil, and juniper berry oil); *Phytex (combined with borotannic acid complex, salicylic acid, and acetic acid); *PR Heat Spray (combined with ethyl nicotinate and camphor).

methysergide A drug that antagonizes the action of the neurotransmitter *serotonin (5-hydroxytryptamine). It is used for preventing attacks in severe recurrent *migraine and other headaches with vascular causes that do not respond to standard treatments. In much higher doses it is used to treat diarrhoea associated with carcinoid syndrome (caused by a tumour that secretes serotonin). Methysergide is available as tablets on *prescription only; patients taking it should be closely monitored in hospitals because of the severity of its side effects.
Side effects: nausea, vomiting, abdominal discomfort, drowsiness, and dizziness often occur at the start of treatment; other side effects include mental and behavioural disturbances, insomnia, fluid retention and weight gain, vasospasm (constriction of the arteries), and – after prolonged treatment – abnormal development of fibrous tissue within the abdomen and elsewhere.
Precautions: methysergide should not be given to people with high blood pressure or heart, lung, liver, or kidney disease, or to women who are pregnant or breastfeeding. It should be used with caution in patients with a history of peptic ulceration.
Interactions with other drugs:

Antibiotics: macrolides and telithromycin increase the risk of toxic effects and should not be given with methysergide.

Antifungal drugs: imidazoles and triazoles increase the risk of toxic effects and should not be given with methysergide.

Antiviral drugs: efavirenz and most protease inhibitors should not be taken with methysergide as they increase the risk of toxic effects.

Cimetidine: increases the risk of toxic effects and should not be given with methysergide.

5HT$_1$ agonists: increase the risk of vasospasm; methysergide should not be started for 6 hours after stopping almotriptan, rizatriptan, sumatriptan, or zolmitriptan, and these drugs should not be started for 24 hours after stopping methysergide; methysergide should not be started for 24 hours after stopping eletriptan or frovatriptan, and these drugs should not be started for 24 hours after stopping methysergide.

Proprietary preparation: Deseril.

metipranolol A *beta blocker used in the form of eye drops for treating chronic (open-angle) *glaucoma in people who are allergic to the preservatives (such as benzalkonium chloride) that are included in similar preparations and people who wear soft contact lenses (who should not use eye drops containing benzalkonium chloride). Metipranolol is available on *prescription only.

Side effects, precautions, and interactions with other drugs: *see* BETA BLOCKERS.

Proprietary preparation: Minims Metipranolol.

metoclopramide A drug that antagonizes the action of *dopamine. It is an *antiemetic used to prevent or treat nausea and vomiting, including that produced by radiotherapy or cytotoxic chemotherapy for cancer, when it is usually given together with other drugs. It is also included in some preparations for the treatment of *migraine, to alleviate the nausea and vomiting that can accompany migraine headaches and to hasten the absorption of analgesic drugs. It is not effective for motion sickness. Metoclopramide also stimulates gastric motility (*see* PROKINETIC DRUGS) and is used for the treatment of various gastrointestinal disorders, including indigestion (apart from that caused by peptic ulceration) and gastro-oesophageal reflux (*see* ACID-PEPTIC DISEASES). It is available, on *prescription only, as tablets, *modified-release capsules, an oral solution, or a solution for intramuscular or intravenous injection.

Side effects: metoclopramide can cause abnormal facial and body movements, such as twisting of the neck (*see* EXTRAPYRAMIDAL REACTIONS); these effects are more common in children and young adults (under 20 years old). Other side effects include raised serum prolactin, which causes breast enlargement and milk production.

Precautions: in people under 20 years old, metoclopramide should only be used for treating vomiting caused by radiotherapy or chemotherapy, severe vomiting of known cause that is resistant to other drugs, or to facilitate the insertion of a nasogastric tube (through the nose to the stomach). It should not be used for 3–4 days after gastrointestinal surgery and should not be taken during breastfeeding. It should be used with caution in people with impaired liver or kidney function, women who are pregnant, and the elderly.

Interactions with other drugs:

Analgesics: the effects of aspirin and paracetamol are enhanced by metoclopramide.

Antipsychotics: the risk of extrapyramidal reactions is increased.

Ciclosporin: its plasma concentration is increased.

Tetrabenazine: the risk of extrapyramidal reactions is increased.

Proprietary preparations: Maxolon; Maxolon High Dose; Maxolon SR (modified-release capsules); MigraMax (combined with aspirin); *Paramax (combined with paracetamol).

Metoject (medac GmbH) *See* METHOTREXATE.

metolazone A thiazide-like diuretic (*see* THIAZIDE DIURETICS) used for the treatment of *hypertension and *oedema. It is available as tablets on *prescription only.
Side effects, precautions, and interactions with other drugs: *see* THIAZIDE DIURETICS.
Proprietary preparation: Metenix 5.
See also ANTIHYPERTENSIVE DRUGS; DIURETICS.

Metopirone (Alliance) *See* METYRAPONE.

metoprolol tartrate A cardioselective *beta blocker used for the treatment and prevention of heart *arrhythmias and migraine and the treatment of *hypertension, *heart failure, and *angina. It is also given after a heart attack to prevent worsening of the condition. It is available as tablets, *modified-release tablets, or an injection on *prescription only.
Side effects and precautions: *see* BETA BLOCKERS.
Interactions with other drugs:
Antidepressants: citalopram, escitalopram, and paroxetine may increase the effect of metoprolol in lowering blood pressure.
Propafenone: increases the plasma concentration of metoprolol.
For other interactions, *see* BETA BLOCKERS.
Proprietary preparations: Betaloc; Lopresor; Lopresor SR (modified-release tablets).
See also ANTI-ARRHYTHMIC DRUGS; ANTIHYPERTENSIVE DRUGS.

Metosyn (GP Pharma) *See* FLUOCINONIDE.

Metrogel (Galderma) *See* METRONIDAZOLE.

Metrolyl (Sandoz) *See* METRONIDAZOLE.

metronidazole An *antibiotic with activity against certain types of bacteria and protozoa. It is used to treat trichomonal vaginitis (a sexually transmitted protozoal infection of the vagina) and bacterial vaginitis. It is also active against *Entamoeba histolytica*, the cause of amoebic dysentry and ulcers of the gut wall, and *Giardia*, which causes diarrhoea. The drug is also used to treat or prevent surgical and gynaecological infections and to treat dental and gum infections (including gingivitis). Metronidazole is effective in the treatment of pseudomembranous colitis, an infection of the large bowel caused by overgrowth of the microbes normally occurring in the gut, which is often caused by the use of broad-spectrum antibiotics. Topical metronidazole is used to prevent the odour associated with infected tumours and to treat rosacea (a chronic inflammatory condition of the face). A *prescription only medicine, it is available as tablets or a suspension for oral use, a solution for *intravenous infusion, and as a gel, cream, or suppositories for topical use.

Side effects: include nausea, vomiting, an unpleasant taste in the mouth, furred tongue, and loss of appetite. Rare side effects are drowsiness, headache, dizziness, rash, and darkening of urine; on prolonged therapy transient epileptic seizures and peripheral neuropathy (causing numbness and tingling of the limbs) may occur. Topical preparations may cause local irritation.
Precautions: alcohol should be avoided during treatment as the combination may lead to vomiting. The drug should be used with caution in women who are pregnant or breastfeeding.
Interactions with other drugs (unlikely with topical preparations):
Anticoagulants: the effects of warfarin and acenocoumarol are enhanced.
Busulfan: its plasma concentrations (and risk of adverse effects) are increased.
Cimetidine: increases plasma concentrations of metronidazole.
Lithium: concentrations of lithium may be increased and cause toxic effects.
Phenytoin: the effects of phenytoin are increased.
Proprietary preparations: Acea (gel); Anabact (gel); Elyzol (gel); Flagyl (tablets and suppositories); Metrogel (gel); Metrolyl (suspension and infusion); Metrosa (gel); Metrotop (gel); Norzol (oral solution); Rosiced (cream); Rozex (cream and gel); Vaginyl (tablets); Zidoval (gel); Zyomet (gel).

Metrosa (Linderma) *See* METRONIDAZOLE.

Metrotop (Medlock) *See* METRONIDAZOLE.

Metvix (Galderma) *See* METHYL AMINOLEVULINATE.

metyrapone A drug that inhibits production by the adrenal glands of the *corticosteroids cortisol and aldosterone (which acts on the kidneys to regulate salt and water balance). It is used to treat Cushing's syndrome or given in combination with glucocorticoids (*see* CORTICOSTEROIDS) to treat resistant *oedema. Metyrapone is available as capsules on *prescription only.
Side effects: include nausea, vomiting, hypotension (low blood pressure), dizziness, and drowsiness.
Precautions: metyrapone should not be taken by people suffering from pituitary disorders or adrenal insufficiency or by women who are pregnant or breastfeeding.
Proprietary preparation: Metopirone.

Mezavant XL (Shire Pharmaceuticals) *See* MESALAZINE.

Mezolar Matrix Transdermal Patches (Sandoz) *See* FENTANYL.

Miacalcic (Novartis) *See* CALCITONIN (SALMON).

mianserin hydrochloride An *antidepressant drug, similar to the *tricyclic antidepressants, used for the treatment of depressive illness, particularly when sedation is required. It is available as tablets on *prescription only.
Side effects: similar to *amitriptyline hydrochloride, but mianserin has fewer

antimuscarinic effects (e.g. dry mouth, difficulty in urinating, blurred vision); it can cause blood disorders and joint pain and arthritis.
Precautions: a full blood count should be taken every four weeks during the first three months of treatment. Treatment should be stopped if signs of infection (e.g. fever, sore throat) develop. *See also* TRICYCLIC ANTIDEPRESSANTS.
Interactions with other drugs: *see* TRICYCLIC ANTIDEPRESSANTS.

micafungin An *antifungal drug used for the treatment of generalized candidiasis and candidiasis of the oesophagus and for the prevention of *Candida* infection in patients undergoing bone marrow transplantation. It is given by intravenous infusion under expert supervision and is available on *prescription only.
Side effects: include nausea, vomiting, abdominal pain, headache, rash, anaemia, low white blood cell counts, and reduced blood concentrations of potassium, magnesium, and calcium.
Precautions: micafungin should not be given to people with severe liver disease. It has been associated with impaired liver function, which should therefore be monitored during treatment. Micafungin may also impair kidney function. It should be avoided in pregnancy and used with caution in breastfeeding women.
Proprietary preparation: Mycamine.

m

Micanol (GP Pharma) *See* DITHRANOL.

Micardis (Boehringer Ingelheim Ltd) *See* TELMISARTAN.

Micardis Plus (Boehringer Ingelheim) A proprietary combination of *telmisartan (an angiotension II inhibitor) and *hydrochlorothiazide (a thiazide diuretic), used for the treatment of *hypertension that has not responded to telmisartan alone. It is available as tablets on *prescription only.
Side effects and precautions: *see* TELMISARTAN; THIAZIDE DIURETICS.
Interactions with other drugs: *see* ACE INHIBITORS; THIAZIDE DIURETICS.

Micolette Micro-enema (Pinewood) A proprietary combination of *sodium citrate (an osmotic laxative), *sodium lauryl sulphoacetate (a wetting agent), and glycerol (*see* GLYCERIN), used for the treatment of constipation. It can be obtained without a prescription, but only from pharmacies.
Precautions: *see* SODIUM CITRATE.

miconazole An imidazole *antifungal drug similar to *ketoconazole. It is used to treat and prevent a wide range of fungal infections, including candidiasis (thrush), especially of the vulva and vagina, tinea (ringworm), and gastrointestinal infections. It may also be used as a solution to wash out the bladder in cases of *Candida* infection. It is available as tablets, vaginal capsules, pessaries, a mouth gel, a cream, a powder, and a spray powder. Tablets, pessaries, and vaginal capsules are available on *prescription only; topical preparations may be bought without a prescription, but only from pharmacies.
Side effects: the tablets may cause nausea, vomiting, and rashes; tablets that

adhere to the gum may cause abdominal pain, altered taste, and itching. Topical preparations may produce skin irritation.
Precautions: miconazole should not be used by people with liver disease and should be used with caution by women who are pregnant or breastfeeding.
Interactions with other drugs:

Anticoagulants: the effects of warfarin and acenocoumarol are enhanced.
Antidiabetic drugs: plasma concentrations of the sulphonylureas are increased; the effect of gliclazide and glipizide in lowering blood pressure is enhanced and they should not be taken with miconazole.
Antipsychotic drugs: pimozide and sertindole should not be taken with miconazole because of the risk of irregular heart rhythms.
Ciclosporin: its plasma concentration may be increased.
Ergot alkaloids: the adverse effects of ergotamine and methysergide may be increased and these drugs should not be taken with miconazole.
Mizolastine: its plasma concentration may be increased and it should not be taken with miconazole.
Phenytoin: its effect is enhanced.
Reboxetine: should not be taken with miconazole.
Simvastatin: should not be taken with miconazole as this combination increases the risk of muscle damage.
Tacrolimus: its plasma concentration may be increased.

Proprietary preparations: Daktarin; Daktarin Oral Gel; Gyno-Daktarin (vaginal cream); Loramyc (tablets that adhere to the gum); *Daktacort (combined with hydrocortisone).

Micralax Micro-enema (UCB Pharma) A proprietary combination of *sodium citrate (an osmotic laxative) and sodium alkylsulphoacetate (a wetting agent) used for the treatment of constipation. It can be obtained without a prescription, but only from pharmacies.
Precautions: *see* SODIUM CITRATE.

Microgynon 30 (Bayer) A proprietary combination of *ethinylestradiol (30 micrograms) and *levonorgestrel used as an *oral contraceptive. **Microgynon 30 ED** contains both active and dummy tablets, so that a tablet is taken each day of a 28-day cycle. Both preparations are available as tablets on *prescription only.
Side effects, precautions, and interactions with other drugs: *see* ORAL CONTRACEPTIVES.

Micronor (Janssen-Cilag) *See* NORETHISTERONE; ORAL CONTRACEPTIVES.

Micropirin (Dexcel Pharma) *See* ASPIRIN.

midazolam A *benzodiazepine that is used to produce sedation in patients about to undergo surgery. It also causes amnesia, so that patients do not remember the preoperative period, and recovery from its effects after surgery is more rapid than with *diazepam. Midazolam is also used to treat status epilepticus (*see* ANTICONVULSANT DRUGS), although it does not have a *licence for this. It is available as an oral liquid or an injection on *prescription only.

Side effects and precautions: high dosages given by intravenous injection may cause profound sedation and depression of breathing. *See also* BENZODIAZEPINES.

Interactions with other drugs:

Antibiotics: clarithromycin, erythromycin, Synercid, and telithromycin inhibit the breakdown of midazolam, increasing its sedative effect.

Antifungal drugs: itraconazole, ketoconazole, fluconazole, and posaconazole inhibit the breakdown of midazolam, causing profound sedation.

Antiviral drugs: atazanavir, efavirenz, ritonavir, indinavir, nelfinavir, and saquinavir increase the risk of profound sedation and should not be used with midazolam; fosamprenavir increases the risk of profound sedation and depression of breathing.

See also BENZODIAZEPINES.

Proprietary preparation: Hypnovel.

Midrid (Manx) A proprietary combination of *paracetamol (an analgesic) and *isometheptene mucate (a vasoconstrictor) in the form of capsules, used for the treatment of *migraine attacks. Packs containing 100 capsules are available on *prescription only, but 15-capsule packs can be obtained from pharmacies without a prescription.

Side effects and precautions: *see* PARACETAMOL; ISOMETHEPTENE MUCATE.

m

Interactions with other drugs: *see* ISOMETHEPTENE MUCATE.

Mifegyne (Exelgyn Laboratories) *See* MIFEPRISTONE.

mifepristone A drug that blocks the action of *progesterone, a hormone that is essential for maintaining a pregnancy. Mifepristone is used to induce abortion up to the 24th week of pregnancy. It is taken by mouth under medical supervision; if the pregnancy is more advanced than 7 weeks *gemeprost or *misoprostol pessaries may need to be given in addition. Mifepristone is also used for softening and dilating the cervix (neck of the uterus) before mechanical termination of pregnancy. It is available as tablets on *prescription only.

Side effects: include stomach cramps, contractions of the uterus, malaise, and vaginal bleeding (sometimes severe); less common side effects are faintness, headache, nausea, vomiting, and rashes.

Precautions: mifepristone should not be used if an ectopic pregnancy is suspected or in women with chronic adrenal failure, severe asthma, or liver or kidney disease, or during breastfeeding.

Proprietary preparation: Mifegyne.

Migard (Menarini) *See* FROVATRIPTAN.

miglustat A drug used for the treatment of Gaucher's disease when *imiglucerase cannot be used and of Niemann-Pick disease, in which lipids accumulate in the bone marrow, brain, liver, and spleen. It works by inhibiting an enzyme involved in the synthesis of lipids. Miglustat is available as capsules on *prescription only.

Side effects: include diarrhoea, abdominal pain, nausea and vomiting, weight changes, dizziness, headache, 'pins and needles', and fatigue.
Precautions: miglustat should not be taken by women who are pregnant or breastfeeding, and men who are taking it should not father a child during or for three months after treatment. It should not be taken by people with severe kidney disease.
Proprietary preparation: Zavesca.

migraine A recurrent headache that is usually throbbing and typically affects one side of the head. Some attacks are preceded by a warning (**aura**) consisting of visual disturbances and numbness and/or weakness of the limbs. The headache is often accompanied by nausea and vomiting. Migraine may be precipitated or exacerbated by certain foods (such as cheese or chocolate), red wine, or stress. It is thought to be caused by changes in the blood vessels around the brain and eyes and in the scalp, which constrict and then become overdilated.

A variety of drugs is available for the treatment of migraine attacks. Analgesics, for pain relief, usually contain *aspirin, *paracetamol, and/or *codeine; if these are ineffective, *tolfenamic acid (an NSAID) may be tried. For people who fail to respond to these analgesics, *$5HT_1$ agonists, such as *sumatriptan or *zolmitriptan, are the recommended treatment for an acute attack. They act by reversing the overdilatation of the blood vessels in the brain. *Ergotamine tartrate also constricts blood vessels, but it is less selective in this action than the $5HT_1$ agonists and has more severe side effects. Antiemetics, such as *metoclopramide, *cyclizine, or *buclizine hydrochloride, may be required to relieve the nausea and vomiting associated with a migraine headache. These may be used alone or combined with an analgesic. *See also* ISOMETHEPTENE MUCATE.

For people who experience frequent migraine attacks (more than one a month), a preventive approach is needed. The drugs used for this purpose include *beta blockers (such as *propranolol, *metoprolol, *nadolol, and *timolol), the antihistamines *pizotifen and *cyproheptadine (which antagonize the effects of *serotonin), and *topiramate. Since long-term treatment with these drugs is not advisable, the patient's condition should be assessed at six-monthly intervals to see if treatment needs to be continued. Some individuals benefit from the herbal remedy feverfew. *See also* METHYSERGIDE.

Migraine Relief (Boots) A proprietary combination of *paracetamol (a non-opioid analgesic) and *codeine phosphate (an opioid analgesic), used for the relief of *migraine and other forms of mild to moderate pain. It is available as capsules without a prescription, but only from Boots pharmacies.
Side effects and precautions: *see* PARACETAMOL; CODEINE.
Interactions with other drugs: *see* OPIOIDS.

Migraleve (McNeil Ltd) A proprietary preparation consisting of a combination of the analgesics *paracetamol and *codeine phosphate and the antiemetic antihistamine *buclizine hydrochloride in the form of **pink**

tablets, packaged with a combination of paracetamol and codeine phosphate (**yellow tablets**), used for the treatment of *migraine. Two pink tablets taken at the start of a migraine attack are followed by two yellow tablets at four-hourly intervals. Migraleve can be obtained without a prescription, but only from pharmacies.
Side effects: Migraleve causes drowsiness.
Precautions: Migraleve should not be taken by children under 10 years old, except under medical supervision. *See also* PARACETAMOL; ANTIHISTAMINES.
Interactions with other drugs: *see* ANTIHISTAMINES; OPIOIDS.

MigraMax (Cephalon) A proprietary combination of lysine acetylsalicylate (which is metabolized to *aspirin) and *metoclopramide (an antiemetic), used for the treatment of headache, nausea, and vomiting associated with migraine. It is available, on *prescription only, as an oral powder to be dissolved in water.
Side effects, precautions, and interactions with other drugs: *see* ASPIRIN; METOCLOPRAMIDE.

Migril (Wockhardt UK) A proprietary combination of *ergotamine tartrate, *cyclizine hydrochloride (an antiemetic antihistamine), and *caffeine hydrate, used for the treatment of *migraine. It is available as tablets on prescription only.
Side effects and precautions: *see* ERGOTAMINE TARTRATE; CYCLIZINE; ANTIHISTAMINES; CAFFEINE.
Interactions with other drugs: *see* ERGOTAMINE TARTRATE; ANTIHISTAMINES.

Mildison Lipocream (Astellas Pharma) *See* HYDROCORTISONE.

Milpar (Merck Consumer Health) A proprietary combination of *liquid paraffin (a faecal softener) and *magnesium hydroxide (an osmotic laxative), used for the treatment of constipation. It is available as a liquid and can be obtained without a prescription, but only from phamacies.
Side effects and precautions: *see* LIQUID PARAFFIN; MAGNESIUM SALTS.
Interactions with other drugs: *see* ANTACIDS.

milrinone A drug, similar to *enoximone, that acts on the heart muscles to strengthen the heartbeat. It is used for the short-term treatment of severe congestive *heart failure, especially in people who have not responded to standard therapy, and acute heart failure occurring after heart surgery. Milrinone is available as an injection on *prescription only.
Side effects, precautions, and interactions with other drugs: *see* ENOXIMONE.
Proprietary preparation: Primacor.

Mimpara (Amgen) *See* CINACALCET.

mineralocorticoids *See* CORTICOSTEROIDS.

Minijet Adrenaline (UCB Pharma) *See* ADRENALINE.

Minijet Aminophylline (UCB Pharma) *See* AMINOPHYLLINE.

Minijet Atropine (UCB Pharma) *See* ATROPINE SULPHATE.

Minijet Calcium Chloride (UCB Pharma) *See* CALCIUM CHLORIDE.

Minijet Naloxone (UCB Pharma) *See* NALOXONE HYDROCHLORIDE.

Minijet Sodium Bicarbonate (UCB Pharma) *See* SODIUM BICARBONATE.

Minims Artificial Tears (Bausch & Lomb UK) A proprietary combination of *sodium chloride and *hydroxyethylcellulose, used as a lubricant for dry eyes. It is available as single-dose eye drops and can be obtained without a prescription, but only from pharmacies.

Minims Atropine Sulphate (Bausch & Lomb UK) *See* ATROPINE SULPHATE.

Minims Chloramphenicol (Bausch & Lomb UK) *See* CHLORAMPHENICOL.

Minims Cyclopentolate (Bausch & Lomb UK) *See* CYCLOPENTOLATE HYDROCHLORIDE.

Minims Dexamethasone (Bausch & Lomb UK) *See* DEXAMETHASONE.

Minims Fluorescein Sodium (Bausch & Lomb UK) *See* FLUORESCEIN SODIUM.

Minims Lidocaine and Fluorescein (Bausch & Lomb UK) A proprietary combination of *lidocaine hydrochloride (a local anaesthetic) and *fluorescein sodium (a dye), used for locating damaged areas of the cornea and foreign bodies in the eye. It is available as single-dose eye drops on *prescription only.

m

Minims Metipranolol (Bausch & Lomb UK) *See* METIPRANOLOL.

Minims Phenylephrine (Bausch & Lomb UK) *See* PHENYLEPHRINE.

Minims Pilocarpine (Bausch & Lomb UK) *See* PILOCARPINE.

Minims Prednisolone (Bausch & Lomb UK) *See* PREDNISOLONE.

Minims Proxymetacaine and Fluorescein (Bausch & Lomb UK) A proprietary combination of proxymetacaine (a *local anaesthetic) and *fluorescein sodium (a dye), used to facilitate minor eye procedures, such as the removal of foreign bodies. It is available as eye drops on *prescription only.

Minims Saline (Bausch & Lomb UK) *See* SODIUM CHLORIDE.

Minims Tetracaine Hydrochloride (Bausch & Lomb UK) *See* TETRACAINE.

Minims Tropicamide (Bausch & Lomb UK) *See* TROPICAMIDE.

Minitran (3M Health Care) *See* GLYCERYL TRINITRATE.

Minocin, Minocin MR (Meda Pharmaceuticals) *See* MINOCYCLINE.

minocycline A tetracycline antibiotic used for the treatment of chronic bronchitis, brucellosis, chlamydial infections, and infections caused by

mycoplasmas and rickettsias (*see* TETRACYCLINES). It is also used to treat gum disease and acne. Unlike most tetracyclines, minocycline does not exacerbate kidney disease and may be used by people with kidney impairment. It is available, on *prescription only, as tablets, capsules, *modified-release capsules, or a gel for oral (topical) application.
Side effects: *see* TETRACYCLINES. In addition, this drug may cause dizziness and vertigo, severe rashes, and pigmentation (sometimes irreversible). Local irritation can occur with topical application.
Precautions: *see* TETRACYCLINES. In addition, liver function should be monitored if this drug is used for more than six months.
Interactions with other drugs: *see* TETRACYCLINES.
Proprietary preparations: Acnamino MR (modified-release capsules); Aknemin (capsules); Dentomycin (gel); Minocin (tablets); Minocin MR (modified-release capsules); Sebact MR (modified-release capsules); Sebomin MR (modified-release capsules).

Minodiab (Pharmacia) *See* GLIPIZIDE.

minoxidil A *vasodilator drug used for the treatment of severe *hypertension and also to promote hair growth in male-pattern baldness (for both men and women). For treating hypertension minoxidil is supplied as tablets on *prescription only; it should be used with a beta blocker and a diuretic. For the treatment of baldness minoxidil is available as a solution for topical application and can be obtained from pharmacies without a prescription; it cannot be prescribed on the NHS.
Side effects: the tablets can cause fluid retention, weight gain, *oedema, excessive hair growth, and an increase in heart rate. These side effects are less likely to occur with the solution as only a small percentage of the drug is absorbed; local side effects include dermatitis.
Precautions: monoxidil tablets should not be taken by people with phaeochromocytoma (a tumour of the adrenal glands that can unpredictably release large amounts of adrenaline or noradrenaline, raising blood pressure). They must be used with caution in pregnant women and people with certain heart conditions. The solution should not be allowed to come into contact with the eyes, mouth, and mucous membranes, or with broken, infected, or inflamed skin.
Proprietary preparations: Loniten (tablets); Regaine (solution).

Mintec (Shire Pharmaceuticals) *See* PEPPERMINT OIL.

Miochol-E (Novartis) *See* ACETYLCHOLINE CHLORIDE.

miotics Drugs that cause the pupil of the eye to contract by constricting the muscle of the iris. This pulls the iris away from the cornea and thus increases the angle between the iris and cornea, through which fluid (aqueous humour) drains from the front chamber of the eye. Miotics are used to improve the outflow of fluid from the eye (and therefore reduce the pressure) in the treatment of *glaucoma. *See* PILOCARPINE.

Mirapexin (Boehringer Ingelheim) *See* PRAMIPEXOLE.

Mircera (Roche Products) *See* ERYTHROPOIETIN.

Mirena (Bayer) *See* LEVONORGESTREL.

mirtazapine An *antidepressant drug that enhances the effects of *serotonin and *noradrenaline in the brain. It has fewer antimuscarinic side effects than the *tricyclic antidepressants and does not cause the nausea and other gastrointestinal upsets associated with *SSRIs; however, sedation can occur at the start of treatment. Mirtazapine is available as tablets and dispersible tablets on *prescription only.
Side effects: include an increase in appetite, weight gain, and drowsiness. Signs of infection (such as fever and sore throat) should be reported to a doctor as this may indicate a blood disorder.
Precautions: mirtazapine is not recommended for women who are pregnant or breastfeeding. It should be used with caution in people with epilepsy, impaired liver or kidney function, heart disease, low blood pressure, diabetes, glaucoma, psychotic illness, or a history of manic depressive illness. Alcohol increases the sedative effect of mirtazapine.
Interactions with other drugs:
Antidepressants: mirtazapine should not be started until two weeks after stopping MAOIs; MAOIs should not be started until two weeks after mirtazapine has been stopped; moclobemide should not be started until at least one week after stopping mirtazepine.
Anxiolytics and hypnotics: enhance the sedative effect of mirtazapine.
Proprietary preparation: Zispin SolTab (dispersible tablets).

misoprostol An *analogue of *prostaglandins that has *cytoprotectant action and is used in the treatment of duodenal, gastric, and *NSAID-induced ulcers (*see* ACID-PEPTIC DISEASES). It is given in combination with NSAIDs to avoid the gastrointestinal problems that these drugs can cause. Misoprostol is available as tablets on *prescription only.
Side effects: include diarrhoea, abdominal pain, indigestion, flatulence, nausea and vomiting, and abnormal vaginal bleeding.
Precautions: misoprostol should not be taken by women who are pregnant, planning to become pregnant, or breastfeeding. It should only be used in premenopausal women if they require NSAID therapy and are at high risk of ulceration induced by NSAIDs; these women must take effective contraception measures.
Proprietary preparations: Cytotec; *Arthrotec (combined with diclofenac sodium); *Napratec (packaged with naproxen).

mitomycin A *cytotoxic antibiotic used for the treatment of cancer of the mouth, oesophagus, and stomach, breast cancer, and recurrent superficial bladder tumours. It is injected intravenously for gastrointestinal or breast cancer and instilled directly into the bladder to treat bladder cancer; it is usually given at six-weekly intervals because it causes delayed *bone marrow

suppression. Mitomycin is available as a form for injection on *prescription only.
Side effects: include bone marrow suppression (long-term use may permanently damage the bone marrow) and damage to the lung and kidneys. *See also* CYTOTOXIC DRUGS.
Precautions: *see* CYTOTOXIC DRUGS. Mitomycin is irritant to the skin and must be handled with caution.
Interactions with other drugs:
Clozapine: there is a risk of agranulocytosis (a blood disorder), and this drug should not be given with mitomycin.
Proprietary preparation: Mitomycin C Kyowa.

Mitomycin C Kyowa (Kyowa Hakko) *See* MITOMYCIN.

mitotane A drug used to relieve the symptoms of cancer of the outer layer (cortex) of the adrenal gland that cannot be surgically removed. It works by suppressing activity of the adrenal cortex and is available as tablets on *prescription only.
Side effects: most common are loss of appetite, nausea, vomiting, stomach pain, impaired function of the testes or ovaries, thyroid disorders, and damage to the central nervous system.
Precautions: mitotane should not be taken by women who are pregnant or breastfeeding or by people with severe kidney disease. It should be used with caution in people with liver disease. A doctor should be consulted if injury occurs or infection or illness develop during treatment.
Interactions with other drugs:
Clozapine: should not be taken with mitotane as this combination increases the risk of agranulocytosis (a blood disorder).
Warfarin: its plasma concentration may be reduced by mitotane.
Proprietary preparation: Lysodren.

mitoxantrone **<mitozantrone>** A *cytotoxic antibiotic used for the treatment of breast *cancer. It is also used for the treatment of leukaemias and lymphomas. Mitoxantrone is available, on *prescription only, as a solution for intravenous infusion.
Side effects: *bone marrow suppression is the most likely side effect; high doses can have adverse effects on the heart. *See also* DOXORUBICIN; CYTOTOXIC DRUGS.
Precautions: *see* DOXORUBICIN; CYTOTOXIC DRUGS.
Proprietary preparation: Onkotrone.

Mixtard 30 (Novo Nordisk) *See* INSULIN.

mizolastine One of the newer (non-sedating) *antihistamines, used to relieve the symptoms of such allergic conditions as hay fever and urticaria (nettle rash). It is available as tablets on *prescription only.
Side effects: *see* ANTIHISTAMINES. Mizolastine may also cause weight gain.
Precautions: mizolastine should not be taken by people with heart disease or

severe liver disease or by women who are pregnant or breastfeeding. *See also* ANTIHISTAMINES.

Interactions with other drugs:

Anti-arrhythmic drugs: amiodarone, disopyramide, flecainide, and propafenone should not be taken with mizolastine, as this increases the risk of ventricular *arrhythmias.

Antibiotics: moxifloxacin and macrolides (such as erythromycin) should not be taken with mizolastine, as this increases the risk of ventricular arrhythmias.

Antifungal drugs: itraconazole and imidazoles inhibit the breakdown of mizolastine and should not be taken with it.

Sotalol: should not be taken with mizolastine, as this increases the risk of ventricular arrhythmias.

Proprietary preparation: Mizollen.

Mizollen (sanofi-aventis) *See* MIZOLASTINE.

Mobic (Boehringer Ingelheim Ltd) *See* MELOXICAM.

Mobiflex (Roche Products) *See* TENOXICAM.

Mobigel Spray (Goldshield) *See* DICLOFENAC SODIUM.

moclobemide A reversible *monoamine oxidase inhibitor (MAOI) used for the treatment of severe depression and social anxiety disorder. It does not have such a severe reaction as most MAOIs when interacting with food and beverages that contain tyramine (including cheese and wine), but people taking moclobemide should still moderate their intake of these foods and drinks and be aware of the potential danger. Moclobemide is available as tablets on *prescription only.

Side effects: include sleep disturbances, dizziness, stomach upsets, headache, agitation, and dry mouth.

Precautions: moclobemide should not be taken by people in confusional states or who are agitated or excited, or by those with phaeochromocytoma (a tumour of the adrenal gland) or by breastfeeding women. *See also* MONOAMINE OXIDASE INHIBITORS.

Interactions with other drugs:

Antidepressants: should not be taken with moclobemide, which should not be started until 1–5 weeks after stopping them; there is an increased risk of adverse effects when moclobemide is given with duloxetine or escitalopram (which should not be taken with it).

$5HT_1$ agonists: there is an increased risk of adverse effects on the central nervous system if moclobemide is taken with rizatriptan or sumatriptan (which should not be started until two weeks after stopping moclobemide) or zolmitriptan (whose dosage should be reduced).

Opioid analgesics: blood pressure may be increased or reduced; dextromethorphan and pethidine should not be given with moclobemide.

Selegiline: should not be taken with moclobemide.

Sympathomimetics: increase the risk of a dangerous rise in blood pressure and should not be taken with moclobemide.

See also MONOAMINE OXIDASE INHIBITORS.

Proprietary preparation: Manerix.

modafinil A drug that acts on the brain as a *stimulant and is used to treat narcolepsy (an extreme tendency to fall asleep) and obstructive sleep apnoea (when breathing stops because the airways are obstructed). It is available as tablets on *prescription only.
Side effects: include loss of appetite, abdominal pain, headache, insomnia, excitation, euphoria, nervousness, dry mouth, palpitations, a fast heart rate, hypertension (high blood pressure), tremor, nausea, stomach discomfort, rashes, and itching.
Precautions: modafinil should not be taken by women who are pregnant or breastfeeding or by people with moderate to severe hypertension or certain heart conditions. It should be used with caution in people with liver or kidney disease. Treatment should be stopped if psychiatric symptoms or a rash develop. Long-term treatment with modafinil may cause *dependence.
Interactions with other drugs:

Ciclosporin: its plasma concentration is reduced.

Oral contraceptives: modafinil reduces their contraceptive effect; alternative methods of contraception should be considered.

Proprietary preparation: Provigil.

m

Modecate (sanofi-aventis) *See* FLUPHENAZINE DECANOATE.

modified-release preparation (**sustained-release preparation**; **continuous-release preparation**) A formulation of a drug taken orally that releases the active component slowly over a long period. Drugs taken by mouth are usually absorbed in minutes or a few hours from the gut into the blood, where they are removed by excretory mechanisms – often via the liver or kidneys. As a result, plasma concentrations of the drug rise and fall, then rise again when the next dose is taken. For some drugs this fluctuating plasma concentration is not desirable. In such cases, modified-release tablets or capsules enable the drug to be released over several hours, so that a relatively constant plasma concentration of the drug can be maintained. The terms 'modified release', 'sustained release', or 'continuous release' are often incorporated into the proprietary names of these preparations in the forms 'MR', 'SR', 'CR', or 'Continus'. 'LA' and 'XL' also indicate modified-release preparations.

Modisal XL, Modisal LA (Sandoz) *See* ISOSORBIDE MONONITRATE.

Modrasone (Teva UK) *See* ALCLOMETASONE DIPROPIONATE.

Modrenal (Bioenvision) *See* TRILOSTANE.

Moduretic (Du Pont Pharmaceuticals) *See* CO-AMILOZIDE.

moexipril hydrochloride An *ACE inhibitor used for the treatment of *hypertension. It is available as tablets on *prescription only.
Side effects, precautions, and interactions with other drugs: *see* ACE INHIBITORS.
Proprietary preparation: Perdix.
See also ANTIHYPERTENSIVE DRUGS.

Mogadon (Roche Products) *See* NITRAZEPAM.

Molaxole (Meda Pharmaceuticals) A proprietary combination of *potassium chloride, *sodium chloride, *sodium bicarbonate, and macrogol '3350' (*see* POLYETHYLENE GLYCOLS), used as an *osmotic laxative. It is available as an oral powder to be dissolved in water and can be obtained without a prescription, but only from pharmacies.

Molcer (Wallace) *See* DOCUSATE SODIUM.

Molipaxin (sanofi-aventis) *See* TRAZODONE.

mometasone furoate A potent *corticosteroid used for the treatment of *psoriasis and for eczema that has not responded to other treatments, for the prevention and treatment of allergic rhinitis, including hay fever, and for the prevention of asthma. It is available, on *prescription only, as a cream, ointment, scalp lotion, metered-dose nasal spray, or powder for use in a metered *inhaler.
Side effects and precautions: *see* CORTICOSTEROIDS; TOPICAL STEROIDS. The nasal spray may cause headache, sore throat, and nasal irritation.
Proprietary preparations: Asmanex Twisthaler (inhaler); Elocon (cream, ointment, or lotion); Nasonex (nasal spray).

monoamine oxidase inhibitors (MAOIs) A class of *antidepressant drugs that act by inhibiting monoamine oxidases, enzymes that break down noradrenaline and serotonin, and thus increase the activity of these neurotransmitters in the brain. Because they also inhibit enzymes that break down certain other chemicals (especially tyramine), they interact, sometimes quite dangerously, with other drugs and certain foods and beverages (see precautions and interactions with other drugs below). For this reason MAOIs are used less often than other types of antidepressants, although they are useful for treating people who do not respond to *tricyclic antidepressants or *SSRIs. They are most commonly given to patients who have depression with hypochondriacal or hysterical features. The MAOIs are *isocarboxazid, *phenelzine, and *tranylcypromine (which is the most hazardous). *Moclobemide is a newer type of MAOI that reversibly inhibits monoamine oxidase type A; it is less likely than traditional MAOIs to cause adverse effects due to tyramine.
Side effects: include a sudden fall in blood pressure on standing (causing faintness), dizziness, drowsiness, insomnia, weakness and fatigue, dryness of the mouth, and constipation and other gastrointestinal disturbances; less

common side effects are headache, oedema, skin rashes, blood disorders, sexual disturbances, jaundice, weight gain, and mania.
Precautions: foods and beverages rich in tyramine (e.g. cheese, hung meat or game, meat or yeast extracts, pickled herrings, flavoured textured vegetable proteins, and wine) should be avoided as they can cause dramatic and dangerous rises in blood pressure. This effect can persist for some two weeks after stopping the MAOI. MAOIs should be stopped gradually at the end of treatment.
Interactions with other drugs:

Analgesics: opioid analgesics (especially pethidine) can cause severe reactions and should not be taken with MAOIs. The non-opioid analgesic nefopam should also be avoided.
Antidepressants: it is dangerous to take MAOIs with other antidepressants, and this should only be done under specialist supervision. Other antidepressants should not be started for two weeks after treatment with MAOIs has stopped, and MAOIs should not be started for at least one week after treatment with other antidepressants has stopped.
Antihypertensive drugs: their effect in lowering blood pressure is enhanced; indoramin should not be taken with MAOIs.
Anti-parkinsonian drugs: entacapone should not be taken with MAOIs; levodopa and rasagiline cause a dangerous rise in blood pressure; levodopa should not be started until two weeks after stopping MAOIs, and MAOIs should not be started until two weeks after stopping rasagiline.
Atomoxetine: should not be started until two weeks after stopping MAOIs, which should not be started until two weeks after stopping atomoxetine.
Bupropion: should not be started until two weeks after stopping MAOIs.
Carbamazepine: there is an increased risk of convulsions.
Clozapine: stimulation of the central nervous system can occur.
$5HT_1$ agonists: there is a risk of adverse effects on the central nervous system if rizatriptan, sumatriptan, or zolmitriptan are taken with MAOIs; rizatriptan and sumatriptan should not be started until two weeks after stopping MAOIs.
Methyldopa: should not be taken with MAOIs.
Sibutramine: there is a risk of adverse effects on the central nervous system, and this drug should not be taken with MAOIs.
Sympathomimetics: cause a dangerous rise in blood pressure if taken with MAOIs; methylphenidate should not be taken until two weeks after stopping MAOIs.
Tetracaine: stimulation of the central nervous system and increased blood pressure can occur.

monoclonal antibody An antibody produced by genetic engineering techniques from a cell clone (i.e. numerous identical cells originally derived from a single parent cell) and therefore consisting of a single type of *immunoglobulin. Monoclonal antibodies have been developed for targeting specific tissues for use in treating certain cancers (*see* ALEMTUZUMAB; CETUXIMAB; PANITUMUMAB; RITUXIMAB; TRASTUZUMAB) and other conditions.

m

See also ABCIXIMAB; ADALIMUMAB; BASILIXIMAB; ECULIZUMAB; IBRITUMONAB TIUXETAN; INFLIXIMAB; OMALIZUMAB; PALIVIZUMAB; PANITUMUMAB; RANIBIZUMAB; USTEKINUMAB.

monofluorophosphate *See* FLUORIDE.

Monomax SR, Monomax XL (Chiesi) *See* ISOSORBIDE MONONITRATE.

Monomil XL (IVAX) *See* ISOSORBIDE MONONITRATE.

Mononine (CSL Behring) *See* FACTOR IX.

Monosorb XL 60 (Dexcel Pharma) *See* ISOSORBIDE MONONITRATE.

montelukast A *leukotriene receptor antagonist used as an *adjunct to an inhaled *corticosteroid for the treatment of mild to moderate *asthma that is not adequately controlled by the usual combination of a corticosteroid and a beta stimulant (such as *salbutamol). It can also be used to prevent an attack of asthma being brought on by exercise, but it should not be used to treat acute attacks. Montelukast is available as tablets, chewable tablets, or granules on *prescription only.
Side effects: include abdominal pain, headache, thirst, diarrhoea, and dizziness.
Precautions: the chewable tablets contain aspartame and should be used with caution by people who have phenylketonuria. Montelukast should be used with caution by women who are pregnant or breastfeeding.
Interactions with other drugs:
Phenobarbital: can reduce the effectiveness of montelukast.
Proprietary preparation: Singulair.

m

moracizine (**moricizine**) A class I *anti-arrhythmic drug used to treat life-threatening *arrhythmias. It is available as tablets on *prescription only.
Side effects: include dizziness, nervousness, 'pins and needles', gastrointestinal upset, dry mouth, sweating, chest pain, muscle pain, sleep disorders, blurred vision.
Precautions: moracizine should not be taken by people with liver or kidney disease, if congestive *heart failure is present, or by pregnant women. *See also* ANTI-ARRHYTHMIC DRUGS.

Morhulin (Actavis) A proprietary combination of cod liver oil (an *emollient) and *zinc oxide (an astringent protective agent) in the form of an ointment, used for the prevention and treatment of napkin rash, pressure sores, and leg ulcers and for the relief of *eczema and minor wounds and abrasions. It is freely available *over the counter.

Morphgesic SR (Amdipharm) *See* MORPHINE.

morphine An opiate that is the most commonly used of the *opioid analgesics for treating severe pain, including that caused by surgery. It is particularly valuable for controlling pain in terminal illnesses; as well as pain relief, it also induces feelings of well-being and mental detachment. Morphine

is also used to control coughing in terminally ill patients. Because it is constipating, low doses of morphine are used in some *antidiarrhoeal preparations. Morphine is a *controlled drug; it is available as tablets, *modified-release tablets or capsules, oral solutions, suppositories, and solutions for injection.
Side effects: nausea and vomiting, drowsiness, and constipation frequently occur (morphine may need to be given with a laxative or an antiemetic); higher doses cause depression of breathing and low blood pressure. Other side effects can include difficulty in passing urine, dry mouth, sweating, constriction of the pupils, a feeling of faintness on standing, palpitations, confusion, and hallucinations.
Precautions: morphine should be used with caution in people with asthma or other respiratory disorders (it can exacerbate asthma and should not be used during an attack), low blood pressure, an underactive thyroid gland, an enlarged prostate gland, liver or kidney disease, or epilepsy, and in women who are pregnant or breastfeeding. It should not be used in people with severely depressed breathing or acute alcoholism, or in those who have a head injury. Treatment with morphine must be stopped gradually in those who have been taking it on a long-term basis in order to avoid withdrawal reactions. *See also* OPIOIDS.
Interactions with other drugs: *see* OPIOIDS.
Proprietary preparations: Depodur (injection); Minijet Morphine Sulphate (injection); Morphgesic SR (modified-release tablets); MST Continus (modified-release tablets or suspension); MXL (modified-release capsules); Oramorph (oral solution); Oramorph SR (modified-release tablets); Sevredol (tablets); Zomorph (modified-release capsules); *Cyclimorph (combined with cyclizine tartrate); *J Collis Browne's Mixture (combined with peppermint oil); *J Collis Browne's Tablets (combined with calcium carbonate and kaolin).

Motens (Boehringer Ingelheim) *See* LACIDIPINE.

Motifene 75 mg (Daiichi Sankyo) *See* DICLOFENAC SODIUM.

Motilium (sanofi-aventis) *See* DOMPERIDONE.

Motrin (McNeil Ltd) *See* IBUPROFEN.

Movelat (Genus Pharmaceuticals) A proprietary combination of *salicylic acid and mucopolysaccharide polysulphate (a *heparinoid), used for the relief of rheumatic, muscular, and mild arthritic pain, sprains, and strains (*see* RUBEFACIENTS). It is available as a cream (which also contains *thymol) and a gel, both of which can be obtained from pharmacies without a prescription.
Side effects and precautions: *see* SALICYLATES.

Movicol (Norgine) A proprietary combination of macrogol '3350' (*see* POLYETHYLENE GLYCOLS), *sodium bicarbonate, *sodium chloride, and *potassium chloride, used as an *osmotic laxative for the treatment of chronic constipation and impacted faeces. **Movicol-Half** and **Movicol Paediatric Plain** (for children aged 2–11 years) are half the strength of Movicol. All these

preparations are available as an oral powder to be dissolved in water and can be obtained without a prescription, but only from pharmacies.
Side effects and precautions: *see* POLYETHYLENE GLYCOLS.

Moviprep (Norgine) A proprietary preparation consisting of *potassium chloride, *sodium chloride, macrogol '3350' (*see* POLYETHYLENE GLYCOLS), and sodium sulphate as an oral powder (sachet A) and sodium ascorbate and ascorbic acid (*see* VITAMIN C) as an oral powder (sachet B). It is used to evacuate the bowel before investigative procedures or surgery; the powders are dissolved in 2 litres of water. Moviprep can be obtained without a prescription, but only from pharmacies.
Side effects and precautions: *see* BOWEL-CLEANSING SOLUTIONS; POLYETHYLENE GLYCOLS. Moviprep causes a watery diarrhoea and can lead to dehydration; a further litre of water should therefore be taken to prevent dehydration.

moxifloxacin A *quinolone antibiotic used for the treatment of acute bacterial sinusitis, acute exacerbations of chronic bronchitis, community-acquired pneumonia, and mild to moderate pelvic inflammatory disease when *first-line treatment has failed to resolve the infection. It is available as tablets on *prescription only.
Side effects: *see* QUINOLONES. Additional side effects include *arrhythmias.
Precautions: *see* QUINOLONES. In addition, moxifloxacin should not be taken by people with impaired liver function or a history of arrhythmias.
Interactions with other drugs: there is an increased risk of ventricular arrhythmias if moxifloxacin is taken with certain other drugs, which should therefore not be used with it. These drugs include antimalarials, phenothiazine, butyrophenone and thioxanthene antipsychotic drugs, atomoxetine, erythromycin (by mouth or infusion), mizolastine, pentamidine, sotalol, and tricyclic antidepressants.
See also QUINOLONES.
Proprietary preparation: Avelox.

moxisylyte **<thymoxamine>** An *alpha blocker taken by mouth for the short-term treatment of Raynaud's syndrome (poor circulation of the hands and feet). Moxisylyte is available, on *prescription only, as tablets.
Side effects: include nausea, diarrhoea, flushing, headache, and dizziness.
Precautions: moxisylyte should not be taken by people with active liver disease or by pregnant women. It should be used with caution in people with diabetes.
Interactions with other drugs:
Alpha blockers and beta blockers: may cause a severe fall in blood pressure on standing.
Proprietary preparation: Opilon (tablets).
See also VASODILATORS.

moxonidine A drug that acts in the brain to reduce activity in the *sympathetic nervous system, causing a fall in the resistance of the blood vessels and a decrease in blood pressure. Thus, it has similar actions to *alpha

m

blockers, but does not cause the side effects of dry mouth and sedation seen with these drugs. It is used for the treatment of mild to moderate *hypertension. It is available as tablets on *prescription only.
Side effects: include headache, weakness, dizziness, dry mouth, sleep disturbances, and nausea.
Precautions: moxonidine should not be taken by patients with certain types of heart disease or with severe liver or kidney disease.
Proprietary preparation: Physiotens.
See also ANTIHYPERTENSIVE DRUGS.

Mozobil (Genzyme Therapeutics) *See* PLERIXAFOR.

MST Continus (Napp Pharmaceuticals) *See* MORPHINE.

Mucoclear 6% (Pari) *See* SODIUM CHLORIDE.

Mucodyne (sanofi-aventis) *See* CARBOCISTEINE.

Mucogel (Chemidex Pharma) *See* CO-MAGALDROX.

mucolytic drugs Agents that dissolve or break down mucus and thus facilitate expectoration. Mucolytics are used to treat chest conditions involving excessive or thickened mucus secretions. *See* ACETYLCYSTEINE; CARBOCISTEINE; DORNASE ALFA; ERDOSTEINE. *Compare* EXPECTORANTS.

m

Multi-Action Actifed Chesty Coughs (McNeil Products Ltd) A proprietary combination of *pseudoephedrine (a decongestant), *triprolidine (an antihistamine), and *guaifenesin (an expectorant), used to relieve the symptoms of coughs, colds, and hay fever. This medicine is available as an oral solution without a prescription, but only from pharmacies. It cannot be prescribed on the NHS.
Side effects and interactions with other drugs: *see* ANTIHISTAMINES; DECONGESTANTS; EPHEDRINE HYDROCHLORIDE; GUAIFENESIN.
Precautions: this medicine should not normally be given to children under two years old. *See also* ANTIHISTAMINES; DECONGESTANTS; EPHEDRINE HYDROCHLORIDE; GUAIFENESIN.

Multi-Action Actifed Dry Coughs (McNeil Products Ltd) A proprietary combination of *dextromethorphan (a cough suppressant), *pseudoephedrine (a decongestant), and *triprolidine (an antihistamine), used for the relief of dry coughs and congestion of the upper airways (including that due to hay fever and similar allergic conditions). It is available without a prescription, but only from pharmacies. It cannot be prescribed on the NHS.
Side effects and interactions with other drugs: *see* ANTIHISTAMINES; DECONGESTANTS; DEXTROMETHORPHAN; EPHEDRINE HYDROCHLORIDE; OPIOIDS.
Precautions: this medicine should not normally be given to children under two years old. *See also* ANTIHISTAMINES; DECONGESTANTS; EPHEDRINE HYDROCHLORIDE; OPIOIDS.

Multi-Action Actifed Tablets (McNeil Products Ltd) *See* PSEUDOEPHEDRINE.

mupirocin A broad-spectrum *antibiotic that is not related to any of the other antibiotics. It is used for treating bacterial skin infections and is especially useful for nasal infections, since it is active against methicillin-resistant *Staphylococcus aureus* (MRSA), a bacterium that is resistant to many antibiotics and may be carried in the nostrils. Mupirocin is available, on *prescription only, as a cream or ointment to be applied to the skin or nostrils.
Side effects: mupirocin may cause stinging on application; contact with the eyes should be avoided.
Precautions: mupirocin should be used with caution by people with kidney disease.
Proprietary preparations: Bactroban Cream; Bactroban Nasal Ointment; Bactroban Ointment.

muscle relaxants Drugs that reduce the tension in skeletal muscles. They are used to treat muscle spasms (involuntary and often painful contractions of muscles caused by injury or disease) and spasticity, in which the muscles are continually in a state of increased tension or rigidity due to such disorders as multiple sclerosis and cerebral palsy.

Muscle relaxants either act centrally (i.e. on the brain or spinal cord), to inhibit the nerve signals that cause the muscles to contract (*see* BACLOFEN; DIAZEPAM; METHOCARBAMOL; TIZANIDINE), or directly on the muscles themselves, to prevent the activity in the cells that cause the muscles to contract (*see* DANTROLENE SODIUM). The dosage of these drugs may need some adjustment to obtain the optimum that controls symptoms but does not cause muscle weakness. Skeletal muscle relaxants should not be stopped abruptly or stiffness may be worse than before treatment.

The muscle relaxants used in surgery during general anaesthesia work in a different way. They act at neuromuscular junctions (where the nerve fibre meets the muscle it supplies) to block the transmission of nerve impulses, either by binding to receptor sites normally occupied by the chemical transmitter *acetylcholine (nondepolarizing muscle relaxants, such as **atracurium besilate**, **pancuronium**, **rocuronium bromide**, and **mivacurium**) or by mimicking the action of acetylcholine, making the muscle no longer receptive to stimulation by this transmitter (depolarizing muscle relaxants, such as **suxamethonium**).

Drugs that relax smooth muscle include *antispasmodics, *bronchodilators, and *vasodilators.

MUSE (Meda Pharmaceuticals) *See* ALPROSTADIL.

MXL (Napp Pharmaceuticals) *See* MORPHINE.

Mycamine (Astellas Pharma Ltd) *See* MICAFUNGIN.

Mycil Foot Spray (Crookes Healthcare) *See* TOLNAFTATE.

Mycil Gold (Crookes Healthcare) *See* CLOTRIMAZOLE.

m

Mycil Ointment (Crookes Healthcare) A proprietary combination of *tolnaftate (an antifungal drug) and *benzalkonium chloride (an antiseptic), used for the treatment of tinea (ringworm), including athlete's foot, and prickly heat. It is freely available *over the counter.

Mycil Powder (Crookes Healthcare) A proprietary combination of *tolnaftate (an antifungal drug) and *chlorhexidine (an antiseptic), used for the treatment of tinea (ringworm), including athlete's foot, and prickly heat. It is freely available *over the counter.

Mycobutin (Pharmacia) *See* RIFABUTIN.

mycophenolate mofetil An *immunosuppressant drug used in conjunction with *ciclosporin and *corticosteroids for the prevention of rejection in kidney transplant patients. It is available, on *prescription only, as capsules, tablets, an oral suspension, or a form for intravenous infusion.
Side effects: include diarrhoea, vomiting, constipation, nausea, abdominal pain, high blood pressure, chest pain, breathlessness, cough, dizziness, insomnia, headache, and tremor.
Precautions: full blood counts must be performed during therapy. Mycophenolate should not be given to patients with active gastrointestinal disease or to women who are pregnant or breastfeeding; women should avoid becoming pregnant for six weeks after treatment stops.
Interactions with other drugs:
Aciclovir: plasma concentrations of both drugs are increased.
Antacids: reduce the absorption of mycophenolate.
Colestyramine: reduces the absorption of mycophenolate.
Rifampicin reduces the plasma concentration of mycophenolate.
Proprietary preparations: CellCept; Myfortic (tablets).

Mycota (Thornton and Ross) *See* UNDECENOIC ACID.

Mydriacyl (Alcon Laboratories) *See* TROPICAMIDE.

Mydrilate (Intrapharm) *See* CYCLOPENTOLATE HYDROCHLORIDE.

Myfortic (Novartis) *See* MYCOPHENOLATE MOFETIL.

Myleran (GlaxoSmithKline) *See* BUSULFAN.

Myocet (Cephalon) *See* DOXORUBICIN.

Myocrisin (sanofi-aventis) *See* SODIUM AUROTHIOMALATE.

Myotonine (Glenwood Laboratories) *See* BETHANECHOL CHLORIDE.

Myozyme (Genzyme Therapeutics) *See* ALGLUCOSIDASE ALFA.

Mysoline (Acorus Therapeutics) *See* PRIMIDONE.

myxoedema *See* THYROID HORMONES.

nabilone A synthetic derivative of cannabis that is used to prevent or treat the nausea and vomiting caused by *cytotoxic drug treatment for cancer. It is used in patients who have not responded to other *antiemetics, but treatment needs to be carefully supervised, since some people can experience disorientation and mood changes as side effects (see below). Nabilone is available as capsules on *prescription only.
Side effects: include drowsiness, vertigo, euphoria, shaky movements, dry mouth, visual disturbances, difficulty in concentrating, sleep disturbances, confusion, disorientation, hallucinations, psychosis, depression, lack of coordination, tremor, a fast heart rate, and loss of appetite. Mood changes and other mental side effects may persist for up to three days after stopping the treatment.
Precautions: nabilone should not be taken by people with severe liver disease or by women who are breastfeeding. It should be used with caution in people with a history of psychiatric disorders, in the elderly, and in pregnant women. Nabilone may affect driving ability, and its sedative effects are increased by alcohol.
Interactions with other drugs:
Anxiolytics and hypnotics: enhance the sedative effects of nabilone.

nabumetone An *NSAID used for the treatment of pain and inflammation in osteoarthritis and rheumatoid arthritis. It is available as tablets or a suspension on *prescription only.
Side effects, precautions, and interactions with other drugs: *see* NSAIDs.
Proprietary preparation: Relifex.

nadolol A *beta blocker used for the treatment and prevention of heart *arrhythmias and *angina. It is also used for the prevention of *migraine and, combined with a diuretic, for the treatment of *hypertension. It is available as tablets on *prescription only.
Side effects, precautions, and interactions with other drugs: *see* BETA BLOCKERS.
Proprietary preparation: Corgard.

nafarelin An analogue of *gonadorelin used to treat *endometriosis and to suppress the release of gonadotrophins by the pituitary gland before inducing ovulation in women undergoing fertility treatment. Nafarelin is available, on *prescription only, as a nasal spray.
Side effects: include transient nasal irritation, hot flushes, loss of libido, vaginal dryness, emotional upset, headache, changes in breast size, breast

tenderness, ovarian cysts, depression, muscle aches, tingling in the fingers or toes, acne, migraine, bouts of palpitation, and blurred vision.
Precautions: *see* BUSERELIN.
Proprietary preparation: Synarel.

naftidrofuryl oxalate A drug used for the treatment of disorders of the peripheral arteries, such as intermittent claudication (poor circulation in the legs giving rise to cramping pain on exercise), and cerebrovascular disease, although its value is not proven. It is available as capsules on *prescription only.
Side effects: include nausea, pains in the stomach region, and rashes.
Proprietary preparation: Praxilene.

Naglazyme (BioMarin) *See* GALSULFASE.

Nalcrom (sanofi-aventis) *See* SODIUM CROMOGLICATE.

nalidixic acid A *quinolone antibiotic, similar to *ciprofloxacin, that is used for the treatment of urinary-tract infections. It is available, on *prescription only, as a suspension.
Side effects and precautions: *see* QUINOLONES.
Interactions with other drugs:
Melphalan: its adverse effects may be increased.
See also QUINOLONES.
Proprietary preparation: Uriben.

n

Nalorex (Bristol-Myers Squibb) *See* NALTREXONE HYDROCHLORIDE.

naloxone hydrochloride A drug that opposes the action of *opioids. It is used to treat overdosage with opioids and also to reverse the depression of breathing caused by the use of opioid analgesics during surgery. Naloxone is available as an injection or intravenous infusion on *prescription only.
Side effects: nausea and vomiting, an increase in heart rate, and abnormal heartbeats may occur.
Precautions: naloxone should be used with caution in patients who are physically dependent on opioids, who have cardiovascular disease, or who are receiving other drugs that can have adverse effects on the heart. When given after surgery, the dosage should be calculated to reverse the respiratory effects of the opioids without interfering with their pain-relieving effects.
Proprietary preparations: Minijet Naloxone; *Suboxone (combined with buprenorphine hydrochloride); *Targinact (combined with oxycodone).

naltrexone hydrochloride A drug that opposes the action of *opioids (such as heroin) and is used to help maintain a drug-free habit in people who were formerly dependent on opioids. Naltrexone is usually started after the individual has abstained from taking opioid drugs for at least 7–10 days. It is available as tablets on *prescription only.
Side effects: include nausea, vomiting, abdominal pain, anxiety, nervousness, difficulties in sleeping, headache, reduced energy, and joint and muscle pain. Less frequently there may be mood changes and decreased potency.

Precautions: naltrexone should not be taken by people who are still dependent on opioids. Liver function should be monitored before and during treatment.
Proprietary preparations: Nalorex; Opizone.

nandrolone decanoate An *anabolic steroid that is sometimes used as an *adjunct in the treatment of aplastic *anaemias (types of anaemia resulting from a failure of the bone marrow to produce blood cells). It is available as a solution for injection on *prescription only.
Side effects: include acne, oedema (accumulation of fluid in the tissues) due to sodium retention, masculinization in women, and high plasma calcium concentrations.
Precautions: nandrolone should not be used during pregnancy or breastfeeding or in men with suspected prostate cancer or breast cancer. It should be used with caution in people with liver or kidney disease, high blood pressure, epilepsy, migraine, or diabetes.
Interactions with other drugs: *see* ANABOLIC STEROIDS.
Proprietary preparation: Deca-Durabolin.

Napratec (Pharmacia) A proprietary preparation consisting of tablets of *naproxen (an NSAID) packaged with tablets of *misoprostol (a prostaglandin analogue). It is used for the treatment of rheumatoid arthritis, osteoarthritis, and ankylosing spondylitis; the misoprostol is included to prevent the bleeding and ulceration of the stomach or duodenum that may result from the use of naproxen alone. Napratec is available on *prescription only.
Side effects and precautions: *see* NSAIDs; MISOPROSTOL.
Interactions with other drugs: *see* NSAIDs.

Naprosyn, Naprosyn EC (Roche Products) *See* NAPROXEN.

naproxen An *NSAID used for the treatment of pain and inflammation in rheumatoid arthritis (including arthritis in children), acute gout, and other disorders of the joints or muscles. It is also used to relieve period pains. Naproxen is available, on *prescription only, as tablets and *enteric-coated tablets.
Side effects: *see* NSAIDs.
Precautions and interactions with other drugs: *see* NSAIDs.
Proprietary preparations: Arthroxen; Feminax Ultra; Naprosyn; Naprosyn EC; Synflex; *Napratec (packaged with misoprostol).

Naramig (GlaxoSmithKline) *See* NARATRIPTAN.

naratriptan A *$5HT_1$ agonist used to treat acute attacks of *migraine. A single dose can relieve a migraine headache at any stage of the attack. Naratriptan is available as tablets on *prescription only.
Side effects: include sensations of tingling, heat, heaviness, pressure, or tightness; if tightness in the chest or throat is severe, treatment should be discontinued. Other side effects may include a slow or fast heart rate, disturbed vision, flushing, dizziness, and weakness.

Precautions: naratriptan should not be taken by people with certain heart conditions, uncontrolled high blood pressure, or disease of the peripheral blood vessels or by those who have previously had a heart attack or a stroke. It should be used with caution by women who are pregnant or breastfeeding and by people with impaired liver or kidney function.
Interactions with other drugs:
Ergot alkaloids: ergotamine and methysergide should not be taken with naratriptan.
St John's wort: increases the risk of adverse effects on the central nervous system and should not be taken with naratriptan.
Proprietary preparation: Naramig.

Nardil (Archimedes Pharma) *See* PHENELZINE.

Nasacort (sanofi-aventis) *See* TRIAMCINOLONE ACETONIDE.

Naseptin (Alliance) A proprietary combination of *chlorhexidine (an antiseptic) and *neomycin sulphate (an antibiotic), used for the treatment of nasal infections caused by bacteria and to eradicate *Staphylococcus* bacteria that may be carried in the nostrils. It is available as a cream on *prescription only.
Side effects: allergic rashes may develop.
Precautions: prolonged use should be avoided.

Nasobec (Teva UK) *See* BECLOMETASONE DIPROPIONATE.

Nasofan (IVAX) *See* FLUTICASONE PROPIONATE.

Nasonex (Schering-Plough) *See* MOMETASONE FUROATE.

natalizumab A *monoclonal antibody used for the treatment of severe relapsing multiple sclerosis (MS) that has not responded to *interferon beta. It is given by intravenous infusion and is available on *prescription only.
Side effects and precautions: side effects include nausea, vomiting, headache, dizziness, sore throat, joint pain, fever, tiredness, and urinary tract infection. More rare side effects are allergic reactions (e.g. rash, itching, difficulty in breathing, chest pain, swelling of the face), liver damage (e.g. yellowing of the skin, darkening of the urine), and progressive multifocal leukoencephopathy (PML), a serious brain disorder with symptoms similar to MS; if any of these reactions or symptoms develop, they should be reported to a doctor.
Proprietary preparation: Tysabri.

Natecal D3 (Chiesi) A proprietary combination of *calcium carbonate and *colecalciferol (vitamin D_3), used to treat *vitamin D deficiency and as an *adjunct in the treatment of osteoporosis. It is available as chewable tablets and can be obtained without a prescription, but only from pharmacies.
Side effects: nausea, vomiting, and other stomach upsets may occur. *See also* VITAMIN D.
Precautions: this medicine should be taken with caution by people with kidney disease or a history of kidney stones.

Interactions with other drugs:
Antiepileptic drugs: carbamazepine, phenobarbital, phenytoin, and primidone reduce the effects of Natecal D3.
Thiazide diuretics: increase the risk of high concentrations of calcium in the blood; *see* VITAMIN D.

nateglinide An *oral hypoglycaemic drug used, in combination with *metformin, for the treatment of type 2 *diabetes mellitus. It works by stimulating the secretion of *insulin. Nateglinide is available as tablets on *prescription only.
Side effects: include low blood glucose levels, abdominal pain, indigestion, diarrhoea, and allergic reactions (e.g. itching, rash).
Precautions: nateglinide should not be taken by people with severe liver disease or by women who are pregnant or breastfeeding.
Interactions with other drugs:
Fluconazole: may increase the effects of nateglinide.
Gemfibrozil: may increase the effects of nateglinide.
Rifampicin: may reduce the effects of nateglinide.
Proprietary preparation: Starlix.

Natracalm (Chefaro UK) A proprietary preparation consisting of an extract of passion flower, a traditional herbal remedy used for the relief of nervous tension and the stress and strain of everyday life. It is freely available *over the counter in the form of tablets.
Precautions: Natracalm should not be taken with antidepressants or by women who are pregnant or breastfeeding or by people who are driving or operating machinery.
Interactions with other drugs:
Sedatives: Natracalm may increase their effects.

Natrasleep (Chefaro UK) A proprietary combination of valerian extract and hop extract, a traditional herbal remedy used to encourage natural sleep. It is freely available *over the counter in the form of tablets.
Precautions: Natrasleep should not be taken with antidepressants or by women who are pregnant or breastfeeding or by people who are driving or operating machinery.
Interactions with other drugs:
Sedatives: Natrasleep may increase their effects.

Natrilix, Natrilix SR (Servier Laboratories) *See* INDAPAMIDE.

Navelbine (Pierre Fabre) *See* VINORELBINE.

Navidrex (Alliance) *See* CYCLOPENTHIAZIDE.

Nebido (Bayer) *See* TESTOSTERONE.

Nebilet (Menarini) *See* NEBIVOLOL.

nebivolol A cardioselective *beta blocker with vasodilating action, used for

the treatment of essential *hypertension and chronic heart failure. It is available as tablets on *prescription only.
Side effects, precautions, and interactions with other drugs: *see* BETA BLOCKERS.

See also ANTIHYPERTENSIVE DRUGS.
Proprietary preparation: Nebilet.

nebulizer A device that forces compressed air through a solution of a drug so that a fine spray is delivered to a face mask and can be inhaled. Nebulizers are often used to administer drugs to children who lack the coordination to use a metered-dose or breath-activated *inhaler.

nedocromil sodium A *chromone drug used to prevent attacks in the treatment of *asthma and for the treatment of allergic conjunctivitis. It is available as a metered-dose aerosol for inhalation, as a pump spray for the nose, and as eye drops. Nedocromil is a *prescription only medicine.
Side effects: with eye drops there may be mild local irritation and taste disturbances. When inhaled it may cause coughing, occasionally headache and stomach upsets, and rarely transient wheezing.
Proprietary preparations: Rapitil (eye drops); Tilade CFC-free Inhaler (aerosol inhaler); Tilarin (nasal spray).

nefopam An *analgesic used for the relief of persistent pain that has not responded to other non-opioid analgesics; the way in which it works is not completely understood. Nefopam is used to treat moderate pain, including that occurring after operations or dental procedures or associated with cancer; it does not reduce fever or inflammation. Nefopam is available as tablets on *prescription only.
Side effects: include nausea, nervousness, dry mouth, urinary retention, and dizziness.
Precautions: nefopam should not be used to relieve the pain of a heart attack and should not be taken by people with epilepsy or other convulsive disorders. It should be used with caution in people with liver or kidney disease or urinary retention, in elderly people, and in women who are pregnant or breastfeeding.
Interactions with other drugs:

MAOIs: should not be taken with nefopam.

Tricyclic antidepressants: may increase the side effects of nefopam.

Proprietary preparation: Acupan.

Negaban (Eumedica) *See* TEMOCILLIN.

nelarabine An *antimetabolite used for the treatment of T-cell acute lymphoblastic leukaemia and T-cell lymphoblastic lymphoma (types of *cancer affecting white blood cells called T cells) that have not responded to or have relapsed following treatment with at least two other chemotherapy drugs. It is available as an intravenous infusion on *prescription only.
Side effects: *see* CYTOTOXIC DRUGS. Additional side effects include loss of

appetite, numbness and 'pins and needles', unsteadiness, tremor, dizziness, headache, blurred vision, wheeze, breathlessness, and fatigue.
Precautions: *see* CYTOTOXIC DRUGS. In addition, nelarabine is associated with nerve damage, and patients should be closely observed for signs and symptoms of this.
Proprietary preparation: Atriance.

nelfinavir A protease inhibitor (*see* ANTIVIRAL DRUGS) that is used in combination with other antiretroviral drugs for the treatment of *HIV infection. It is available, on *prescription only, as tablets.
Side effects: include diarrhoea, flatulence, nausea, rashes, reduced white-blood-cell count, and hepatitis.
Precautions: nelfinavir should not be taken by women who are breastfeeding. It should be used with caution in people with kidney or liver disease, haemophilia, or diabetes and in pregnant women.
Interactions with other drugs: nelfinavir is a potent inhibitor of several enzyme systems in the liver that are involved in metabolizing drugs; it therefore has the potential to interact with many drugs. A doctor should be consulted before taking nelfinavir with any other drug.
Proprietary preparation: Viracept.

NeoClarityn (Schering-Plough) *See* DESLORATADINE.

Neo-Cytamen (UCB Pharma) *See* HYDROXOCOBALAMIN.

Neo-Mercazole (Amdipharm) *See* CARBIMAZOLE.

neomycin sulphate An *aminoglycoside antibiotic that is used to sterilize the bowel before surgery. Given by mouth a few hours before surgery, it acts locally on the gut but is not absorbed. It is also used to treat infections of the skin, ears, and eyes but is too toxic to be injected. Available on *prescription only, it is administered orally as tablets or topically as a cream, nose, ear, or eye drops, an ear or eye ointment, or by nasal spray.
Side effects, precautions, and interactions with other drugs: similar to those of *gentamicin, but as very little of the drug is absorbed into the body problems rarely occur.
Proprietary preparations: Nivemycin (tablets); *Neosporin (combined with polymyxin B sulphate); *Betnesol-N and *Betnovate-N (combined with betamethasone); *Dermovate-NN (combined with clobetasol and nystatin); *Maxitrol (combined with dexamethasone); *Naseptin (combined with chlorhexidine); *Neosporin (combined with polymyxin B and gramicidin); *Otomize (combined with dexamethasone); *Otosporin (combined with polymyxin B sulphate and hydrocortisone); *Predsol-N (combined with prednisolone); *Synalar N (combined with fluocinolone acetonide).

Neo-Naclex-K (Goldshield) A proprietary combination of *bendroflumethiazide (a thiazide diuretic) and *potassium chloride, used for the treatment of *hypertension and *oedema associated with heart failure,

liver disease, or kidney disease. It is available as *modified-release tablets on *prescription only.
Side effects, precautions, and interactions with other drugs: *see* THIAZIDE DIURETICS.

See also ANTIHYPERTENSIVE DRUGS; DIURETICS.

Neoral (Novartis) *See* CICLOSPORIN.

NeoRecormon (Roche Products) *See* ERYTHROPOIETIN.

Neosporin (Teva UK) A proprietary combination of *gramicidin, *neomycin, and *polymyxin B sulphate, used for the treatment of bacterial infections of the eye and for the prevention of infection after eye surgery. It is available as eye drops on *prescription only.
Side effects, precautions, and interactions with other drugs: *see* NEOMYCIN SULPHATE.

neostigmine An *anticholinesterase drug used for the treatment of myasthenia gravis. It is also injected by anaesthetists after surgery to reverse the action of drugs that have been used to paralyse or relax muscles during surgical procedures; for this purpose it is used in conjunction with *glycopyrronium bromide or (less commonly) *atropine sulphate. Neostigmine is available as tablets or an injection on *prescription only.
Side effects: nausea and vomiting, increased salivation, diarrhoea, and abdominal cramps are the most common side effects. Overdosage worsens these effects and can cause slowing of the heart rate and low blood pressure.
Precautions: neostigmine should not be given to people with intestinal or urinary obstruction or to those with asthma. It should be used with caution in those with low blood pressure, peptic ulcers, epilepsy, Parkinson's disease, or kidney disease.
Interactions with other drugs:

Antibiotics: aminoglycosides, clindamycin, and colistin antagonize the action of neostigmine.
Chloroquine: increases the symptoms of myasthenia gravis and thus diminishes the effect of neostigmine.
Hydroxychloroquine: increases the symptoms of myasthenia gravis and thus diminishes the effect of neostigmine.
Lithium: antagonizes the effect of neostigmine.
Propafenone: may antagonize the action of neostigmine.
Propranolol: antagonizes the action of neostigmine.

Neotigason (Actavis) *See* ACITRETIN.

nepafenac An *NSAID used for the treatment of postoperative pain and inflammation associated with cataract surgery. It is available as eye drops on *prescription only.
Side effects and precautions: headache, blurred vision, and a dry eye may occur. Nepafenac may cause corneal thinning, ulceration, or perforation; if there is any evidence of these, the drops should be discontinued and a doctor

consulted. Nepafenac should be used with caution in people with pre-existing corneal problems. It may cause temporary visual disturbance, which should be allowed to resolve completely before driving or operating machinery.
Proprietary preparation: Nevanac.

Nerisone, Nerisone Forte (Meadow) *See* DIFLUCORTOLONE VALERATE.

Neulactil (Winthrop Pharmaceuticals) *See* PERICYAZINE.

Neulasta (Amgen) *See* PEGFILGRASTIM.

Neupogen (Amgen) *See* FILGRASTIM.

Neupro (UCB Pharma) *See* ROTIGOTINE.

NeuroBloc (Eisai) *See* BOTULINUM TOXIN TYPE B.

neuroleptic drugs *See* ANTIPSYCHOTIC DRUGS.

Neurontin (Pfizer) *See* GABAPENTIN.

Neutrogena Norwegian Formula Dermatological Cream (Johnson & Johnson) *See* GLYCERIN.

Neutrogena T/Gel Therapeutic Shampoo (Johnson & Johnson) *See* COAL TAR.

Nevanac (Alcon) *See* NEPAFENAC.

nevirapine A non-nucleoside *antiviral drug that inhibits reverse transcriptase by binding directly to the enzyme, thus blocking the synthesis of retroviral DNA and preventing viral replication. It is used in combination therapy for the treatment of infections in patients with advanced or progressive *HIV disease. Nevirapine is available as tablets or a suspension on *prescription only.
Side effects: include rash (which should be reported to a doctor), nausea, fatigue, fever, headache, somnolence, and hepatitis.
Precautions: nevirapine should not be taken by people with severe liver disease or by women who are breastfeeding. It should be used with caution in all women.
Interactions with other drugs:
Antifungal drugs: nevirapine reduces the plasma concentration of ketoconazole and the two drugs should not be taken together; fluconazole increases the plasma concentration of nevirapine.
Antiviral drugs: the plasma concentrations of atazanavir and etravirine may be reduced by nevirapine and should not be taken with it.
Aripiprazole: its plasma concentration may be reduced and its dosage should therefore be increased.
Oral contraceptives: their contraceptive effect is reduced.
Rifampicin: reduces the plasma concentration of nevirapine and should not be taken with it.

St John's wort: reduces the plasma concentration of nevirapine and should not be taken with it.
Warfarin: its anticoagulant effect may be enhanced or reduced.
Proprietary preparation: Viramune.

Nexavar (Bayer) *See* SORAFENIB.

Nexium (AstraZeneca) *See* ESOMEPRAZOLE.

Niaspan (Abbott) *See* NICOTINIC ACID.

Nicam (Dermal Laboratories) *See* NICOTINAMIDE.

nicardipine A class II *calcium antagonist used for the prevention of chronic stable *angina and the treatment of *hypertension. It is available as capsules and *modified-release capsules on *prescription only.
Side effects: *see* CALCIUM ANTAGONISTS.
Precautions: nicardipine should not be used to treat unstable or acute angina or to treat patients who have had a heart attack during the previous month. It should not be taken by women who are pregnant or breastfeeding. *See also* CALCIUM ANTAGONISTS.
Interactions with other drugs:
Ciclosporin: its plasma concentration is increased by nicardipine.
Digoxin: its plasma concentration is increased by nicardipine.
Phenytoin: reduces the effects of nicardipine.
Rifampicin: may reduce the effects of nicardipine.
See also CALCIUM ANTAGONISTS.
Proprietary preparations: Cardene; Cardene SR (modified-release capsules).
See also ANTIHYPERTENSIVE DRUGS.

nicorandil A *potassium channel activator that is used for the prevention and long-term treatment of *angina. It is available as tablets on *prescription only.
Side effects: include headache (especially at the start of treatment), flushing, nausea, vomiting, dizziness, and weakness. High dosages of nicorandil may cause a fall in blood pressure and/or an increase in heart rate.
Precautions and interactions with other drugs: nicorandil should not be taken by people with low blood pressure or heart failure or by breastfeeding women. It should be used with caution in people with certain types of heart or lung disease and in women who are pregnant. Nicorandil's effects in lowering blood pressure may be increased if it is taken with alcohol, tricyclic antidepressants, or vasodilators. These effects are significantly increased by sildenafil, tadalafil, and vardenafil, which should not be taken with nicorandil.
Proprietary preparation: Ikorel.

Nicorette, Nicorette Inhalator, Nicorette Invisi, Nicorette Microtab, Nicorette Nasal Spray (McNeil Ltd) *See* NICOTINE.

nicotinamide A vitamin of the B group (*see* VITAMIN B COMPLEX). It is a derivative of *nicotinic acid, another B vitamin, and both forms of the vitamin

are equally active in the body, being required for many metabolic reactions. Deficiency can lead to pellagra, symptoms of which include dermatitis. Supplements of nicotinamide in the form of multivitamin preparations are used to treat or prevent deficiency; most of them are available without a prescription. Nicotinamide is also used for the *topical treatment of mild to moderate inflamed acne; it is available as a gel and can be obtained without a prescription, but only from pharmacies.
Side effects: the gel may cause dryness, itching, redness, or irritation of the skin.
Precautions: the gel should not be applied near the eyes, nostrils or mouth.
Proprietary preparations: Freederm (gel); Nicam (gel); *Pabrinex (combined with other B vitamins and vitamin C); *Yeast-Vite (combined with thiamine, riboflavin, and caffeine).

nicotine An *alkaloid that occurs in tobacco and is absorbed into the body when tobacco is chewed or smoked, causing an increase in blood pressure and heart rate and stimulating the brain and central nervous system. The effects of nicotine are responsible for the psychological *dependence of regular smokers on cigarettes; heavy smokers can experience withdrawal symptoms if they stop smoking abruptly.

Various nicotine products are available to help smokers give up the habit. Such products contain nicotine in precise amounts and are used to replace the nicotine usually obtained from cigarettes when a person is trying to give up smoking. The dosage of nicotine can then be reduced in a controlled manner to avoid the problem of withdrawal. Nicotine products in the form of chewing gum, inhalators ('mock cigarettes'), *transdermal (skin) patches, and *sublingual tablets can be obtained from pharmacies without a prescription; they cannot be prescribed on the NHS. A nasal spray is available on *prescription only.
Side effects: include nausea, dizziness, headache, influenza-like symptoms, palpitations, indigestion, insomnia and vivid dreams, and muscle aches. Skin patches may cause local reactions. Sprays can cause throat and nasal irritation, nose bleeds, watery eyes, and sensations in the ear. Gums can irritate the throat and cause mouth ulcers and sometimes swelling of the tongue. Inhalators can cause a sore mouth or throat, mouth ulcers, a swollen tongue, cough, running nose, and sinusitis.
Precautions: nicotine products should not be used by people with severe heart disease or after a heart attack or a recent stroke, or by women who are pregnant or breastfeeding. Patches are not suitable for occasional smokers and should never be placed on broken skin. People should not smoke while they are using nicotine products.
Interactions with other drugs:

Theophylline: nicotine products may reduce the effectiveness of theophylline.

Proprietary preparations: Boots NicAssist (chewing gum, inhalator, skin patches); Nicorette (chewing gum, skin patches); Nicorette Inhalator; Nicorette Invisi (skin patches); Nicorette Microtab (sublingual tablets);

Nicorette Nasal Spray; Nicotinell (chewing gum, lozenges, skin patches); NiQuitin (chewing gum, lozenges, skin patches).

Nicotinell (Novartis) *See* NICOTINE.

nicotinic acid A member of the *vitamin B complex. Nicotinic acid functions as a *lipid-lowering drug and is used as an adjunct to *statin: it reduces concentrations of *cholesterol and *triglycerides in the blood and increases HDL-cholesterol (*see* LIPOPROTEINS). However, it causes *vasodilatation and other side effects that may limit its use. Nicotinic acid is available as *modified-release tablets; it is a *prescription only medicine if used as a lipid-lowering drug.

Nicotinic acid derivatives are used as *vasodilators to treat peripheral vascular disease and other disorders of circulation, including Raynaud's syndrome (*see* INOSITOL NICOTINATE). They can reduce concentrations of fibrinogen (an agent involved in the clotting of blood) and lower blood viscosity (the fluidity of the blood). The nicotinic acid derivative *acipimox is used as a lipid-lowering drug.
Side effects: include flushing, dizziness, headache, nausea and vomiting, palpitations, and itching.
Precautions and interactions with other drugs: nicotinic acid should not be taken by women who are breastfeeding or by people with peptic ulcers, and it should be used with caution in people with diabetes, gout, liver or kidney disease, unstable *angina or in those who have had a heart attack and in pregnant women. It should also be used with caution if taken with statins, since the combination of these two types of lipid-lowering drugs can affect the muscles.
Proprietary preparations: Niaspan; *Tredaptive (combined with laropiprant).

nicoumalone *See* ACENOCOUMAROL.

nifedipine A class II *calcium antagonist used for the prevention of *angina and the treatment of *hypertension. It is also used to treat Raynaud's phenomenon (pallor and numbness of the fingers). A *prescription only medicine, it is available as capsules or tablets, some of which are *modified-release formulations.
Side effects: *see* CALCIUM ANTAGONISTS.
Precautions: nifedipine should not be used to treat unstable angina and should not be given to patients who have had a heart attack in the previous month. *See also* CALCIUM ANTAGONISTS.
Interactions with other drugs:

Antibiotics: rifampicin reduces the effects of nifedipine; Synercid increases the plasma concentration of nifedipine.

Beta blockers: may cause a profound fall in blood pressure and heart failure.

Digoxin: its plasma concentration may be increased by nifedipine.

Magnesium (injections): cause a profound fall in blood pressure.

Phenytoin: reduces the effects of nifedipine.

Tacrolimus: its plasma concentration may be increased by nifedipine.
See also CALCIUM ANTAGONISTS.

Proprietary preparations: Adalat (capsules); Adalat LA (modified-release tablets); Adalat Retard (modified-release tablets); Adipine MR (modified-release tablets); Adipine XL (modified-release tablets); Coracten SR, Coracten XL (modified-release capsules); Fortipine LA 40 (modified-release tablets); Hypolar Retard (modified-release tablets); Nifedipress MR (modified-release tablets); Tensipine MR (modified-release tablets); Valni XL (modified-release tablets); *Beta-Adalat (combined with atenolol); *Tenif (combined with atenolol).
See also ANTIHYPERTENSIVE DRUGS.

Nifedipress MR (Dexcel Pharma) *See* NIFEDIPINE.

Niferex, Niferex Drops (Tillomed Laboratories) *See* POLYSACCHARIDE–IRON COMPLEX.

Night Nurse (GlaxoSmithKline) A proprietary combination of *paracetamol (an analgesic and antipyretic), *promethazine hydrochloride (an antihistamine that induces drowsiness), and *dextromethorphan (a cough suppressant), taken at night to relieve the symptoms of colds, chills, and influenza. It is available as a liquid or capsules and can be obtained without a prescription, but only from pharmacies.
Side effects: *see* DEXTROMETHORPHAN; ANTIHISTAMINES.
Precautions: Night Nurse should not be given to children under six years old except on medical advice. *See also* PARACETAMOL; ANTIHISTAMINES; OPIOIDS.
Interactions with other drugs: *see* ANTIHISTAMINES; OPIOIDS.

n

nilotinib A *tyrosine kinase inhibitor used for the treatment of chronic myeloid leukaemia (*see* CANCER) that has failed to respond to at least one other therapy, including *imatinib. It is available as capsules on *prescription only.
Side effects: include abdominal pain, constipation, diarrhoea, indigestion, weight changes, *arrhythmias, flushing, cough, breathlessness, headache, fatigue, insomnia, dry skin, and rash.
Precautions: nilotinib should not be taken by breastfeeding women and should be used with caution in people susceptible to arrhythmias, in those with liver disease, and in pregnant women. *See also* CYTOTOXIC DRUGS.
Interactions with other drugs:
Antibiotics: rifampicin reduces the plasma concentration of nilotinib and should not be taken with it. Clarithromycin, moxifloxacin, and telithromycin should not be taken with nilotinib.
Antifungal drugs: itraconazole, ketoconazole, and voriconazole increase the plasma concentration of nilotinib and should not be taken with it.
Clozapine: increases the risk of agranulocytosis (a blood disorder) and should not be taken with nilotinib.
Ritonavir: should not be taken with nilotinib.
Proprietary preparation: Tasigna.

nimodipine A class II *calcium antagonist that relaxes the cerebral arteries,

which supply blood to the brain. It is used to prevent spasm of these arteries following a subarachnoid haemorrhage (bleeding into the spaces around the brain caused by a rupture of one of the cerebral arteries), and thus prevents further interruption of the blood supply to the brain. Nimodipine is available, as tablets or a solution for infusion, on *prescription only.
Side effects: include low blood pressure, flushing, headache, and gastrointestinal upset (including nausea).
Precautions: nimodipine should not be taken by people with unstable *angina or within one month of a heart attack. It should be used with caution in patients with swelling of the brain, raised pressure within the brain, or poor kidney function. *See also* CALCIUM ANTAGONISTS.
Interactions with other drugs:
Rifampicin: reduces the plasma concentration of nimedipine.
See also CALCIUM ANTAGONISTS.
Proprietary preparation: Nimotop.

Nimotop (Bayer) *See* NIMODIPINE.

Nipent (Hospira) *See* PENTOSTATIN.

NiQuitin (GlaxoSmithKline) *See* NICOTINE.

nitisinone A drug used in the treatment of hereditary tyrosinaemia type 1 (HT-1) in combination with dietary restriction of tyrosine and phenylalanine. HT-1 is a genetic disorder of protein metabolism in which an enzyme deficiency causes the build-up of the amino acid tyrosine in the blood and tissues, resulting in severe kidney and liver failure. Nitisinone works by preventing the accumulation of toxic metabolites of tyrosine in the tissues. It is taken as capsules under expert supervision and is available on *prescription only.
Side effects: include low counts of white blood cells and platelets, cloudiness and inflammation of the cornea, conjunctivitis, intolerance of the eye to light, and eye pain.
Precautions: regular eye and liver function tests should be carried out before and during treatment, and platelet and white cell counts should be monitored. Nitisinone should not be given to women who are pregnant or breastfeeding.
Proprietary preparation: Orfadin.

nitrates *Vasodilator drugs used in the treatment of *angina, and also as adjuncts to *cardiac glycosides and *diuretics in the treatment of congestive *heart failure. Nitrates dilate large veins, which reduces the amount of blood returning to the heart and therefore decreases the workload on the heart. The drugs in this group are *isosorbide mononitrate, *isosorbide dinitrate, and *glyceryl trinitrate. Nitrates are available in a variety of formulations: sublingual tablets (which dissolve in the mouth when placed under the tongue), buccal tablets (which dissolve when inserted between teeth and cheek), oral tablets (which are swallowed), *modified-release tablets and capsules, chewable tablets, a sublingual spray (which is absorbed across the

lining of the mouth), ointment or skin patches (both of which are applied to the chest wall and absorbed through the skin), and intravenous solutions. The choice of product depends on the onset and duration of action required.
Side effects: headache, flushing, and dizziness are the most common side effects; less commonly fainting may occur. Side effects decrease with long-term use.
Precautions: some patients on long-acting nitrates or transdermal patches rapidly develop *tolerance. Therefore longer acting tablets and modified-release preparations are usually administered so that there is a 'nitrate-free' period at night, and transdermal patches should be removed for several consecutive hours during each 24 hours. This helps to avoid tolerance and increases the efficacy of the nitrate in preventing angina attacks.
Interactions with other drugs:
Antihypertensive drugs: can cause a further lowering of blood pressure.
Sildenafil, tadalafil, and vardenafil: cause significant lowering of blood pressure and should not be used with nitrates.

nitrazepam A long-acting *benzodiazepine used for the short-term treatment of insomnia. It is available as tablets or an oral suspension on *prescription only; certain proprietary preparations cannot be prescribed on the NHS.
Side effects and precautions: *see* BENZODIAZEPINES; DIAZEPAM.
Interactions with other drugs: *see* BENZODIAZEPINES.
Proprietary preparations: Mogadon; Remnos; Somnite.

n

Nitrocine (UCB Pharma) *See* GLYCERYL TRINITRATE.

Nitro-Dur (Schering-Plough) *See* GLYCERYL TRINITRATE.

nitrofurantoin An *antibiotic used for the treatment of urinary-tract infections and to prevent infection during surgery of the genitourinary tract. It is especially useful for treating kidney infections that are resistant to other antibiotics. It is available, on *prescription only, as tablets, capsules, *modified-release capsules, or a suspension.
Side effects: include gastrointestinal upset, breathing difficulties, rash, and itching. Rare side effects are jaundice, inflammation of the liver, and blood disorders. The drug should be withdrawn if signs of breathing problems, jaundice, or liver problems occur.
Precautions: nitrofurantoin should not be taken by people with impaired kidney function or by women at the end of pregnancy or who are breastfeeding.
Interactions with other drugs:
Magnesium trisilicate: reduces absorption of nitrofurantoin.
Probenecid: increases the potential toxicity of nitrofurantoin.
Proprietary preparations: Furadantin; Macrobid; Macrodantin.

Nitrolingual Pumpspray (Merck Serono) *See* GLYCERYL TRINITRATE.

Nitromin (Egis) *See* GLYCERYL TRINITRATE.

Nitronal (Merck Serono) *See* GLYCERYL TRINITRATE.

Nivaquine (sanofi-aventis) *See* CHLOROQUINE.

Nivemycin (Sovereign Medical) *See* NEOMYCIN SULPHATE.

nizatidine An *H_2-receptor antagonist used in the treatment of duodenal or gastric ulcers, ulcers caused by use of *NSAIDs, and gastro-oesophageal reflux disease, and for the prevention of ulcer recurrence (*see* ACID-PEPTIC DISEASES). It is available as capsules or an injection on *prescription only. Packs containing no more than two weeks' supply of capsules, for the treatment and prevention of indigestion and heartburn in those over 16 years old, can be obtained from pharmacies without a prescription.
Side effects: include anaemia, sweating, itching, hepatitis, and jaundice. *See also* H_2-RECEPTOR ANTAGONISTS.
Precautions: nizatidine should be used with caution by people with liver or kidney disease and by women who are pregnant or breastfeeding.
Proprietary preparation: Axid.

Nizoral (Janssen-Cilag) *See* KETOCONAZOLE.

Nocutil *See* DESMOPRESSIN.

Nolvadex Forte (AstraZeneca) *See* TAMOXIFEN.

Non-Drowsy Sinutab (McNeil Ltd) A proprietary combination of *pseudoephedrine (a decongestant) and *paracetamol (an analgesic and antipyretic), used for the relief of upper airways infections, including colds, coughs, and nasal congestion. It is available as tablets and can be obtained without a prescription, but only from pharmacies.
Side effects and interactions with other drugs: *see* EPHEDRINE HYDROCHLORIDE; DECONGESTANTS.
Precautions: *see* PARACETAMOL; DECONGESTANTS; EPHEDRINE HYDROCHLORIDE.

Non-Drowsy Sudafed Children's Syrup (McNeil Ltd) *See* PSEUDOEPHEDRINE.

Non-Drowsy Sudafed Congestion and Headache Capsules (McNeil Ltd) A proprietary combination of *paracetamol (an analgesic and antipyretic), *caffeine (a stimulant), and *phenylephrine (a decongestant), used for the relief of sinusitis, nasal congestion, and fever. It is freely available *over the counter.
Side effects and interactions with other drugs: *see* PHENYLEPHRINE.
Precautions: *see* PARACETAMOL; CAFFEINE; PHENYLEPHRINE.

Non-Drowsy Sudafed Congestion, Cold and Flu Tablets (McNeil Ltd) A proprietary combination of *paracetamol (an analgesic and antipyretic) and *pseudoephedrine (a decongestant), used for the relief of sinusitis, nasal congestion, and fever. It is available without a prescription, but only from pharmacies.

Side effects and interactions with other drugs: *see* EPHEDRINE HYDROCHLORIDE; DECONGESTANTS.
Precautions: *see* PARACETAMOL; DECONGESTANTS; EPHEDRINE HYDROCHLORIDE.

Non-Drowsy Sudafed Congestion Relief Capsules (McNeil Ltd) *See* PHENYLEPHRINE.

Non-Drowsy Sudafed Decongestant Elixir (McNeil Ltd) *See* PSEUDOEPHEDRINE.

Non-Drowsy Sudafed Decongestant Nasal Spray (McNeil Ltd) *See* XYLOMETAZOLINE.

Non-Drowsy Sudafed Dual Relief Max (McNeil Ltd) A proprietary combination of *ibuprofen (an NSAID) and *pseudoephedrine (a decongestant), used for the relief of sinusitis, headache, and fever. It is available as tablets without a prescription, but only from pharmarcies.
Side effects and interactions with other drugs: *see* NSAIDs; EPHEDRINE HYDROCHLORIDE; DECONGESTANTS.
Precautions: *see* NSAIDs; DECONGESTANTS.

Non-Drowsy Sudafed Expectorant (McNeil Ltd) A proprietary combination of *guaifenesin (an expectorant) and *pseudoephedrine (a decongestant), used to relieve the symptoms of infection of the upper airways associated with a productive cough and sinusitis. It is available without a prescription, but only from pharmacies.
Side effects, precautions and interactions with other drugs: *see* EPHEDRINE HYDROCHLORIDE; DECONGESTANTS; GUAIFENESIN.

Non-Drowsy Sudafed Inhalant Oil (McNeil Ltd) An inhalant oil consisting of racemic *camphor, *eucalyptus oil, *menthol, and *peppermint oil, used for the relief of nasal congestion. Vapours from the oil are inhaled. It is freely available *over the counter.

Non-Drowsy Sudafed Linctus (McNeil Ltd) A proprietary combination of *pseudoephedrine (a decongestant) and *dextromethorphan (a cough suppressant), used for the relief of upper airways infections, including colds, coughs, and nasal congestion. It is available without a prescription, but only from pharmacies.
Side effects and interactions with other drugs: *see* DEXTROMETHORPHAN; EPHEDRINE HYDROCHLORIDE; DECONGESTANTS.
Precautions: *see* OPIOIDS; EPHEDRINE HYDROCHLORIDE; DECONGESTANTS.

nonoxinol-9 (**nonoxynol-9**) A drug that kills sperm and is the active ingredient of *spermicidal contraceptives. It is freely available *over the counter in the form of a cream.
Side effects: *see* SPERMICIDAL CONTRACEPTIVES.
Proprietary preparation: Gygel.

non-steroidal anti-inflammatory drugs *See* NSAIDs.

nonylic acid vanillylamide A drug that is used as a *rubefacient for the relief of muscular aches and pains. It is an ingredient of a cream that is freely available *over the counter.
Side effects and precautions: *see* RUBEFACIENTS.
Proprietary preparation: *Pain Relief Balm (combined with ethyl nicotinate and glycol salicylate).

Nootropil (UCB Pharma) *See* PIRACETAM.

noradrenaline (**norepinephrine**) A substance that transmits messages in the *sympathetic nervous system. It acts on *adrenoceptors to have effects on the heart, blood vessels, intestines, lungs, salivary glands, and bladder. It is also available as a drug, **noradrenaline acid tartrate** (**norepinephrine bitartrate**), which is used in an emergency to restore dangerously low blood pressure or to treat cardiac arrest. Noradrenaline is given by intravenous infusion (for low blood pressure) or by rapid injection into a vein or the heart (for cardiac arrest). Available on *prescription only, it is only used in a hospital setting.
Side effects: include hypertension (high blood pressure), headache, and arrhythmias (irregular heartbeat).
Precautions: noradrenaline should not be given to people with hypertension or to pregnant women. It should be used with caution in patients with thrombosis, diabetes, thyroid disease, or following a heart attack.
Interactions with other drugs:

Antidepressants: MAOIs and moclobemide may cause severe hypertension; hypertension and arrhythmias may occur if noradrenaline is given to patients who are taking tricyclic antidepressants.
Antiparkinsonian drugs: entacapone may increase the effects of noradrenaline; rasagiline may cause severe hypertension.
Beta blockers: may cause severe hypertension and a slow heart rate.
Dopexamine: may increase the effect of noradrenaline.

Proprietary preparation: Levophed.

Norditropin (Novo Nordisk) *See* SOMATROPIN.

norelgestromin *See* EVRA.

norepinephrine *See* NORADRENALINE.

norethisterone A synthetic *progestogen. Combined with *oestrogens it is used in *oral contraceptives, and as an *adjunct to oestrogens it is used as part of *hormone replacement therapy (HRT). It can be used alone as a progestogen-only contraceptive pill and – but only for a limited period – to delay menstruation, to treat heavy or painful periods, or to relieve premenstrual tension. Norethisterone is also used as a *depot contraceptive, which is given by intramuscular injection and lasts for up to eight weeks. It is also used to treat certain cancers. Norethisterone is available, on *prescription only, as tablets, skin patches, or as a solution for injection.

Side effects, precautions, and interactions with other drugs: *see* ORAL CONTRACEPTIVES; PROGESTOGENS.
Proprietary preparations: Micronor (contraceptive pill); Noriday (contraceptive pill); Noristerat (depot contraceptive); Primolut N (tablets); Utovlan (tablets); *BiNovum (combined with ethinylestradiol); *Brevinor (combined with ethinylestradiol); *Climagest (packaged with estradiol valerate); *Climesse (combined with estradiol valerate); *Clinorette (combined with estradiol); *Elleste Duet (packaged with estradiol); *Elleste Duet Conti (combined with estradiol); *Evorel Conti (combined with estradiol); *Evorel Sequi (combined with estradiol); *Kliofem (combined with estradiol); *Kliovance (combined with estradiol); *Loestrin 20 and Loestrin 30 (combined with ethinylestradiol); *Norimin (combined with ethinylestradiol); *Norinyl-1 (combined with mestranol); *Ovysmen (combined with levonorgestrel); *Novofem (combined with estradiol); *Synphase (combined with ethinylestradiol); *TriNovum (combined with ethinylestradiol); *Trisequens (combined with estradiol).

norfloxacin A *quinolone antibiotic, similar to *ciprofloxacin, that is used for the treatment and prevention of urinary-tract infections. It is available as tablets on *prescription only.
Side effects, precautions, and interactions with other drugs: *see* QUINOLONES.
Proprietary preparation: Utinor.

Norgalax Micro-enema (Norgine) *See* DOCUSATE SODIUM.

n

norgestimate A synthetic *progestogen used as an ingredient in combined *oral contraceptives. It is available on *prescription only.
Side effects, precautions, and interactions with other drugs: *see* ORAL CONTRACEPTIVES.
Proprietary preparation: *Cilest (combined with ethinylestradiol).

Norgeston (Bayer) *See* LEVONORGESTREL; ORAL CONTRACEPTIVES.

Noriday (Pharmacia) *See* NORETHISTERONE; ORAL CONTRACEPTIVES.

Norimin (Pharmacia) A proprietary combination of *ethinylestradiol and *norethisterone used as an *oral contraceptive. It is available as tablets on *prescription only.
Side effects, precautions, and interactions with other drugs: *see* ORAL CONTRACEPTIVES.

Norimode (Tillomed Laboratories) *See* LOPERAMIDE HYDROCHLORIDE.

Norinyl-1 (Pharmacia) A proprietary combination of *mestranol and *norethisterone used as an *oral contraceptive. It is available as tablets on *prescription only.
Side effects, precautions, and interactions with other drugs: *see* ORAL CONTRACEPTIVES.

Noristerat (Bayer) *See* NORETHISTERONE.

Normacol (Norgine) *See* STERCULIA.

Normacol Plus (Norgine) A proprietary combination of *sterculia and frangula (both *bulk-forming laxatives), used for treating constipation and for encouraging bowel movement after haemorrhoidectomy. It is freely available *over the counter in the form of granules.
Side effects and precautions: *see* ISPAGHULA HUSK.

normal immunoglobulin *See* IMMUNOGLOBULINS.

Normasol (Medlock) *See* SODIUM CHLORIDE.

Normax (UCB Pharma) *See* CO-DANTHRUSATE.

Norphyllin SR (Napp Pharmaceuticals) *See* AMINOPHYLLINE.

Norprolac (Ferring Pharmaceuticals) *See* QUINAGOLIDE.

nortriptyline A *tricyclic antidepressant drug used for the treatment of depressive illness and also bedwetting in children; it is less sedative than *amitriptyline. It is available as tablets on *prescription only.
Side effects, precautions, and interactions with other drugs: *see* AMITRIPTYLINE HYDROCHLORIDE; TRICYCLIC ANTIDEPRESSANTS.
Proprietary preparation: Allegron.

Norvir (Abbott) *See* RITONAVIR.

Norzol (Rosemont Pharmaceuticals) *See* METRONIDAZOLE.

Novgos (Genus Pharmaceuticals) *See* GOSERELIN.

Novofem (Novo Nordisk) A proprietary preparation of *estradiol tablets and combined estradiol/*norethisterone tablets, used as sequential combined *hormone replacement therapy for the relief of menopausal symptoms and prevention of osteoporosis in women who have not had a hysterectomy. It is available on *prescription only.
Side effects, precautions, and interactions with other drugs: *see* HORMONE REPLACEMENT THERAPY.

NovoMix 30 (Novo Nordisk) *See* INSULIN.

NovoRapid (Novo Nordisk) *See* INSULIN.

NovoSeven (Novo Nordisk) *See* FACTOR VIIA.

Noxafil (Schering-Plough) *See* POSACONAZOLE.

Nozinan (sanofi-aventis) *See* LEVOMEPROMAZINE.

NSAIDs (non-steroidal anti-inflammatory drugs) A large group of drugs that reduce inflammation. NSAIDs act by inhibiting the enzymes (cyclo-oxygenases: COX-1 and COX-2) required for the production of *prostaglandins, which are involved in inflammation. They also have *analgesic (pain-relieving) activity. NSAIDs are used for the long-term treatment of inflammatory rheumatic diseases and back pain; they are particularly appropriate for the relief of chronic pain and stiffness in inflammatory diseases of the joints, such as rheumatoid arthritis. NSAIDs are also used to relieve acute pain, such as that occurring after operations or associated with acute gout or heavy periods (in which they reduce the production of prostaglandins that are thought to be responsible for the increased blood flow and painful contractions of the uterus). In cancer patients, NSAIDs may reduce the need for *opioid analgesics; they are particularly suitable for the pain associated with secondary tumours (metastases) in bones.

Many of the side effects of NSAIDs are related to their suppression of prostaglandins, which – in addition to their role in the inflammatory response – also protect the lining of the stomach against attack by gastric acid (*see* ACID-PEPTIC DISEASES). Therefore many NSAIDs have adverse effects on the stomach and intestines (see Side effects below). However, these effects vary in severity with different NSAIDs; there is also considerable variation in how individuals respond to the different drugs in this group. It may therefore take a period of 'trial and error' before the NSAID that suits a particular individual is found. **COX-2 inhibitors** are a subgroup of NSAIDs that selectively inhibit cyclo-oxygenase 2 (COX-2) and appear to cause less severe adverse effects on the stomach and intestines. They include *celecoxib, *etoricoxib, and *parecoxib.

NSAIDs are available in a variety of forms, including tablets, capsules, *modified-release formulations, injections, and suppositories. Some are also available as gels or creams to be applied to the skin to relieve sprains, strains, aches, and pains. Most preparations are *prescription only medicines, but some can be obtained without a prescription.

n

See ACECLOFENAC; ACEMETACIN; AZAPROPAZONE; BENZYDAMINE HYDROCHLORIDE; DEXKETOPROFEN; DICLOFENAC SODIUM; ETODOLAC; FELBINAC; FENBUFEN; FENOPROFEN; FLURBIPROFEN; IBUPROFEN; INDOMETACIN; KETOPROFEN; KETOROLAC TROMETAMOL; MEFENAMIC ACID; MELOXICAM; NABUMETONE; NAPROXEN; NEPAFENAC; PIROXICAM; SULINDAC; TENOXICAM; TIAPROFENIC ACID; TOLFENAMIC ACID.

Side effects: gastrointestinal effects can include indigestion, nausea, diarrhoea, and occasionally bleeding and ulceration. Indigestion can be prevented by taking NSAIDs with milk or food; to reduce the likelihood of bleeding and ulceration, NSAIDs can be taken with an *antacid, *H_2-receptor antagonist, or *proton pump inhibitor, or with *misoprostol. NSAIDs can cause allergic reactions, such as rashes, an asthma attack, or (rarely) swelling of the face and constriction of the airways (*see* ANAPHYLAXIS). Other side effects may include headache, dizziness, vertigo, tinnitus (the sensation of noises in the ear), and sensitivity to sunlight (especially with topical preparations).

Precautions: NSAIDs should not be taken by people who have had allergic reactions to aspirin or other NSAIDs (including an asthma attack, itching, or a running nose) or by people who have peptic ulcers, except on medical advice. They should not be taken by women who are pregnant or breastfeeding.

NSAIDs should only be prescribed for people with a history of peptic ulcers and for elderly people after other treatments have been carefully considered. NSAIDs should be used with caution in people who have liver, kidney, or heart disease. Topical NSAIDs are usually not recommended for children. They should not come into contact with the eyes, lips, or other mucous membranes or with broken skin. Prolonged exposure of treated skin to sunlight should be avoided.

Interactions with other drugs:

ACE inhibitors: NSAIDs may reduce the effect of ACE inhibitors in lowering blood pressure.

Analgesics: aspirin should not be taken with other NSAIDs and two or more NSAIDs should not be taken together, since this is likely to increase their gastrointestinal side effects.

Antibiotics: NSAIDs may increase the risk of convulsions with quinolones.

Anticoagulants: the risk of bleeding may be increased if anticoagulants are taken with NSAIDs.

Antidepressants: the risk of bleeding is increased if SSRIs or venlafaxine are taken with NSAIDs.

Antidiabetic drugs: NSAIDs may enhance the effects of the sulphonylureas.

Ciclosporin: there is an increased risk of kidney damage if ciclosporin is taken with NSAIDs.

Diuretics: the risk of kidney damage is increased if diuretics are taken with NSAIDs.

Erlotinib: increases the risk of bleeding if taken with NSAIDs.

Lithium: its excretion is reduced by NSAIDs, so that it builds up in the bloodstream and is more likely to cause adverse effects.

Methotrexate: its excretion is reduced by NSAIDs, so that it builds up in the bloodstream and is more likely to cause adverse effects.

Phenytoin: its effects may be increased if taken with NSAIDs.

Probenecid: may increase the effects of NSAIDs.

Tacrolimus: there may be increased risk of kidney damage if this drug is taken with NSAIDs.

nucleoside analogues *See* ANTIVIRAL DRUGS.

Nuelin SA (Meda Pharmaceuticals) *See* THEOPHYLLINE.

Nurofen, Nurofen for Children (Reckitt Benckiser) *See* IBUPROFEN.

Nurofen Plus (Reckitt Benckiser) A proprietary combination of *ibuprofen (an NSAID) and *codeine phosphate (an opioid analgesic), used for the relief of migraine, tension headaches, toothache, period pains, sciatica, lumbago, and rheumatism. It is available as tablets and can be obtained without a prescription, but only from pharmacies.

Side effects, precautions, and interactions with other drugs: *see* IBUPROFEN; NSAIDs; CODEINE; OPIOIDS.

Nu-Seals Aspirin (Alliance) *See* ASPIRIN.

Nutraplus (Galderma) *See* UREA.

Nutrizym 10, Nutrizym 22 (Merck Serono) *See* PANCREATIN.

NutropinAq (Ipsen) *See* SOMATROPIN.

NuvaRing (Organon Laboratories) A proprietary combination of *etonogestrel and *ethinylestradiol, used as a *depot contraceptive in the form of a vaginal ring. The ring is inserted into the vagina on day 1 of each menstrual cycle and removed on day 22, after which breakthrough bleeding occurs. It is available on *prescription only.
Side effects, precautions, and interactions with other drugs: *see* ORAL CONTRACEPTIVES.

Nuvelle Continuous (Bayer) A proprietary preparation of *estradiol and *norethisterone, used as continuous combined *hormone replacement therapy for the relief of menopausal symptoms and the prevention of osteoporosis in women who have not had a hysterectomy. It is available as tablets on *prescription only.
Side effects, precautions, and interactions with other drugs: *see* HORMONE REPLACEMENT THERAPY.

Nyogel (Novartis) *See* TIMOLOL MALEATE.

Nystaform (Typharm) A proprietary combination of *nystatin (an antifungal drug) and *chlorhexidine (an antiseptic), used for the treatment of skin infections. It is available as a cream on *prescription only.
Side effects and precautions: *see* NYSTATIN.

n

Nystaform-HC (Typharm) A proprietary combination of *nystatin (an antifungal agent), *chlorhexidine (an antiseptic), and *hydrocortisone (a corticosteroid), used for the treatment of a variety of skin conditions in which infection is present or suspected. It is available as a cream or ointment on *prescription only.
Side effects and precautions: *see* TOPICAL STEROIDS.

Nystan (Bristol-Myers Squibb) *See* NYSTATIN.

nystatin An *antifungal drug that is particularly effective in treating candidiasis (thrush). Since it is not absorbed from the gastrointestinal tract, it is particularly useful for treating candidiasis of the mouth, throat, and gut, as well as the genital area. As it is too toxic to be administered intravenously, it is not suitable for treating systemic (generalized) infections. Nystatin is available, on *prescription only, as a suspension and a cream.
Side effects: high doses may cause nausea, vomiting, and diarrhoea. Oral preparations may cause local irritation and (rarely) allergic reactions, and a rash may rarely occur after topical application.
Precautions: nystatin should be used with caution by women who are pregnant or breastfeeding.
Proprietary preparations: Nystan; *Dermovate-NN (combined with clobetasol and neomycin); *Nystaform (combined with chlorhexidine);

*Nystaform-HC (combined with chlorhexidine and hydrocortisone); *Timodine (combined with hydrocortisone, benzalkonium chloride and dimeticone); *Trimovate (combined with clobetasone butyrate and oxytetracycline).

Nytol (GlaxoSmithKline) *See* DIPHENHYDRAMINE.

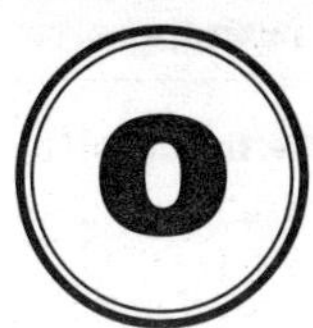

obesity The condition in which excess fat has accumulated in the body (mostly in the tissues beneath the skin), which is usually caused by the consumption of more food than is required for producing enough energy for daily activities. Obesity is usually considered to be present when a person is 20% above the recommended weight for his or her height and build. It is measured by means of the body mass index (BMI), which is calculated by dividing a person's weight by the square of their height. A BMI of 18.5–25 kg/m^2 is regarded as within the normal range; someone with a BMI of over 25 would be considered to be overweight, and a BMI of 30 or more indicates clinical obesity.

Obesity is the most common nutritional disorder of Western societies and predisposes to many health problems, including heart disease and diabetes. The main treatment is dietary restriction; drug treatment (if considered necessary) should only be used in conjunction with a carefully controlled diet. Anti-obesity drugs that act on the digestive tract include *orlistat and *methylcellulose; *sibutramine acts on the brain to suppress appetite.

Occlusal (Alliance) *See* SALICYLIC ACID.

octafonium chloride <**octaphonium chloride**> An antiseptic, similar to *cetrimide, that is an ingredient of an ointment for the treatment of minor wounds, cuts, grazes, burns, scalds, and blisters.
Proprietary preparation: *Germolene Antiseptic Ointment (combined with zinc oxide, methyl salicylate, and phenol).

Octagam (Octapharma) *See* IMMUNOGLOBULINS.

Octanate (Octapharma) *See* FACTOR VIII.

Octaplas SPC (Octapharma) A proprietary preparation made from frozen plasma, which contains clotting factors and other proteins necessary for blood clotting. It is used to replace clotting factor deficiencies occurring, for example, in liver failure or massive blood transfusion, and to reverse the effects of *warfarin. It is administered by intravenous infusion and is available on *prescription only.
Side effects: include fever, chills, nausea, vomiting, back pain, and (rarely) *anaphylaxis.
Precautions: Octaplas should be used with caution in people with heart failure or pulmonary *oedema and in pregnant women.

Octaplex (Octapharma) *See* PROTHROMBIN COMPLEX.

Octim (Ferring Pharmaceuticals) *See* DESMOPRESSIN.

octocog alfa *See* FACTOR VIII.

octreotide A long-acting *analogue of somatostatin, a hormone that is produced in the brain, gastrointestinal tract, and pancreas and inhibits the release of *growth hormone. It is used for the treatment of acromegaly (a conditon due to excessive secretion of growth hormone by a tumour in the pituitary gland), either in the short term for patients awaiting pituitary surgery and for the long-term treatment of those individuals with acromegaly who do not respond to surgery, *dopamine antagonists, or radiotherapy. It may also be used until radiotherapy is effective. Octreotide is also used to inhibit the secretions (and thus relieve the symptoms) of hormone-secreting tumours of the gastrointestinal tract. It is available as a solution for injection on *prescription only.
Side effects: include pain, stinging, and swelling at the injection site and gastrointestinal upsets, such as loss of appetite, nausea, vomiting, and abdominal pain; gallstones may develop with long-term treatment.
Precautions: octreotide should be used with caution in women who are pregnant or breastfeeding. Diabetic patients may need to reduce their dosage of insulin or oral antidiabetic drugs. Gall bladder function should be monitored throughout treatment. The drug should be stopped gradually at the end of treatment.
Interactions with other drugs:
Antidiabetic drugs: doses of these may need to be reduced (see Precautions).
Ciclosporin: octreotide reduces the plasma concentration of ciclosporin.
Cimetidine: octreotide may delay the absorption of cimetidine.
Proprietary preparations: Sandostatin; Sandostatin Lar (depot injection).

Ocufen (Allergan) *See* FLURBIPROFEN.

Oculotect (Novartis) *See* POVIDONE.

Ocusan (Agepha) *See* SODIUM HYALURONATE.

oedema Excessive accumulation of fluid in the body tissues. The resultant swelling may be local, as occurs after injury or with inflammation, or it may be more general, as in *heart failure. In generalized oedema there may be accumulation of fluid within the chest cavity (pleural effusion) or abdomen (ascites). Oedema can also occur within the spaces of the lungs (**pulmonary oedema**). Other causes of oedema include varicose veins, cirrhosis of the liver, acute inflammation of the kidney or other kidney disease, starvation, and (rarely) diabetes. Allergic reactions may be accompanied by local oedema. It can also be produced in response to some drugs. In all these cases the kidneys can be stimulated to excrete more urine by using a *diuretic. Temporary oedema can occur before menstruation or on long-haul flights, when it typically affects the legs, ankles, and feet.

oestradiol *See* ESTRADIOL.

oestriol *See* ESTRIOL.

Oestrogel (Ferring Pharmaceuticals) *See* ESTRADIOL; HORMONE REPLACEMENT THERAPY.

oestrogen antagonists (**anti-oestrogens**) Drugs that oppose the action of oestrogens, the female sex hormones. The main anti-oestrogens are *clomifene citrate, *tamoxifen, and *toremifene. In the brain, oestrogen normally prevents the release of *gonadotrophins from the pituitary gland. Oestrogen antagonists block this action, so that the pituitary is stimulated to produce greater amounts of gonadotrophins, which (in women) stimulate the ovaries to produce egg cells. Anti-oestrogens are therefore used in the treatment of infertility in women. Tamoxifen, *fulvestrant, and toremifene can also block the action of oestrogen in other cells of the body, including cancer cells, and are therefore also used to treat tumours that require oestrogen for their continued growth. *See also* AROMATASE INHIBITORS.

oestrogens A group of steroid hormones, including *estradiol, *estriol, and *estrone, that control female sexual development, promoting growth and function of the female sex organs and female secondary sex characteristics (such as breast development and growth of pubic hair). Oestrogens are synthesized mainly by the ovaries; small amounts are produced by the adrenal glands, testes, and placenta. Naturally occurring oestrogens and **conjugated oestrogens** (mixtures of natural oestrogens obtained from the urine of pregnant mares) are used mainly to treat a deficiency of these hormones (resulting in lack of sexual development and absence of periods) and symptoms of the menopause (*see* HORMONE REPLACEMENT THERAPY). Synthetic oestrogens (*see* ETHINYLESTRADIOL; MESTRANOL) are used mainly in *oral contraceptives, in which they are combined with *progestogens, but some preparations are used in HRT (*see also* ESTROPIPATE). Oestrogens are also used to treat some menstrual disorders and certain types of prostate and breast cancer.
Side effects: include nausea and vomiting, swelling and tenderness of the breasts, weight gain due to fluid and salt retention, abdominal cramps, headache and dizziness, and irregular vaginal bleeding. There may be changes in libido and depression, and contact lenses may irritate.
Precautions: prolonged treatment with oestrogens alone may increase the risk of cancer of the endometrium (lining of the uterus). For this reason women with an intact uterus who are undergoing hormone replacement therapy are usually given oestrogens in combination with a progestogen. Oestrogens should not be used during pregnancy or breastfeeding or by women with cancer of the breast, uterus, or genital tract (or a history of these oestrogen-dependent cancers), thrombosis, liver disorders, or undiagnosed vaginal bleeding. Oestrogens should be used with caution by women with a history of migraine (or migraine-like headaches) or breast lumps. Oestrogens can increase the size of existing fibroids and exacerbate the symptoms of *endometriosis.
Interactions with other drugs:
ACE inhibitors: their effect in lowering blood pressure is reduced.

Antibiotics: ampicillin, tetracyclines, rifabutin, and rifampicin reduce the effects of oestrogens.
Anticoagulants: the effects of warfarin and acenocoumarol may be enhanced or reduced; the effects of phenindione are antagonized.
Antiepileptic drugs: carbamazepine, oxcarbazepine, phenobarbital, phenytoin, primidone, rufinamide, and topiramate reduce the effects of oestrogens.
Antifungal drugs: griseofulvin, fluconazole, itraconazole, and ketoconazole can reduce the effects of oestrogens.
Antiviral drugs: nelfinavir, nevirapine, and ritonavir reduce the effects of oestrogen; atazanavir increases the plasma concentration of ethinylestradiol and should not be used with it.
Aprepitant: may reduce the effects of oestrogens.
Beta blockers: their effect in lowering blood pressure is reduced.
Bile acids: oestrogens increase the elimination of cholesterol in bile.
Bosentan: may reduce the effects of oestrogens.
Ciclosporin: oestrogens increase the plasma concentration (and therefore side effects) of ciclosporin.
Modafinil: reduces the effects of oestrogens.
St John's wort: reduces the effects of oestrogens and should not be used with them.

oestrone *See* ESTRONE.

ofloxacin A *quinolone antibiotic, similar to *ciprofloxacin, that is used for the treatment of infections of the urinary tract, respiratory tract, and skin. It is also used to treat infections of the genital tract (including gonorrhoea and nongonococcal urethritis) and bacterial infections of the eye. It is available, on *prescription only, as tablets, a solution for *intravenous infusion, or eye drops.
Side effects, precautions, and interactions with other drugs: *see* QUINOLONES.
Proprietary preparations: Exocin (eye drops); Tarivid.

Oftaquix (Kestrel) *See* LEVOFLOXACIN.

Oilatum Cream (GlaxoSmithKline) *See* ARACHIS OIL.

Oilatum Emollient, Oilatum Junior Emollient (GlaxoSmithKline) *See* LIQUID PARAFFIN.

Oilatum Plus (GlaxoSmithKline) A proprietary combination of *benzalkonium chloride and *triclosan (both antiseptics) and *liquid paraffin (an emollient), to be added to the bath for the treatment of *eczema, particularly if there is a risk of this becoming infected. It is also available as a shower gel. Oilatum Plus is freely available *over the counter.

ointment A greasy preparation that is applied to the skin or mucous membranes; it may or may not contain pharmacologically active ingredients. Ointments are usually insoluble in water and not easily removed from the surface to which they are applied (*compare* CREAM). Skin ointments commonly contain soft paraffin and/or liquid paraffin. *See* EMOLLIENTS.

olanzapine An atypical *antipsychotic drug used for the treatment of schizophrenia and mania. It is available as tablets, dispersible tablets, or a form for injection on *prescription only.
Side effects: include weight gain, dizziness, low blood pressure on standing (which can cause fainting in some people), drowsiness, increased appetite, and mild antimuscarinic effects (*see* CHLORPROMAZINE HYDROCHLORIDE). Occasionally olanzapine causes blood disorders.
Precautions: olanzapine should not be taken by people with acute glaucoma or by women who are breastfeeding. It should be used with caution by pregnant women, men with an enlarged prostate gland, and by anyone with liver or kidney disease, a low white blood cell count, or bone marrow suppression.
Interactions with other drugs:
Anaesthetics: their effect in lowering blood pressure is enhanced.
Antidepressants: there is an increased risk of antimuscarinic effects and arrhythmias if olanzapine is taken with tricyclic antidepressants; fluvoxamine increases the plasma concentration of olanzapine.
Antiepileptic drugs: their anticonvulsant effects are antagonized by olanzapine; carbamazepine reduces the effects of olanzapine; valproate increases the risk of low blood counts of neutrophils (a type of white blood cell).
Ritonavir: may increase the effects of olanzapine.
Sedatives: the sedative effects of olanzapine are increased if it is taken with anxiolytic or hypnotic drugs, or any other drug that causes sedation.
Sibutramine: increases the risk of adverse effects on the central nervous system.
Proprietary preparations: ZypAdhera (injection); Zyprexa.

Olbas Oil (Lane Health Products) A proprietary combination of *eucalyptus oil, *menthol, *cajuput oil, *clove oil, *juniper berry oil, and *methyl salicylate. It can be inhaled (from a handkerchief or dissolved in hot water) to relieve bronchial and nasal congestion due to colds, influenza, catarrh, and hay fever or applied topically to relieve muscular aches and pains or stiffness due to backache, sciatica, lumbago, or fibrositis. Olbas Oil is freely available *over the counter.
Precautions: Olbas Oil is not recommended for children under two years old.

Olbas Pastilles (Lane Health Products) A proprietary combination of *eucalyptus oil, *menthol, *peppermint oil, *clove oil, *juniper berry oil, and *methyl salicylate, used for the relief of colds, coughs, catarrh, sore throats, influenza, nasal congestion, and catarrhal headaches. These pastilles are freely available *over the counter.
Precautions: Olbas Pastilles are not recommended for children under seven years old.

Olbetam (Pharmacia) *See* ACIPIMOX.

olmesartan An *angiotensin II inhibitor used for the treatment of essential *hypertension. It is available as tablets on *prescription only.
Side effects: *see* ANGIOTENSIN II INHIBITORS. There may also be stomach upsets, chest pain, and swelling of the ankles.
Precautions: olmesartan should not be taken by pregnant women or by people with an obstructed bile duct or severe liver or kidney disease. *See also* ANTIHYPERTENSIVE DRUGS.
Interactions with other drugs: *see* ACE INHIBITORS; ANTIHYPERTENSIVE DRUGS.
Proprietary preparations: Olmetec, *Olmetec Plus (combined with hydrochlorothiazide); *Sevikar (combined with amlodipine).

Olmetec (Daiichi Sankyo UK Ltd) *See* OLMESARTAN.

Olmetec Plus (Daiichi Sankyo UK Ltd) A proprietary combination of *olmesartan) (an angiotensin II inhibitor) and *hydrochlorothiazide (a thiazide diuretic), used in the treatment of essential *hypertension. It is available as tablets on *prescription only.
Side effects and precautions: *see* OLMESARTAN; THIAZIDE DIURETICS; ANTIHYPERTENSIVE DRUGS.
Interactions with other drugs: *see* ACE INHIBITORS; THIAZIDE DIURETICS; ANTIHYPERTENSIVE DRUGS.

olopatadine An *antihistamine used for the treatment of seasonal allergic conjunctivitis. It is available as eye drops on *prescription only.
Side effects: include eye pain and irritation.
Precautions: olopatadine should not be used while wearing contact lenses, and should be used with caution by women who are pregnant or breastfeeding. It may cause temporary blurring of vision, affecting the ability to drive or use machinery.
Proprietary preparation: Opatanol.

olsalazine sodium An *aminosalicylate used for the treatment of mild ulcerative colitis and to maintain patients in remission from it. It is available as capsules or tablets on *prescription only.
Side effects: include diarrhoea and joint pains; *see also* AMINOSALICYLATES.
Precautions: *see* AMINOSALICYLATES.
Proprietary preparation: Dipentum.

Omacor (Solvay Healthcare) *See* OMEGA-3 FATTY ACID COMPOUNDS.

omalizumab A *monoclonal antibody used for the treatment of severe allergic asthma that is not controlled by inhaled beta agonists and corticosteroids. It acts by binding to a specific type of *immunoglobulin that is involved in the allergic response. Omalizumab is given by subcutaneous injection and is available on *prescription only.
Side effects: include headache and reactions at the injection site.
Precautions: omalizumab should not be given to breastfeeding women and

should be used with caution in people with autoimmune disease and liver or kidney disease and in pregnant women.
Proprietary preparation: Xolair.

omega-3 fatty acid compounds Preparations of fish oils that are rich in certain essential fatty acids. They reduce plasma concentrations of *triglycerides and are used in treating people with high plasma triglyceride concentrations. These compounds are available as capsules or a liquid in two forms – **omega-3 acid ethylesters** and **omega-3 marine triglycerides** – and can be obtained from pharmacies without a prescription.
Side effects: fish oils can cause occasional nausea, belching, or other gastrointestinal upsets.
Precautions: fish oils should be used with caution by people who have bleeding disorders and by those who are taking anticoagulants. Esters should not be taken by breastfeeding women.
Proprietary preparations: Maxepa (triglycerides); Omacor (esters).

omeprazole A *proton pump inhibitor used for the treatment of reflux oesophagitis, gastric and duodenal ulcers (including those associated with *Helicobacter pylori* infection and the use of *NSAIDs), Zollinger-Ellison syndrome, and other kinds of *acid-peptic disease. It is available as capsules, tablets, dispersible tablets, and a form for intravenous injection or infusion on *prescription only.
Side effects: include nausea, headache, diarrhoea, constipation, dizziness, itching, rashes, allergic reactions, sensitivity of the skin to sunlight, and 'pins and needles'.
Precautions: *see* PROTON PUMP INHIBITORS.
Interactions with other drugs:
Antifungal drugs: the absorption of ketoconazole and itraconazole may be reduced by omeprazole.
Antiplatelet drugs: the effects of clopidogrel and prasugrel may be reduced and these drugs should not be taken with omeprazole.
Antiviral drugs: omeprazole reduces the plasma concentrations of atazanavir and nelfinavir (which should not be used with it); omeprazole increases the plasma concentration of raltegravir and should not be used with it; tipranavir reduces the plasma concentration of omeprazole.
Cilostazol: its plasma concentration (and possibly adverse effects) are increased and it should not be used with omeprazole.
Digoxin: its plasma concentration may be increased by omeprazole.
Phenytoin: its effect may be enhanced by omeprazole.
Warfarin: its effect is enhanced by omeprazole.
Proprietary preparations: Losec; Losec MUPS (dispersible tablets); Mepradec (capsules).

Omnitrope (Sandoz) *See* SOMATROPIN.

Oncovin (Baxter Healthcare) *See* VINCRISTINE SULPHATE.

ondansetron An *antiemetic used for the prevention or treatment of

nausea and vomiting associated with *cytotoxic chemotherapy or radiotherapy or occurring after surgery. It acts by opposing the action of the neurotransmitter 5-hydroxytryptamine (*serotonin) at receptors in the central nervous system and in the gut. It is available, on *prescription only, as tablets, suppositories, syrup, or an intramuscular or intravenous injection.
Side effects: include headache, constipation, a sense of flushing or warmth, and hiccups.
Precautions: ondansetron should be used with caution by people with liver disease or certain types of *arrhythmia and by women who are pregnant or breastfeeding.
Proprietary preparations: Ondemet; Zofran; Zofran Melt (dispersible tablets).

Ondemet (Beacon Pharmaceuticals) *See* ONDANSETRON.

One Alpha (Leo Pharmaceuticals) *See* ALFACALCIDOL.

Onkotrone (Baxter Healthcare) *See* MITOXANTRONE.

Opatanol (Alcon) *See* OLOPATADINE.

opiates *See* OPIOIDS.

Opilon (Archimedes Pharma) *See* MOXISYLYTE.

opioids A group of *analgesics that includes the **opiates** – naturally occurring compounds, such as *morphine, found in the opium poppy (*Papaver somniferum*) and their derivatives – together with synthetic drugs that have similar effects. Opioids are extremely effective pain-killers, but people are often reluctant to use them because of fears of addiction and associations with illicit 'street drugs'. When taken repeatedly, opioids can cause *dependence, and *tolerance to their action may develop, so that increased doses are required to produce the same analgesic effect (see side effects and precautions below). However, when used in a clinical setting for the control of acute pain, there is little risk of opioids causing dependence.

Opioids are classified as **weak opioids** or **strong opioids**. Weak opioids, such as *codeine, and *dihydrocodeine, are used for the treatment of mild to moderate pain. Strong opioids, which include morphine, *diamorphine, *fentanyl, *alfentanil, and *oxycodone, are particularly useful in controlling severe pain, such as that associated with major surgery or advanced cancer. For chronic pain, treatment will often start with weak opioids (usually in combination with other analgesics) and then progress to strong opioids, either alone or in combination with other analgesics. The advantage of including other analgesics is to reduce the dosages and therefore the side effects of the opioids.

Some opioids are used to suppress coughing and to treat diarrhoea. Opioid *cough suppressants include codeine, *dextromethorphan, and *pholcodine (the last two have no analgesic activity). Opioids used as *antidiarrhoeal drugs include codeine, morphine, *loperamide hydrochloride, and **diphenoxylate hydrochloride** (combined with atropine in *co-phenotrope).

Because of their potential for abuse, many opioids are *controlled drugs, i.e. their prescription and use is strictly regulated.
Side effects and precautions: the most common side effects of opioids are nausea and vomiting, constipation, and drowsiness (which may affect driving ability and the performance of other skilled tasks. The effects of alcohol may be enhanced by opioids. People taking opioids should be warned that there may be withdrawal symptoms (including sweating, hallucinations, and strange dreams) when the drug is stopped, particularly if high dosages have been used. *See also* MORPHINE.
Interactions with other drugs: because the effects of opioids can be additive, opioids should not be used in combination with each other. Opioids enhance the sedative effects of anxiolytic drugs, hypnotics, and antipsychotics.

Antidepressants: MAOIs may have severe effects on blood pressure; opioids should therefore not be taken with MAOIs or for two weeks after stopping MAOIs; moclobemide can raise or lower blood pressure.
Antihistamines: their sedative effects are increased.
Sodium oxybate: its effects are enhanced and it should not be used with opioids.
Details of specific interactions are listed at entries for individual opioids.

Opizone (Britannia Pharmaceuticals) *See* NALTREXONE HYDROCHLORIDE.

Opticrom (sanofi-aventis) *See* SODIUM CROMOGLICATE.

Optilast (Meda Pharmaceuticals) *See* AZELASTINE HYDROCHLORIDE.

Optimax (Merck Serono) *See* TRYPTOPHAN.

Optivate (Bio Products Laboratory) A proprietary combination of *Factor VIII and *von Willebrand factor (both blood-clotting factors), used for treating haemophilia A (*see* HAEMOSTATIC DRUGS). It is available as a form for injection on *prescription only.
Side effects: *see* FACTOR VIII.

Optive (Allergan) A proprietary combination of *carmellose sodium (a tear thickener and strengthener) and *glycerin (an emollient), used for the relief of dry eyes. It is available *over the counter in the form of eye drops.

Optrex (Crookes Healthcare) *See* HAMAMELIS.

Optrex Allergy Eye Drops (Crookes Healthcare) *See* SODIUM CROMOGLICATE.

Orabase (ConvaTec) A proprietary combination of *carmellose sodium (a protective agent) and pectin and gelatine (which thicken the preparation and encourage its adherence to the lining of the mouth). It is used to protect mouth sores and ulcers against abrasions and the action of saliva. Orabase is available as an ointment and can be obtained without a prescription, but only from pharmacies.

Oragard-B (Colgate-Palmolive) *See* BENZOCAINE.

oral Taken by mouth. *Compare* PARENTERAL.

oral antidiabetic drugs *See* ORAL HYPOGLYCAEMIC DRUGS.

Oralbalance (Anglian Pharma) A proprietary combination of *xylitol (a sugar) and oxidase enzymes (to replace normal salivary enzymes), used as an artificial saliva for the relief of dry mouth, which occurs, for example, after radiotherapy. It is freely available *over the counter in the form of a gel.

oral contraceptives Tablets consisting of one or more synthetic female sex hormones taken by women to prevent pregnancy. Most oral contraceptives are **combined pills** (known colloquially as 'the pill'), consisting of an *oestrogen and a *progestogen, which suppress ovulation by, respectively, blocking the release of follicle-stimulating hormone and blocking the release of luteinizing hormone from the pituitary gland (*see* GONADOTROPHINS). Progestogens also alter the lining of the uterus and the viscosity of mucus in the cervix, so that conception is less likely. The oestrogens used in combined pills are *ethinylestradiol, *mestranol (which is converted to ethinylestradiol in the body), and *estradiol; a variety of progestogens are used, including *desogestrel, *etonogestrel, *gestodene, *levonorgestrel, *norgestimate, and *norethisterone. **Biphasic** and **triphasic pills** are taken in two or three phases during the menstrual cycle. The tablets in each phase contain different amounts of oestrogen and progestogen to be taken on different days of the cycle; therefore the pills must be taken in the right order: packaging usually makes this a simple procedure. Phasic pills are designed to reduce the total amount of hormones taken, but still retain the same efficacy. Combined pills are usually taken for 21 days, with a gap of 7 days before starting the next cycle during which the 'period' occurs. Some combined pills, known as **everyday (ED) pills**, are packaged with placebo (dummy) pills for these 7 days so that a tablet is taken every day and thus the need to remember when to start the next pack is eliminated. It is best to take combined pills at the same time every day to maintain their efficacy. A pill that is taken more than 12 hours late is regarded as 'missed', and the normal cycle of pill taking should be resumed as soon as possible by taking the missed pill and continuing with the rest of the pack; in addition, extra contraception should be used for 7 days. If the 7 days of extra precautions run past the end of a pack, a new pack should be started immediately; i.e. without the usual 7-day gap in pill taking or without taking the 7 dummy pills in ED preparations. Most of the side effects of the pill (see below) are related to the oestrogen content. There is a small risk that blood clots may form in the veins, especially the deep veins of the legs (deep-vein *thrombosis), which may be carried in the bloodstream and block a blood vessel in another part of the body (thromboembolism), most often in the lungs. This risk is greater with some oral contraceptives than with others, depending on which progestogen is used in the preparation. However, the risk of a thromboembolism is actually higher during pregnancy.

Progestogen-only pills contain only a synthetic progestogen and no oestrogen. In some women these pills suppress ovulation completely; in others the normal menstrual cycle occurs. Because they cause fewer side effects than the combined pill, progestogen-only pills are more acceptable to some women, especially those who are breastfeeding, who have diabetes, who are at risk of developing thromboembolism (see precautions below), or who cannot take oestrogens. These pills should be taken every day of the cycle, at the same time each day – preferably several hours before intercourse. A pill should be regarded as missed if only 3 hours late, in which case the pills should be resumed as soon as possible and extra contraception should be used for the following week.

A progestogen-only pill containing a high dose of levonorgestrel is available for postcoital (emergency) contraception – the so-called 'morning-after pill'.

Oral contraceptives may also be given to regulate the menstrual cycle, to relieve very heavy or painful periods, and to treat premenstrual tension. They are available on *prescription only.

Side effects: with combined pills, these include breast enlargement, fluid retention with a bloated feeling, weight gain, cramps and pains in the legs, headache, nausea, vomiting, depression, loss of libido, vaginal discharge, skin changes (including brown patches on the face), and breakthrough bleeding. There may be changes in libido, depression, an increase in blood pressure, and irritation from contact lenses. The occurrence of a migraine-like headache for the first time, frequent severe headaches, or visual disturbance should be reported immediately to a doctor. For side effects of progestogen-only pills, *see* PROGESTOGENS.

Precautions: combined pills should not be used during breastfeeding or by women with a history of thrombosis, heart disease, or angina, sickle-cell anaemia, a history of jaundice during pregnancy or any liver disease, breast or genital cancer, or undiagnosed vaginal bleeding; they should not be taken during pregnancy and must be stopped if pregnancy occurs. Combined pills should be used with caution by women with high blood pressure, Raynaud's syndrome, diabetes, varicose veins, asthma, severe depression, or multiple sclerosis and by those on dialysis. The risk of thombosis is increased with age, smoking, and obesity. Breast examination should be carried out before and during treatment. For precautions with progestogen-only pills, *see* PROGESTOGENS.

Interactions with other drugs (of combined pills):

ACE inhibitors: their effect in lowering blood pressure is reduced.

Antibiotics: ampicillin, tetracycline, rifabutin, and rifampicin reduce the contraceptive effect of combined pills. Additional contraception should be used while taking a short course of broad-spectrum antibiotics and for 7 days after stopping treatment; for women taking rifampicin, additional contraception should be continued for 4–8 weeks after stopping this drug. Women taking a longer course of these antibiotics are advised to use an oral contraceptive containing a higher dose (50 micrograms) of ethinylestradiol; for women taking a longer course of rifampicin, an alternative method of contraception may be advised.

Anticoagulants: the effects of warfarin, acenocoumarol, and phenindione are antagonized.

Antiepileptic drugs: carbamazepine, oxcarbazepine, phenobarbital,

phenytoin, primidone, rufinamide, and topiramate reduce the contraceptive effect of combined pills. Additional contraception should be used while taking a short course of these drugs and for 7 days after stopping treatment. Women taking a longer course of these drugs are advised to use an oral contraceptive containing a higher dose (50 micrograms) of ethinylestradiol.
Antifungal drugs: griseofulvin, fluconazole, itraconazole, and ketoconazole can reduce the contraceptive effect of combined pills. Additional contraception should be used while taking a short course of these drugs and for 7 days after stopping treatment. Women taking a longer course of these drugs are advised to use an oral contraceptive containing a higher dose (50 micrograms) of ethinylestradiol.
Aprepitant: reduces the contraceptive effect of combined pills.
Antiviral drugs: reduce the contraceptive effect of combined pills.
Bosentan: reduces the contraceptive effect of combined pills.
Ciclosporin: combined pills increase the plasma concentration (and therefore side effects) of ciclosporin.
Modafinil: reduces the contraceptive effect of combined pills.
St John's wort: reduces the contraceptive effect of combined pills and should not be taken with them.

Proprietary preparations: see table.

See also DEPOT CONTRACEPTIVES.

Oral contraceptives

Proprietary preparation	Ingredients	Formulation (per 28-day pack)
Combined pills		
Brevinor	†ethinylestradiol norethisterone	21 active tablets
Cilest	ethinylestradiol norgestimate	21 active tablets
Femodene	ethinylestradiol gestodene	21 active tablets
Femodene ED	ethinylestradiol gestodene	21 active tablets + 7 dummy tablets
Femodette	ethinylestradiol gestodene	21 active tablets
Loestrin 20	ethinylestradiol (20 mcg) norethisterone	21 active tablets
Loestrin 30	ethinylestradiol (30 mcg) norethisterone	21 active tablets
Marvelon	ethinylestradiol desogestrel	21 active tablets
Mercilon	ethinylestradiol (20 mcg) desogestrel	21 active tablets

Proprietary preparation	Ingredients	Formulation (per 28-day pack)
Microgynon 30	ethinylestradiol levonorgestrel	21 active tablets
Microgynon 30 ED	ethinylestradiol levonorgestrel	21 active tablets + 7 dummy tablets
Norimin	ethinylestradiol norethisterone	21 active tablets
Norinyl-1	mestranol (50 mcg) norethisterone	21 active tablets
Ovranette	ethinylestradiol levonorgestrel	21 active tablets
Ovysmen	ethinylestradiol norethisterone	21 active tablets
Qlaira	estradiol dienogest	21 active tablets
Sunya 20/75	ethinylestradiol gestodene	21 active tablets
Yasmin	ethinylestradiol drospirenone	21 active tablets
Phasic combined pills		
BiNovum	ethinylestradiol norethisterone	2 phases (7 + 14) of active tablets
Logynon	ethinylestradiol levonorgestrel	3 phases (6 + 5 + 10) of active tablets
Logynon ED	ethinylestradiol levonorgestrel	3 phases (6 + 5 + 10) of active tablets + 7 dummy tablets
Synphase	ethinylestradiol norethisterone	3 phases (7 + 9 + 5) of active tablets
Triadene	ethinylestradiol gestodene	3 phases (6 + 5 + 10) of active tablets
TriNovum	ethinylestradiol norethisterone	3 phases (7 + 7 + 7) of active tablets
Progestogen-only pills		
Cerazette	desogestrel	28 active tablets
Femulen	ethynodiol diacetate	28 active tablets
Micronor	norethisterone	28 active tablets
Norgeston	levonorgestrel	28 active tablets
Noriday	norethisterone	28 active tablets

† doses of ethinylestradiol/mestranol are 30–35 mcg (standard strength) except where otherwise stated

Oraldene (McNeil Ltd) *See* HEXETIDINE.

oral hypoglycaemic drugs (**oral antidiabetic drugs**) Drugs that are taken by mouth to reduce the concentration of glucose (sugar) in the blood; they act in various ways. Oral hypoglycaemic drugs are usually prescribed for people with type II (noninsulin-dependent) *diabetes mellitus, in whom there is still some natural insulin production by the pancreas. The main oral hypoglycaemic drugs used are the *sulphonylureas and *metformin hydrochloride (a biguanide). Others include *acarbose, *exenatide, *nateglinide, *pioglitazone and *rosiglitazone (the thiazolidinediones), *repaglinide, *sitagliptin, and *vildagliptin.

oral rehydration therapy (**ORT**) Solutions designed to replace fluids and *electrolytes lost in cases of dehydration, especially caused by diarrhoea. ORT solutions contain salts, such as *sodium chloride, *potassium chloride, *sodium citrate, and *sodium bicarbonate, together with glucose or other forms of carbohydrate, which enhance their absorption. ORT preparations are available as powders or effervescent tablets to be dissolved in water and taken by mouth; they can be obtained without a prescription, but only from pharmacies.
Proprietary preparations: *Dioralyte Natural (glucose, sodium chloride, potassium chloride, and disodium hydrogen citrate); *Dioralyte Relief (sodium chloride, potassium chloride, sodium citrate, and precooked rice powder); *Electrolade (sodium chloride, potassium chloride, sodium bicarbonate, and glucose).

O

Oramorph (Boehringer Ingelheim) *See* MORPHINE.

Orap (Janssen-Cilag) *See* PIMOZIDE.

orciprenaline sulphate A *sympathomimetic drug that stimulates beta *adrenoceptors in the airways and – to a lesser extent – in the heart. It was formerly quite widely used as a *bronchodilator in the treatment of *asthma, but has now largely been replaced by other bronchodilators with fewer adverse effects. Orciprenaline is available as a syrup on *prescription only.
Side effects: similar to those of *salbutamol, but orciprenaline is more likely to have adverse effects on the heart.
Precautions and interactions with other drugs: *see* SALBUTAMOL.
Proprietary preparation: Alupent.

Orelox (sanofi-aventis) *See* CEFPODOXIME.

Orencia (Bristol-Myers Squibb) *See* ABATACEPT.

Orfadin (Swedish Orphan International) *See* NITISINONE.

Orgalutran (Organon Laboratories) *See* GANIRELIX.

Orgaran (Organon Laboratories) *See* DANAPAROID SODIUM.

Original Andrews Salts (GlaxoSmithKline) A proprietary combination of *sodium bicarbonate, *magnesium sulphate, and *citric acid, used as an

*antacid for the relief of stomach upset and indigestion, and as a laxative. It is freely available *over the counter in the form of an effervescent powder.
Side effects and interactions with other drugs: *see* ANTACIDS.
Precautions: Andrews Salts are not recommended for children under three years old.

Orlept (Wockhardt UK) *See* SODIUM VALPROATE.

orlistat A drug that inhibits pancreatic lipases, digestive enzymes that are secreted by the pancreas and break down dietary fat so that it can be absorbed. Orlistat acts in the stomach and small intestine to prevent the absorption of up to one-third of the dietary intake of fat. It is used in conjunction with a low-calorie diet in the treatment of *obesity, but it should only be taken by people who are clinically obese or by those who are severely overweight in whom obesity is causing medical problems, such as diabetes. People taking orlistat must demonstrate that they have previously been able to adhere to a low-calorie diet and other weight-reducing measures for a period of at least three months, which has failed to achieve the desired weight loss. Orlistat is available as capsules on *prescription only; a lower-strength preparation can be obtained from *pharmacies without a prescription.
Side effects: include the frequent passage of copious liquid oily stools, flatulence, and stomach upset (all of which are less marked if fat intake is reduced), headache, menstrual irregularity, anxiety, and fatigue.
Precautions: orlistat should not be taken by women who are breastfeeding, by people with obstructed bile ducts or other conditions in which secretion of bile into the intestine is reduced, or by those in whom absorption from the intestine is reduced. Orlistat should be used with caution by people with epilepsy and in pregnant women.
Interactions with other drugs:
Acarbose: should not be used with orlistat.
Amiodarone: its plasma concentration may be reduced.
Ciclosporin: its absorption may be reduced.
Vitamin supplements: orlistat may impair the absorption of fat-soluble vitamins (A, D, E, and K), therefore multivitamin preparations should not be taken for at least two hours after taking orlistat.
Proprietary preparations: Alli (low strength); Xenical.

orphenadrine An *antimuscarinic drug that has pronounced skeletal *muscle relaxant properties. It is used for the treatment of Parkinson's disease and the reversal of drug-induced *extrapyramidal reactions (*see* ANTIPARKINSONIAN DRUGS). A *prescription only medicine, it is available as tablets and an oral solution.
Side effects: include dry mouth, gastrointestinal disturbances, dizziness, and blurred vision; less common side effects are difficulty in urinating, slow heart rate, nervousness, euphoria, and insomnia. In high doses and in susceptible individuals, mental confusion, excitement, and psychiatric disturbances can occur.

Precautions and interactions with other drugs: *see* TRIHEXYPHENIDYL HYDROCHLORIDE.
Proprietary preparations: Biorphen; Disipal.

ORT *See* ORAL REHYDRATION THERAPY.

Ortho-Gynest (Janssen-Cilag) *See* ESTRIOL.

Orudis, Orudis Suppositories (sanofi-aventis) *See* KETOPROFEN.

Oruvail (sanofi-aventis) *See* KETOPROFEN.

oseltamivir An *antiviral drug used for the treatment and prevention of influenza. It is most effective when taken within two days of the symptoms first appearing (for treatment) or of exposure to influenza (for prevention). Oseltamivir acts by reducing replication of the virus. It is available as capsules or an oral suspension on *prescription only.
Side effects: common side effects include headache, nausea, vomiting, abdominal pain, diarrhoea, dizziness, and general fatigue.
Precautions: oseltamivir should be used with caution in people with kidney disease and in women who are pregnant or breastfeeding.
Proprietary preparation: Tamiflu.

Osmanil (Winthrop Pharmaceuticals) *See* FENTANYL.

osmotic laxatives *Laxatives that act by retaining water in the colon (large bowel). Osmotic laxatives include magnesium salts (such as *magnesium hydroxide and *magnesium sulphate) and *lactulose, which are taken orally for the treatment of constipation; *phosphate laxatives, which are given as suppositories or enemas for constipation or for clearing the bowel before surgery or examination; and *sodium citrate, which is given rectally to treat constipation. *See also* BOWEL-CLEANSING SOLUTIONS.

Osvaren (Frefenius Medical Care) A proprietary combination of *calcium acetate and *magnesium carbonate, used as an *antacid for the relief of heartburn, indigestion, and trapped wind (*see* ACID-PEPTIC DISEASES). It is available as tablets without a prescription.
Side effects, precautions, and interactions with other drugs: *see* ANTACIDS.

OTC *See* OVER THE COUNTER.

Otex (Diomed Developments) *See* UREA HYDROGEN PEROXIDE.

Otomize (GlaxoSmithKline) A proprietary combination of *dexamethasone (a corticosteroid), *acetic acid, and *neomycin sulphate (an antibiotic), used for the treatment of inflammation and infections of the outer ear. It is available as a pump-action spray on *prescription only.
Side effects: there may be transient stinging or burning on application.
Precautions: Otomize should not be used on perforated eardrums or by pregnant women.

Otosporin (GlaxoSmithKline) A proprietary combination of *polymyxin B

sulphate and *neomycin sulphate (both antibiotics) and *hydrocortisone (a corticosteroid), used for the treatment of bacterial infections and inflammation of the outer ear. It is available as ear drops on *prescription only.
Side effects: a secondary infection may occur (*see* CORTICOSTEROIDS).
Precautions: long-term use of these drops in infants should be avoided. Otosporin should not be used by people with perforated eardrums or untreated viral, fungal, or tuberculous infections.

Otrivine (Novartis) *See* XYLOMETAZOLINE.

Otrivine-Antistin (Novartis) A proprietary combination of *xylometazoline (a sympathomimetic drug) and *antazoline (an antihistamine), used for the treatment of allergic conjunctivitis. It is available as eye drops without a prescription, but only from a *pharmacy.
Side effects: include transient stinging, headache, drowsiness, blurred vision, and rebound congestion (*see* DECONGESTANTS).
Precautions: the drops should not to be used by people with acute glaucoma or by wearers of contact lenses.

over the counter Denoting or relating to drugs that can be obtained without a *prescription. There are two legal categories of such drugs: those that can only be bought from a pharmacy when a registered pharmacist is present – these pharmacy medicines are designated P; and those that can be bought from the self-service displays of pharmacies or from any other retail outlet, designated GSL (general sales list). For some OTC drugs there may be a restriction on the quantity that can be purchased from a GSL outlet or at one time. The term 'over the counter' can be applied to either P drugs or GSL drugs, although it is more properly restricted to GSL items (in this dictionary described as "freely available over the counter"). Some drugs may be classified as GSL or P at low doses, but as POM (*prescription only medicine) at higher doses. A medical practitioner can prescribe OTC medicines, although some are restricted and cannot be prescribed at NHS expense.

Ovestin (Organon Laboratories) *See* ESTRIOL.

Ovex (McNeill Ltd) *See* MEBENDAZOLE.

Ovitrelle (Serono) *See* HUMAN CHORIONIC GONADOTROPHIN.

Ovranette (Pfizer) A proprietary combination of *ethinylestradiol and *levonorgestrel used as an *oral contraceptive. It is available as tablets on *prescription only.
Side effects, precautions, and interactions with other drugs: *see* ORAL CONTRACEPTIVES.

Ovysmen (Janssen-Cilag) A proprietary combination of *ethinylestradiol and *norethisterone used as an *oral contraceptive. It is available as tablets on *prescription only.

Side effects, precautions, and interactions with other drugs: *see* ORAL CONTRACEPTIVES.

Oxactin (Discovery Pharmaceuticals) *See* FLUOXETINE.

oxaliplatin A *cytotoxic drug that is an *analogue of *cisplatin but is less toxic. It is used, together with 5-fluorouracil and folinic acid, as an *adjunct for the treatment of colorectal and colon cancer. It is given under expert supervision by intravenous infusion and is available on *prescription only.
Side effects: include diarrhoea, nausea, vomiting, peripheral neuropathy (causing numbness and tingling of the limbs), and ear damage.
Precautions: *see* CISPLATIN; CYTOTOXIC DRUGS. Oxaliplatin should not be given to people with *bone marrow suppression or peripheral neuropathy.
Interactions with other drugs: *see* CISPLATIN.
Proprietary preparation: Eloxatin.

oxazepam A short-acting *benzodiazepine used for short-term treatment of anxiety. It is available as tablets on *prescription only.
Side effects and precautions: *see* DIAZEPAM; BENZODIAZEPINES.
Interactions with other drugs: *see* BENZODIAZEPINES.

oxcarbazepine An *anticonvulsant drug used to treat partial epileptic seizures. It is available as tablets or an oral suspension on *prescription only.
Side effects: include dizziness, drowsiness, blurred vision, nausea, vomiting, and headache.
Precautions: there is a small risk of blood, liver, or skin disorders in those taking oxcarbazepine, and if symptoms such as bleeding, bruising, fever, sore throat, lethargy, confusion, muscle twitching, rash, or blistering develop, a doctor should be consulted.
Interactions with other drugs:

Antidepressants: reduce the effect of oxcarbazepine and therefore increase the risk of convulsions. St John's wort should not be taken with oxcarbazepine.

Antimalarial drugs: quinine, hydroxychloroquine, and mefloquine increase the risk of convulsions.

Antipsychotics: reduce the effect of oxcarbazepine and therefore increase the risk of convulsions.

Imatinib: oxcarbazepine reduces its plasma concentration and should not be taken with it.

Oral contraceptives: their effects are reduced.

Proprietary preparation: Trileptal.

oxerutins Naturally occurring compounds used for the relief of heavy aching legs, night cramp, and other symptoms associated with poor circulation, although their value is not proven. They are available as capsules and can be obtained without a prescription, but only from pharmacies.
Side effects: include gastrointestinal upset, flushes, and headache.
Proprietary preparation: Paroven.

Oxis Turbohaler (AstraZeneca) *See* FORMOTEROL FUMARATE.

oxpentifylline *See* PENTOXIFYLLINE.

oxprenolol hydrochloride A *beta blocker used to treat *angina, *arrhythmias, and anxiety. It is also used as a *modified-release formulation for the treatment of *hypertension. It is available as tablets or modified-release tablets on *prescription only.
Side effects, precautions, and interactions with other drugs: *see* BETA BLOCKERS.
Proprietary preparations: Trasicor; Slow-Trasicor (modified-release tablets); *Trasidrex (combined with cyclopenthiazide).
See also ANTIHYPERTENSIVE DRUGS; ANTI-ARRHYTHMIC DRUGS.

Oxyal (Kestrel) *See* SODIUM HYALURONATE.

oxybuprocaine *See* LOCAL ANAESTHETICS.

oxybutynin hydrochloride An *antimuscarinic drug used to treat abnormal frequency and urgency in passing urine, urinary incontinence, and bedwetting. It acts by reducing instability in the muscle of the bladder wall. However, oxybutynin has a high level of side effects, and the dosage must be carefully assessed in older people. It is available as tablets, *modified-release tablets, an *elixir, or skin patches on *prescription only; the modified-release tablets and skin patches reduce the side effects.
Side effects: include dry mouth, constipation, blurred vision, nausea, abdominal discomfort, flushing (more marked in children), difficulty in passing urine, headache, dizziness, drowsiness, dry skin, rash, increased sensitivity to sunlight, diarrhoea, restlessness, disorientation, hallucination, and convulsions. Children are more susceptible to the disorientating or hallucinatory effects of oxybutynin.
Precautions: oxybutynin should not be taken by people with obstruction of the gut or severe ulcerative colitis, or by people in whom the outlet of the bladder is obstructed (for example, by an enlarged prostate gland). It should be used with caution in frail elderly people, in people with liver or kidney disease, some types of heart disease, an overactive thyroid gland, or glaucoma and in women who are pregnant or breastfeeding.
Interactions with other drugs: *see* ANTIMUSCARINIC DRUGS.
Proprietary preparations: Cystrin; Ditropan (tablets or elixir); Kentera (skin patches); Lyrinel XL (modified-release tablets).

oxycodone An *opioid analgesic that is used mainly for the relief of pain in patients who are terminally ill. A *controlled drug, it is available as a solution for injection or infusion, an oral solution, capsules, or modified-release tablets.
Side effects and precautions: *see* MORPHINE; OPIOIDS.
Interactions with other drugs: *see* OPIOIDS.
Proprietary preparations: OxyContin (modified-release tablets); OxyNorm; *Targinact (combined with naloxone hydrochloride).

OxyContin (Napp Pharmaceuticals) *See* OXYCODONE.

oxymetazoline A *sympathomimetic drug that constricts blood vessels and is used as a nasal *decongestant. It is available as a nasal spray without a prescription.
Side effects, precautions, and interactions with other drugs: *see* XYLOMETAZOLINE; DECONGESTANTS.
Proprietary preparations: Boots Nasal Spray; Vicks Sinex.

OxyNorm (Napp Pharmaceuticals) *See* OXYCODONE.

oxytetracycline A tetracycline antibiotic used for the treatment of chronic bronchitis, brucellosis, chlamydial infections, and infections caused by mycoplasmas and rickettsias (*see* TETRACYCLINES). It is also used to treat mouth ulcers and *acne. It is available, on *prescription only, as tablets.
Side effects, precautions, and interactions with other drugs: *see* TETRACYCLINES.

oxytocin A hormone produced by the pituitary gland that causes contractions of the uterus during labour and also stimulates milk production in nursing mothers. It is used therapeutically to induce labour and to prevent or treat bleeding from the uterus after childbirth. Since high doses may overstimulate the uterus, posing a threat to the fetus, oxytocin should only be used to induce labour under medical supervision. It may also be used in certain cases to assist abortion. Oxytocin is available, on *prescription only, as a solution for slow intravenous injection or infusion; it is usually used only in hospitals.
Side effects: include spasm of the uterus, nausea, vomiting, irregular heart rhythms, and rashes or other allergic reactions.
Precautions: oxytocin should not be used when there is any mechanical obstruction to delivery or when a vaginal delivery is not appropriate or in women with severe cardiovascular disease. It should be used with caution in women who are over 35 years old or who have had a previous Caesarean section.
Interactions with other drugs:
Anaesthetics: may possibly reduce the effect of oxytocin; inhaled anaesthetics increase the risk of low blood pressure and *arrhythmias.
Prostaglandins: enhance the effect of oxytocin.
Vasoconstrictor sympathomimetic drugs: their effects in constricting blood vessels and increasing blood pressure are enhanced.
Proprietary preparations: Syntocinon; *Syntometrine (combined with ergometrine maleate).

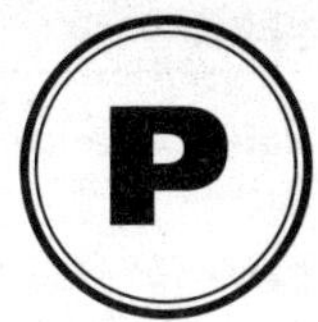

P (pharmacy medicine) *See* OVER THE COUNTER.

Pabal (Ferring Pharmaceuticals) *See* CARBETOCIN.

Pabrinex (Link Pharmaceuticals) A proprietary combination of *thiamine hydrochloride, *nicotinamide, *pyridoxine hydrochloride, and *riboflavin (all of which are B vitamins) and ascorbic acid (*see* VITAMIN C), used for the treatment of severe vitamin B deficiency states, such as those caused by alcoholism or occurring after acute infections, surgery, or in some psychiatric conditions. It may also be needed by people undergoing kidney dialysis. Pabrinex is available as an intramuscular or intravenous injection on *prescription only.
Side effects and precautions: since severe allergic reactions can occur during or after injection, Pabrinex should be reserved for those patients unable to take the vitamins by mouth. When given intravenously, the injection should be slow (over 10 minutes).

paclitaxel A *taxane that is used in conjunction with *cisplatin for the treatment of primary ovarian *cancer; it is used alone for treating ovarian cancer that has spread to other parts of the body and has not responded to platinum-containing drugs. It is also used for treating advanced breast cancer when standard therapy has failed. Paclitaxel may cause severe allergic reactions: drugs to prevent this, including *corticosteroids and *antihistamines, are therefore usually given before treatment starts. Paclitaxel is available as a solution for intravenous infusion on *prescription only.
Side effects: include severe allergic reactions (see above), a fall in blood pressure, slowing of heart rate, *bone marrow suppression, hair loss, muscle pain, nerve damage, nausea, and vomiting. *See also* CYTOTOXIC DRUGS.
Precautions: paclitaxel should not be given to pregnant or breastfeeding women or people with severe liver disease. *See also* CYTOTOXIC DRUGS.
Interactions with other drugs:

Clozapine: there is an increased risk of agranulocytosis (a blood disorder), and this drug should not be used with paclitaxel.

Proprietary preparations: Abraxane; Taxol.

Pain Relief Balm (Boots) A proprietary combination of the rubefacients *glycol salicylate, *ethyl nicotinate, and *nonylic acid vanillylamide, used for the relief of muscular pain and stiffness. It is available *over the counter in the form of a cream, but only from Boots stores.
Side effects and precautions: *see* RUBEFACIENTS; SALICYLATES.

paint A liquid preparation that is applied to the skin or mucous membranes. Paints usually contain antiseptics, astringents, caustics, or analgesics.

Paldesic (Rosemont Pharmaceuticals) *See* PARACETAMOL.

palifermin A drug used to treat mouth sores and ulcers in people with leukaemia or lymphoma (*see* CANCER) who are receiving high-dose chemo- and radiotherapy. It is available as a form for injection on *prescription only.
Side effects: include altered taste, thickening and discoloration of the tongue, fluid retention, rash, and itching.
Precautions: palifermin is not recommended for pregnant or breastfeeding women.
Proprietary preparation: Kepivance.

paliperidone An atypical *antipsychotic drug used in the treatment of schizophrenia. It is available as *modified-release tablets on *prescription only.
Side effects: include weight gain, dizziness, low blood pressure on standing (which may cause fainting), abdominal pain, dry mouth, increased salivation, drowsiness, headache, and a fast or slow heart rate.
Precautions: paliperidone should not be taken by women who are breastfeeding or by elderly patients with dementia. It should be used with caution in people with impaired liver or kidney function, Parkinson's disease, or blockage of the intestinal tract.
Interactions with other drugs:

Anaesthetics: the effect of general anaesthetics in lowering blood pressure is enhanced.
Antiepileptic drugs: their anticonvulsant effect is antagonized.
Ritonavir: may increase the plasma concentration of paliperidone.
Sibutramine: there is an increased risk of adverse effects on the central nervous system.
Tricyclic antidepressants: their plasma concentrations (and risk of adverse effects) are increased.

Proprietary preparation: Invega.

palivizumab A *monoclonal antibody used for the prevention of serious lung disease in children caused by the respiratory syncytial virus, which would require hospitalization. It is prescribed under specialist supervision and given by intramuscular injection.
Side effects: include fever and reactions at the injection site.
Proprietary preparation: Synagis.

Palladone, Palladone SR (Napp Pharmaceuticals) *See* HYDROMORPHONE HYDROCHLORIDE.

palonosetron An *antiemetic used to prevent nausea and vomiting induced by chemotherapy drugs. It acts by inhibiting the action of the neurotransmitter *serotonin at specific receptors in the central nervous system and gut. It is available in injectable form on *prescription only.

Side effects: include diarrhoea, constipation, headache, dizziness, indigestion, and abdominal pain.
Precautions: palonosetron should be used with caution in people with a history of constipation or intestinal obstruction, those who are taking drugs known to cause arrhythmias, and in pregnant or breastfeeding women.
Proprietary preparation: Aloxi.

Paludrine (AstraZeneca) *See* PROGUANIL HYDROCHLORIDE.

Paludrine/Avloclor (AstraZeneca) A proprietary preparation consisting of 14 tablets of *chloroquine phosphate packaged with 98 tablets of *proguanil hydrochloride (the recommended dosages), used for the prevention of malaria. It is available without a prescription, but only from pharmacies.
Side effects, precautions, and interactions with other drugs: *see* CHLOROQUINE; PROGUANIL HYDROCHLORIDE.

Pamergan P100 (Martindale Pharmaceuticals) A proprietary combination of *pethidine hydrochloride (an opioid analgesic) and *promethazine hydrochloride (a sedating antihistamine), used for pain relief during labour and before, during, or after surgery. A *controlled drug, it is available as an injection.
Side effects: *see* PETHIDINE HYDROCHLORIDE; PROMETHAZINE HYDROCHLORIDE.
Precautions: *see* ANTIHISTAMINES; MORPHINE.
Interactions with other drugs: *see* ANTIHISTAMINES; PETHIDINE HYDROCHLORIDE.

pamidronate disodium *See* DISODIUM PAMIDRONATE.

Panadol (GlaxoSmithKline) *See* PARACETAMOL.

Panadol Extra (GlaxoSmithKline) A proprietary combination of *paracetamol (an analgesic and antipyretic) and *caffeine (a stimulant), used for the relief of headache (including migraine), toothache, neuralgia, rheumatic pain, backache, period pains, and the symptoms of influenza and colds. It is available as tablets or soluble tablets and can be obtained without a prescription, but larger packs are only available from pharmacies.
Precautions: Panadol Extra should not be given to children, except on medical advice. *See also* PARACETAMOL; CAFFEINE.

Panadol Night (GlaxoSmithKline) A proprietary combination of *paracetamol (an analgesic) and *diphenhydramine (a sedative antihistamine), used for the short-term treatment of pains that are disturbing sleep, such as rheumatic and muscle pain, backache, neuralgia, toothache, migraine, and period pains. It is available as tablets and can be obtained without a prescription, but only from pharmacies.
Side effects: *see* ANTIHISTAMINES.
Precautions: Panadol Night should not be taken for more than seven consecutive nights without medical advice; it is not recommended for children except on medical advice. *See also* PARACETAMOL; ANTIHISTAMINES.
Interactions with other drugs: *see* ANTIHISTAMINES.

Panadol Ultra (GlaxoSmithKline) A proprietary combination of *paracetamol (a non-opioid analgesic) and *codeine (an opioid analgesic), used for the relief of rheumatic pains, sciatica, lumbago, strains and sprains, neuralgia, and migraine. It is available as tablets and can be obtained without a prescription, but only from pharmacies.
Side effects: *see* CODEINE.
Precautions: Panadol Ultra should not be given to children under 12 years old. *See also* PARACETAMOL.
Interactions with other drugs: *see* OPIOIDS.

Pancrease HL (Janssen-Cilag) *See* PANCREATIN.

pancreatin An extract of the pancreas (usually obtained from pigs) that contains the pancreatic enzymes amylase, lipase, and protease, which aid the digestion and absorption of starch, fat, and protein. Pancreatin is used as replacement therapy when the body's natural pancreatic enzymes are lacking. A lack of enzymes may be due to inherited conditions, such as cystic fibrosis, or disease, such as chronic pancreatitis, or it may occur following surgical removal of the pancreas. Pancreatin should be taken before or with meals and the dosage adjusted according to absorption of food – judged by the size, number, and consistency of stools and lack of diarrhoea. Preparations should be swallowed without chewing; if they are mixed with food, the food should not be too hot, since the enzymes may be inactivated. Pancreatin is available as granules, capsules, tablets, or powder; some preparations are *enteric-coated, which enables a higher concentration of enzymes to reach the duodenum. Pancreatin preparations of standard strength can be obtained from pharmacies without a prescription; higher-strength preparations are *prescription only medicines.
Side effects: include nausea, vomiting, and abdominal discomfort. Irritation of the mouth or anal region can occur if the enzymes are taken without food or are used in excessive dosage.
Precautions: a high intake of fluids must be maintained, particularly in those taking higher-strength preparations. Individuals taking high dosages should report unusual abdominal symptoms to a doctor.
Proprietary preparations: Creon; Creon 10 000; Creon 25 000 (high-strength); Creon 40 000 (highest strength); Creon Micro (granules); Nutrizym 10; Nutrizym 22 (high-strength); Pancrease HL (high-strength); Pancrex; Pancrex V.

Pancrex, Pancrex V (Paines & Byrne) *See* PANCREATIN.

panitumumab A *monoclonal antibody used for the treatment of advanced colorectal cancer that is stimulated to proliferate by a protein, epidermal growth factor (EGF). It acts by binding to receptors for EGF. Panitumumab is given by intravenous infusion and is available on *prescription only.
Side effects: include rash, reddening and flaking of the skin, dry skin, diarrhoea, nausea, vomiting, fatigue, and headache.

Precautions: panitumumab should not be given to people with lung disease or to women who are pregnant or breastfeeding.
Proprietary preparation: Vectibix.

PanOxyl (Stiefel Laboratories) *See* BENZOYL PEROXIDE.

panthenol *See* VITAMIN B COMPLEX.

pantoprazole A *proton pump inhibitor used for the treatment of duodenal or gastric ulcers, moderate to severe reflux oesophagitis, and Zollinger-Ellison syndrom (*see* ACID-PEPTIC DISEASES). It is available, on *prescription only, as *enteric-coated tablets or an injection.
Side effects: include headache, diarrhoea, rashes, itching, dizziness, nausea and vomiting, and constipation.
Precautions: *see* PROTON PUMP INHIBITORS.
Interactions with other drugs:
Atazanavir: its plasma concentration is reduced.
Clopidogrel: its effect may be reduced.
Warfarin: its anticoagulant effect may be enhanced.
Proprietary preparation: Protium.

pantothenic acid *See* VITAMIN B COMPLEX.

papaveretum An *opioid analgesic consisting of a mixture of *morphine hydrochloride, *papaverine hydrochloride, and *codeine hydrochloride in fixed amounts. It is used for the treatment of pain following surgery and also as part of premedication for the control of existing pain before surgery. Papaveretum was formerly known by the proprietary name **Omnopon**. A combination of papaveretum and *hyoscine hydrobromide is also used in premedication. Both preparations are available as injections; they are *controlled drugs.
Side effects and precautions: *see* MORPHINE; OPIOIDS.
Interactions with other drugs: *see* OPIOIDS.

papaverine An alkaloid, derived from opium, that relaxes smooth muscle. It is an ingredient of *papaveretum. Alone, papaverine is used in the treatment of impotence, being injected directly into the penis to achieve an erection, although it does not have a *licence for this purpose. Papaverine is available as a solution for injection on *prescription only.
Side effects and precautions: there may be a burning pain and bruising at the injection site. An erection that lasts for longer than four hours is a medical emergency and requires prompt treatment (by withdrawing blood from the penis followed, if necessary, by injections of phenylephrine or adrenaline).

paracetamol A drug that relieves pain (*see* ANALGESICS) and also reduces fever (but has no anti-inflammatory activity). Paracetamol provides effective relief of mild to moderate pain, including headache, toothache, period pains, backache, and rheumatic pains, and is useful for reducing high temperatures in colds, influenza, and other feverish conditions. Unlike *aspirin, it does not irritate the stomach lining and is preferred to aspirin for elderly people and

young children (under 12 years old). Paracetamol is available as tablets, soluble tablets, capsules, solutions, suppositories, and a solution for intravenous infusion; there are also suspensions and solutions specially formulated for babies and young children, often as flavoured sugar-free syrups. Paracetamol can be obtained without a prescription, but because it can have serious effects in overdosage (see below) there are restrictions on the quantities of tablets or capsules that can be supplied. Packs containing 16 tablets or capsules are freely available *over the counter; packs containing up to 32 (or exceptionally up to 100) tablets or capsules can only be obtained from pharmacies. Larger quantities are available on *prescription only. Paracetamol is combined with aspirin, codeine, or other ingredients in a variety of compound analgesic preparations and cold remedies. *See also* CO-CODAMOL; CO-DYDRAMOL; CO-PROXAMOL.
Side effects and precautions: side effects of recommended doses (up to 8 tablets/capsules a day in adults) are rare, but rashes or other allergic reactions may rarely occur; pancreatitis has been reported after prolonged use. In higher than recommended doses paracetamol causes liver damage, which may not be apparent for two days or more and can be fatal unless treated immediately with the antidote (methionine or acetylcysteine). For this reason it is important not to mix preparations containing paracetamol, in case the recommended dose is accidentally exceeded, and paracetamol should be taken with caution by people with liver disease.
Proprietary preparations: Alvedon (suppositories); Anadin Paracetamol; Boots Cold & Flu Relief Hot Blackcurrant, Hot Lemon; Boots Paracetamol Capsules/Suspension; Boots Paracetamol and Codeine Extra Capsules; Calpol; Disprol; Fennings Children's Cooling Powders; Hedex; Medinol; Paldesic; Panadol; Panadol Soluble; Perfalgan (infusion). For details of these and other preparations of which paracetamol is an ingredient, see Appendix 1.

p

Paracetamol and Codeine Caplets (Boots) *See* CO-CODAMOL.

Paracodol (Bayer Plc) *See* CO-CODAMOL.

Paradote (Penn Pharmaceuticals) A proprietary combination of *paracetamol (an analgesic and antipyretic) and *methionine (its antidote); this mixture is called **co-methiamol**. Paradote is used to relieve pain and reduce fever; the methionine is included in an attempt to prevent liver damage caused by overdosage of paracetamol. It is available as tablets without a prescription, but only from pharmacies.
Side effects and precautions: *see* PARACETAMOL; METHIONINE.

paraldehyde An *anticonvulsant drug used to treat status epilepticus, a medical emergency in which epileptic seizures occur repeatedly without the person recovering consciousness between them. Paraldehyde is available on *prescription only; it is given as an enema.
Side effects: paraldehyde may cause rashes, and the enema may irritate the rectum.
Precautions: paraldehyde should be used with caution in people with disease

of the airways, lungs, or liver and in women who are pregnant or breastfeeding.

Paramax (sanofi-aventis) A proprietary combination of *paracetamol (an analgesic) and *metoclopramide (an antiemetic), used for the relief of migraine. It is available as tablets or effervescent powder on *prescription only.
Side effects, precautions, and interactions with other drugs: *see* PARACETAMOL; METOCLOPRAMIDE.

Paramol (SSL International) A proprietary combination of *paracetamol (an analgesic and antipyretic) and *dihydrocodeine (an opioid analgesic), used for the relief of headache, migraine, fevers, period pains, toothache, backache, and other muscular aches and pains. It is available as tablets and can be obtained without a prescription, but only from pharmacies.
Side effects: *see* MORPHINE.
Precautions: Paramol is not recommended for children. *See also* PARACETAMOL; MORPHINE.
Interactions with other drugs: *see* OPIOIDS.

parasympathetic nervous system A part of the nervous system that works in conjunction with another series of nerves (the *sympathetic nervous system) to control certain functions of the heart, lungs, intestines and pancreas, salivary glands, bladder, and genitalia. In general, the actions of the parasympathetic nervous system oppose those of the sympathetic nervous system. Both the parasympathetic and sympathetic nervous systems function automatically – we are not aware of their actions and have no voluntary control over them.

The substance that relays information in the parasympathetic nervous system is *acetylcholine, which acts on very small specialized areas of the cells of the target tissues called receptors. Many drugs act on the parasympathetic nervous system, either by mimicking the actions of acetylcholine (*see* CHOLINERGIC DRUGS) or by opposing them (*see* ANTIMUSCARINIC DRUGS).

parasympathomimetic drugs *See* CHOLINERGIC DRUGS.

parathyroid hormone (**parathormone**) A hormone that is synthesized and released by the parathyroid glands, situated at the base of the neck behind the thyroid gland, in response to low concentrations of *calcium in the blood. It acts in opposition to calcitonin to control the distribution of calcium and phosphate in the body (*see* CALCITONIN (SALMON). Parathyroid hormone promotes the transfer of calcium from the bones to the blood; it also converts *vitamin D to its active form, which increases absorption of calcium from the intestine. A deficiency of parathyroid hormone results in reduced concentrations of calcium in the blood, causing tetany (spasm and twitching of the muscles). This condition may be treated with forms of vitamin D.

A genetically engineered form of parathyroid hormone is used for the treatment of osteoporosis in postmenopausal women who are at high risk of fractures of the spine. It is available as a form for subcutaneous injection on *prescription only. *See also* TERIPARATIDE.

Side effects: include nausea, vomiting, indigestion, constipation, diarrhoea, palpitations, headache, dizziness, and muscle cramps.
Precautions: parathyroid hormone should not be given to women with high blood-calcium levels, metabolic bone disease (e.g. Paget's disease), or severe liver or kidney disease, or who are pregnant or breastfeeding.
Proprietary preparations: Preotact.

Pardelprin (Actavis) *See* INDOMETACIN.

parecoxib A COX-2 inhibitor (*see* NSAIDs) used for the relief of pain after surgery. It is available as a form for intramuscular or intravenous injection on *prescription only.
Side effects: *see* NSAIDs. There may also be low or high blood pressure, indigestion, itching, and back pain.
Precautions: *see* NSAIDs. Parecoxib should not be taken by people who have had allergic reactions to drugs or have inflammatory bowel disease.
Interactions with other drugs: *see* NSAIDs.
Proprietary preparation: Dynastat.

parenteral Introduced into the body by any way other than through the mouth. The term is applied, for example, to administration of drugs by injection.

paricalcitol A *vitamin D analogue used to prevent or reduce excessive secretion of *parathyroid hormone in people with chronic kidney failure. It is available as capsules or a form for injection on *prescription only.
Side effects: *see* VITAMIN D. There may also be indigestion, taste disturbances, breast tenderness, and acne.
Precautions: *see* VITAMIN D. Blood concentrations of calcium, phosphate, and parathyroid hormone should be monitored during treatment.
Interactions with other drugs: *see* VITAMIN D.
Proprietary preparation: Zemplar.

p

Pariet (Eisai) *See* RABEPRAZOLE SODIUM.

Parkinson's disease *See* ANTIPARKINSONIAN DRUGS.

Parlodel (Meda Pharmaceuticals) *See* BROMOCRIPTINE.

Paroven (Novartis) *See* OXERUTINS.

paroxetine An *antidepressant drug of the *SSRI group. It is used for the treatment of depressive illness, obsessive-compulsive disorder, panic disorder, post-traumatic stress disorder, and anxiety disorders. Paroxetine is available as tablets or liquid on *prescription only.
Side effects: *see* SSRIs. In addition, yawning and *extrapyramidal reactions may occur.
Precautions: *see* SSRIs.
Interactions with other drugs:
Antipsychotic drugs: paroxetine may inhibit the breakdown of aripiprazole,

whose dosage should therefore be reduced; the plasma concentrations of clozapine and sertindole are increased by paroxetine.
Phenytoin: reduces the plasma concentration of paroxetine.
Selegiline: increases the risk of adverse effects on the central nervous system and high blood pressure; paroxetine should not be taken until two weeks after stopping selegiline, which should not be started until two weeks after stopping paroxetine.
Sumatriptan: increases the risk of adverse effects on the central nervous system.
Tamoxifen: the breakdown to its active form may be inhibited and paroxetine should not be taken with tamoxifen.
See also SSRIs.
Proprietary preparation: Seroxat.

Partobulin SDF (Baxter Healthcare) *See* ANTI-D (RH_0) IMMUNOGLOBULIN.

Parvolex (UCB Pharma) *See* ACETYLCYSTEINE.

paste A medicinal preparation of a thick and stiff consistency, which is applied to the skin. It contains a high proportion of insoluble powder (e.g. zinc oxide or starch) in an *ointment base.

pastille A medicinal tablet that contains gelatine and glycerin (and is therefore soft); it is usually coated with sugar. Pastilles should be sucked, so that the medication is applied to the mouth and throat.

Pavacol-D (Alliance) *See* PHOLCODINE.

peanut oil *See* ARACHIS OIL.

Pedea (Orphan Europe) *See* IBUPROFEN.

pediculicides *See* LICE.

pegaptanib sodium A drug used for the treatment of wet age-related macular degeneration, a disorder of the eye affecting the area of greatest visual acuity (the macula). It works by binding to and inhibiting *vascular endothelial growth factor, and therefore it prevents the proliferation of blood vessels around the macula. Pegaptanib is given by injection into the vitreous fluid of the eye under expert supervision and is available on *prescription only.
Side effects: include raised pressure in the eye, a running nose, headache, and eye pain.
Precautions: pegaptanib should not be given to people with eye infections, and it should be used with caution in women who are pregnant or breastfeeding. Pressure in the eye should be monitored following the injection.
Proprietary preparation: Macugen.

Pegasys (Roche Products) *See* PEGINTERFERON ALFA.

pegfilgrastim pegylated recombinant human granulocyte-colony

stimulating factor: a form of *granulocyte-colony stimulating factor derived from *filgrastim. It is used for the treatment of neutropenia (a decrease in the number of neutrophils, a type of white blood cell) induced by *cytotoxic drug treatment for cancer. Pegfilgrastim is available as a form for subcutaneous injection on *prescription only; its use is restricted to specialist units.
Side effects and precautions: *see* FILGRASTIM.
Proprietary preparation: Neulasta.

peginterferon alfa A derivative of *interferon alfa used for the treatment of chronic hepatitis C (often in combination with *ribavirin) and chronic hepatitis B. It is available as a form for injection on *prescription only.
Side effects and interactions with other drugs: *see* INTERFERON ALFA.
Precautions: *see* INTERFERON ALFA. Peginterferon alfa should not be given to women who are breastfeeding.
Proprietary preparations: Pegasys; PegIntron.

PegIntron (Schering-Plough) *See* PEGINTERFERON ALFA.

pegvisomant A drug that reduces the action of *growth hormone and is used for the treatment of acromegaly. It is given by subcutaneous injection (the injection site is changed regularly to prevent a build-up of fatty tissue) and is available on *prescription only.
Side effects: common side effects include dizziness, headache, nausea, diarrhoea, joint pain, and hypertension.
Precautions: pegvisomant should not be given to women who are pregnant or breastfeeding and should be used with caution in people with liver disease or diabetes.
Proprietary preparation: Somavert.

pemetrexed An *antimetabolite that is used, in combination with *cisplatin, for the treatment of malignant pleural mesothelioma (cancer of the membrane lining the lungs) that cannot be treated surgically and advanced non-small-cell lung cancer. It is available as an injectable form on *prescription only.
Side effects: *see* CYTOTOXIC DRUGS. Additional side effects include skin disorders.
Precautions: *see* CYTOTOXIC DRUGS.
Proprietary preparation: Alimta.

Penbritin (Chemidex Pharma) *See* AMPICILLIN.

penciclovir A nucleoside analogue (*see* ANTIVIRAL DRUGS) used for the treatment of cold sores. It is available as a cream.
Side effects: there may be transient burning or stinging.
Precautions: penciclovir should be used with caution by those whose immune systems are functioning poorly (due to disease or drug therapy) and by women who are pregnant or breastfeeding. The cream should not come into contact with the eyes or mucous membranes.

Proprietary preparations: Fenistil (pharmacy medicine); Vectavir (prescription only medicine).

penicillamine A drug used for the treatment of active progressive rheumatoid arthritis and having similar actions to gold (*see* SODIUM AUROTHIOMALATE). Side effects are frequent, which may restrict its use. It must be started at a low dosage, which is gradually increased over months; improvement may not be seen for 6–12 weeks after treatment starts. Penicillamine is also used for the treatment of Wilson's disease (in which copper accumulates in the body), chronic active (autoimmune) hepatitis, and cystinuria (a kidney disease). It is available as tablets on *prescription only.
Side effects: include nausea at the start of treatment, which resolves with further use; loss of appetite and taste and nerve damage; and fever, rash, and bloody or cloudy urine (which should all be reported to a doctor).
Precautions and interactions with other drugs: blood counts and urine examination must be performed in the early stages of treatment. Concurrent treatment with gold, chloroquine, hydroxychloroquine, or immunosuppressants should be avoided; clozapine should also be avoided and it increases the risk of agranulocytosis (a blood disorder). Penicillamine should be used with caution in people with kidney disease and in women who are pregnant or breastfeeding.
Proprietary preparation: Distamine.

penicillins A group of bactericidal beta-lactam *antibiotics that act by interfering with bacterial cell wall synthesis. They penetrate well into most body tissues and fluids, but do not enter the cerebrospinal fluid (surrounding the brain and spinal cord) unless there is inflammation of cerebrospinal tissues. Some penicillins are broken down by enzymes called beta-lactamases (or penicillinases), which are produced by some types of bacteria, so they are sometimes given with *clavulanic acid or *tazobactam, which inhibit these enzymes; alternatively, penicillinase-resistant penicillins must be used. The ability of a drug to resist attack by these enzymes is an important factor in determining which drug is effective against specific types of bacteria.

The most important side effect of penicillins is hypersensitivity (allergy), which can cause rashes and occasionally an extreme and potentially fatal allergic reaction (*see* ANAPHYLAXIS). If an individual is allergic to one type of penicillin he or she will be allergic to all penicillins. It is important, therefore, that anyone with known sensitivity always tells a doctor who is prescribing antibiotics. Otherwise penicillins are relatively free from severe side effects, but they may cause diarrhoea. Penicillins are classified according to their spectrum of antibacterial activity; for example **broad-spectrum penicillins** are active against a wide range of bacteria.

See AMOXICILLIN; AMPICILLIN; BENZYLPENICILLIN (PENICILLIN G); CO-AMOXICLAV; CO-FLUAMPICIL; FLUCLOXACILLIN; PHENOXYMETHYLPENICILLIN (PENICILLIN V); PIPERACILLIN; PIVMECILLINAM HYDROCHLORIDE; TEMOCILLIN; TICARCILLIN.

Pennsaid (Dimethaid International) *See* DICLOFENAC SODIUM.

p

Pentacarinat (sanofi-aventis) *See* PENTAMIDINE ISETHIONATE.

pentamidine isethionate A drug used for the treatment of pneumonia caused by *Pneumocystis jirovecii* (*carinii*), especially in people who cannot tolerate, or have not responded to, *co-trimoxazole. Pentamidine has also been used for treating certain other serious infections, such as leishmaniasis. It has the potential for causing severe side effects, including a dangerous fall in blood pressure (see below), and should therefore only be used by specialists. Pentamidine is available, on *prescription only, as a form for injection or as a solution to be used in a *nebulizer.
Side effects: when given by injection pentamidine can have serious side effects, including severe hypotension (low blood pressure), low blood glucose (*see* HYPOGLYCAEMIA), *arrhythmias, and reduced numbers of white blood cells and platelets. Other side effects include nausea, vomiting, dizziness, fainting, flushing, rash, taste disturbances, and pain or other reactions at the injection site. If given by inhalation side effects are reduced because less of the drug is absorbed, but there may be constriction of the airways, cough, wheezing, and shortness of breath.
Precautions: pentamidine should be used with caution in women who are pregnant or breastfeeding and in people with high or low blood pressure, high or low blood sugar, or blood disorders.
Interactions with other drugs: pentamidine should not be given to (or should be used with caution in) patients who are taking amiodarone, the antipsychotic drugs amisulpride or droperidol, ivabradine, the antibiotics erythromycin or moxifloxacin, or the tricyclic antidepressants, since these drugs increase the risk of arrhythmias occurring.
Proprietary preparation: Pentacarinat.

Pentasa (Ferring Pharmaceuticals) *See* MESALAZINE.

pentazocine An *opioid analgesic used for the treatment of moderate to severe pain. When injected, it is more potent than dihydrocodeine or codeine but has additional side effects and is not suitable for some patients (see below). Pentazocine is a *controlled drug; it is available as tablets, capsules, or an injection.
Side effects: *see* MORPHINE. In addition, it may cause hallucinations.
Precautions: pentazocine should not be given to patients who are regularly taking other opioids, since it antagonizes their action and can cause withdrawal symptoms; it should not be used in people who have had a heart attack or who have heart failure. *See also* MORPHINE.
Interactions with other drugs: *see* OPIOIDS.
Proprietary preparation: Fortral.

Pentostam (GlaxoSmithKline UK) *See* SODIUM STIBOGLUCONATE.

pentostatin A *cytotoxic drug that is highly effective in the treatment of hairy cell leukaemia (*see* CANCER). It is available as an injection on *prescription only and is most usually used in specialist centres.

Side effects: include *bone marrow suppression and decreased activity of the immune system, which reduces the body's resistance to infection.
Precautions: *see* CYTOTOXIC DRUGS. In addition, pentostatin should not be given to patients with kidney disease.
Interactions with other drugs:
Clozapine: should not be given with pentostatin since this increases the risk of agranulocytosis (a blood diorder).
Cytotoxic drugs: the adverse effects of fludarabine on the lungs are increased if it is taken with pentostatin; high-dose cyclophosphamide should not be given with pentostatin since this increases the risk of adverse effects.
Proprietary preparation: Nipent.

pentoxifylline <**oxpentifylline**> A *xanthine used in the treatment of peripheral vascular disease, such as Raynaud's syndrome. It is available as *modified-release tablets on *prescription only.
Side effects: include gastrointestinal disturbances, dizziness, and headache. *See also* XANTHINES.
Precautions: pentoxifylline should not be taken by people with the acute porphyrias, cerebral haemorrhage (bleeding into the brain), bleeding in the retina, or a heart attack or by women who are pregnant or breastfeeding.
Interactions with other drugs:
Ketorolac: increases the risk of gastrointestinal bleeding and should not be taken with pentoxifylline.
Theophylline: its plasma concentration is increased.
Proprietary preparation: Trental.

Pentrax (Alliance) *See* COAL TAR.

Pepcid (Merck Sharp & Dohme) *See* FAMOTIDINE.

PepcidTwo (McNeil Ltd) A proprietary combination of *famotidine (an H_2-receptor antagonist) and *calcium carbonate and *magnesium sulphate (antacids), used to treat the symptoms of gastro-oesophageal reflux (*see* ACID-PEPTIC DISEASES). It is available as chewable tablets on *prescription only.
Side effects, precautions, and interactions with other drugs: *see* FAMOTIDINE; ANTACIDS.

Peppermint Indigestion Tablets (Boots) A proprietary combination of the *antacids *calcium carbonate, *sodium bicarbonate, *magnesium trisilicate, and *magnesium carbonate, used for the treatment of indigestion. It is available *over the counter but only from Boots stores.
Side effects, precautions, and interactions with other drugs: *see* ANTACIDS.

peppermint oil An oil extracted from the peppermint plant, used for its *antispasmodic effect on the gut to relieve the symptoms of irritable bowel syndrome, especially abdominal colic. It is also included as an ingredient in many *antacid preparations and in preparations to relieve nasal congestion. Peppermint oil is available as *enteric-coated capsules or *modified-release

capsules, which can be obtained without a prescription, but only from pharmacies.
Side effects: peppermint oil may cause heartburn and (rarely) allergic reactions.
Proprietary preparations: Colpermin (modified-release capsules); Mintec (enteric-coated capsules); plus many other proprietary preparations of which it is an ingredient.

Peptac (IVAX) A proprietary combination of sodium alginate (*see* ALGINIC ACID), *sodium bicarbonate, and *calcium carbonate, used as an antacid in the treatment of heartburn and reflux (*see* ACID-PEPTIC DISEASES). It is available as a sugar-free suspension and can be obtained without a prescription, but only from pharmacies.
Side effects, precautions, and interactions with other drugs: *see* ANTACIDS.

peptic ulcers *See* ACID-PEPTIC DISEASES.

Pepto-Bismol (Procter & Gamble) *See* BISMUTH SUBSALICYLATE.

Percutol (Teva UK) *See* GLYCERYL TRINITRATE.

Perdix (UCB Pharma) *See* MOEXIPRIL HYDROCHLORIDE.

Perfalgan (Bristol-Myers Squibb) *See* PARACETAMOL.

pergolide A *dopamine receptor agonist, similar to *bromocriptine, used alone or as an *adjunct to *levodopa in the treatment of Parkinson's disease. It is available as tablets on *prescription only.
Side effects: include hallucinations, confusion, involuntary abnormal movements, somnolence, abdominal pain, nausea, dyspepsia, double vision, breathlessness, lung problems, and insomnia.
Precautions: pergolide should not be taken by people with heart-valve disease and should be used with caution in people with abnormal heart rhythms (*see* ARRHYTHMIA) or a history of confusion or hallucinations and in women who are pregnant or breastfeeding (it stops production of breast milk). Dosage should be reduced gradually at the end of treatment.
Interactions with other drugs:
Antipsychotics: antagonize the effect of pergolide.
Metoclopramide: antagonizes the effect of pergolide.
Proprietary preparation: Celance.

Pergoveris (Merck Serono) A proprietary combination of *follitropin alfa and *lutropin alfa (both gonadotrophins), used in the treatment of fertility disorders. It is available as a solution for subcutaneous injection on *prescription only.
Side effects and precautions: *see* FOLLITROPIN; LUTROPIN ALFA.

Periactin (Merck Sharp & Dohme) *See* CYPROHEPTADINE HYDROCHLORIDE.

pericyazine A phenothiazine *antipsychotic drug used for the treatment of schizophrenia and as an *adjunct for the short-term treatment of severe

anxiety or agitation and violent or dangerously impulsive behaviour. It is available as tablets or a syrup on *prescription only.
Side effects: as for *chlorpromazine, but pericyazine is more sedating, has more pronounced antimuscarinic effects (e.g. dry mouth, constipation, difficulty in passing urine, blurred vision) but fewer *extrapyramidal reactions, and may depress breathing. Low blood pressure may occur at the start of treatment.
Precautions and interactions with other drugs: *see* CHLORPROMAZINE HYDROCHLORIDE.
Proprietary preparation: Neulactil.

Perinal (Dermal Laboratories) A proprietary combination of *hydrocortisone (a corticosteroid) and *lidocaine hydrochloride (a local anaesthetic), used for the relief of pain or itching in or around the anus. It is available in a metered-dose spray and can be obtained without a prescription, but only from pharmacies.
Side effects: *see* CORTICOSTEROIDS.
Precautions: Perinal should not be used when viral or fungal infection is present; prolonged use should be avoided. Perinal is not recommended for children under 14 years old.

perindopril An *ACE inhibitor used as an adjunct to *diuretics for the treatment of *heart failure and to prevent further heart damage after a heart attack; it is also licensed for use in the treatment of *hypertension. It is available as tablets in two forms, **perindopril erbumine** and **perindopril arginine**, on *prescription only.
Side effects, precautions, and interactions with other drugs: *see* ACE INHIBITORS.
Proprietary preparations: Coversyl Arginine; *Coversyl Arginine Plus (combined with indapamide).

Periogard (Colegate-Palmolive) *See* CHLORHEXIDINE.

Periostat (Alliance) *See* DOXYCYCLINE.

permethrin A pesticide that is used clinically to treat infestations of crab *lice and *scabies. It is available as a cream and can be obtained without a prescription, but only from pharmacies.
Side effects: permethrin may cause itching, redness, and stinging of the skin.
Precautions: permethrin should not be applied near the eyes or on broken skin; treatment of children under two years old should be supervised by a doctor.
Proprietary preparations: Lyclear Creme Rinse; Lyclear Dermal Cream.

Permitabs (Alliance) *See* POTASSIUM PERMANGANATE.

Peroxyl (Colgate-Palmolive) *See* HYDROGEN PEROXIDE.

perphenazine A phenothiazine *antipsychotic drug used for the treatment of schizophrenia and mania and for the short-term management of severe

p

anxiety or agitation and violent or dangerously impulsive behaviour. It is also used as an *antiemetic to treat severe nausea and vomiting. Perphenazine is available as tablets on *prescription only.
Side effects: as for *chlorpromazine, but perphenazine is less sedating and has fewer antimuscarinic effects, and *extrapyramidal reactions are more frequent.
Precautions: perphenazine should not be used to treat agitated elderly patients. *See also* CHLORPROMAZINE HYDROCHLORIDE.
Interactions with other drugs: *see* CHLORPROMAZINE HYDROCHLORIDE.

Persantin, Persantin Retard (Boehringer Ingelheim) *See* DIPYRIDAMOLE.

Peru balsam (**balsam of Peru**) A balsam exuded from the trunk of the tree *Myroxylon balsamum.* It has mild antiseptic properties by virtue of its content of cinnamic acid and *benzoic acid. Peru balsam can be used diluted with castor oil to soothe bedsores and chronic venous ulcers, and it is included as an ingredient in some topical preparations for the treatment of *eczema and in preparations to relieve the pain and itching of *haemorrhoids.
Proprietary preparations: *Anugesic-HC (combined with zinc oxide, bismuth oxide, hydrocortisone acetate, and benzyl benzoate); *Anugesic-HC Suppositories (combined with zinc oxide, bismuth oxide, bismuth subgallate, pramocaine hydrochloride, and hydrocortisone acetate); *Anusol (combined with zinc oxide, bismuth subgallate, and bismuth oxide); *Anusol-HC (combined with zinc oxide, bismuth subgallate, bismuth oxide, hydrocortisone acetate, and benzyl benzoate).

pessary (**vaginal suppository**) A bullet-shaped plug containing a drug that is administered by insertion into the vagina. Pessaries are used when the drug needs to be delivered to the vaginal wall or the cervix; examples of drugs administered as pessaries are antibiotics used in the treatment of vaginal infections or prostaglandins used to induce labour or abortion.

pethidine hydrochloride An *opioid analgesic used for the treatment of moderate to severe pain and for pain relief during labour and before, during, or after surgery. Pethidine is a *controlled drug; it is available as tablets or an injection.
Side effects: *see* MORPHINE. In addition, there may be adverse effects on the nervous system and overdosage may cause convulsions.
Precautions: *see* MORPHINE.
Interactions with other drugs:

MAOIs: should not be taken with pethidine or for two weeks after stopping pethidine.
Moclobemide: may cause high or lower blood pressure and should not be taken with pethidine.
Rasagiline: increases the risk of adverse effects on the central nervous system; pethidine should not be taken until two weeks after stopping rasagiline.

Ritonavir: increases the plasma concentration of pethidine; these two drugs should not be taken together.
Selegiline: should not be taken with pethidine as the combination of these two drugs can cause a high fever and have severe effects on the central nervous system.
See also OPIOIDS.

Proprietary preparations: *Pamergan P100 (combined with promethazine).

petroleum jelly *See* WHITE SOFT PARAFFIN; YELLOW SOFT PARAFFIN.

Pevaryl (Janssen-Cilag) *See* ECONAZOLE NITRATE.

pharmacy medicine *See* OVER THE COUNTER.

Pharmaton Vitality Capsules (Boehringer Ingelheim) A proprietary combination of ginseng extract, *vitamin A, cyanocobalamin, biotin, nicotinamide, ascorbic acid, folic acid, the *vitamin B complex, *vitamin C, *vitamin D_3, and *vitamin E, and various minerals (including selenium). It is used to relieve fatigue and to supplement dietary intake of vitamins. Pharmaton is freely available *over the counter in the form of capsules.

Pharmorubicin (Pharmacia) *See* EPIRUBICIN.

phenelzine A *monoamine oxidase inhibitor used for the treatment of depressive illness. It is available as tablets on *prescription only.
Side effects and interactions with other drugs: *see* MONOAMINE OXIDASE INHIBITORS.
Precautions: *see* MONOAMINE OXIDASE INHIBITORS. In addition, phenelzine should not be taken by people with liver disease or by those who have had a stroke.
Proprietary preparation: Nardil.

p

Phenergan (sanofi-aventis) *See* PROMETHAZINE HYDROCHLORIDE.

phenindione An oral *anticoagulant used for the prevention and treatment of deep-vein *thrombosis and pulmonary embolism and for the prevention of embolism in people with atrial fibrillation (*see* ARRHYTHMIA) and in those who have received an artificial heart valve. It is available as tablets on *prescription only.
Side effects: *see* WARFARIN SODIUM. Phenindione is more likely than warfarin to cause allergic reactions, such as rashes, fever, blood disorders, diarrhoea, and damage to the liver or kidneys.
Precautions: *see* WARFARIN SODIUM.
Interactions with other drugs:
Amiodarone: enhances the anticoagulant effect of phenindione.
Anabolic steroids: enhance the anticoagulant effect of phenindione.
Antiplatelet drugs: clopidogrel and dipyridamole enhance the anticoagulant effect of phenindione.
Lipid-lowering drugs: the anticoagulant effect of phenindione is enhanced

by rosuvastatin and the fibrates; the effect of phenindione is altered by colestyramine.
NSAIDs: enhance the anticoagulant effect of phenindione; diclofenac and ketorolac should not be taken with phenindione.
Oral contraceptives: reduce the anticoagulant effect of phenindione.
Ritonavir: may enhance the anticoagulant effect of phenindione.
Testosterone: enhances the anticoagulant effect of phenindione.
Tetracyclines: may enhance the anticoagulant effect of phenindione.
Thyroid hormones: enhance the anticoagulant effect of phenindione.
Vitamin K: reduces the anticoagulant effect of phenindione.

phenobarbital <**phenobarbitone**> A *barbiturate that is used mainly as an *anticonvulsant drug for the treatment of all forms of epilepsy (including status epilepticus) except absence seizures, although newer antiepileptics are now usually preferred. It has a sedating effect in adults and may cause behavioural problems in children. A *controlled drug, it is available as tablets or an elixir for oral use and as a form for injection (to treat status epilepticus).
Side effects: include drowsiness, lethargy, mental depression, and allergic skin reactions. Paradoxical excitement, restlessness, and confusion can occur in the elderly and hyperactivity in children.
Precautions: phenobarbital should be used with caution in people who have liver or kidney disease and in women who are pregnant or breastfeeding; women who are planning to become pregnant should seek specialist advice.
Interactions with other drugs:
Antidepressants: the plasma concentration of mianserin is reduced by phenobarbital; St John's wort should not be taken with phenobarbital.
Antiepileptic drugs: phenobarbital may reduce their anticonvulsant actions.
Antifungal drugs: the plasma concentrations of itraconazole, posaconazole, and voriconazole may be reduced by phenobarbital, which should not be taken with voriconazole.
Antipsychotic drugs: reduce the anticonvulsive actions of phenobarbital; the plasma concentration of aripiprazole may be reduced by phenobarbital and its dosage should therefore be increased.
Eplerenone: its plasma concentration is reduced and it should not be taken with phenobarbital.
Stiripentol: increases the plasma concentration of phenobarbital.
Tacrolimus: its plasma concentration is reduced by phenobarbital.
Telithromycin: its plasma concentration is reduced and it should not be taken during and for two weeks after treatment with phenobarbital.
See also BARBITURATES.

phenobarbitone *See* PHENOBARBITAL.

phenol A *disinfectant that is used in diluted solutions as an ingredient in some *antiseptic preparations. Oily phenol is used in *sclerotherapy for treating *haemorrhoids; it is available as a solution for injection on *prescription only.

Side effects: injection of phenol may cause local irritation and if it leaks from the injection site it may damage surrounding tissue.
Proprietary preparations: *Blistex Relief Cream (combined with ammonia); *Germolene Antiseptic Cream (combined with chlorhexidine); *Germolene Antiseptic Ointment (combined with methyl salicylate, octafonium chloride, and zinc oxide); *TCP Antiseptic Liquid (halogenated phenols).

phenothiazines A group of chemically related compounds that are used mainly as *antipsychotic drugs, although some of them have other uses as well (for example, as *antiemetics). *See* CHLORPROMAZINE HYDROCHLORIDE; FLUPHENAZINE DECANOATE; PERICYAZINE; PERPHENAZINE; PIPOTIAZINE PALMITATE; PROCHLORPERAZINE; PROMAZINE HYDROCHLORIDE; TRIFLUOPERAZINE.

phenoxybenzamine hydrochloride A powerful *alpha blocker that is used in conjunction with a *beta blocker to treat episodes of *hypertension associated with phaeochromocytoma, a tumour of the adrenal gland that unpredictably secretes large amounts of adrenaline and noradrenaline, causing sudden attacks of raised blood pressure. Phenoxybenzamine is available, on *prescription only, as capsules or a form for intravenous infusion.
Side effects: include low blood pressure on standing (with dizziness and a fast heart rate), tiredness, nasal congestion, constriction of the pupils, and failure of ejaculation; decreased sweating and a dry mouth can occur after infusion.
Precautions: phenoxybenzamine should not be given to people who have had a stroke or are recovering from a heart attack. It should be used with caution in the elderly, in people with heart failure or other heart disease or kidney disease, and in pregnant women.
Interactions with other drugs: *see* ALPHA BLOCKERS.
Proprietary preparation: Dibenyline (capsules).

phenoxymethylpenicillin (**penicillin V**) A *penicillin that has a similar spectrum of action to *benzylpenicillin but is less active and is therefore not used for serious infections. It has the advantage that it can be taken by mouth. It is available as tablets or a syrup on *prescription only.
Side effects: include diarrhoea, nausea, and allergic reactions (*see* BENZYLPENICILLIN).
Precautions: *see* BENZYLPENICILLIN; PENICILLINS.
Interactions with other drugs: *see* BENZYLPENICILLIN.

phentolamine An *alpha blocker used for the treatment of episodes of hypertension in phaeochromocytoma, a tumour of the adrenal gland that can release large amounts of noradrenaline and adrenaline unpredictably and thereby cause raised blood pressure. It is available as a solution for injection on *prescription only.
Side effects, precautions, and interactions with other drugs: *see* ALPHA BLOCKERS.
Proprietary preparation: Rogitine.
See also ANTIHYPERTENSIVE DRUGS.

phenylephrine A *sympathomimetic drug that constricts blood vessels. It is widely used as a nasal *decongestant and is an ingredient in many cough and cold preparations. It is also used in eye drops to dilate the pupils in order to facilitate ophthalmic examinations and is combined with local anaesthetics in topical preparations to restrict the action of the anaesthetic to the area of application. Phenylephrine can be administered by injection or intravenous infusion to increase blood pressure and is sometimes used for this purpose in emergencies until blood or plasma transfusions can be given although it does not have a *licence for this. Phenylephrine for injection or infusion is a *prescription only medicine; other preparations are available without a prescription.
Side effects: include headache and high blood pressure, changes in heart rate, vomiting, and tingling and coolness of the skin.
Precautions: phenylephrine should not be taken by people with an overactive thyroid gland. *See also* NORADRENALINE.
Interactions with other drugs:
Guanethidine: phenylephrine antagonizes its effect in lowering blood pressure.
MAOIs: may cause a dangerous rise in blood pressure.
Proprietary preparations: Boots Congestion Relief Capsules; Non-Drowsy Sudafed Congestion Relief Capsules; Minims Phenylephrine (eye drops); *Beechams All-in-One (combined with guaifenesin and paracetamol); *Beechams Flu-Plus Caplets (combined with paracetamol and caffeine); *Beechams Flu-Plus Hot Lemon, Beechams Flu-Plus Hot Berry Fruits (combined with paracetamol); *Beechams Powders Capsules (combined with paracetamol and caffeine); *Boots Cold and 'Flu Relief Tablets (combined with caffeine, paracetamol, and ascorbic acid); *Boots Maximum Strength Cold & Flu Relief Direct Dose Lemon/Blackcurrant (combined with paracetamol); *Boots Max Strength Cold & Flu Capsules (combined with paracetamol and caffeine); *Boots Max Strength Sinus Relief Capsules (combined with paracetamol and caffeine); *Lemsip Cold & Flu Capsules (combined with caffeine and paracetamol); *Lemsip Cold & Flu Lemon (combined with paracetamol and vitamin C); *Non-Drowsy Sudafed Congestion and Headache Capsules (combined with paracetamol and caffeine).

phenytoin An *anticonvulsant used to orally treat epilepsy (major and partial seizures) and status epilepticus (repeated seizures with no recovery of consciousness between them) and to control or prevent seizures following neurosurgery or head injury. It is also used to treat trigeminal neuralgia. **Fosphenytoin sodium**, a drug that is converted to phenytoin in the body, is given by intravenous infusion or intramuscular injection to treat status epilepticus and seizures following surgery or head injury when oral phenytoin cannot be used. Phenytoin is available on *prescription only, either as an injection or infusion for use under medical supervision or as tablets, chewable tablets, capsules, or a suspension for oral use.
Side effects: include nausea, vomiting, headache, tremor, nervousness, and insomnia; less common effects are unsteadiness, shakiness, slurred speech,

acne, increased growth of body hair, overgrowth of the gums, and rashes (if rashes develop the treatment should be discontinued). Rapid involuntary eye movements and blurred vision are signs of overdosage.

Precautions: phenytoin should be used with caution in women who are pregnant or breastfeeding and in people with impaired liver function. Women who are planning to become pregnant should seek specialist advice. Symptoms of blood or skin disorders (e.g. fever, sore throat, rashes, mouth ulcers, bruising) should be reported to a doctor. When given intravenously, continuous monitoring of the electrocardiogram is essential and resuscitative equipment should be available.

Interactions with other drugs:

Analgesics: the plasma concentration of phenytoin is increased by azapropazone (which should not be taken with phenytoin); the effects of phenytoin are enhanced by aspirin and possibly by other NSAIDs; the effects of methadone are reduced by phenytoin.

Anti-arrhythmic drugs: amiodarone increases the plasma concentration of phenytoin; the plasma concentration of disopyramide is reduced by phenytoin.

Antibiotics: the plasma concentration of phenytoin is increased by chloramphenicol, cycloserine, isoniazid, metronidazole, and trimethoprim and reduced by rifampicin. The plasma concentration of telithromycin is reduced by phenytoin, which should be avoided during and for two weeks after treatment with phenytoin.

Anticoagulants: the metabolism of warfarin and acenocoumarol is increased by phenytoin, which may reduce their anticoagulant effect (but in some cases has enhanced it).

Anticonvulsants: taking two or more anticonvulsants together may enhance their adverse effects: phenytoin often reduces plasma concentrations of clonazepam, carbamazepine, lamotrigine, topiramate (which increases the plasma concentration of phenytoin), and sodium valproate and increases the plasma concentration of ethosuximide and phenobarbital; stiripentol increases the plasma concentration of phenytoin.

Antidepressants: antagonize the anticonvulsant effect of phenytoin. Fluoxetine and fluvoxamine increase the plasma concentration of phenytoin; the plasma concentrations of mianserin, mirtazapine, paroxetine, and tricyclic antidepressants are reduced by phenytoin.

Antifungal drugs: fluconazole, miconazole, and voriconazole increase the plasma concentration of phenytoin; the plasma concentrations of itraconazole, ketoconazole, and posaconazole are reduced by phenytoin (itraconazole should not be taken with phenytoin).

Antimalarial drugs: chloroquine, hydroxychloroquine, mefloquine, and pyrimethamine antagonize the anticonvulsant effect of phenytoin; the antifolate effect of pyrimethamine is enhanced by phenytoin.

Antipsychotics: antagonize the anticonvulsant effect of phenytoin; the plasma concentrations of aripiprazole, clozapine, quetiapine, and

sertindole are reduced by phenytoin (the dosage of aripiprazole should be increased).
Calcium antagonists: diltiazem increases the plasma concentration of phenytoin; phenytoin reduces the effects of felodipine, isradipine, and verapamil and probably also of nicardipine, nifedipine, and diltiazam.
Ciclosporin: its plasma concentration is reduced by phenytoin.
Corticosteroids: their effects are reduced by phenytoin.
Disulfiram: inhibits the breakdown of phenytoin and therefore increases the risk of its toxic effects.
Eplerenone: its plasma concentration is reduced and it should not be taken with phenytoin.
Indinavir: its plasma concentration may be reduced.
Oral contraceptives: their contraceptive effect is reduced by phenytoin.
Sulfinpyrazone: increases the plasma concentration of phenytoin.
Theophylline: the plasma concentrations of both drugs are reduced.
Ulcer-healing drugs: cimetidine increases the plasma concentration of phenytoin; sucralfate reduces the absorption of phenytoin; esomeprazole increases the effects of phenytoin.

Proprietary preparations: Epanutin; Epanutin Infatabs (chewable tablets); Epanutin Ready-Mixed Parenteral; Pro-Epanutin (fosphenytoin).

Phillips' Milk of Magnesia (Bayer) *See* MAGNESIUM HYDROXIDE.

pholcodine A weak *opioid that acts as a *cough suppressant but has no appreciable analgesic activity. It is therefore used for the treatment of dry or painful coughs and is available as a linctus and as an ingredient of many cough medicines. Pholcodine is usually freely available *over the counter, although some preparations can be bought only from a pharmacy, depending on the other ingredients.

Side effects: as for *codeine, but side effects are rare. Pholcodine is not addictive.

Precautions: *see* CODEINE.

Interactions with other drugs: *see* OPIOIDS.

Proprietary preparations: Benylin Children's Dry Coughs; Boots Daytime Cough Relief; Famel Linctus; Galenphol, Galenphol Paediatric, and Galenphol Strong; Hill's Balsam Dry Cough Syrup; Pavacol-D; Tixylix Dry Cough; *Boots Children's 1 Year Plus Night Time Cough Syrup (combined with diphenhydramine); *Boots Day Cold Comfort (combined with paracetamol and pseudoephedrine); *Boots Night Cold Comfort (combined with paracetamol, diphenhydramine, and pseudoephedrine); *Boots Night-time Cough Relief Syrup 2 Years Plus (combined with diphenhydramine); *Boots Nirolex Night Time Cough Relief Linctus (combined with diphenhydramine); *Day Nurse (combined with paracetamol and pseudoephedrine); *Tixylix Cough & Cold (combined with chlorphenamine and pseudoephedrine); *Tixylix Night Cough (combined with promethazine).

Phosex (Vitaline Pharmaceuticals) *See* CALCIUM ACETATE.

PhosLo (Frefenius Medical Care) *See* CALCIUM ACETATE.

phosphate-binding agents Drugs, including aluminium- and calcium-containing salts, that are used to bind to phosphates in the diet and stop them from being absorbed. This is important in people who have kidney disease, especially those who are on kidney dialysis, since high concentrations of phosphate in the blood can cause bone disease. Phosphate-binding agents, which are taken before food, include *aluminium hydroxide, *calcium carbonate, *calcium acetate, *lanthanum, and *sevelamer.

phosphate laxatives A group of phosphate salts used as *osmotic laxatives to evacuate the bowel before abdominal X-ray examinations or before investigative procedures or surgery of the bowel. They are also used to relieve postoperative constipation and in obstetrics. The common phosphate laxatives are *sodium acid phosphate and **sodium phosphate** which are available as enemas or suppositories and can be obtained without a prescription, but only from pharmacies. **Sodium dihydrogen phosphate dihydrate** and **disodium phosphate dodecahydrate** are ingredients in *bowel-cleansing solutions.
Side effects: there may be local irritation.
Precautions: phosphates should be used with caution in elderly people and should not be used in patients with acute gastrointestinal disorders.

Phosphate-Sandoz (HK Pharma) A proprietary combination of *sodium acid phosphate, *sodium bicarbonate, and *potassium bicarbonate, used as a *phosphate supplement. It is also occasionally used to reduce high plasma calcium concentrations that result from overproduction of *parathyroid hormone by the parathyroid gland or occur with certain cancers. Phosphate-Sandoz is available as effervescent tablets and can be obtained without a prescription, but only from pharmacies.
Side effects and precautions: *see* PHOSPHATE SUPPLEMENTS. When used to reduce plasma calcium, this medicine may bind to calcium to form calcium phosphate in the tissues, leading to kidney impairment and the formation of kidney stones.

phosphate supplements Preparations containing phosphate salts (usually *sodium acid phosphate) used to treat conditions of phosphate deficiency. Supplementary phosphate may be required in addition to *vitamin D for treating patients with a type of rickets or osteomalacia in which plasma phosphate concentrations are very low. A lack of phosphate is occasionally also seen in people with diabetic ketoacidosis (a condition that can occur in poorly controlled *diabetes mellitus) and in alcoholics. Phosphate supplements are usually taken by mouth, but infusions may be required for treating severe cases of phosphate depletion.
Side effects: diarrhoea is the most common side effect.
Precautions: plasma concentrations of electrolytes should be monitored during phosphate therapy.

phosphodiesterase inhibitors Compounds that inhibit the enzyme phosphodiesterase and thereby allow the accumulation of the substance cAMP (cyclic adenosine monophosphate). cAMP is produced when the *sympathetic nervous system is stimulated (among other circumstances). Thus an accumulation of cAMP has a similar effect to stimulating the sympathetic nervous system (*see* SYMPATHOMIMETIC DRUGS). There are two types of phosphodiesterase (PDE) inhibitor: the *xanthines, which are *bronchodilators used for treating asthma; and the PDE type III inhibitors (such as *enoximone and *milrinone), which have been used in the treatment of congestive *heart failure.

Photofrin (Axcan Pharma) *See* PORFIMER SODIUM.

Phyllocontin Continus (Napp Pharmaceuticals) *See* AMINOPHYLLINE.

Physeptone (Martindale Pharmaceuticals) *See* METHADONE HYDROCHLORIDE.

Physiotens (Solvay Healthcare) *See* MOXONIDINE.

Phytex (Wynlit Laboratories) A proprietary combination of the antifungal agent borotannic acid complex (consisting of tannic acid and boric acid), *salicylic acid, *methyl salicylate, and *acetic acid, used for the treatment of fungal infections of the skin and nails. It is available as a solution for painting on the nails and can be obtained without a prescription, but only from pharmacies.
Precautions: Phytex should not be used during pregnancy.

phytomenadione (vitamin K$_1$) A form of *vitamin K that is used in the prevention and treatment of haemorrhage (severe bleeding) in low-birth-weight babies. Phytomenadione is available as a solution for intramuscular injection or for oral administration on *prescription only.
Proprietary preparations: Konakion MM; Konakion MM Paediatric.

Picolax (Ferring Pharmaceuticals) A proprietary combination of *sodium picosulfate (a stimulant laxative) and *magnesium citrate (an osmotic laxative), used to evacuate the bowel before radiological procedures, investigation, or surgery. It is available as an oral powder to be dissolved in water and can be obtained without a prescription, but only from pharmacies.
Side effects and precautions: *see* BOWEL-CLEANSING SOLUTIONS.

piles *See* HAEMORRHOIDS.

pilocarpine A *cholinergic drug that is used (in the form of drops or gel) to improve the drainage of fluid from the front chamber of the eye (*see* MIOTICS) in the treatment of *glaucoma. Because it stimulates the salivary glands, pilocarpine is also used (as tablets) to prevent the dry mouth caused by radiation treatment and to treat dry eyes and dry mouth in Sjögren's syndrome (which affects the salivary and tear-producing glands). It is available, on *prescription only, as eye drops, eye gel, or tablets.
Side effects: eye formulations commonly cause temporary blurring of vision, and there may be brow ache and headache. The tablets (and rarely the eye

formulations) may cause watering eyes, sweating, chills, diarrhoea, nausea, abdominal pain, and increased frequency of urination.
Precautions: eye formulations should not be used by people with inflammation of the iris or by those who wear soft contact lenses. Pilocarpine tablets should not be used by people with heart or circulatory disease, asthma, or lung disease, or inflammation of the iris or by women who are pregnant or breastfeeding.
Interactions with other drugs:
Beta blockers: the risk of abnormal heart rhythms is increased.
Proprietary preparations: Minims Pilocarpine (preservative-free single-dose eye drops); Pilogel (eye gel); Salagen (tablets).

Pilogel (Alcon Laboratories) *See* PILOCARPINE.

pimecrolimus A drug that affects the immune response, used in the treatment of mild to moderate *eczema when topical *corticosteroids cannot be given. It works by modulating the inflammatory chemicals secreted by some white blood cells. Pimecrolimus is available as a cream on *prescription only.
Side effects: include skin irritation, itching, and skin infection.
Precautions: the cream should not be applied to skin that is infected, reddened, or flaking or to skin tumours. It should not be used by people with immune deficiency. Excessive exposure to sunlight or sun lamps and consumption of alcohol should be avoided as these can cause skin irritation. Pimecrolimus is not recommended for children under two years of age.
Proprietary preparation: Elidel.

pimozide An *antipsychotic drug used for the treatment of schizophrenia and some other psychoses. It is available as tablets on *prescription only.
Side effects: as for *chlorpromazine but pimozide is less sedating, has more pronounced *extrapyramidal reactions, and can cause serious abnormalities in heart rhythm (*arrhythmias).
Precautions: pimozide should not be taken by women who are breastfeeding or by people who have, or have had, heart arrhythmias. People who are being treated with pimozide will need periodic heart monitoring.
Interactions with other drugs: pimozide should not be used with other antipsychotic drugs or with certain other drugs (see below), as this increases the risk of serious effects on the heart.
Anaesthetics: their effect in lowering blood pressure is enhanced.
Anti-arrhythmic drugs: amiodarone and disopyramide should not be taken with pimozide.
Antibiotics: pimozide should not be taken with clarithromycin, erythromycin, moxifloxacin, or telithromycin.
Antidepressants: tricyclic antidepressants and SSRIs should not be taken with pimozide.
Antiepileptic drugs: their anticonvulsant effects are antagonized by pimozide.

Antifungal drugs: the imidazoles and triazoles should not be taken with pimozide.
Antimalarial drugs: pimozide should not be taken with mefloquine or quinine.
Antipsychotic drugs: atazanavir, efavirenz, indinavir, nelfinavir, ritonavir, and saquinavir should not be taken with pimozide.
Aprepitant: should not be taken with pimozide.
Atomoxetine: increases the risk of arrhythmias.
Diuretics: should not be taken with pimozide.
Ivabradine: increases the risk of arrhythmias.
Methadone: increases the risk of arrhythmias.
Sedatives: the sedative effects of pimozide are increased if it is taken with anxiolytic or hypnotic drugs, or any other drug that causes sedation.
Sotalol: increases the risk of arrhythmias.

Proprietary preparation: Orap.

pindolol A non-cardioselective *beta blocker used for the treatment of *angina and *hypertension. It is available as tablets on *prescription only.
Side effects, precautions, and interactions with other drugs: *see* BETA BLOCKERS.
Proprietary preparations: Visken; *Viskaldix (combined with clopamide).
See also ANTIHYPERTENSIVE DRUGS.

pioglitazone An *oral hypoglycaemic drug used in the treatment of type 2 *diabetes mellitus, either alone or in combination with *metformin hydrochloride, a *sulphonylurea, or both. It appears to act by reducing the body's resistance to insulin, which leads to a reduction in blood-glucose levels. Pioglitazone is available as tablets on *prescription only.
Side effects: include visual disturbance, upper airways infections, weight increase, sinusitis, and insomnia.
Precautions: pioglitazone should not be taken by people with heart failure or a history of heart failure, by those with impaired liver function, or by women who are pregnant or breastfeeding.
Proprietary preparations: Actos; *Competact (combined with metformin hydrochloride).

piperacillin A broad-spectrum *penicillin that is active against *Pseudomonas* and *Proteus* bacteria. It is used for the treatment of systemic and local infections (such as infected wounds or burns) and respiratory, urinary-tract, abdominal, or skin infections. Given by injection or infusion in combination with *tazobactam, it is available on *prescription only.
Side effects, precautions, and interactions with other drugs: *see* BENZYLPENICILLIN.
Proprietary preparation: *Tazocin (combined with tazobactam).

piperazine An *anthelmintic that acts by paralysing intestinal worms so that they can be eliminated from the body. It is used for the treatment of roundworm and threadworm infestations. Piperazine is available as an elixir

and as a powder combined with sennosides (to aid elimination of the worms) and can be obtained without a prescription, but only from pharmacies.
Side effects: include nausea, vomiting, colic, diarrhoea, allergic reactions (including itching), and rarely visual disturbances, vertigo, and dizziness.
Precautions: piperazine should be used with caution by people with liver disease, kidney disease, or epilepsy and by women who are pregnant or breastfeeding.
Proprietary preparation: *Pripsen (combined with sennosides).

Piportil Depot (sanofi-aventis) *See* PIPOTIAZINE PALMITATE.

pipotiazine palmitate **<pipothiazine palmitate>** A phenothiazine *antipsychotic drug used for the maintenance treatment of schizophrenia and other psychoses. It is available as a *depot injection on *prescription only.
Side effects, precautions, and interactions with other drugs: *see* CHLORPROMAZINE HYDROCHLORIDE.
Proprietary preparation: Piportil Depot.

piracetam An *anticonvulsant drug used to treat myoclonus – a sudden spasm of the muscles that occurs in people with certain other neurological illnesses. It is available, on *prescription only, as tablets or an oral solution.
Side effects: include weight gain, nervousness, somnolence, and depression.
Precautions: piracetam should not be taken by people who have liver or kidney disease or bleeding into the brain or by women who are pregnant or breastfeeding. The drug should be withdrawn gradually at the end of treatment.
Proprietary preparation: Nootropil.

Piriteze Allergy Syrup, Piriteze Allergy Tablets (GlaxoSmithKline) *See* CETIRIZINE HYDROCHLORIDE.

Piriton (GlaxoSmithKline) *See* CHLORPHENAMINE MALEATE.

piroxicam An *NSAID used for the treatment of pain and inflammation in rheumatoid arthritis (including arthritis in children) and other disorders of the joints and muscles and to relieve the pain of acute gout. It is available, on *prescription only, as tablets, dispersible tablets, capsules, and a gel for topical application (a gel formulation can be obtained from pharmacies without a prescription).
Side effects: *see* NSAIDs. There is an increased risk of bleeding in the gastrointestinal tract and of skin reactions.
Precautions: *see* NSAIDs.
Interactions with other drugs: *see* NSAIDs. In addition:

Ritonavir: should not be used with piroxicam since it increases plasma concentrations of piroxicam to an extent that might cause toxic effects.

Proprietary preparations: Feldene; Feldene Gel; Feldene Melt (tablets that readily dissolve in the mouth).

Pitressin (Goldshield) *See* VASOPRESSIN.

pivmecillinam hydrochloride A *penicillin-type antibiotic used mainly for the treatment of urinary tract infections. It is available as tablets on *prescription only.
Side effects: include nausea, vomiting, and indigestion. *See also* BENZYLPENICILLIN.
Precautions: pivmecillinam should not be taken by people with narrowing of the oesophagus or obstruction of the intestines. *See also* BENZYLPENICILLIN.
Interactions with other drugs: *see* BENZYLPENICILLIN.
Proprietary preparation: Selexid.

pizotifen An *antihistamine that also opposes the action of *serotonin; it is used for the prevention of *migraine or recurrent vascular headaches. Pizotifen is available as tablets or an elixir on *prescription only.
Side effects: include drowsiness, increased appetite, and weight gain.
Precautions: drowsiness may affect driving performance or other skilled tasks. Pizotifen should be used with caution by people with glaucoma, urinary retention, or kidney disease and by women who are pregnant or breastfeeding.
Proprietary preparation: Sanomigran.

placebo A medicine that is ineffective but may help to relieve a condition because the patient has faith in its powers. New drugs are tested against placebos in clinical trials: the drug's effect is compared with the **placebo response**, which occurs even in the absence of any pharmacologically active substance in the placebo.

Plaquenil (sanofi-aventis) *See* HYDROXYCHLOROQUINE SULPHATE.

Plavix (sanofi-aventis) *See* CLOPIDOGREL.

p

Plendil (AstraZeneca) *See* FELODIPINE.

plerixafor A drug that, in combination with *granulocyte-colony stimulating factor, facilitates the release of stem cells from the bone marrow into the bloodstream in people with lymphoma and multiple myeloma (cancers of the lymph nodes and bone marrow). The stem cells are then extracted and used for transplantation. Plerixafor is available as a form for subcutaneous injection on *prescription only.
Side effects: include diarrhoea, nausea, vomiting, stomach discomfort, reactions at the injection site, insomnia, dizziness, sweating, joint pain, and fatigue.
Precautions: plerixafor is not recommended for women who are pregnant or breastfeeding. White blood cell and platelet counts should be monitored during treatment.
Proprietary preparation: Mozobil.

Pletal (Otsuka Pharmaceuticals) *See* CILOSTAZOL.

podophyllotoxin A caustic agent (*see* KERATOLYTICS) that is the main active constituent of *podophyllum. It is used to treat and dissolve warts affecting

the penis or female genitalia. It is available, on *prescription only, as a solution or cream for topical application.
Side effects: local irritation may occur.
Precautions: podophyllotoxin should not be used on open wounds or by women who are pregnant or breastfeeding. It is very irritant to the eyes.
Proprietary preparations: Condyline; Warticon.

podophyllum A caustic resin (*see* KERATOLYTICS) that is used in the form of a compound ointment **podophyllin paint** for treating warts on the sole of the foot. It is available without a prescription, but only from pharmacies.
Side effects and precautions: if many warts are to be treated, only a few should be treated at any one time, since podophyllum is extremely toxic if absorbed. It should not be applied to healthy skin (skin surrounding the wart should be protected during application) or to open wounds, and should not come into contact with the face (it is very irritant to the eyes). It should not be used by women who are pregnant or breastfeeding.
Proprietary preparation: *Posalfilin (combined with salicylic acid).

Politid XL (Actavis) *See* VENLAFAXINE.

Pollenshield Hayfever, Pollenshield Hayfever Relief (Actavis) *See* CETIRIZINE HYDROCHLORIDE.

polyacrylic acid *See* CARBOMER.

polyethylene glycols (**macrogols**) Polymers that are hydrophilic and are used as bases for ointments. Macrogol '3350' (polyethylene glycol '3350') is an *osmotic laxative that is used, in combination with other ingredients, for treating chronic constipation or clearing the bowel (*see* BOWEL-CLEANSING SOLUTIONS).
Side effects: macrogols can cause abdominal distension and pain and nausea.
Precautions: preparations containing macrogols should not be used in people with perforated or obstructed intestines and severe inflammatory bowel disease (such as Crohn's disease or ulcerative colitis). They should be used with caution during pregnancy and breastfeeding.
Proprietary preparations: Idrolax; *Klean-Prep (combined with sodium sulphate, sodium bicarbonate, sodium chloride, and potassium chloride); *Laxido Orange (combined with sodium bicarbonate, sodium chloride, and potassium chloride); *Molaxole (combined with sodium bicarbonate, sodium chloride, and potassium chloride); *Movicol (combined with sodium chloride, sodium bicarbonate, and potassium chloride); *Moviprep (combined with sodium sulphate, sodium chloride, and potassium chloride).

Polyfax (Teva UK) A proprietary combination of the antibiotics *polymyxin B sulphate and *bacitracin zinc, used to treat styes, conjunctivitis, and inflammation of the eyelids and to prevent infection after eye surgery or removal of foreign bodies. It is also used for treating skin infections, impetigo, and burns. Polyfax is available as separate ointments for the eyes and skin on *prescription only.

Side effects: there may be local irritation due to allergic reactions.
Precautions: if large areas of skin are treated the ointment may be absorbed, giving rise to hearing impairment. This is more likely to occur in children, the elderly, and people with kidney disease.

polymyxin B sulphate An antibacterial drug that is used in combination with a variety of other *antibiotics to treat a wide range of bacterial infections.
Side effects, precautions, and interactions with other drugs: see entries for individual combined preparations.
Proprietary preparations: *Maxitrol (combined with dexamethasone, hypromellose, and neomycin sulphate); *Neosporin (combined with neomycin sulphate); *Otosporin (combined with neomycin sulphate and hydrocortisone); *Polyfax (combined with bacitracin).

polysaccharide–iron complex A combination of *iron and a polysaccharide (a complex sugar) used for the treatment of iron-deficiency anaemia. It is available as an *elixir and can be obtained without a prescription, but only from pharmacies. A formulation for use in children can be prescribed on the NHS, but only for treating premature babies.
Side effects, precautions, and interactions with other drugs: *see* IRON.
Proprietary preparations: Niferex; Niferex Drops (for children).

Polytar (Stiefel Laboratories) A proprietary combination of *tar, *coal tar extract, *arachis oil, *cade oil, coal tar solution, and oleyl alcohol, used for the treatment of scaly and itching scalp disorders, including *psoriasis, *eczema, and dandruff. It is freely available *over the counter in the form of a liquid.
Side effects and precautions: *see* COAL TAR.

Polytar AF (Stiefel Laboratories) A proprietary combination of *tar, *coal tar extract, *arachis oil, *cade oil, coal tar solution, pine tar, and pyrithione zinc, used for the treatment of scaly scalp disorders, including *psoriasis, *eczema, and dandruff. It is freely available *over the counter in the form of a shampoo.
Side effects and precautions: *see* COAL TAR.

Polytar Plus (Stiefel Laboratories) A proprietary combination of *tar, *coal tar extract, *arachis oil, cade oil, coal tar solution, oleyl alcohol, and hydrolysed animal protein, used for the treatment of scaly and itching scalp disorders, including *psoriasis, *eczema, and dandruff. It is freely available *over the counter in the form of a liquid.
Side effects and precautions: *see* COAL TAR.

polyvinyl alcohol An agent that is used in the treatment of dry eyes to thicken the natural film of tears that covers the eyes. It is available as eye drops and can be obtained without a prescription, but only from pharmacies.
Side effects: there may be transient stinging and blurred vision on application.
Precautions: polyvinyl alcohol should not be used with soft contact lenses.
Proprietary preparations: Liquifilm Tears; Refresh Ophthalmic Solution; Sno Tears.

POM *See* PRESCRIPTION ONLY MEDICINE.

Ponstan (Chemidex Pharma) *See* MEFENAMIC ACID.

poractant alfa A synthetic pulmonary *surfactant that is used to treat breathing difficulties in premature babies who are receiving mechanical ventilation (*see* VENTILATOR). It is also used to prevent breathing difficulties in premature babies. Poractant alfa is available, on *prescription only, as a suspension that is administered through a tube placed in the trachea (windpipe).
Precautions: constant monitoring of heart rate and blood gases is necessary during treatment as poractant alfa can cause a rapid improvement in the baby's condition and high concentrations of oxygen in the tissues have toxic effects.
Proprietary preparation: Curosurf.

porfimer sodium A drug used for the treatment of a type of lung cancer and oesophageal cancer. It is injected into the bloodstream, accumulates in the cancer cells, and is then activated by laser light to destroy these cells. Porfimer sodium is available on *prescription only.
Side effects: *see* CYTOTOXIC DRUGS. There may also be swelling, itching, and blistering of the skin and constipation.
Precautions: *see* CYTOTOXIC DRUGS. This treatment makes the skin and eyes sensitive to light, and sunlight or bright indoor light should be avoided for at least 30 days after treatment. Porfimer sodium should not be given to people with porphyria or severe liver disease or to pregnant or breastfeeding women.
Proprietary preparation: Photofrin.

posaconazole A triazole *antifungal drug used for the treatment of fungal infections that have not responded to other agents, including generalized aspergillosis, candidiasis of the throat and pharynx, and coccidioidomycosis. It is taken as an oral solution under expert supervision and is available on *prescription only.
Side effects: include drowsiness, headache, dizziness, nausea, vomiting, abdominal pain, and diarrhoea.
Precautions: posaconazole should not be taken by women who are pregnant or breastfeeding or by people with porphyria. It should be used with caution in people with *arrhythmias, a slow heart rate, or some forms of heart disease.
Interactions with other drugs: pimozide and Riamet should not be taken with posaconazole since they increase the risk of ventricular arrhythmias.

Antidepressants: the plasma concentrations (and therefore adverse effects) of midazolam and reboxetine are increased; reboxetine should not be taken with posaconazole.

Cimetidine: reduces the plasma concentration of posaconazole.

Efavirenz: reduces the plasma concentration of posaconazole.

Ergot alkaloids: the plasma concentrations (and therefore toxic effects) of ergotamine and methysergide are increased, and these drugs should not be taken with posaconazole.

Immunosuppressants: the plasma concentrations (and therefore adverse effects) of ciclosporin, sirolimus, and tacrolimus are increased.

Phenytoin: reduces the plasma concentration of posaconazole.
Rifabutin: reduces the plasma concentration of posaconazole and its plasma concentration is increased.
Statins: the risk of muscle damage is increased when atorvastatin and simvastatin are taken with posaconazole, and these drugs should not be used with it.
Proprietary preparation: Noxafil.

Posalfilin (Norgine) A proprietary combination of *salicylic acid (a keratolytic) and *podophyllum resin (a caustic agent), used for the treatment of verrucas. It is available as an ointment and can be obtained without a prescription, but only from pharmacies.
Side effects and precautions: *see* SALICYLIC ACID; PODOPHYLLUM.

postcode prescribing The practice in the National Health Service of blacklisting certain expensive drugs in some regions, although doctors in other regions may be allowed to prescribe them. Thus whether or not a patient can benefit from these drugs may depend on their postcode.

Potaba (Glenwood Laboratories) *See* POTASSIUM AMINOBENZOATE.

potassium A mineral element necessary for the functioning of all cells of the body (*see* ELECTROLYTE). Together with *sodium, it is essential for the conduction of impulses in nerves and the functioning of muscles. Low concentrations of potassium can cause weakness, confusion, and in severe cases abnormal heart rhythms (*see* ARRHYTHMIA). **Potassium supplements** are salts of potassium given to prevent or treat potassium deficiency. This is particularly necessary during treatment with *anti-arrhythmic drugs or *digoxin, when low concentrations of potassium in the blood may induce irregularities in heart rhythm; in patients with certain kidney diseases, cirrhosis of the liver, or heart failure; and in cases of severe or chronic diarrhoea. Potassium supplements may also be required by the elderly and by people taking *corticosteroids or certain *diuretics, but in the latter case a *potassium-sparing diuretic may be given instead of a potassium supplement. Potassium supplements are given in the form of oral *potassium chloride, but if potassium depletion is severe potassium chloride can be given intravenously.
Side effects: include nausea and vomiting.
Precautions: potassium salts may cause ulceration of the bowel or oesophagus (gullet) and should be discontinued if there is discomfort or bleeding. They should generally not be used by people with severe kidney disease or those taking ACE inhibitors (see below), except in rare cases under specialist supervision, and should be used with caution by those with mild or moderate kidney disease. *Modified-release preparations must always be swallowed whole and never chewed or broken up.
Interactions with other drugs:
ACE inhibitors: can cause high concentrations of potassium in the blood.

Angiotensin II inhibitors: can cause high concentrations of potassium in the blood.
Ciclosporin: can cause high concentrations of potassium in the blood.
Potassium-sparing diuretics: can cause high concentrations of potassium in the blood.
Tacrolimus: can cause high concentrations of potassium in the blood.

potassium aminobenzoate The potassium salt of *aminobenzoic acid, one of the B group vitamins. It is used for the treatment of various disorders associated with excessive thickening or scarring of connective tissue, such as scleroderma, but its therapeutic value is doubtful. Potassium aminobenzoate is available as capsules, tablets, or sachets of powder to be dissolved in water; it can be obtained from pharmacies without a prescription.
Proprietary preparation: Potaba.

potassium bicarbonate A *potassium salt that is an ingredient of oral potassium supplements and other preparations (in which it provides effervescence) and of some *antacid preparations.
Side effects, precautions, and interactions with other drugs: *see* POTASSIUM.
Proprietary preparations: *Gaviscon Advance (combined with sodium alginate); *Phosphate-Sandoz (combined with sodium bicarbonate and sodium acid phosphate); *Resolve (combined with paracetamol, citric acid, sodium bicarbonate, sodium carbonate, and vitamin C); *Sando-K (combined with potassium chloride).

potassium channel activators A new class of drugs that dilate both veins and arteries. They are used for the prevention and long-term treatment of *angina. The main drug in this class is *nicorandil.

potassium chloride A salt of *potassium used as a potassium supplement. It may be combined with *diuretics to maintain potassium balance. Potassium chloride is available as tablets or a syrup without a prescription, but some preparations can only be obtained from pharmacies. *Modified-release tablets of potassium chloride should be swallowed whole with plenty of water while sitting or standing. Preparations for intravenous infusions are available on *prescription only.
Side effects, precautions, and interactions with other drugs: *see* POTASSIUM.
Proprietary preparations: Kay-Cee-L (syrup); Slow-K (modified-release tablets); *Boots Dual Action Diarrhoea Relief (sachets: combined with sodium chloride, sodium citrate, citric acid, and glucose); *Dioralyte Natural, Blackcurrent and Citrus GSL (combined with glucose, sodium chloride, and disodium hydrogen citrate); *Dioralyte Relief (combined with sodium chloride, sodium citrate, and precooked rice powder); *Diumide-K Continus (combined with furosemide); *Electrolade (combined with sodium chloride, sodium bicarbonate, and glucose); *Klean-Prep (combined with macrogol '3350', sodium sulphate, sodium bicarbonate, and sodium chloride); *Laxido Orange (combined with macrogol '3350', sodium chloride, and sodium bicarbonate); *Molaxole (combined with macrogol '3350', sodium chloride,

and sodium bicarbonate); *Movicol (combined with polyethylene glycol, sodium bicarbonate, and sodium chloride); *Moviprep (combined with macrogol '3350', sodium sulphate, sodium ascorbate, and ascorbic acid); *Neo-Naclex-K (combined with bendroflumethiazide); *Sando-K (combined with potassium bicarbonate); *Sensodyne (combined with sodium fluoride and triclosan).

potassium citrate A drug used for the treatment of cystitis: it acts by making the urine alkaline. It is available, without a prescription, as an oral solution or effervescent tablets.
Side effects: there may be stomach irritation and increased urine production.
Precautions: potassium citrate should be used with caution by people with kidney disease.
Interactions with other drugs:
Potassium-sparing diuretics: there is a risk of increased plasma concentrations of *potassium.
Proprietary preparations: Cymalon Cranberry Liquid; Effercitrate (tablets).

potassium hydroxyquinoline sulphate A drug with *antifungal, antibacterial, and deodorant properties. It is used, often in conjunction with *benzoyl peroxide, in the *topical treatment of fungal infections, minor bacterial infections, and acne.
Proprietary preparation: *Quinoderm (combined with benzoyl peroxide).

potassium iodate A drug used to prevent the uptake of radioactive iodine by the thyroid gland, for example after a nuclear accident. It is available as tablets on *prescription only.
Side effects: include rash, headache, nausea, vomiting, diarrhoea, stomach discomfort, spasm of the bronchi, and over- or underactivity of the thyroid gland.
Precautions and interactions with other drugs: potassium iodate should not be taken by people with kidney failure, a form of vasculitis (inflammation of blood vessels), or dermatitis herpetiformis (a type of itchy rash). Drugs increasing plasma potassium levels, including potassium-sparing diuretics and ACE inhibitors, should be used with caution with potassium iodate.
Proprietary preparation: Potassium Iodate Tablets (Cambridge Laboratories).

potassium permanganate A salt of potassium that forms a purple solution with *antiseptic and *astringent properties. It is used to cleanse and deodorize the skin in people with weeping *eczema and to cleanse wounds. Potassium permanganate is available as a solution or as tablets to be dissolved in water; it can be obtained without a prescription, but only from pharmacies.
Side effects: potassium permanganate can irritate mucous membranes; it also stains skin and clothing.
Proprietary preparation: Permitabs (tablets).

potassium-sparing diuretics (**K^+-sparing diuretics**) A class of mild *diuretics that act on the kidneys to promote loss of water. They are different

from other diuretics in that they do not cause the loss of *potassium ions (thus there is no need for potassium supplements) and they do not worsen diabetes or gout. They are often combined with other types of diuretics to offset or prevent potassium loss in the treatment of *hypertension. They are also used (rarely) in the treatment of nephrotic syndrome (a kidney disease characterized by protein loss in the urine and *oedema) and oedema that has not responded to other diuretics. The effect of these diuretics lasts for several hours and therefore they should not be taken during the late afternoon or early evening or there may be a need to pass urine during the night. *See* AMILORIDE HYDROCHLORIDE; SPIRONOLACTONE; TRIAMTERENE.
Side effects: potassium may be retained in the body, causing muscle weakness and abnormal heartbeat. Nausea and gastrointestinal upsets are quite common. For more specific side effects, see entries individual drugs.
Precautions: potassium-sparing diuretics should be used with great caution in people taking *ACE inhibitors, preferably under close medical supervision. They should not be given to people taking potassium supplements. Patients taking potassium-sparing diuretics should be warned not to use potassium-containing salt substitutes as this could lead to high blood concentrations of potassium.
Interactions with other drugs:
ACE inhibitors: increase the risk of severely raised blood concentrations of potassium (see above).
Angiotensin II inhibitors: increase the risk of raised blood concentrations of potassium.
Antihypertensive drugs: increase the effect of these diuretics in lowering blood pressure.
Ciclosporin: increases the risk of raised concentrations of potassium.
Lithium: its plasma concentration is increased.

povidone A drug used for the treatment of dry eyes in people with tear deficiency. It is available as eye drops without a prescription.
Proprietary preparation: Oculotect.

povidone–iodine An *antiseptic used for the treatment of minor skin infections and to disinfect the skin before surgery. It works by slowly releasing *iodine. For skin infections, or to disinfect the skin before surgery, the drug is available in varying strengths as an alcoholic tincture, an antiseptic solution, and a surgical scrub. It is also available as a powder or an ointment that can be applied to the skin to treat infections or ulcers or to dress cuts and abrasions. Povidone–iodine can be obtained without a prescription.
Side effects: rarely, the drug may cause allergic reactions.
Precautions: providone–iodine should be used with caution in people with certain kidney diseases, in women who are pregnant or breastfeeding, and on broken skin.
Proprietary preparations: Betadine; Savlon Dry; Videne.

Powergel (Menarini) *See* KETOPROFEN.

Pradaxa (Boehringer Ingelheim) *See* DABIGATRAN ETEXILATE.

pramipexole A *dopamine receptor agonist used alone or as an *adjunct to *levodopa in the treatment of Parkinson's disease (*see* ANTIPARKINSONIAN DRUGS). It is also licensed for use in restless legs syndrome. Pramipexole is available as tablets on *prescription only.
Side effects: include visual hallucinations, movement disorders, impulsive behaviour, somnolence and suddenly falling asleep, a fall in blood pressure, nausea, and constipation.
Precautions: pramipexole should not be taken by women who are pregnant or breastfeeding. It should be used with caution in people with psychotic disorders, kidney disease, or severe cardiovascular disease. People taking pramipexole should avoid driving and operating machinary. Dosage should be reduced gradually at the end of treatment.
Interactions with other drugs:
Antipsychotics: antagonize the effect of pramipexole.
Cimetidine: increases the plasma concentration of pramipexole.
Methyldopa: antagonizes the effect of pramipexole.
Proprietary preparation: Mirapexin.

pramocaine hydrochloride <**pramoxine hydrochloride**> A *local anaesthetic that is included as an ingredient in preparations for relieving the pain and itching associated with minor skin conditions and *haemorrhoids.
Side effects: pramocaine may cause initial burning or stinging.
Precautions: preparations containing pramocaine should not be applied to the eyes or nose.
Proprietary preparations: *Anugesic-HC (combined with zinc oxide, hydrocortisone acetate, Peru balsam, and benzyl benzoate); *Anugesic-HC Suppositories (combined with zinc oxide, hydrocortisone acetate, Peru balsam, bismuth subgallate, bismuth oxide, and benzyl benzoate); *Proctofoam HC (combined with hydrocortisone acetate).

pramoxine hydrochloride *See* PRAMOCAINE HYDROCHLORIDE.

Prandin (Daiichi Sankyo UK Ltd) *See* REPAGLINIDE.

prasugrel hydrochloride An *antiplatelet drug used, in combination with *aspirin, to prevent strokes and heart attacks in people who have angina or have already had a heart attack and are undergoing surgery to open up blocked arteries in the heart. It is available as tablets on *prescription only.
Side effects: include excessive bleeding.
Precautions: prasugrel should not be taken by people with bleeding peptic ulcers or bleeding from any other site or by people who have had a stroke. It is not recommended for pregnant or breastfeeding women. Prasugrel should be used with caution in people at risk of bleeding (e.g. from recent surgery or in those taking anticoagulant drugs), in people with liver or kidney disease, and in the elderly.
Interactions with other drugs:

p

Proton pump inhibitors: esomeprazole, lansoprazole, and omeprazole may reduce the effects of prasugrel and should not be taken with it.
Proprietary preparation: Efient.

pravastatin A *statin used for the treatment of primary hypercholesterolaemia (*see* HYPERLIPIDAEMIA) that has not responded to dietary measures. It is also used to prevent the progression of *atherosclerosis in patients with coronary artery disease and to reduce the incidence of coronary thrombosis in those at risk. It is available as tablets on *prescription only.
Side effects and precautions: *see* STATINS.
Interactions with other drugs:
Clarithromycin: increases the plasma concentration of pravastatin.
See also STATINS.
Proprietary preparation: Lipostat.

Praxilene (Merck Serono) *See* NAFTIDROFURYL OXALATE.

prazosin An *alpha blocker that produces peripheral *vasodilatation. It is used to treat *hypertension, congestive *heart failure, and Raynaud's syndrome (poor circulation in the hands and feet). It is also used as an *adjunct in the treatment of the symptoms of urinary obstruction due to an enlarged prostate gland. Because it can cause a dramatic drop in blood pressure, the initial doses are low and should be given while the patient is lying down. Doses are then increased as necessary. Prazosin is available as tablets on *prescription only.
Side effects and interactions with other drugs: *see* ALPHA BLOCKERS.
Precautions: alcohol may increase the side effects of this drug. Driving and hazardous work should be undertaken with caution until people are aware of whether or not the drug causes them to feel dizzy or faint.
Proprietary preparation: Hypovase.
See also ANTIHYPERTENSIVE DRUGS; VASODILATORS.

Predfoam (Forrest Laboratories) *See* PREDNISOLONE.

Pred Forte (Allergan) *See* PREDNISOLONE.

prednisolone A *corticosteroid with anti-inflammatory and anti-allergic activity. It is used to treat *asthma, inflammatory bowel disease, rheumatic disease, and inflammatory conditions of the eyes and ears. Prednisolone is widely used in *cancer treatment, as it has a marked effect against some types of leukaemia, Hodgkin's disease, and non-Hodgkin's lymphomas. It is also active in hormone-sensitive breast cancer and has a role in the palliative care of patients in the terminal stages of cancer, in whom it may produce a sense of wellbeing. Prednisolone is available, on *prescription only, as tablets, *enteric-coated tablets, an enema or suppositories, eye or ear drops, or as a solution for local injection into joints or around tendons.
Side effects: *see* CORTICOSTEROIDS; TOPICAL STEROIDS.
Precautions and interactions with other drugs: *see* CORTICOSTEROIDS.

Proprietary preparations: Deltacortril; Deltastab (injection); Minims Prednisolone (eye drops); Predfoam (rectal foam); Pred Forte (eye drops); Predsol (eye or ear drops, enema, suppositories); *Predsol-N (combined with neomycin sulphate); *Scheriproct (combined with cinchocaine hydrochloride).

Predsol (UCB Pharma) *See* PREDNISOLONE.

Predsol-N (UCB Pharma) A proprietary combination of *prednisolone (a corticosteroid) and *neomycin sulphate (an antibiotic), used for the treatment of inflammation of the outer ear with infection and eczema and inflammation of the eye. It is available as drops on *prescription only.
Side effects: there may be local irritation due to allergic reactions.
Precautions: prolonged use of the drops should be avoided.

pregabalin An *anticonvulsant drug used for the treatment of pain associated with nerve damage, partial epilepsy, and generalized anxiety disorder. It is available as capsules on *prescription only.
Side effects: include dry mouth, drowsiness, shaky movements, fatigue, headache, nausea and vomiting, blurred or double vision, eye irritation, *oedema, weight gain, changes in appetite, euphoria, and attention disturbance.
Precautions: pregabalin should be avoided by women who are breastfeeding and used with caution by pregnant women and by people with congestive heart failure or kidney disease. Dosages should be reduced gradually at the end of treatment.
Proprietary preparation: Lyrica.

Pregaday (UCB Pharma) A proprietary combination of *ferrous fumarate and *folic acid, used to prevent deficiencies of iron and folic acid during pregnancy. It is available as tablets and can be obtained without a prescription, but only from pharmacies.
Side effects, precautions, and interactions with other drugs: *see* IRON.

Pregnyl (Organon Laboratories) *See* HUMAN CHORIONIC GONADOTROPHIN.

Premarin (Pfizer) *See* HORMONE REPLACEMENT THERAPY.

Premique (Pfizer) A proprietary combination of conjugated *oestrogens and *medroxyprogesterone used as continuous combined *hormone replacement therapy for the relief of menopausal symptoms and prevention of osteoporosis in women who have not had a hysterectomy and who have not had a period for a year. **Premique Low Dose** is less than half the strength of Premique and used for the relief of menopausal symptoms only. Both preparations are available as tablets on *prescription only.
Side effects, precautions, and interactions with other drugs: *see* HORMONE REPLACEMENT THERAPY.

Premique Cycle (Pfizer) A proprietary preparation of conjugated *oestrogen tablets and *medroxyprogesterone tablets used as sequential

combined *hormone replacement therapy for the relief of menopausal symptoms and the prevention of osteoporosis in women who have not had a hysterectomy. It is available on *prescription only.
Side effects, precautions, and interactions with other drugs: *see* HORMONE REPLACEMENT THERAPY.

Prempak-C (Pfizer) A proprietary preparation of conjugated *oestrogen tablets and *levonorgestrel tablets used as sequential combined *hormone replacement therapy for the relief of menopausal symptoms and prevention of osteoporosis in women who have not had a hysterectomy. The tablets, which are available on *prescription only, must be taken in the prescribed order.
Side effects, precautions, and interactions with other drugs: *see* HORMONE REPLACEMENT THERAPY.

Preotact (Nycomed UK) *See* PARATHYROID HORMONE.

Preparation H (Pfizer) A proprietary combination of shark liver oil and yeast cell extract, used to relieve the discomfort of *haemorrhoids and anal itching and also as a lubricant for easing painful bowel movements. It is freely available *over the counter in the form of an ointment or suppositories.

Prescal (Novartis) *See* ISRADIPINE.

prescription A document giving the details of a medication, including the dosage and quantity, to be dispensed by a pharmacist for an identified patient. A prescription must be signed in ink by a registered medical practitioner, although a few items may now be prescribed by certain nurses. A drug that can only be issued on prescription has the legal category of **prescription only medicine** (**POM**), which must be stated on the packaging. Medical practitioners may also prescribe items that do not legally require a prescription (*see* OVER THE COUNTER). Some 'blacklisted' drugs cannot be prescribed on the National Health Service; if they fall in the POM category they must be issued on a private prescription. *See also* POSTCODE PRESCRIBING.

prescription only medicine (**POM**) A legal category denoting a drug that can only be dispensed with a *prescription.

Preservex (Almirall) *See* ACECLOFENAC.

Prestim (Meda Pharmaceuticals) A proprietary combination of *timolol maleate (a beta blocker) and *bendroflumethiazide (a thiazide diuretic), used in the treatment of mild to moderate *hypertension. It is available as tablets on *prescription only.
Side effects, precautions, and interactions with other drugs: *see* BETA BLOCKERS; THIAZIDE DIURETICS.

See also ANTIHYPERTENSIVE DRUGS; DIURETICS.

Prezista (Janssen-Cilag) *See* DARUNAVIR.

PR Heat Spray (Crookes Healthcare) A proprietary combination of *methyl

salicylate, *ethyl nicotinate, and *camphor, used as a *rubefacient for the relief of muscular and rheumatic pains and stiffness, including backache, sciatica, lumbago, and fibrositis, bruises, sprains, and chilblains. It is freely available *over the counter.
Side effects and precautions: *see* RUBEFACIENTS.

Priadel (sanofi-aventis) *See* LITHIUM CARBONATE; LITHIUM CITRATE.

Prialt (Eisai) *See* ZICONOTIDE ACETATE.

prilocaine A *local anaesthetic that is similar to *lidocaine and has similar uses. It is available as an injection and is combined with lidocaine in a topical preparation.
Side effects and precautions: *see* LIDOCAINE. In addition, high doses can cause methaemoglobinaemia (the presence in the blood of an abnormal form of haemoglobin that cannot carry oxygen around the body), and prilocaine should not be given to patients with anaemia. It should be used with caution in patients with severe hypertension or heart disease.
Proprietary preparations: Citanest (injection; prescription only medicine); *Emla (combined with lidocaine; pharmacy medicine).

Primacor (sanofi-aventis) *See* MILRINONE.

primaquine A drug that is used in the treatment of benign *malaria; it is given after *chloroquine has been used to eliminate the malaria parasites that may still be present in the liver. Primaquine is available as tablets on special order since it does not currently have a *licence.
Side effects: include nausea, vomiting, and abdominal pain.
Precautions: primaquine should be used with caution by women who are pregnant or breastfeeding and by people with rheumatoid arthritis.
Interactions with other drugs:
Mepacrine: increases the risk of side effects from primaquine.
Riamet: should not be taken with primaquine.

Primaxin (Merck Sharp & Dohme) *See* IMIPENEM.

primidone An *anticonvulsant drug that may be used for the treatment of all forms of epilepsy except absence seizures. It is converted to *phenobarbital in the body. A *prescription only medicine, it is available for oral use as tablets.
Side effects: *see* BARBITURATES.
Precautions: women who are pregnant, or who are planning to become pregnant, should seek specialist advice. *See also* BARBITURATES.
Interactions with other drugs: taking two or more anticonvulsants together may increase their adverse effects. Other interactions are those of barbiturates used for treating epilepsy (*see* BARBITURATES).
Proprietary preparation: Mysoline.

Primolut N (Bayer) *See* NORETHISTERONE.

Pripsen (Thornton and Ross) A proprietary combination of *piperazine (an

anthelmintic) and sennosides (a laxative; *see* SENNA), used to treat infestations of roundworms or threadworms; sennosides are included to aid elimination of the worms. It is available as an oral powder to be mixed with water or milk and can be obtained without a prescription, but only from pharmacies.
Side effects and precautions: *see* PIPERAZINE.

Privigen (CSL Behring) *See* IMMUNOGLOBULINS.

Pro-Banthine (Archimedes Pharma) *See* PROPANTHELINE BROMIDE.

probenecid A drug used for the prevention of kidney damage caused by treatment with *cidofovir. It is available as tablets on *prescription only.
Side effects: these are infrequent but may include nausea and vomiting. Occasionally allergic rashes may occur.
Precautions: people taking probenecid must maintain an adequate fluid intake (at least 2 litres a day) to prevent crystals of uric acid being passed in the urine (which can cause pain and bleeding). Probenecid should not be taken by people with kidney stones, kidney disease, a history of blood disorders, or acute gout and it should be used with caution in those with peptic ulcers.
Interactions with other drugs:
Antibacterials: probenecid increases plasma concentrations of penicillins, cephalosporins, and quinolones.
Antiviral drugs: probenecid increases plasma concentrations of aciclovir, famciclovir, ganciclovir, and zidovudine and may cause toxic effects.
Aspirin: antagonizes the effect of probenecid.
Methotrexate: probenecid increases plasma concentrations of methotrexate and may cause toxic effects.
NSAIDs: probenecid increases plasma concentrations of dexketoprofen, indometacin, ketoprofen, ketorolac (which should not be taken with it), and naproxen.

procarbazine A *cytotoxic drug used for the treatment of Hodgkin's disease (*see* CANCER). It is available as capsules on *prescription only.
Side effects: include nausea and *bone marrow suppression (*see* CYTOTOXIC DRUGS); if an allergic rash develops, treatment should be discontinued.
Precautions: *see* CYTOTOXIC DRUGS. In addition, procarbazine should not be taken by people with severe liver or kidney disease. Alcohol should not be taken with procarbazine as this combination may result in a severe reaction (including a throbbing headache, palpitation, nausea, and vomiting).
Interactions with other drugs:
Clozapine: should not be taken with procarbazine as this combination increases the risk of agranulocytosis (a blood disorder).

prochlorperazine A phenothiazine *antipsychotic drug used for the treatment of schizophrenia and other psychoses and mania and for the short-term management of severe anxiety. It is also used as an *antiemetic to treat severe nausea and vomiting, especially that produced by chemotherapy or radiotherapy or associated with migraine, and to treat and prevent the vertigo

and nausea caused by Ménière's disease or other disorders of the middle ear. Prochlorperazine is available, on *prescription only, as tablets, *buccal tablets, a syrup, or an injection.
Side effects: as for *chlorpromazine, but prochlorperazine is less sedating, produces fewer antimuscarinic effects, and has more pronounced *extrapyramidal reactions.
Precautions and interactions with other drugs: *see* CHLORPROMAZINE HYDROCHLORIDE.
Proprietary preparations: Buccastem (buccal tablets); Stemetil.

Procoralan (Servier Laboratories) *See* IVABRADINE.

Proctofoam HC (Meda Pharmaceuticals) A proprietary combination of *hydrocortisone acetate (a corticosteroid) and *pramocaine hydrochloride (a local anaesthetic), used in the treatment of *haemorrhoids, inflammation of the bowel, and anal fissures. It is available as a foam in an aerosol on *prescription only.
Side effects: *see* CORTICOSTEROIDS.
Precautions: Proctofoam should not be used when viral or fungal infection is present and should not be used for longer than seven days. Proctofoam is not recommended for children.

Proctosedyl (sanofi-aventis) A proprietary combination of *hydrocortisone (a corticosteroid) and *cinchocaine hydrochloride (a local anaesthetic), used for the treatment of *haemorrhoids and anal inflammation and itching. It is available as an ointment or suppositories on *prescription only.
Side effects: *see* CORTICOSTEROIDS.
Precautions: Proctosedyl should not be used when viral or fungal infection is present and should not be used for longer than seven days.

procyclidine An *antimuscarinic drug used for the treatment of Parkinson's disease and for the reversal of drug-induced *extrapyramidal reactions (*see* ANTIPARKINSONIAN DRUGS). It is available as tablets, a syrup, or an injection on *prescription only.
Side effects, precautions, and interactions with other drugs: *see* TRIHEXYPHENIDYL HYDROCHLORIDE.
Proprietary preparations: Arpicolin; Kemadrin.

Pro-Epanutin (Pfizer) *See* PHENYTOIN.

Proflex (Novartis) *See* IBUPROFEN.

progesterone A steroid hormone secreted by the ovaries and placenta and also in small amounts by the adrenal glands and the testes. It is responsible for preparing the lining of the uterus (endometrium) for pregnancy. If fertilization occurs progesterone maintains the pregnancy and inhibits the further release of eggs from the ovaries. It is used therapeutically to treat abnormal vaginal bleeding, premenstrual syndrome, and postnatal depression. It is also used to maintain early pregnancies and to treat infertility in *in vitro* fertilization procedures. Progesterone is used as an *adjunct to

oestrogens in *hormone replacement therapy (HRT). Progesterone is available, on *prescription only, as a solution for intramuscular injection, a vaginal gel, capsules, or *pessaries. Synthetic versions of progesterone have a variety of therapeutic uses and are major ingredients of hormonal contraceptives (*see* PROGESTOGENS).
Side effects: include acne, urticaria (nettle rash), fluid retention, weight changes, stomach upsets, changes in libido, breast discomfort, premenstrual symptoms, menstrual disturbances, pigmentation of the face, depression, fever, insomnia, sleepiness, loss of hair on the head, and increase in body hair. Local reactions can occur on injection; diarrhoea and flatulence can occur with rectal administration.
Precautions: progesterone should not be given to women with undiagnosed vaginal bleeding, a history of liver tumours, or severe liver disease and should be used with caution in women with diabetes or epilepsy and in those who suffer from migraine.
Interactions with other drugs: *see* PROGESTOGENS.
Proprietary preparations: Crinone (vaginal gel for infertility); Cyclogest (pessaries); Gestone (injection); Utrogestan (capsules for HRT).

progestogens A group of steroids that includes the naturally occurring hormone *progesterone, which maintains the normal course of pregnancy, and synthetic equivalents of progesterone: the term is usually restricted to synthetic forms. Synthetic progestogens are used to treat menstrual disorders, including heavy, painful, or irregular periods. Because they prevent the release of egg cells from the ovary, they are major constituents of *oral contraceptives, either alone (in progestogen-only pills) or combined with an *oestrogen. They are also used in other forms of hormonal contraception (*see* DEPOT CONTRACEPTIVES) and in *hormone replacement therapy, and some are used in the treatment of breast and endometrial cancer and *endometriosis. Synthetic progestogens may be taken by mouth, by injection, by implants, or as skin patches. The commonly used progestogens are *desogestrel, *dydrogesterone, *etynodiol diacetate, *gestodene, *levonorgestrel, *medroxyprogesterone, *norethisterone, and *norgestimate.
Side effects: include irregular menstrual bleeding, breast discomfort, acne, cysts in the ovary, headache, nausea, and weight gain; there may be changes in libido.
Precautions: progestogens should not be taken by women with a history of heart disease, arterial disease, thrombosis, undiagnosed vaginal bleeding, a history of liver tumours, severe liver disease, breast or genital cancer, or previous ectopic pregnancy. They should not be taken during pregnancy. They should be used with caution by women with high blood pressure, ovarian cysts, or migraine.
Interactions with other drugs:

Antibiotics: rifampicin and rifabutin reduce the contraceptive effects of progestogens. *See* ORAL CONTRACEPTIVES.

Anticoagulants: the effect of warfarin may be reduced or enhanced; the effect of phenindione is reduced.

Antiepileptic drugs: carbamazepine, oxcarbazepine, phenobarbital, phenytoin, primidone, rufinamide, and topiramate reduce the contraceptive effects of progestogens (*see* ORAL CONTRACEPTIVES); the plasma concentration of lamotrigine is increased.
Aprepitant: may reduce the contraceptive effects of progestogens. *See* ORAL CONTRACEPTIVES.
Bosentan: may reduce the contraceptive effects of progestogens. *See* ORAL CONTRACEPTIVES.
Ciclosporin: progestogens increase the plasma concentration (and therefore side effects) of ciclosporin.
Griseofulvin: reduces the effects of progestogens. *See* ORAL CONTRACEPTIVES.
Nevirapine: reduces the effects of progestogens.
St John's wort: reduces the contraceptive effects of progestogens and should not be taken with them.

Prograf (Astellas Pharma) *See* TACROLIMUS.

proguanil hydrochloride A drug used, usually in combination with *chloroquine, for the prevention of *malaria. It is also used in combination with *atovaquone for the treatment of falciparum malaria and for the prevention of this in areas where there is resistance to melfloquine or chloroquine. Proguanil is available as tablets.
Side effects: these are rare, but may include mild stomach upsets and diarrhoea and, occasionally, mouth ulcers and soreness, rashes, and hair loss.
Precautions: proguanil should be used with caution in people with impaired kidney function. Pregnant women should take folic acid supplements.
Interactions with other drugs:
Riamet: should not be taken with proguanil.
Warfarin: the anticoagulant effect of this drug may be enhanced.
Proprietary preparations: Paludrine (pharmacy medicine); *Malarone and Malarone Paediatric (combined with atovaquone; prescription only medicine); *Paludrine/Avloclor (packaged with chloroquine; pharmacy medicine).

Progynova, Progynova TS (Bayer) *See* ESTRADIOL; HORMONE REPLACEMENT THERAPY.

prokinetic drugs A group of drugs that act on the gut to stimulate the emptying of the stomach. They therefore prevent reflux of acid and stomach contents (which can cause heartburn) and they also increase the motility of the oesophagus. The common drugs in this group are *metoclopramide and *domperidone, which are *dopamine receptor antagonists.

Proleukin (Novartis) *See* ALDESLEUKIN.

promazine hydrochloride A phenothiazine *antipsychotic drug used as an *adjunct for the short-term treatment of moderate or severe agitation, including agitation and restlessness in elderly patients. It is available, on *prescription only, as tablets, or a suspension.

Side effects, precautions, and interactions with other drugs: *see* CHLORPROMAZINE HYDROCHLORIDE.

promethazine hydrochloride One of the original (sedating) *antihistamines, used to relieve the symptoms of such allergic conditions as hay fever and urticaria. It is also used as an *antiemetic and as a *hypnotic drug for the short-term treatment of insomnia. Promethazine is available as tablets or an elixir that can be bought from pharmacies without a *prescription, and as a solution for injection on *prescription only.
Side effects: *see* ANTIHISTAMINES; promethazine may also cause EXTRAPYRAMIDAL REACTIONS.
Precautions and interactions with other drugs: *see* ANTIHISTAMINES.
Proprietary preparations: Phenergan; Sominex (tablets for insomnia); *Day and Night Nurse (combined with paracetamol, pseudoephedrine, pholcodine, and dextromethorphan); *Medised (combined with paracetamol); *Night Nurse (combined with paracetamol and dextromethorphan); *Pamergan P100 (combined with pethidine); *Tixylix Night Cough (combined with pholcodine).

promethazine teoclate An *antihistamine used for the treatment of nausea, vomiting, vertigo, and motion sickness. It is available as tablets without a *prescription.
Side effects: drowsiness is the most common side effect; *see* ANTIHISTAMINES.
Precautions and interactions with other drugs: *see* ANTIHISTAMINES.
Proprietary preparation: Avomine.

Promixin (Profile Pharma) *See* COLISTIN.

propafenone hydrochloride A class I *anti-arrhythmic drug that is also a *beta blocker; it is used in the prevention and treatment of *arrhythmias. It is available as tablets on *prescription only.
Side effects: include dizziness, nausea, vomiting, bitter taste, constipation, blurred vision, dry mouth, diarrhoea, headache, fatigue, and allergic skin reactions.
Precautions: therapy should be initiated under hospital supervision. Propafenone should be used with caution in patients with airways disease (including asthma), liver or kidney disease, or heart failure. *See also* ANTI-ARRHYTHMIC DRUGS.
Interactions with other drugs:

Anti-arrhythmic drugs depression of heart function is increased.

Anticoagulants: the effects of warfarin and acenocoumarol are enhanced by propafenone.

Antidepressants: there is an increased risk of arrhythmias if tricyclic antidepressants are taken with propafenone.

Antipsychotic drugs: some antipsychotics increase the risk of arrhythmias.

Antiviral drugs: ritonavir and fosamprenavir should not be taken with propafenone as these drugs increase the plasma concentration of propafenone, which increases the risk of arrhythmias.

Beta blockers depression of heart function is increased.
Cimetidine: increases the plasma concentration of propafenone.
Digoxin: propafenone increases the plasma concentration of digoxin, whose dosage will therefore need to be reduced.
Mizolastine: there is an increased risk of arrhythmias and this drug should not be taken with propafenone.
Rifampicin: reduces the plasma concentration (and therefore effect) of propafenone.

Proprietary preparation: Arythmol.

propamidine isethionate An *antibiotic used for the treatment of conjunctivitis and infections of the eyelids caused by bacteria; it is especially useful in treating acanthamoeba keratitis, a sight-threatening infection caused by inadequately cleaned contact lenses Propamidine is available as eye drops or ointment and can be obtained without a prescription, but only from pharmacies.

Proprietary preparations: Brolene (eye drops or ointment); Golden Eye (drops); Golden Eye Ointment.

propantheline bromide An *antimuscarinic drug used mainly for the relief of gut spasms (*see* ANTISPASMODICS). It is available as tablets on *prescription only.

Side effects and precautions: *see* ANTIMUSCARINIC DRUGS.

Proprietary preparation: Pro-Banthine.

Propecia (Merck Sharp & Dohme) *See* FINASTERIDE.

Propess (Ferring Pharmaceuticals) *See* DINOPROSTONE.

p

Propine (Allergan) *See* DIPIVEFRINE.

propiverine hydrochloride An *antimuscarinic drug used to treat urinary incontinence and abnormal frequency or urgency in passing urine. It is available as tablets or *modified-release capsules on *prescription only.

Side effects: include dry mouth, blurred vision, and (less frequently) nausea, abdominal discomfort, low blood pressure, drowsiness, difficulty in passing urine, and fatigue. A fast heart rate, restlessness, irritability, hot flushes, and rash are rare side effects.

Precautions: propiverine should not be taken by people with obstruction of the gut, severe ulcerative colitis, impaired liver function, or by people in whom the outlet of the bladder is obstructed (for example by an enlarged prostate gland), or by women who are pregnant or breastfeeding. It should be used with caution in frail elderly people and in people with heart disease, glaucoma, kidney disease, an overactive thyroid gland, or reflux oesophagitis caused by a hiatus hernia.

Interactions with other drugs: *see* ANTIMUSCARINIC DRUGS.

Proprietary preparations: Detrunorm; Detrunorm XL.

propranolol hydrochloride A non-cardioselective *beta blocker used for the treatment and prevention of heart *arrhythmias and *angina and for the

treatment of *hypertension. It is used after a heart attack to prevent worsening of the condition. It is also used for the prevention of *migraine, the treatment of anxiety, and to relieve the acute symptoms of hyperthyroidism before surgery. It is available, on *prescription only, as tablets, *modified-release capsules, an oral solution, or a solution for injection.
Side effects and precautions: *see* BETA BLOCKERS; ANTIHYPERTENSIVE DRUGS.
Interactions with other drugs:
Anti-arrhythmic drugs: the adverse effects of lidocaine are increased if it is taken with propranolol. *See also* BETA BLOCKERS.
Bupivacaine: its adverse effects may be increased.
Chlorpromazine: the plasma concentrations of both drugs may be increased if they are taken together.
Rifampicin: reduces the plasma concentration of propranolol.
For other interactions, *see* BETA BLOCKERS.
Proprietary preparations: Angilol (tablets); Bedranol SR (modified-release capsules); Beta-Prograne (modified-release capsules); Inderal; Inderal LA (modified-release capsules); Half-Inderal LA (half the strength of Inderal LA); Syprol (oral solution).

proprietary name The trade name of a drug: the name assigned to it by the company who manufactures it. For example, Zantac is a proprietary name for ranitidine. When drugs are first introduced by a pharmaceutical company they are under patent and may only be dispensed or sold under the trade name. On expiry of the patent (usually after ten years) any other company may manufacture the drug, although they will still need a *licence, granted by the Medicines and Healthcare products Regulatory Agency, in order to sell the drug under its generic name. Most generic drugs are cheaper than the corresponding proprietary preparations. This is particularly apparent with *over the counter medicines, such as aspirin and paracetamol.

propylthiouracil An antithyroid drug similar to *carbimazole. It is used to treat thyrotoxicosis (overproduction of *thyroid hormones) and also to reduce hormone concentrations before surgery to remove part of an overactive thyroid gland. Propylthiouracil is available as tablets on *prescription only.
Side effects and precautions: *see* CARBIMAZOLE.

Proscar (Merck Sharp & Dohme) *See* FINASTERIDE.

prostaglandins A large group of hormone-like substances that exert their effects close to where they are produced. They are produced by many organs and tissues and have a wide range of actions. For example, they cause contraction of smooth muscle, such as the uterus or intestines, and dilatation of blood vessels, and they are mediators of the inflammatory response (*aspirin and other *NSAIDs act by blocking their production). They are also involved in the production of mucus in the stomach, which provides protection against gastric acid. Synthetic forms (*analogues) of prostaglandins are used for the treatment of peptic ulcers (*see* MISOPROSTOL), to induce labour and abortion and to treat bleeding after childbirth (*see*

CARBOPROST; DINOPROSTONE; GEMEPROST), and to treat men with erectile dysfunction and babies with congenital heart disease (*see* ALPROSTADIL) and people with glaucoma (*see* BIMATOPROST; LATANOPROST; TRAVOPROST).

Prostap SR, Prostap 3 (Takeda) *See* LEUPRORELIN.

Prostin E2 (Pharmacia) *See* DINOPROSTONE.

Prostin VR (Pharmacia) *See* ALPROSTADIL.

Prosulf (Wockhardt UK) *See* PROTAMINE SULPHATE.

protamine sulphate A drug used to counteract overdosage with *heparin and low molecular weight heparins. It is available as a solution for injection on *prescription only.
Side effects: include nausea, vomiting, flushing, low blood pressure, slow heart rate, and breathlessness.
Precautions: there can be allergic reactions, for example in people who have had previous treatment with protamine *insulin or who are allergic to fish.
Proprietary preparation: Prosulf.

protease inhibitors *See* ANTIVIRAL DRUGS.

Protelos (Servier Laboratories) *See* STRONTIUM RANELATE.

Prothiaden (Teofarma) *See* DOSULEPIN HYDROCHLORIDE.

prothrombin complex A medicine prepared from human plasma and containing several blood clotting factors (including *Factor IX). It is used for the treatment and prevention during surgery of bleeding due to deficiency of any of these factors, either congenital or acquired (e.g. caused by treatment with warfarin). It is available as a powder and solvent for slow intravenous infusion on *prescription only.
Precautions: there is a risk of thrombosis, and this medicine should not be given to people with angina or to those who have recently had a heart attack. It should be used with caution in people with a history of coronary artery disease.
Proprietary preparations: Beriplex; Octaplex.

p

protirelin Thyrotrophin-releasing hormone, which is secreted by the hypothalamus (in the brain) and controls the secretion of thyrotrophin, a hormone that is secreted by the pituitary gland and acts on the thyroid gland to stimulate production of *thyroid hormones. Protirelin is given intravenously to assess the function of the thyroid gland, although its use has largely been superseded by other techniques. Failure of protirelin to produce a rise in plasma thyrotrophin concentrations indicates hyperthyroidism (excessive production of thyroid hormones). Protirelin is available as an injection on *prescription only.
Side effects: an increased desire to pass urine, flushing, dizziness, nausea, and a strange taste in the mouth can occur after rapid injection.
Precautions: protirelin should be used with caution in pregnant women, and

in people with an underactive pituitary gland, asthma, chronic bronchitis, or certain heart conditions.
Proprietary preparation: Protirelin Ampoules.

Protirelin Ampoules (Cambridge Laboratories) *See* PROTIRELIN.

Protium (Nycomed UK) *See* PANTOPRAZOLE.

proton pump inhibitors Drugs that inhibit gastric (stomach) acid secretion and are used for the treatment of gastric and duodenal ulcers, reflux oesophagitis, and other types of *acid-peptic disease. They act by inhibiting the movements of hydrogen and potassium ions in the stomach – the so-called proton pump, which causes acid secretion. Proton pump inhibitors produce a more rapid response and promote ulcer healing at a faster rate than *H_2-receptor antagonists. In combination with antibiotics, they are used to eradicate *Helicobacter pylori*, a common cause of ulcers. *See* ESOMEPRAZOLE; LANSOPRAZOLE; OMEPRAZOLE; PANTOPRAZOLE; RABEPRAZOLE SODIUM.
Side effects: diarrhoea, rash, and headache are among the most common side effects. More details are provided in entries for individual drugs.
Precautions: proton pump inhibitors should be used with caution in women who are pregnant or breastfeeding and in people with liver disease. They should not be used in patients in whom stomach cancer is a possibility without further investigation.
Interactions with other drugs: see entries for individual drugs.

Protopic (Astellas Pharma Ltd) *See* TACROLIMUS.

Provera (Pharmacia) *See* MEDROXYPROGESTERONE.

Provigil (Cephalon) *See* MODAFINIL.

Pro-Viron (Bayer) *See* MESTEROLONE.

proxymetacaine *See* LOCAL ANAESTHETICS.

Prozac (Eli Lilly & Co) *See* FLUOXETINE.

pseudoephedrine A *sympathomimetic drug that constricts blood vessels. It is used mainly as a *decongestant and is included in many oral proprietary preparations for treating colds and coughs. It is similar in action to *ephedrine. Most preparations containing pseudoephedrine can be bought from pharmacies without a prescription.
Side effects, precautions, and interactions with other drugs: *see* DECONGESTANTS; EPHEDRINE HYDROCHLORIDE.
Proprietary preparations: Boots Decongestant Tablets; Contac (capsules); Galpseud (tablets and liquid); Meltus Decongestant (liquid); Multi-Action Actifed Tablets; Non-Drowsy Sudafed Children's Syrup; Non-Drowsy Sudafed Decongestant Elixir; *Adult Meltus Chesty Coughs with Congestion (combined with guaifenesin and menthol); *Benadryl Plus Capsules (combined with acrivastine); *Benylin Day & Night Tablets (day tablets: combined with paracetamol); *Benylin Four Flu (combined with

p

diphenhydramine and paracetamol); *Boots Catarrh Syrup for Children (combined with diphenhydramine); *Boots Cough and Decongestion Syrup 2 Years Plus (combined with guaifenesin); *Boots Decongestant Tablets with Paracetamol (combined with paracetamol); *Boots Night Cold Comfort (combined with diphenhydramine, paracetamol, and pholcodine); *Boots Nirolex Chesty Cough and Congestion Relief Linctus (combined with guaifenesin); *Day Nurse (combined with pholcodine and paracetamol); *Day and Night Nurse (combined with paracetamol, pholcodine, promethazine hydrochloride, and dextromethorphan); *Junior Meltus Dry Coughs with Congestion (combined with dextromethorphan); *Lemsip Flu 12 Hr (combined with ibuprofen); *Lemsip Max Flu Lemon (combined with paracetamol); *Meltus Dry Cough (combined with dextromethorphan); *Multi-Action Actifed Chesty Coughs (combined with triprolidine and guaifenesin); *Multi-Action Actifed Dry Coughs (combined with dextromethorphan and triprolidine); *Non-Drowsy Sinutab (combined with paracetamol); *Non-Drowsy Sudafed Congestion, Cold and Flu Tablets (combined with paracetamol); *Non-Drowsy Sudafed Dual Relief Max (combined with ibuprofen); *Non-Drowsy Sudafed Expectorant (combined with guaifenesin); *Non-Drowsy Sudafed Linctus (combined with dextromethorphan); *Robitussin Chesty Cough with Congestion (combined with guaifenesin); *Tixylix Cough & Cold (combined with chlorphenamine and pholcodine). *Vicks Cold & Flu Care Medinite Complete (combined with dextromethorphan, doxylamine, and paracetamol).

psoriasis A chronic skin disease in which scaly pink patches form on the elbows, knees, scalp, and other parts of the body, often causing itching. Its cause is not known, but the disorder often runs in families: it most commonly starts in adolescence. Psoriasis sometimes occurs in association with arthritis (psoriatic arthropathy). Occasionally the disease may be very severe, affecting much of the skin and causing considerable disability. While psychological stress may cause an exacerbation of psoriasis, the only significant event that precipitates the disease is a preceding streptococcal infection. Drugs, such as lithium or beta blockers, may occasionally be responsible.

Although there is as yet no cure, treatment of psoriasis has improved greatly in recent years. *Emollients provide relief of symptoms and may be the only treatment required for mild psoriasis. For mild to moderate psoriasis, *dithranol, *coal tar, and *salicylic acid are often effective; *topical steroids may also be used. The *vitamin D analogues *calcipotriol, *calcitriol, and *tacalcitol and the *retinoid *tazarotene are newer *topical treatments for moderately severe disease. *Systemic therapy, with drugs such as *methotrexate, *acitretin, or *ciclosporin, is reserved for the worst cases.

Psoriderm (Dermal Laboratories) *See* COAL TAR.

Psorin (LPC) A proprietary combination of *coal tar and *salicylic acid (keratolytics) and *dithranol, used for the treatment of chronic *psoriasis. It is available as a ointment and can be obtained without a prescription, but only from pharmacies.

Precautions: Psorin should not come into contact with the eyes and should not be used with topical steroids. Exposure of treated skin to direct sunlight should be avoided.

Psorin Scalp Gel (LPC) A proprietary combination of *dithranol and *salicylic acid (a keratolytic), used for the treatment of chronic *psoriasis of the scalp. It can be obtained without a prescription, but only from pharmacies.
Precautions: the gel should not come into contact with the eyes and should not be used with topical steroids. Exposure of the treated scalp to direct sunlight should be avoided. The gel should be washed off after one hour.

Pulmicort Inhaler (AstraZeneca) *See* BUDESONIDE.

Pulmicort Respules (AstraZeneca) *See* BUDESONIDE.

Pulmicort Turbohaler (AstraZeneca) *See* BUDESONIDE.

Pulmo Bailly (DDD) A proprietary combination of *codeine (a cough suppressant) and guaiacol (an *expectorant), used to relieve the symptoms of coughs, colds, bronchial catarrh, and other infections of the upper airways, such as pharyngitis or laryngitis. It is available as a liquid without a prescription, but only from pharmacies.
Side effects, precautions, and interactions with other drugs: *see* CODEINE.

pulmonary embolism *See* THROMBOSIS.

Pulmozyme (Roche Products) *See* DORNASE ALFA.

Pulvinal Beclometasone (Chiesi) *See* BECLOMETASONE DIPROPIONATE.

Pulvinal Salbutamol (Chiesi) *See* SALBUTAMOL.

pumilio pine oil An aromatic oil obtained by distillation of the leaves of a pine tree, *Pino murgo pumilio.* It is used in combination with other aromatic oils in inhalations to relieve coughs and nasal congestion. Pumilio pine oil is also used as a *rubefacient.
Proprietary preparation: *Karvol (combined with other aromatic substances and chlorobutanol).

Puregon (Organon Laboratories) *See* FOLLITROPIN.

purgatives *See* LAXATIVES.

Puri-Nethol (GlaxoSmithKline) *See* MERCAPTOPURINE.

Pyralvex (Norgine) A proprietary combination of anthraquinone glycosides (anti-inflammatory agents) and *salicylic acid (a keratolytic), used for the treatment of mouth ulcers and sores caused by ill-fitting dentures. It is available as a solution and can be obtained without a prescription, but only from pharmacies.
Precautions: Pyralvex is not recommended for children. *See also* SALICYLIC ACID.

pyrazinamide A bactericidal *antibiotic drug used in combination with other drugs for the treatment of *tuberculosis, although it does not have a *licence for this. It is effective only during the first two or three months but is particularly useful in treating tuberculous meningitis. It is available as tablets on *prescription only.
Side effects: pyrazinamide may have adverse effects on the liver, including fever, loss of appetite, liver enlargement, and jaundice; other possible side effects are nausea, vomiting, muscle aches, and itching.
Precautions: people taking pyrazinamide should report symptoms of liver toxicity, such as persistent nausea and vomiting, malaise, and jaundice, to their doctor.
Interactions with other drugs:
Probenecid: its effects are antagonized by pyrazinamide.
Sulfinpyrazone: the effect of this drug in treating gout is reduced.
Proprietary preparation: *Rifater (combined with rifampicin and isoniazid).

pyridostigmine An *anticholinesterase drug used for the treatment of myasthenia gravis. It is less powerful but longer acting than *neostigmine and may be preferable as dosing is less frequent. Pyridostigmine is available as tablets on *prescription only.
Side effects: nausea and vomiting, increased salivation, diarrhoea, and abdominal cramps are the most common side effects.
Precautions: pyridostigmine should not be taken by people with intestinal or urinary obstruction and should be used with caution in those with asthma, low blood pressure, peptic ulcers, epilepsy, Parkinson's disease, or kidney disease.
Interactions with other drugs:
Antibiotics: aminoglycosides, clindamycin, and colistin antagonize the action of pyridostigmine.
Propranolol: antagonizes the action of pyridostigmine.
Proprietary preparation: Mestinon.

pyridoxine **(vitamin B$_6$)** A vitamin of the B group (*see* VITAMIN B COMPLEX) used as a vitamin supplement and to prevent the nerve damage that can occur in those receiving *isoniazid therapy. It is also used to treat a certain type of *anaemia (sideroblastic anaemia). In the form of **pyridoxine hydrochloride** it is freely available *over the counter as tablets or *modified-release tablets; these cannot be prescribed on the NHS.
Precautions: pyridoxine may have adverse effects on the nervous system in high dosages; prolonged use at these dosages is not recommended.
Proprietary preparation: *Vigranon B (combined with other B vitamins).

pyrimethamine A drug that prevents the replication of the parasite that causes *malaria. It is used in combination with sulfadoxine (a *sulphonamide) for the treatment of malaria. Pyrimethamine may also be used in the treatment of toxoplasmosis, but it does not have a *licence for this. It is available as tablets on *prescription only.
Side effects: include rashes and insomnia; because pyrimethamine interferes

with folic acid metabolism (the antifolate effect) there is a risk of anaemia or other blood disorders. *See also* CO-TRIMOXAZOLE.

Precautions: pyrimethamine should be used with caution in people with liver or kidney disease and in women who are breastfeeding. Pregnant women should take folate supplements. *See also* CO-TRIMOXAZOLE.

Interactions with other drugs:

Antibiotics: co-trimoxazole and trimethoprim enhance the antifolate effect of pyrimethamine.

Methotrexate: enhances the antifolate effect of pyrimethamine.

Phenytoin: enhances the antifolate effect of pyrimethamine and its anticonvulsant effect is antagonized by pyrimethamine.

See also CO-TRIMOXAZOLE.

Proprietary preparation: Daraprim.

Qlaira (Bayer) A proprietary combination of *estradiol and dienogest (a *progestogen agonist), used as an *oral contraceptive. It is available as tablets on *prescription only.
Side effects, precautions, and interactions with other drugs: *see* ORAL CONTRACEPTIVES.

Questran, Questran Light (Bristol-Myers Squibb) *See* COLESTYRAMINE.

quetiapine An atypical *antipsychotic drug that is used for the treatment of schizophrenia. It reduces both the positive symptoms (e.g. delusions) and the negative symptoms (e.g. apathy) of the disease without causing *extrapyramidal reactions. It is also used for treating episodes of mania. Quetiapine is available as tablets and *modified-release tablets on *prescription only.
Side effects: include weight gain, dizziness, low blood pressure on standing (which can cause fainting in some people), sleepiness, indigestion, constipation, dry mouth, a running nose, and a fast heart rate. Quetiapine may prolong a certain phase of the heartbeat (the QT interval), which can lead to *arrhythmias, and reduce the numbers of certain white blood cells.
Precautions: quetiapine should not be taken by women who are breastfeeding. It should be used with caution in pregnant women and in people with cardiovascular disease, a history of stroke or epilepsy, Parkinson's disease, or liver or kidney impairment. It should also be used with care in people taking other drugs that prolong the QT interval (such as atomoxetine, methadone, and tricyclic antidepressants).
Interactions with other drugs:
Anaesthetics: their effect in lowering blood pressure is increased.
Antidepressants: there is an increased risk of antimuscarinic effects and arrhythmias if quetiapine is taken with tricyclic antidepressants.
Antiepileptic drugs: quetiapine antagonizes the effects of these drugs in controlling seizures; phenytoin increases the metabolism of quetiapine, whose dosage may therefore need to be increased.
Ritonavir: may increase the effects of quetiapine.
Sedatives: the sedative effects of quetiapine are increased if it is taken with anxiolytic or hypnotic drugs, or any other drug that causes sedation.
Sibutramine: there is an increased risk of adverse effects on the central nervous system.
Proprietary preparations: Seroquel; Seroquel XL (modified-release tablets.

quinagolide A *dopamine receptor agonist, very similar to *bromocriptine, used to reduce elevated prolactin concentrations in certain types of infertility. It is available as tablets on *prescription only.

Side effects: include nausea, headache, dizziness, fatigue, loss of appetite, gastrointestinal disturbances, insomnia, oedema (swelling), flushing, nasal congestion, and low blood pressure.
Precautions: quinagolide should not be taken by people with kidney or liver impairment and should be used with caution in those who have a history of psychiatric disorders. Women should stop taking the drug if they become pregnant.
Interactions with other drugs:
Dopamine antagonists: may reduce its effect.
Proprietary preparation: Norprolac.

quinalbarbitone *See* SECOBARBITAL.

quinapril An *ACE inhibitor used as an adjunct to *diuretics for the treatment of *heart failure. It is also used to treat all grades of *hypertension. It is available as tablets on *prescription only.
Side effects, precautions, and interactions with other drugs: *see* ACE INHIBITORS.
Proprietary preparations: Accupro; *Accuretic (combined with hydrochlorothiazide).
See also ANTIHYPERTENSIVE DRUGS.

quinine A drug used to treat falciparum *malaria and malarias in which the causative species of *Plasmodium* is not known. Quinine is also used, at a much lower dosage, to prevent leg cramps at night. It is available, on *prescription only, as tablets (quinine sulphate) or an injection (quinine dihydrochloride).
Side effects: at dosages used to treat malaria, side effects include tinnitus (ringing in the ears), headache, hot flushed skin, nausea, abdominal pain, rashes, disturbed vision, confusion, allergic reactions, blood disorders, acute kidney failure, *arrhythmias and other cardiovascular effects, and (especially after injection) low blood sugar.
Precautions: quinine is extremely toxic in overdosage: immediate advice must be sought from a poisons centre. Quinine must not be taken by people with certain blood disorders, optic neuritis (inflammation of the optic nerve), or tinnitus. It should be used with caution by women who are pregnant or breastfeeding and by people with atrial fibrillation (*see* ARRHYTHMIA) or certain other heart conditions.
Interactions with other drugs:
Amiodarone: should not be used with quinine because the risk of ventricular arrhythmias is increased.
Antipsychotic drugs: droperidol and pimozide should not be used with quinine because the risk of ventricular arrhythmias is increased.
Cimetidine: increases the plasma concentration (and possibly side effects) of quinine.
Digoxin: quinine increases the plasma concentration of digoxin, whose dosage may therefore need to be reduced.
Flecainide: quinine increases the plasma concentration of flecainide.
Mefloquine: there is an increased risk of convulsions.

Moxifloxacin: should not be taken with quinine because the risk of ventricular arrhythmias is increased.
Riamet: there is an increased risk of ventricular arrhythmias.

Quinoderm (Ferndale) A proprietary combination of *benzoyl peroxide (a keratolytic) and *potassium hydroxyquinoline sulphate (an antibacterial and antifungal drug), used for the treatment of acne and infected hair follicles. It is available as a cream and can be obtained without a prescription, but only from pharmacies.
Side effects and precautions: *see* BENZOYL PEROXIDE.

quinolones (**4-quinolones**) A group of bactericidal *antibiotic drugs that are used mainly to treat infections that are resistant to *penicillin. They act by inhibiting enzymes that maintain the structure of bacterial DNA and are active against a wide range of bacteria. *See* CIPROFLOXACIN; LEVOFLOXACIN; MOXIFLOXACIN; NALIDIXIC ACID; NORFLOXACIN; OFLOXACIN.
Side effects: include nausea, vomiting, abdominal pain, diarrhoea, indigestion, and flatulence. More rare side effects are antibiotic-associated inflammation of the bowel, headache, dizziness, sleep disorders, rash, itching, fever, skin sensitivity to light, joint and muscle aches, and blood disorders.
Precautions: quinolones are not recommended for children or growing adolescents or for pregnant women. They should be discontinued if mental disturbance, allergic reactions (such as rashes), or sensitivity to sunlight occur. Quinolones should be used with caution in people with a history of epilepsy or convulsions. Driving ability may be impaired and the effects of alcohol are enhanced in people taking these drugs.
Interactions with other drugs:
Antacids: reduce the absorption of ciprofloxacin, levofloxacin, moxifloxacin, norfloxacin, and ofloxacin.
Anti-arrhythmic drugs: there is an increased risk of ventricular arrhythmias if levofloxacin or moxifloxcin is given with amiodarone or moxifloxcin is given with disopyramide, and these drugs should therefore not be used together.
Anticoagulants: the anticoagulant effects of warfarin and acenocoumarol are increased by ciprofloxacin, nalidixic acid, norfloxacin, and ofloxacin.
Ciclosporin: there is an increased risk of kidney toxicity.
NSAIDs: there is an increased risk of convulsions.
Theophylline: its plasma concentration is enhanced by ciprofloxacin and norfloxacin.
Tizanidine: its plasma concentration (and risk of adverse effects) is increased by ciprofloxacin and norfloxacin; ciprofloxacin should not be taken with tizanidine.

quinupristin *See* SYNERCID.

Qvar, Qvar Autohaler, Qvar Easi-Breath (IVAX) *See* BECLOMETASONE DIPROPRIONATE.

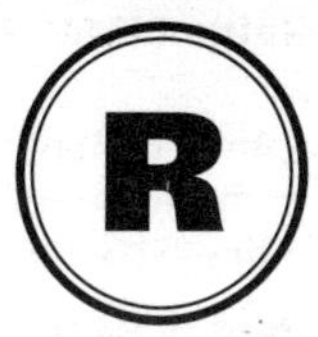

rabeprazole sodium A *proton pump inhibitor used for the treatment of gastric or duodenal ulcers (including those associated with *Helicobacter pylon* infection), gastro-oesophageal reflux disease, and Zollinger-Ellison syndrome (*see* ACID-PEPTIC DISEASES). It is available as *enteric-coated tablets on *prescription only.
Side effects: include headache, diarrhoea, rashes, itching, dizziness, nausea and vomiting, constipation, flatulence, muscle and joint pain, chest pain, inflammation of the mouth lining, cough, and a running nose.
Precautions: *see* PROTON PUMP INHIBITORS.
Interactions with other drugs:
Atazanavir: its plasma concentration is reduced.
Clopidogrel: its effect may be reduced and it should not be taken with rabeprazole.
Proprietary preparation: Pariet.

Radian-B Heat Spray (Roche Products) *See* RADIAN-B MUSCLE LOTION.

Radian-B Muscle Lotion (Roche Products) A proprietary combination of *camphor, *menthol, ammonium *salicylate, and *salicylic acid, used as a *rubefacient for the relief of muscular and rheumatic aches, pains, and stiffness, including pulled muscles, tennis elbow, and golf shoulder. **Radian-B Heat Spray** is an aerosol formulation. Both preparations are freely available *over the counter.
Side effects and precautions: *see* RUBEFACIENTS; SALICYLATES.

Radian-B Muscle Rub (Roche Products) A proprietary combination of *camphor, *menthol, *methyl salicylate, and capsicin (*see* CAPSICUM OLEORESIN) in the form of a cream, used as a *rubefacient for the relief of muscular and rheumatic aches, pains, and stiffness. It is freely available *over the counter.
Side effects and precautions: *see* RUBEFACIENTS; SALICYLATES.

Ralgex Cream (SSL International) A proprietary combination of glycol monosalicylate (*see* GLYCOL SALICYLATE), *methyl nicotinate, and *capsicum oleoresin, used as a *rubefacient for the relief of muscular and rheumatic aches, pains and stiffness. It is freely available *over the counter.
Side effects and precautions: *see* RUBEFACIENTS; SALICYLATES.

Ralgex Freeze Spray (SSL International) A proprietary combination of glycol monosalicylate (*see* GLYCOL SALICYLATE) in a propellant of isopentane and dimethylether that provides a cooling action on the skin (*see* RUBEFACIENTS). It is used for the relief of muscular and rheumatic pain and

sprains and stiffness, including backache, sciatica, and lumbago. It is freely available *over the counter.
Side effects and precautions: *see* RUBEFACIENTS; SALICYLATES.

Ralgex Heat Spray (SSL International) A proprietary combination of glycol monosalicylate (*see* GLYCOL SALICYLATE) and *methyl nicotinate, used as a *rubefacient for the relief of muscular and rheumatic aches, pains, and stiffness, including backache, sciatica, and lumbago. It is freely available *over the counter .
Side effects and precautions: *see* RUBEFACIENTS; SALICYLATES.

raloxifene A drug that acts selectively on *oestrogen receptors in the body: it mimics the action of oestrogen in the bones, heart, and arteries, but does not have oestrogenic effects in the uterus and breast. As a result, raloxifene can increase bone density and therefore protect against osteoporosis, which often develops after the menopause, without increasing the risk of cancer of the uterus or breast. Raloxifene is used to prevent fractures of the bones in the spine caused by osteoporosis in postmenopausal women. However, it does not relieve hot flushes and other symptoms of the menopause. Raloxifene is available as tablets on *prescription only.
Side effects: include hot flushes, leg cramps, and swelling (oedema) of the ankles. There is a risk of blood clots forming in the veins (*see* THROMBOSIS).
Precautions: raloxifene should not be taken by women with a history of venous thrombosis or by those with liver disease, severe kidney disease, cancer of the breast or lining of the uterus, or undiagnosed vaginal bleeding.
Interactions with other drugs:
Anticoagulants: raloxifene opposes the anticoagulant effects of warfarin and acenocoumarol.
Colestyramine: reduces the absorption of raloxifene.
Proprietary preparation: Evista.

r

raltegravir An antiretroviral drug (*see* ANTIVIRAL DRUGS) used, in combination with other antiretrovirals, for the treatment of *HIV infection that has failed to respond to many drugs. It is available as tablets on *prescription only.
Side effects: include abnormal dreams, insomnia, dizziness, headache, vertigo, nausea, vomiting, diarrhoea, abdominal pain, flatulence, rash, and fatigue. Death of bony tissue may occur.
Precautions: raltegravir is not recommended for pregnant or breastfeeding women or for children under 16 years old. It should be used with caution in people with liver disease.
Interactions with other drugs:
Proton pump inhibitors: may increase the plasma concentration of raltegravir; omeprazole should not be taken with it.
Rifampicin: reduces the plasma concentration of raltegravir.
Proprietary preparation: Isentress.

raltitrexed An *antimetabolite used for the palliative treatment of advanced

*cancers of the colon and rectum. It is usually given when *fluorouracil has not been effective or well tolerated or is inappropriate. Raltitrexed is available as an injection on *prescription only.
Side effects: include nausea and vomiting, diarrhoea, *bone marrow suppression, weight loss, dehydration, rash, weakness, fever, pain, and headache. *See also* CYTOTOXIC DRUGS.
Precautions: raltitrexed should not be given to patients with severe liver or kidney disease or to women who are pregnant or breastfeeding. *See also* CYTOTOXIC DRUGS.
Proprietary preparation: Tomudex.

ramipril An *ACE inhibitor used as an adjunct to *diuretics for the treatment of *heart failure. It is also used to treat mild to moderate *hypertension, is given after heart attacks to prevent disease progression in patients with heart failure, and is used to prevent strokes. It is available as capsules or tablets on *prescription only.
Side effects, precautions, and interactions with other drugs: *see* ACE INHIBITORS.
Proprietary preparations: Tritace; *Triapin (combined with felodipine).
See also ANTIHYPERTENSIVE DRUGS.

Ranexa (Menarini) *See* RANOLAZINE.

ranibizumab A *monoclonal antibody used in the treatment of wet age-related macular degeneration, a disorder of the eyes affecting the area of greatest visual acuity (the macula). It works by binding to and inhibiting *vascular endothelial growth factor and therefore it prevents the proliferation of blood vessels around the macula. Ranibizumab is given by injection into the vitreous fluid of the eye under specialist supervision and is available on *prescription only.
Side effects: include headache, nausea, cough, raised pressure in the eye, visual disturbances, eye inflammation, and other eye disorders.
Precautions: ranibizumab should not be given to people with infections or inflammation of the eye, and it should be used with caution in women who are pregnant or breastfeeding. Pressure in the eye should be monitored following the injection. Temporary visual disturbances are possible and patients should be warned of the dangers of operating machinery or driving.
Proprietary preparation: Lucentis.

ranitidine An *H_2-receptor antagonist used in the treatment of gastric and duodenal ulcers, chronic indigestion, reflux oesophagitis, and ulcers caused by the use of *NSAIDs (*see* ACID-PEPTIC DISEASES). It is available, as tablets, effervescent tablets, a sugar-free syrup, or an injection, on *prescription only. Packs containing no more than two weeks' supply of tablets, for the relief of indigestion and heartburn in people over 16 years old, can be obtained from pharmacies without a prescription.
Side effects: include diarrhoea, dizziness, rash, tiredness, and reversible liver changes; rare side effects are reversible confusion, blood disorders, and

muscle or joint pain. In high doses ranitidine can cause breast enlargement in men.
Precautions: ranitidine should be used with caution by people who have poor kidney function and by women who are pregnant or breastfeeding.
Interactions with other drugs:

Antifungal drugs: the absorption of itraconazole and ketoconazole are reduced.

Proprietary preparations: Zantac; Zantac Effervescent.

ranolazine A drug used as an *adjunct for treating angina when *first-line treatment is unsuccessful or cannot be tolerated. It is available as *modified-release tablets on *prescription only.
Side effects: include constipation, nausea and vomiting, headache, and weakness.
Precautions: ranolazine should not be taken by women who are breastfeeding or by people with liver or kidney disease. It should be used with caution in people with severe heart failure or certain *arrhythmias, in those who weigh less than 60 kg, and in the elderly.
Interactions with other drugs:

Antibiotics: clarithromycin and telithromycin may increase the plasma concentration of ranolazine and should not be taken with it; rifampicin reduces the plasma concentration of ranolazine and should not be taken with it.

Antifungal drugs: itraconazole, ketoconazole, posaconazole, and voriconazole may increase the plasma concentration of ranolazine and should not be taken with it.

Disopyramide: should not be taken with ranolazine.

Protease inhibitors: may increase the plasma concentration of ranolazine and should not be taken with it.

Sotalol: should not be taken with ranolazine.

Proprietary preparation: Ranexa.

Rapamune (Pfizer) *See* SIROLIMUS.

Rapifen (Janssen-Cilag) *See* ALFENTANIL.

Rapilysin (Actavis) *See* RETEPLASE.

Rapitil (sanofi-aventis) *See* NEDOCROMIL SODIUM.

Rapydan (EUSA Pharma) A proprietary combination of the local anaesthetics *tetracaine and *lidocaine, used for pain relief during minor surgery. It is applied as a plaster 30 minutes before the procedure and is available on *prescription only.
Side effects and precautions: *see* TETRACAINE.

rasagiline An inhibitor of monoamine oxidase B, an enzyme that breaks down *dopamine and therefore increases levels of dopamine in the brain. It is used for the treatment of Parkinson's disease (*see* ANTIPARKINSONIAN DRUGS),

either alone or in combination with *levodopa. Rasagiline is available as tablets on *prescription only.
Side effects: include headache, flu-like symptoms, malaise, neck pain, allergic reactions, fever, indigestion, loss of appetite, joint pain, vertigo, hallucinations, rhinitis, conjunctivitis, and urgency in passing urine.
Precautions: rasagiline should not be taken by people with severely impaired liver function. It should be used with caution in pregnant and breastfeeding women.
Interactions with other drugs:
Analgesics: rasagiline should not be used with dextromethorphan or pethidine.
Antidepressants: the use of rasagiline with fluoxetine, fluvoxamine, and MAOIs should be avoided; they should not be started until two weeks after stopping rasagiline, and rasagiline should not be started until five weeks after stopping fluoxetine.
Sympathomimetics: should not be taken with rasagiline.
Proprietary preparation: Azilect.

rasburicase A genetically engineered form of an enzyme that breaks down uric acid. It is used to lower uric acid levels in the blood in patients with leukaemia or lymphoma who are receiving chemotherapy. Rasburicase is available as a form for intravenous infusion on *prescription only.
Side effects: include fever.
Precautions: rasburicase should not be given to pregnant or breastfeeding women or to people with metabolic disorders that cause the breakdown of red blood cells. There is a risk of allergic reactions and patients should be monitored for signs of these.
Proprietary preparation: Fasturtec.

Rasilez (Novartis) *See* ALISKIREN.

Ratiograstim (Ratiopharm UK) *See* FILGRASTIM.

Rebetol (Schering-Plough) *See* RIBAVIRIN.

Rebif (Merck Serono) *See* INTERFERON BETA.

reboxetine A drug that inhibits the reuptake of the neurotransmitter *noradrenaline and thus prolongs its action in the brain. It is used for the treatment of depression (*see* ANTIDEPRESSANT DRUGS). Reboxetine is available as tablets on *prescription only.
Side effects: include insomnia, sweating, low blood pressure on standing up, dizziness, difficulties in passing urine, impotence, dry mouth, constipation, and a fast heart rate.
Precautions: reboxetine is not recommended for women who are pregnant or breastfeeding. It should be used with caution in people with severe kidney or liver impairment, a history of epilepsy or cardiovascular disease, bipolar disorder, urinary retention, an enlarged prostate gland, or glaucoma.
Interactions with other drugs: reboxetine should not be taken with

fluvoxamine, imidazoles and triazoles (antifungal drugs), macrolide antibiotics, or Riamet (an antimalarial drug).

MAOIs: reboxetine should not be started until two weeks after stopping MAOIs; MAOIs should not be started until at least one week after reboxetine has been stopped.

Sibutramine: there is an increased risk of adverse effects on the central nervous system and this drug should not be taken with reboxetine.

Proprietary preparation: Edronax.

Rectogesic (ProStrakan) *See* GLYCERYL TRINITRATE.

Redoxon (Roche Products) *See* VITAMIN C.

Reductil (Abbott) *See* SIBUTRAMINE.

ReFacto AF (Pfizer) *See* FACTOR VIII.

Refludan (Celgene Ltd) *See* LEPIRUDIN.

reflux oesophagitis *See* ACID-PEPTIC DISEASES.

Refolinon (Pharmacia) *See* FOLINIC ACID.

Refresh Ophthalmic Solution (Allergan) *See* POLYVINYL ALCOHOL.

Regaine (McNeil Ltd) *See* MINOXIDIL.

Regranex (Janssen-Cilag) *See* BECAPLERMIN.

Regulan (Procter & Gamble) *See* ISPAGHULA HUSK.

Regulose (Novartis) *See* LACTULOSE.

Regurin (Speciality European Pharma) *See* TROSPIUM CHLORIDE.

Relaxit Micro-enema (Crawford Pharmaceuticals) A proprietary combination of *sodium citrate (an osmotic laxative) and *sodium lauryl sulphoacetate (a wetting agent), used for the treatment of constipation. It can be obtained without a prescription, but only from pharmacies.

Precautions: *see* SODIUM CITRATE.

Relenza (GlaxoSmithKline) *See* ZANAMIVIR.

Relestat (Allergan) *See* EPINASTINE HYDROCHLORIDE.

Relifex (Meda Pharmaceuticals) *See* NABUMETONE.

Relistor (Pfizer) *See* METHYLNALTREXONE BROMIDE.

Relpax (Pfizer) *See* ELETRIPTAN.

Remedeine (Napp Pharmaceuticals) A proprietary combination of *paracetamol (a non-opioid analgesic) and *dihydrocodeine tartrate (a weak opioid analgesic), used for the relief of mild to moderate pain. It is available as tablets or effervescent tablets; **Remedeine Forte** contains higher doses of dihydrocodeine. Both preparations are available on *prescription only.

Side effects and precautions: *see* PARACETAMOL; MORPHINE. Remedeine preparations are not recommended for children, and the dosage of Remedeine Forte should be reduced for elderly people.
Interactions with other drugs: *see* OPIOIDS.

Remegel (SSL International) *See* CALCIUM CARBONATE.

Remicade (Schering-Plough) *See* INFLIXIMAB.

remifentanil A strong *opioid with a rapid onset and very short duration of action, used for pain relief during surgical operations. Remifentanil is a *controlled drug that is given by intravenous infusion (an initial dose may be given by intravenous injection).
Side effects and precautions: *see* MORPHINE.
Interactions with other drugs: *see* OPIOIDS.
Proprietary preparation: Ultiva.

Reminyl, Reminyl XL (Shire Pharmaceuticals) *See* GALANTAMINE.

Remnos (DDSA Pharmaceuticals) *See* NITRAZEPAM.

Renagel (Genzyme Therapeutics) *See* SEVELAMER.

Rennie (Bayer) A proprietary combination of the antacids *calcium carbonate and *magnesium carbonate, used for the relief of indigestion, heartburn, flatulence, and stomach upset (*see* ACID-PEPTIC DISEASES). It is freely available *over the counter in the form of chewable tablets.
Side effects and interactions with other drugs: *see* ANTACIDS.
Precautions: Rennies are not recommended for children under six years old.

Rennie Deflatine (Bayer) A proprietary combination of *magnesium carbonate and *calcium carbonate (antacids) and activated *dimeticone (an antifoaming agent), used for the relief of indigestion, heartburn, stomach upset, uncomfortable bloating, flatulence, and painful trapped wind (*see* ACID-PEPTIC DISEASES). It is freely available *over the counter in the form of chewable tablets.
Side effects, precautions, and interactions with other drugs: *see* ANTACIDS.

Rennie Rap-Eze (Bayer) *See* CALCIUM CARBONATE.

ReoPro (Eli Lilly & Co) *See* ABCIXIMAB.

repaglinide An oral antidiabetic drug that acts by stimulating the release of *insulin; it is taken shortly before meals. Repaglinide is used for the treatment of type 2 (noninsulin-dependent) *diabetes mellitus that has not responded to dieting; it can also be given with *metformin when the diabetes is inadequately controlled by metformin alone. Repaglinide is available as tablets on *prescription only.
Side effects: include abdominal pain, constipation, diarrhoea, nausea and vomiting, and (more rarely) allergic reactions (such as rashes).
Precautions: repaglinide should not be taken by people with severe liver disease or by women who are pregnant or breastfeeding.

Interactions with other drugs:

Antibiotics: clarithromycin and trimethoprin may increase the plasma concentration (and therefore effects) of repaglinide; rifampicin may reduce the plasma concentration (and therefore effects) of repaglinide.

Gemfibrozil: may cause a severe fall in blood pressure and should not be taken with repaglinide.

Itraconazole: may increase the plasma concentration (and therefore effects) of repaglinide.

Lapatinib: should not be taken with repaglinide.

Proprietary preparation: Prandin.

Replagal (Shire Pharmaceuticals) *See* AGALSIDASE.

Replenine (Bio Products Laboratory) *See* FACTOR IX.

Replens (Ethical Research Marketing) A proprietary non-hormonal vaginal preparation consisting of purified water with other ingredients that increase its acidity. Providing a high moisture content in the vagina, it is used to relieve the vaginal dryness, itching, and discomfort that can occur at the menopause; its effects last for 2–3 days. Replens is freely available *over the counter as a liquid in prefilled applicators.

Requip, Requip XL (GlaxoSmithKline) *See* ROPINIROLE.

Resolve (SSL International) A proprietary combination of *paracetamol (an analgesic); *citric acid; *sodium bicarbonate, *potassium bicarbonate, and sodium carbonate (antacids); and *vitamin C, used for the relief of headache and overindulgence in food and/or drink. It is available without a prescription as effervescent granules.

Precautions: *see* PARACETAMOL.

Resonium-A (sanofi-aventis) *See* SODIUM POLYSTYRENE SULPHONATE.

Respontin (Allen & Hanburys) *See* IPRATROPIUM BROMIDE.

Restandol (Organon Laboratories) *See* TESTOSTERONE.

Retacrit (Hospira) *See* ERYTHROPOIETIN.

retapamulin An antibacterial drug used for the short-term treatment of impetigo and other superficial skin infections. It is available as an ointment on *prescription only.

Side effects: include skin irritation, pain, itching, and redness.

Precautions: the ointment should be kept away from the eyes and mucous membranes.

Proprietary preparation: Altargo.

reteplase A *fibrinolytic drug used to dissolve blood clots in the coronary arteries (which supply the heart) in people who have had a heart attack; treatment should be started within 12 hours of the attack. Reteplase is available in a form for intravenous injection on *prescription only.

Side effects, precautions, and interactions with other drugs: *see* FIBRINOLYTIC DRUGS.
Proprietary preparation: Rapilysin.

Retin-A (Janssen-Cilag) *See* TRETINOIN.

retinoids A group of drugs derived from vitamin A. On the skin they act to cause drying, peeling, and a reduction in the production of sebum (oil). These effects can be useful in the treatment of *acne, *psoriasis, and other skin disorders. Severe conditions may be treated with retinoids given by mouth, but this must be under hospital supervision. Retinoids include *acitretin, *alitretinoin, *tretinoin, *isotretinoin, and *tazarotene. They are available as capsules or topical preparations on *prescription only. Retinoids can cause abnormalities in the fetus. They should therefore not be taken during pregnancy, and precautions should be taken to avoid becoming pregnant during (and for some retinoids up to two years after) treatment. Breastfeeding should also be avoided during treatment as retinoids can have adverse effects on the babies of breastfeeding mothers.

retinol *See* VITAMIN A.

Retrovir (GlaxoSmithKline) *See* ZIDOVUDINE.

Revatio (Pfizer) *See* SILDENAFIL.

reverse transcriptase inhibitors *See* ANTIVIRAL DRUGS.

Revlimid (Celgene Ltd) *See* LENALIDOMIDE.

Reyataz (Bristol-Myers Squibb) *See* ATAZANAVIR.

Rheumox (Goldshield) *See* AZAPROPAZONE.

Rhinocort Aqua (AstraZeneca) *See* BUDESONIDE.

Rhophylac (CSL Behring) *See* ANTI-D (RH_0) IMMUNOGLOBULIN.

Rhumalgan CR (Sandoz) *See* DICLOFENAC SODIUM.

Riamet (Novartis) A proprietary combination of artemether and lumefantrine (antimalarial drugs derived from *Artemisia* (wormwood) species), used for the treatment of falciparum *malaria. It is available as tablets on *prescription only.
Side effects: include abdominal pain, diarrhoea, nausea, vomiting, cough, headache, sleep disturbance, *arrhythmias, and 'pins and needles'.
Precautions and interactions with other drugs: Riamet should not be taken by people with a history of arrhythmias or congestive heart failure or by breastfeeding women. It should be used with caution in people with liver or kidney disease, in pregnant women, and in combination with other drugs that may cause arrhythmias or have other effects on the heart. These include anti-arrhythmic drugs, other antimalarial drugs, macrolide and quinolone antibiotics, antidepressants, antipsychotics, imidazole and triazole antifungal drugs, sotalol, metoprolol, and cimetidine.

ribavirin <**tribavirin**> An *antiviral drug that is used in the treatment of severe infection caused by the respiratory syncytial virus in infants and children and (in combination with an *interferon) chronic hepatitis C infection. A *prescription only medicine, it is available as tablets, capsules, an oral solution, or an aerosol for inhalation.
Side effects: oral treatment may cause infection, anaemia, loss of appetite, depression, anxiety, insomnia, headache, dizziness, dry mouth, cough, breathlessness, diarrhoea, vomiting, nausea, abdominal pain, itching, rash, hair loss, and muscle and joint pain. Inhalation may worsen the respiratory condition and cause bacterial pneumonia and anaemia.
Precautions: women who are pregnant or attempting to become pregnant should avoid exposure to the aerosol. Ribavirin taken by mouth can cause abnormalities in the fetus, and women who are pregnant or breastfeeding should not use it. Effective contraception should be used during and for four months (for women) and seven months (for men) after treatment. Ribavirin taken by mouth should not be used by women who are breastfeeding and should be used with caution in people with liver, kidney, or heart disease, gout, or eye disorders.
Interactions with other drugs (when taken by mouth):
Antiviral drugs: didanosine increases the risk of side effects and zidovudine increases the risk of anaemia; these drugs should not be taken with ribavirin.
Proprietary preparations: Copegus (tablets); Rebetol (capsules or oral solution); Virazole (inhalation).

riboflavin (<**riboflavine**>; **vitamin B_2**) A vitamin of the B group (*see* VITAMIN B COMPLEX). It is an ingredient of vitamin B and multivitamin preparations to treat vitamin deficiency.
Proprietary preparations: *Pabrinex (combined with other B vitamins and vitamin C); *Vigranon B (combined with other B vitamins); *Yeast-Vite (combined with thiamine, nicotinamide, and caffeine).

rifabutin An *antibiotic used for the prevention of infection in immunocompromised patients and also for the treatment of *tuberculosis and other infections caused by species of *Mycobacterium*. It is available as capsules on *prescription only.
Side effects: include gastrointestinal upset, blood disorders, and discoloration of skin and urine.
Precautions: rifabutin should be used with caution in people with liver or kidney impairment and in women who are pregnant or breastfeeding.
Interactions with other drugs:
Anti-arrhythmic drugs: plasma concentrations of disopyramide and propafenone are reduced.
Antibiotics: clarithromycin and macrolides increase the risk of the toxic effects of rifabutin, whose dosage should therefore be reduced.
Anticoagulants: the effects of warfarin and acenocoumarol are reduced.

Antidiabetic drugs: the effects of chlorpropramide, tolbutamide, and the sulphonylureas are reduced.
Antiepileptic drugs: the effects of carbamazepine and phenytoin are reduced.
Antifungal drugs: fluconazole and possibly other triazoles, posaconazole, and voriconazole increase the effects of rifabutin, whose dosage should therefore be reduced; the plasma concentration of itraconazole is reduced and it should not be taken with rifabutin.
Antiviral drugs: rifabutin should not be taken with indinavir. Atazanavir, darunavir, fosamprenavir, nelfinavir, ritonavir, and tipranavir increase the effects of rifabutin, whose dosage should therefore be reduced.
Aripiprazole: rifabutin reduces the plasma concentration of aripiprazole, whose dosage should therefore be increased.
Atovaquone: its plasma concentration is reduced.
Corticosteroids: the effects of these drugs are reduced.
Lapatinib: should not be taken with rifabutin.
Oral contraceptives: their contraceptive effect is reduced.
Sirolimus: its plasma concentration is reduced and it should not be taken with rifabutin.

Proprietary preparation: Mycobutin.

Rifadin (sanofi-aventis) *See* RIFAMPICIN.

rifampicin An *antibiotic that is especially useful in the treatment of *tuberculosis, when it is used in combination with other antituberculosis drugs, such as *isoniazid and *pyrazinamide. It is also used in the treatment of leprosy, brucellosis, legionnaires' disease, and serious staphylococcal infections. Rifampicin is used to prevent meningitis in carriers of the infecting organisms. It is available, on *prescription only, as capsules or a syrup for oral use and as a solution for intravenous infusion.

Side effects: transient disturbances of liver function may occur, but these do not normally require the treatment to be stopped. Other possible side effects are gastrointestinal disturbances, including nausea, vomiting, and diarrhoea. Intermittent therapy may cause influenza-like symptoms (fever, chills, dizziness, bone pain), wheezing and breathlessness, anaemia, kidney failure, flushing, urticaria and rashes, oedema, muscular weakness, blood disorders, and menstrual disturbances. Urine, saliva, and other body fluids may become coloured orange-red, but this is harmless; discoloration of contact lenses may occur.

Precautions: rifampicin should not be taken by patients with jaundice and must be used with caution in those with impairment of liver or kidney function and in women who are pregnant or breastfeeding. Symptoms of liver disorders (e.g. persistent nausea and vomiting, jaundice) should be reported to a doctor.

Interactions with other drugs:

Anti-arrhythmic drugs: plasma concentrations of disopyramide and propafenone are reduced.

Anticoagulant drugs: the effects of warfarin and acenocoumarol are reduced.
Antidiabetic drugs: the effects of rosiglitazone, tolbutamide, and the sulphonylureas are reduced.
Antiepileptic drugs: the effects of lamotrigine and phenytoin are reduced.
Antifungal drugs: rifampicin reduces the plasma concentrations of fluconazole, itraconazole, ketoconazole, posaconazole, terbinafine, and voriconazole (which should not be taken with it).
Antipsychotic drugs: the plasma concentrations of aripiprazole and haloperidol are reduced; the dosage of aripiprazole should be increased.
Antiviral drugs: rifampicin reduces the plasma concentrations of the following drugs and should not be taken with them: atazanavir, darunavir, fosamprenavir, Kaletra, indinavir, nelfinaquir, nevirapine, saquinavir, and tipranavir; the plasma concentrations of maraviroc and raltegravir are also reduced.
Atovaquone: its effects are reduced by rifampicin.
Bosentan: its plasma concentration is reduced and it should not be taken with rifampicin.
Calcium antagonists: the effects of diltiazem, isradipine, nicardipine, nifedipine, nimodipine, and verapamil are reduced by rifampicin.
Ciclosporin: plasma concentrations of ciclosporin are reduced.
Corticosteroids: the effects of these drugs are reduced.
Cytotoxic drugs: rifampicin reduces the plasma concentrations of dasatinib, imatinib, nilotinib, and temsirolimus, which should therefore not be taken with it.
Eplerenone: its plasma concentration is reduced and it should not be taken with rifampicin.
Mefloquine: its plasma concentration is reduced and it should not be taken with rifampicin.
Mycophenolate: its plasma concentration is reduced.
Oral contraceptives: their contraceptive effect is reduced; extra contraception is required by women who take them.
Ranolazine: its plasma concentration is reduced and it should not be taken with rifampicin.
Sirolimus: its plasma concentration is reduced and it should not be taken with rifampicin.
Tacrolimus: its plasma concentration is reduced.
Telithromycin: its plasma concentration is reduced and it should not be started until two weeks after stopping treatment with rifampicin.

Proprietary preparations: Rifadin; Rimactane; *Rifater (combined with isoniazid and pyrazinamide); *Rifinah (combined with isoniazid).

Rifater (sanofi-aventis) A proprietary combination of *isoniazid, *pyrazinamide, and *rifampicin, used for the treatment of *tuberculosis. It is available as tablets on *prescription only.
Side effects, precautions, and interactions with other drugs: *see* ISONIAZID; PYRAZINAMIDE; RIFAMPICIN.

Rifinah (sanofi-aventis) A proprietary combination of *isoniazid and *rifampicin, used for the treatment of tuberculosis. It is available as tablets on *prescription only.
Side effects, precautions, and interactions with other drugs: *see* ISONIAZID; RIFAMPICIN.

Rilutek (sanofi-aventis) *See* RILUZOLE.

riluzole A drug used in the treatment of motor neurone disease. It can only be used under specialist supervision. Riluzole is available as tablets on *prescription only.
Side effects: include weakness, nausea, vomiting, a fast heart rate, abdominal pain, dizziness, somnolence, tingling.
Precautions: riluzole should not be taken by people with liver or kidney disease or by women who are pregnant or breastfeeding.
Proprietary preparation: Rilutek.

Rimacid (Norton Healthcare; Ranbaxy) *See* INDOMETACIN.

Rimacillin (Ranbaxy) *See* AMPICILLIN.

Rimactane (Sandoz) *See* RIFAMPICIN.

Rimafen (Ranbaxy) *See* IBUPROFEN.

Rimapam (Ranbaxy) *See* DIAZEPAM.

Rimapurinol (Ranbaxy) *See* ALLOPURINOL.

rimexolone A *corticosteroid used to reduce inflammation after eye surgery and for the short-term treatment of inflammatory eye disorders. It is available as eye drops on *prescription only.
Side effects: include eye pain, blurred vision, thinning of the cornea, and raised pressure inside the eye.
Precautions: *see* TOPICAL STEROIDS.
Proprietary preparation: Vexol.

Rimso-50 (Britannia Pharmaceuticals) *See* DIMETHYL SULFOXIDE.

Rinatec (Boehringer Ingelheim) *See* IPRATROPIUM BROMIDE.

ringworm *See* ANTIFUNGAL DRUGS.

Rinstead Adult Gel (Schering-Plough) A proprietary combination of *benzocaine (a local anaesthetic) and *chloroxylenol (an antiseptic), used for the treatment of mouth ulcers, sores caused by dentures, and general soreness of the mouth. It can be obtained without a prescription, but only from pharmacies.
Precautions: this medicine is not recommended for children under 12 years old.

Rinstead Sugar Free Pastilles (Schering-Plough) A proprietary combination of *chloroxylenol (an antiseptic) and *menthol (a soothing

agent), used for the relief of mouth ulcers, sore spots caused by dentures, and soreness in the mouth. It is freely available *over the counter.
Precautions: these pastilles are not recommended for children.

risedronate sodium A *bisphosphonate used for the prevention and treatment of osteoporosis in postmenopausal women and the treatment of Paget's disease (in which the bones become deformed and fracture easily). It is available as tablets on *prescription only.
Side effects: include headache, constipation, indigestion, nausea, abdominal pain, diarrhoea, and pain in the muscles and joints.
Precautions: risedronate should be taken on an empty stomach to prevent food and drink interfering with its absorption in the gut. Therefore the tablets should be swallowed whole, with a full glass of water, at least 30 minutes before breakfast. The patient should then remain standing or sitting upright for at least 30 minutes and not lie down until after eating breakfast. The tablets should not be taken at bedtime or before rising. Risedronate should not be taken by anyone with low plasma-calcium levels or impaired kidney function or by women who are pregnant or breastfeeding. It should be used with caution by people with disorders of the oesophagus.
Interactions with other drugs: *see* ALENDRONIC ACID.
Proprietary preparations: Actonel (daily tablets); Actonel Once a Week (weekly tablets); *Actonel Combi (packaged with calcium carbonate and colecalciferol).

Risperdal, Risperdal Consta, Risperdal Quicklet (Janssen-Cilag) *See* RISPERIDONE.

risperidone An atypical *antipsychotic drug used for the treatment of acute and chronic psychoses, including schizophrenia: it controls both the positive symptoms (e.g. delusions) and the negative symptoms (e.g. apathy) of the disease. It is also used to treat mania and persistent aggression. Risperidone is available as tablets, dispersible tablets, a liquid, or a *depot injection on *prescription only.
Side effects: include weight gain, dizziness, low blood pressure on standing (which can cause fainting in some people), insomnia, agitation, anxiety, headache, drowsiness, lack of concentration, constipation, indigestion, nausea and vomiting, blurred vision, menstrual irregularities, and sexual dysfunction.
Precautions: risperidone should be used with caution in elderly patients, pregnant and breastfeeding women, and in people with liver, heart, or kidney disease, epilepsy, or Parkinson's disease. Drowsiness can affect skilled tasks.
Interactions with other drugs:

Anaesthetics: their effect in lowering blood pressure is enhanced.
Antidepressants: fluoxetine increases the plasma concentration of risperidone; there is an increased risk of antimuscarinic effects and arrhythmias if risperidone is taken with tricyclic antidepressants.
Antiepileptic drugs: their anticonvulsant effects are antagonized by risperidone; carbamazepine reduces the effects of risperidone.

Clozapine: should not be taken with injections of risperidone.
Ritonavir: may increase the effects of risperidone.
Sedatives: the sedative effects of risperidone are increased if it is taken with anxiolytic or hypnotic drugs, or any other drug that causes sedation.
Sibutramine: there is an increased risk of adverse effects on the nervous system and this drug should not be taken with risperidone.

Proprietary preparations: Risperdal; Risperdal Consta (injection); Risperdal Quicklet (dispersible tablets).

Ritalin (Novartis) *See* METHYLPHENIDATE HYDROCHLORIDE.

ritodrine A *sympathomimetic drug that acts on the beta *adrenoceptors to cause relaxation of the muscles of the uterus. It is used to prevent premature labour in women who are 24–33 weeks pregnant. Ritodrine is given by intravenous injection followed by tablets to prevent further episodes during the pregnancy; it is available on *prescription only.
Side effects: include a fast heart rate in the mother and the fetus, anxiety, tremor, flushing, sweating, nausea, vomiting, chest pain, a rise in blood glucose, low blood pressure, and a fall in blood *potassium concentrations. Ritodrine may cause accumulation of fluid in the lungs and heart damage, in which case it should be discontinued immediately. Long-term therapy may produce a large baby.
Precautions: ritodrine should not be given to women who have eclampsia, pre-eclampsia, infection of the uterus or heart disease or to those who have lost a baby during a previous pregnancy. It must be used with caution in multiple pregnancies and in women with diabetes, suspected heart disease, or hyperthyroidism.
Interactions with other drugs:

Antidepressants: there is an increased risk of a dangerous rise in blood pressure if MAOIs or moclobemide are given with ritodrine.
Corticosteroids: increase the risk of low concentrations of potassium in the blood.
Diuretics: increase the risk of low concentrations of potassium in the blood.
Rasagiline: should not be used with ritodrine.
Theophylline: increases the risk of low concentrations of potassium in the blood.

Proprietary preparation: Yutopar.

ritonavir A protease inhibitor (*see* ANTIVIRAL DRUGS), similar to *indinavir, used in combination with other antiretroviral drugs for the treatment of *HIV disease. It is available as capsules or a solution on *prescription only.
Side effects: include stomach and bowel upsets, disturbances of taste, tingling around the mouth or in the fingers and toes, and headache.
Precautions: ritonavir should not be taken by women who are breastfeeding. It should be used with caution in people with liver or kidney disease, diabetes, diarrhoea, and haemophilia and in pregnant women.
Interactions with other drugs: ritonavir is a potent inhibitor of several enzyme systems in the liver that are involved in metabolizing drugs; it

therefore has the potential to interact with many drugs. A doctor should be consulted before ritonavir is taken with any other drug.
Proprietary preparations: Norvir; *Kaletra (combined with lopinavir).

rituximab A *monoclonal antibody that specifically destroys B-lymphocytes (a type of white blood cell). Rituximab is used to treat a type of non-Hodgkin's lymphoma (*see* CANCER) that affects B-lymphocytes and is resistant to standard *cytotoxic drugs. Since the drug acts relatively selectively against the cancerous B-lymphocytes, the widespread adverse effects associated with other cytotoxic drugs do not occur. Rituximab is also used, in combination with *methotrexate, to treat severe rheumatoid arthritis that has not responded to other *disease-modifying antirheumatic drugs. The side effects of rituximab occur during infusion, mostly during the first course of treatment (see below); an analgesic and an antihistamine may need to be given before each infusion to reduce the severity of the side effects. Rituximab is available as a form for infusion on *prescription only.
Side effects: fever, chills, nausea, vomiting, allergic reactions (such as rash, itching, constriction of the airways, breathlessness, and a transient fall in blood pressure), flushing, and tumour pain commonly occur during infusion. The infusion may need to be stopped temporarily in order to treat these effects.
Precautions: rituximab should not be used in women who are breastfeeding or in people with severe infection and should be used with caution in pregnant women and in people with a history of heart disease. Treatment should be carefully monitored under the supervision of a specialist.
Proprietary preparation: MabThera.

rivaroxaban A drug that inhibits Factor Xa (one of the factors involved in blood clotting). It is used as an *anticoagulant to prevent venous thromboembolism (*see* THROMBOSIS) after knee or hip replacement surgery. It is available as tablets on *prescription only.
Side effects: include nausea and bleeding. *See also* ANTICOAGULANTS.
Precautions: rivaroxaban should not be taken by people with active bleeding (e.g. from a peptic ulcer) or by women who are pregnant or breastfeeding. It should be used with caution in people with bleeding disorders or liver or kidney disease and in those who have recently had surgery.
Interactions with other drugs:

Ketoconazole: increases the plasma concentration of rivaroxaban with increased risk of bleeding, and should therefore not be taken with rivaroxaban.

NSAIDs: diclofenac and ketorolac increase the risk of bleeding and should not be taken with rivaroxaban.

Protease inhibitors: increase the plasma concentration of rivaroxaban with increased risk of bleeding, and should therefore not be used with rivaroxaban.

Proprietary preparation: Xarelto.

rivastigmine An *acetylcholinesterase inhibitor that increases the amounts

of acetylcholine in the brain. It is used to treat the symptoms of mild to moderate dementia (including short-term memory loss) that occur in people with Alzheimer's disease or Parkinson's disease. It is available as capsules, an oral solution, or skin patches on *prescription only, and treatment should be supervised by a specialist.
Side effects: include loss of appetite, nausea, vomiting, indigestion, abdominal pain, diarrhoea, weight loss, dizziness, sleepiness, agitation, confusion, and depression.
Precautions: rivastigmine should not be taken by women who are breastfeeding and it should be used with caution in pregnant women, people with liver or kidney disease, certain heart diseases, or peptic ulcers, and in people with a history of asthma or other obstructive lung diseases.
Interactions with other drugs:
Muscle relaxants: rivastigmine either increases or reduces the effects of muscle relaxants used in surgery to paralyse muscles.
Proprietary preparation: Exelon.

Rivotril (Roche Products) *See* CLONAZEPAM.

rizatriptan A *5HT$_1$ agonist used to treat acute attacks of *migraine. A single dose can relieve a migraine headache at any stage of the attack. Rizatriptan is available as tablets or wafers on *prescription only.
Side effects: include sensations of tingling, heat, heaviness, pressure, or tightness; if tightness in the chest or throat is severe, treatment should be discontinued. Other side effects include flushing, dizziness, drowsiness, weakness, indigestion, diarrhoea, palpitations, a fast heart rate, breathlessness, headache, blurred vision, itching, and rash.
Precautions: rizatriptan should not be taken by people with certain heart conditions, uncontrolled high blood pressure, severe kidney disease, or disease of the peripheral blood vessels, or by those who have previously had a stroke. It should be used with caution by women who are pregnant or breastfeeding and by people with impaired liver or kidney function.
Interactions with other drugs:
Antidepressants: MAOIs and moclobemide cause restlessness and other signs of overactivity of the central nervous system if taken with rizatriptan, which should therefore not be started for two weeks after stopping MAOIs or moclobemide.
Other antimigraine drugs: the risk of spasm of the blood vessels, which can have serious consequences, is increased if ergotamine or methysergide are taken with rizatriptan. Ergotamine or methysergide should not be started for 6 hours after stopping rizatriptan, and rizatriptan should not be started for 24 hours after stopping ergotamine.
Propranolol: may increase the plasma concentration of rizatriptan, whose dosage should therefore be reduced.
Proprietary preparations: Maxalt; Maxalt Melt (wafers).

Roaccutane (Roche Products) *See* ISOTRETINOIN.

Robaxin (Almirall) *See* METHOCARBAMOL.

Robinul (Goldshield) *See* GLYCOPYRRONIUM BROMIDE.

Robitussin Chesty Cough (Pfizer) *See* GUAIFENESIN.

Robitussin Chesty Cough with Congestion (Pfizer) A proprietary combination of *pseudoephedrine (a decongestant) and *guaifenesin (an expectorant), used to relieve the symptoms of productive coughs and nasal congestion. It is available as a liquid without a prescription, but only from pharmacies. It cannot be prescribed on the NHS.
Side effects and interactions with other drugs: *see* GUAIFENESIN; EPHEDRINE HYDROCHLORIDE; DECONGESTANTS.
Precautions: this medicine is not recommended for children under two years old. *See also* GUAIFENESIN; EPHEDRINE HYDROCHLORIDE; DECONGESTANTS.

Robitussin Dry Cough (Pfizer) *See* DEXTROMETHORPHAN.

Rocaltrol (Roche Products) *See* CALCITRIOL.

Rocephin (Roche Products) *See* CEFTRIAXONE.

rocuronium bromide *See* MUSCLE RELAXANTS.

Roferon-A (Roche Products) *See* INTERFERON ALFA.

Rogitine (Alliance) *See* PHENTOLAMINE.

ropinirole A *dopamine receptor agonist, similar to *bromocriptine, used for the treatment of Parkinson's disease and restless legs syndrome. It is available as tablets and *modified-release tablets on *prescription only.
Side effects: include nausea, somnolence and suddenly falling asleep, oedema (swelling), abdominal pain, vomiting, and fainting. Occasionally slow heart rate and low blood pressure may occur.
Precautions: ropinirole should not be taken by women who are pregnant or breastfeeding and should be used with caution in people who have liver or kidney disease, severe cardiovascular disease, or psychotic disorders.
Proprietary preparations: Adartrel; Requip; Requip XL (modified-release tablets).

Rosiced (Pierre Fabre) *See* METRONIDAZOLE.

rosiglitazone An *oral hypoglycaemic drug used in the treatment of type 2 *diabetes mellitus, either alone or in combination with *metformin hydrochloride, a *sulphonylurea, or both. It appears to act by reducing the body's resistance to insulin, which leads to a reduction in blood-glucose levels. It is available as tablets on *prescription only.
Side effects: include anaemia, raised levels of blood lipids, weight increase, increased appetite, reduced blood flow to the heart, and bone fractures.
Precautions: rosiglitazone should not be taken by people with heart failure or a history of heart failure, by those with impaired liver function, or by women who are pregnant or breastfeeding.

Interactions with other drugs:
Gemfibrozil: increases the plasma concentration of rosiglitazone.
Rifampicin: reduces the plasma concentration of rosiglitazone.
Proprietary preparations: Avandia; *Avandamet (combined with metformin hydrochloride).

rosuvastatin A *statin used for the treatment of primary hypercholesterolaemia or mixed hyperlipidaemia (*see* HYPERLIPIDAEMIA) that has not responded to dietary measures or exercise. It is available as tablets on *prescription only.
Side effects: *see* STATINS.
Precautions: *see* STATINS. In addition, the maximum dosage should be reduced for people at risk of developing rhabdomyolysis (e.g. those with a history of muscle disorders), and rosuvastatin should be used with caution in people with kidney disease.
Interactions with other drugs:
Antacids: reduce the absorption of rosuvastatin.
Anticoagulants: the effects of oral anticoagulants are increased.
Erythromycin: reduces the plasma concentration of rosuvastatin.
Protease inhibitors: increase the plasma concentration of rosuvastatin, and therefore the risk of muscle damage, and should not be taken with it.
See also STATINS.
Proprietary preparation: Crestor.

rotigotine A *dopamine agonist used alone or as an *adjunct to *levodopa to treat Parkinson's disease. It is also used in the treatment of restless legs syndrome. Rotigotine is available as skin patches on *prescription only.
Side effects: include a fall in blood pressure, somnolence and suddenly falling asleep, hallucinations, local skin irritation, nausea, and vomiting.
Precautions: rotigotine should not be used by women who are pregnant or breastfeeding and should be used with caution in people with liver disease. The patches should not be exposed to heat. People taking rotigotine must not drive or operate machinery. Dosage should be reduced gradually at the end of treatment.
Proprietary preparation: Neupro.

Rowachol (Rowa Pharmaceuticals) A proprietary combination of essential oils (menthol, pinene, menthone, camphene, borneol, and cineole) that has been used as an *adjunct to *bile acids for the dispersal of gallstones. Its value has been questioned. Rowachol is available as capsules on *prescription only.
Interactions with other drugs:
Anticoagulants: the effects of warfarin and acenocoumarol may be reduced.

Rowatinex (Rowa Pharmaceuticals) A proprietary combination of terpenes (volatile oils), including pinene, camphene, and borneol, that is claimed to be of benefit in helping to dissolve and pass kidney stones. It is available as capsules on *prescription only.

Rozex (Galderma) *See* METRONIDAZOLE.

rubefacients (**counterirritants**) Substances that, when rubbed into the skin, cause the blood vessels to dilate, producing redness and a feeling of warmth. This sensation competes with, and to some extent blocks, pain in underlying muscles and joints, since both feelings are conveyed by the same nerves. This action is called **counterirritation**. Rubefacients are used for the relief of muscular aches and pains, rheumatism, and the pain associated with sprains and strains. Common rubefacients include *methyl salicylate, *ethyl salicylate, *glycol salicylate, *capsaicin, *capsicum oleoresin, *methyl nicotinate, and **benzyl nicotinate**. *Menthol and *camphor are also counterirritants, but act by cooling, rather than warming, the skin.
Side effects: when used in large amounts or constantly, rubefacients may irritate the skin.
Precautions: rubefacients are usually not recommended for children and should be avoided during pregnancy and breastfeeding. They should not be covered with dressings and should not come into contact with the eyes, lips, or other mucous membranes, or broken or inflamed skin, where they can cause stinging or burning. Hands should be washed after use to avoid transmission to sensitive areas.

rufinamide An antiepileptic drug (*see* ANTICONVULSANT DRUGS) used as an *adjunct in the treatment of Lennox-Gastraut syndrome (a form of epilepsy). It is available as tablets on *prescription only.
Side effects: include dizziness, sleepiness, unsteady gait, nausea, vomiting, constipation, abdominal pain, weight loss, insomnia, fatigue, and allergic reactions.
Precautions: rufinamide should not be taken by women who are breastfeeding and should be used with caution in people with liver disease and in pregnant women. There is a risk of severe allergic reactions (including fever and rash), and patients should be monitored for signs of these.
Interactions with other drugs:
Antidepressants: may reduce the anticonvulsant effects of rufinamide.
Antimalarial drugs: mefloquine, chloroquine, and hydroxychloroquine antagonize the anticonvulsant effects of rufinamide.
Oral contraceptives: their effect is reduced by rufinamide.
Proprietary preparation: Inovelon.

Rupafin (GlaxoSmithKline) *See* RUPATADINE.

rupatadine An *antihistamine used to treat allergic rhinitis and urticaria (nettle rash). It is available as tablets on *prescription only.
Side effects: include sleepiness, headache, fatigue, dizziness, and dry mouth.
Precautions: rupatadine is not recommended for people with liver or kidney disease. *See also* ANTIHISTAMINES.
Interactions with other drugs:
Erythromycin: increases the plasma concentration of rupatadine.
Ketoconazole: increases the plasma concentration of rupatadine.

See also ANTIHISTAMINES.
Proprietary preparation: Rupafin.

Rusyde (Cox Pharmaceuticals; CP Pharmaceuticals) *See* FUROSEMIDE.

Rynacrom (sanofi-aventis) *See* SODIUM CROMOGLICATE.

Rythmodan, Rythmodan Retard (sanofi-aventis) *See* DISOPYRAMIDE.

Sabril (sanofi-aventis) *See* VIGABATRIN.

Saflutan (Merck Sharp & Dohme Limited) *See* TAFLUPROST.

St John's wort A herbal remedy consisting of an extract of St John's wort (*Hypericum perforatum*), used for treating mild depression. It is freely available *over the counter as capsules and other formulations.
Side effects: the most common side effects are dry mouth, dizziness, stomach upsets, increased sensitivity to sunlight, and fatigue.
Precautions: St John's wort should not be taken by women who are pregnant or breastfeeding. It should not be used to treat moderate or severe depression.
Interactions with other drugs: St John's wort is a potent inducer of an enzyme system involved in metabolizing many drugs, thereby reducing their plasma concentrations. These drugs should therefore not be taken with St John's wort. They include antiepileptic drugs, several antiretroviral drugs (the protease inhibitors, efavirenz, etravirine, maraviroc, nevirapine), ciclosporin, digoxin, oral contraceptives, telithromycin, voriconazole, and warfarin.

Antidepressants: their toxic effects are increased and they should not be taken with St John's wort.

$5HT_1$ agonists: their toxic effects are increased and they should not be taken with St John's wort.

A doctor should be consulted before St John's wort is taken with any other drug.

Saizen (Merck Serono) *See* SOMATROPIN.

Salactol (Dermal Laboratories) A proprietary combination of *salicylic acid and *lactic acid (both keratolytics), used for the treatment of warts, verrucas, corns, and calluses. It is available as a paint and can be obtained without a prescription, but only from pharmacies.
Side effects and precautions: *see* SALICYLIC ACID.

Salagen (Novartis) *See* PILOCARPINE.

Salamol (IVAX) *See* SALBUTAMOL.

Salatac (Dermal Laboratories) A proprietary combination of *salicylic acid and *lactic acid (both keratolytics), used for the treatment of warts, verrucas, corns, and calluses. It is available as a gel and can be obtained without a prescription, but only from pharmacies.
Side effects and precautions: *see* SALICYLIC ACID.

Salazopyrin, Salazopyrin EN-Tabs (Pharmacia) *See* SULFASALAZINE.

Salbulin Novolizer (Meda) *See* SALBUTAMOL.

salbutamol A *sympathomimetic drug that stimulates beta *adrenoceptors in the airways. It is used mainly as a *bronchodilator, to relieve constriction in the airways during attacks of asthma and to alleviate the symptoms of chronic bronchitis and emphysema. Salbutamol has its maximum effect 30–60 minutes after use; its duration of action is 3–6 hours. It also relaxes the muscles of the uterus and may be used intravenously to prevent premature labour. Salbutamol is available, on *prescription only, as tablets, *modified-release tablets or capsules, or a liquid for oral use, as an aerosol or powder for inhalation, as a solution for use in a *nebulizer or a ventilator, and as a solution for injection or infusion.
Side effects: fine tremor (particularly of the hands), restlessness, anxiety, and headache are the most common side effects; less likely are palpitation, dilatation of blood vessels in the extremities, increased heart rate, and muscle cramps. If salbutamol is injected, there may be pain at the injection site.
Precautions: salbutamol should be used with caution by people with an overactive thyroid gland, high blood pressure, certain heart conditions, or diabetes mellitus (particularly if the drug is given intravenously) and by women who are pregnant (unless salbutamol is used to delay labour) or breastfeeding. It is important not to exceed the stated dose; if a previously effective dose does not provide at least three hours relief, a doctor's advice should be sought.
Interactions with other drugs:
Corticosteroids: there is an increased risk of low *potassium concentrations in the blood.
Diuretics: there is an increased risk of low potassium concentrations in the blood.
Methyldopa: may cause low blood pressure when given with salbutamol infusions.
Theophylline: there is an increased risk of low potassium concentrations in the blood.
Proprietary preparations: Airomir (inhaler); Asmasal Clickhaler (breath-activated metered-dose powder inhaler); Pulvinal Salbutamol (inhaler); Salamol Easi-Breathe (aerosol inhalation); Salamol Steri-Neb (nebulizer solution); Salbulin Novolizer (breath-activated metered-dose powder inhaler); Ventmax SR (modified-release capsules); Ventolin (syrup, injection, solution for infusion, aerosol inhalation, solution for respirator); Ventolin Accuhaler (breath-activated aerosol inhaler); Ventolin Evohaler (aerosol inhalation); Ventolin Nebules (ampoules for use in a nebulizer); Volmax (tablets); *Combivent (combined with ipratropium bromide).

salcatonin *See* CALCITONIN (SALMON).

salicylates A group of drugs that are chemically related to *salicylic acid; they are *analgesics that also reduce fever and inflammation. *Aspirin (acetylsalicylic acid) is a salicylate that is taken by mouth to relieve pain, fever, and inflammation. Several salicylates are applied to the skin in the form of

creams, ointments, sprays, or other *topical formulations to relieve pain and stiffness in muscles, joints, and ligaments. These salicylates, which are common ingredients of *rubefacient preparations, include *methyl salicylate (oil of wintergreen), *glycol salicylate, *ethyl salicylate, **ammonium salicylate**, **salicylamide**, and **tetrahydrofurfuryl salicylate**. *Choline salicylate is used as a gel to treat painful conditions of the mouth and gums.
Side effects and precautions: salicylates should not be given to children under 16 years old. Salicylates taken by mouth can irritate the stomach lining and may cause gastric ulceration and bleeding (*see* ASPIRIN). As a result of their wide use and ready availability, salicylates (mainly aspirin) are sometimes a cause of poisoning. Symptoms of mild chronic poisoning (**salicylism**) include headache, dizziness, ringing in the ears, and difficulty in hearing, which can be resolved by reducing the dosage. Topical preparations may cause skin irritation (*see also* RUBEFACIENTS). Excessive or prolonged use of topical preparations containing salicylates should be avoided as these drugs can be absorbed into the body and may cause adverse *systemic effects.

salicylic acid A *salicylate that has *keratolytic properties and is used topically, often in combination with *coal tar or other keratolytics, to remove surface skin in such conditions as dandruff, seborrhoeic *eczema, scaling of the skin, *psoriasis, and acne. It is also used to remove dead skin and promote healing of ulcers, sores, burns, or traumatic injuries and is included in some *rubefacient preparations. Higher concentrations can be used for the removal of hard skin associated with corns and calluses, warts, and verrucas. Salicylic acid is available, alone or in combination with other ingredients, as a liquid, cream, ointment, or shampoo. It can be obtained without a prescription but usually only from pharmacies (depending on the other ingredients).
Side effects: it may cause irritation and drying of the skin.
Precautions: salicylic acid should not be used on facial or genital warts or warts around the anus. It should not be applied to large areas of healthy skin or to broken skin and contact with the eyes should be avoided. High concentrations of salicylic acid should not be used by people with diabetes.
See also SALICYLATES.
Proprietary preparations: Acnisal (liquid for acne); Boots Corn Removal Plasters; Carnation Corn Caps; Carnation Verruca Care; Corn Removal Pads; Corn Removal Plasters; Occlusal (liquid for warts); Soft Corn Removal Pads; Thwart; Verruca Removal System; Verrugon (ointment for verrucas); *Bazuka Gel (combined with lactic acid); *Boots Verruca Removal Gel (combined with camphor); *Capasal (combined with coal tar; *Cocois (combined with coal tar and sulphur); *Corn and Callus Removal Liquid (combined with camphor); *Cuplex (combined with lactic acid and copper acetate); *Diprosalic (combined with betamethasone); *Duofilm (combined with lactic acid); *Meted (combined with sulphur); *Movelat (combined with mucopolysaccharide polysulphate); *Phytex (combined with borotannic complex, methyl salicylate, and acetic acid); *Posalfilin (combined with podophyllum resin); *Pyralvex (combined with anthroquinone glycosides);

*Salactol (combined with lactic acid); *Seal and Heal Verruca Removal Gel (combined with camphor).

Saline Steri-Neb (Teva UK) *See* SODIUM CHLORIDE.

Saliva Orthana (A.S Pharma) A proprietary combination of mucin (a constituent of mucus) obtained from the stomach of pigs and *xylitol (a sugar), used as an artificial saliva for the relief of dry mouth (which occurs, for example, after radiotherapy). It is freely available *over the counter in the form of a mouth spray or lozenges.

Saliveze (Wyvern Medical) A proprietary combination of carboxymethylcellulose (a protective agent; *see* CARMELLOSE) and salts of calcium, potassium magnesium and sodium (*see* ELECTROLYTE), used as an artificial saliva for the relief of dry mouth (which occurs, for example, after radiotherapy). It is freely available *over the counter in the form of a mouth spray.

Salivix (KoGEN) A proprietary combination of *malic acid, acacia, and other ingredients, used as an artificial saliva for the relief of dry mouth (caused, for example, by radiotherapy). It is freely available *over the counter in the form of sugar-free pastilles.

salmeterol A *sympathomimetic drug that stimulates beta *adrenoceptors. It is used as a *bronchodilator in the treatment of asthma, bronchitis, and emphysema. Salmeterol has a longer duration of action than *salbutamol and is therefore taken less frequently. It is used to prevent asthma attacks during the night or induced by exercise; it is not suitable for the relief of acute attacks of asthma since it has a slower onset of action than salbutamol. Salmeterol is used mostly in conjunction with long-term prophylactic therapy, such as *corticosteroids or *chromones. It is available, on *prescription only, as an aerosol or powder for inhalation.
Side effects, precautions, and interactions with other drugs: *see* SALBUTAMOL.
Proprietary preparations: Serevent Accuhaler (breath-activated inhaler for powder); Serevent Diskhaler (inhaler for discs containing powder blisters); Serevent Evohaler (metered-dose aerosol inhalation); *Seretide (combined with fluticasone propionate).

S

Salofalk (Dr Falk Pharma) *See* MESALAZINE.

Samsca (Pharmaceuticals (UK) Ltd) *See* TOLVAPTAN.

Sandimmun (Novartis) *See* CICLOSPORIN.

Sandocal 400 (Novartis) A proprietary combination of *calcium lactate gluconate and *calcium carbonate, used as a *calcium supplement. **Sandocal 1000** is a stronger formulation. Both preparations are available as effervescent tablets and can be obtained without a prescription, but only from pharmacies.
Side effects, precautions, and interactions with other drugs: *see* CALCIUM.

Sandocal + D 600 (Novartis) A proprietary combination of *calcium lactate gluconate, *calcium carbonate, and *colecalciferol (vitamin D_3), used to treat *vitamin D deficiency and as an *adjunct in the treatment of osteoporosis. It is available as effervescent tablets and can be obtained from pharmacies without a prescription.
Side effects, precautions, and interactions with other drugs: *see* CALCIUM; VITAMIN D.

Sandoglobulin (CSL Behring) *See* IMMUNOGLOBULINS.

Sando-K (HK Pharma) A proprietary combination of *potassium chloride and *potassium bicarbonate used as a *potassium supplement. It is available as tablets that dissolve in water to produce an effervescent drink and can be obtained without a prescription, but only from pharmacies.
Side effects, precautions, and interactions with other drugs: *see* POTASSIUM.

Sandostatin (Novartis) *See* OCTREOTIDE.

Sandrena (Organon Laboratories) *See* ESTRADIOL; HORMONE REPLACEMENT THERAPY.

Sanomigran (Novartis) *See* PIZOTIFEN.

sapropterin A drug used as an *adjunct to dietary measures in the treatment of phenylketonuria, a metabolic disease causing an excess of the amino acid phenylalanine in the blood, which damages the nervous system. It is available as dispersible tablets on *prescription only.
Side effects: include diarrhoea, vomiting, abdominal pain, nasal congestion, and cough.
Precautions: sapropterin should not be taken by women who are breastfeeding and should be used with caution in people who are liable to have convulsions or who have liver or kidney disease.
Proprietary preparation: Kuvan.

S

saquinavir A protease inhibitor (*see* ANTIVIRAL DRUGS), similar to *indinavir, used in combination with other antiretrovirals for the treatment of *HIV disease. It is available as capsules on *prescription only.
Side effects: include diarrhoea, dry mouth, abdominal discomfort, nausea, headache, peripheral neuropathy (causing tingling and numbness in the limbs), breathlessness, increased appetite, loss of hair, and rashes.
Precautions: saquinavir should be used with caution by people with impaired kidney or liver function or haemophilia and by pregnant women. It should not be used during breastfeeding.
Interactions with other drugs: saquinavir interacts with a number of drugs, including those listed below, and it is therefore important to inform a doctor before taking any other medicines with saquinavir.

Antiepileptic drugs: primidone, phenobarbital, phenytoin, and carbamazepine can reduce the plasma concentration (and therefore effectiveness) of saquinavir.

Antimigraine drugs: the toxic effects of ergotamine and methysergide may be increased.
Antipsychotic drugs: saquinavir can increase the plasma concentration (and therefore side effects) of pimozide and sertindole, which should therefore not be taken with it.
Antiviral drugs: the plasma concentration (and therefore side effects) of maraviroc are increased by saquinavir; ritonavir increases the plasma concentration of saquinavir and tipranavir reduces it.
Ciclosporin: the plasma concentrations of both drugs are increased.
Cilostazol: its plasma concentration may be increased and it should not be used with saquinavir.
Midazolam: its plasma concentration is increased, causing profound sedation, and it should not be taken with saquinavir.
Ranolazine: its plasma concentration may be increased and it should not be used with saquinavir.
Rifampicin and rifabutin: can reduce the plasma concentration (and therefore effectiveness) of saquinavir and should not be used with it.
Statins: rosuvastatin and simvastatin should not be taken with saquinavir as this increases the risk of muscle damage.
Tacrolimus: its plasma concentration is increased and therefore its dosage may need to be reduced.
Proprietary preparation: Invirase.

Savene (TopoTarget) *See* DEXRAZOXANE.

Savlon Antiseptic Cream, Savlon Antiseptic Liquid (Novartis) Proprietary combinations of the antiseptics *chlorhexidine gluconate and *cetrimide, used for cleansing and disinfecting all types of minor skin disorders and wounds. They are freely available *over the counter.
Side effects: *see* CETRIMIDE.

Savlon Antiseptic Wound Wash (Novartis) *See* CHLORHEXIDINE.

Savlon Dry (Novartis) *See* POVIDONE–IODINE.

scabicides *See* SCABIES.

S

scabies A skin disease caused by infestation with the mite *Sarcoptes scabei.* A scabies infestation causes severe itching (particularly at night); commonly infected areas are the nipples, penis, and the skin between the fingers. Scratching to relieve the itch may lead to secondary infection. Treatment is by application of a **scabicide** (a drug that kills the mite), usually *permethrin or *malathion; it should be applied to all parts of the skin from the neck down. *Benzyl benzoate can also be used but it causes irritation. *Calamine or *crotamiton may be used to relieve itching that persists after the mites have been destroyed. All members of a family need to treated but clothing and bedding do not need to be disinfested.

Scheriproct (Meda Pharmaceuticals) A proprietary combination of *prednisolone hexanoate (a corticosteroid) and *cinchocaine hydrochloride (a

local anaesthetic), used for the short-term relief of the discomfort and pain of *haemorrhoids and itching of the anus. It is available as an ointment or suppositories on *prescription only.
Side effects: *see* CORTICOSTEROIDS.
Precautions: Scheriproct should not be used when viral or fungal infection is present; prolonged use should be avoided.

sclerotherapy The injection of an irritant substance into a vein, which causes scarring and hardening so that the vein eventually closes up. Sclerotherapy using *ethanolamine oleate or *sodium tetradecyl sulphate is used in the treatment of varicose veins; *phenol is used as a sclerosant to treat *haemorrhoids.

Scopoderm TTS (Novartis) *See* HYOSCINE HYDROBROMIDE.

scopolamine *See* HYOSCINE BUTYLBROMIDE; HYOSCINE HYDROBROMIDE.

Seal and Heal Verruca Removal Gel (SSL International) A proprietary combination of *salicylic acid (a keratolytic) and *camphor, used for the treatment of warts and verrucas. It is freely available *over the counter.
Precautions: this preparation is not recommended for children.

Sea-Legs (SSL International) *See* MECLOZINE HYDROCHLORIDE.

Sebact MR (Dexcel Pharma Ltd) *See* MINOCYCLINE.

Sebomin MR (Actavis) *See* MINOCYCLINE.

secobarbital **<quinalbarbitone>** An intermediate-acting *barbiturate used, in combination with *amobarbital, for the short-term treatment of severe insomnia in people who are already taking barbiturates. A *controlled drug, it is available as capsules.
Side effects, precautions, and interactions with other drugs: *see* BARBITURATES.
Proprietary preparation: *Tuinal (combined with amobarbital).

S

Sectral (sanofi-aventis) *See* ACEBUTOLOL.

Securon (Abbott) *See* VERAPAMIL HYDROCHLORIDE.

sedatives *See* ANXIOLYTIC DRUGS.

Select-A-Jet Dopamine (UCB Pharma) *See* DOPAMINE HYDROCHLORIDE.

selective serotonin reuptake inhibitors *See* SSRIs.

selegiline An inhibitor of monoamine oxidase type B, an enzyme that breaks down *dopamine and therefore increases dopamine concentrations in the brain (*compare* MONOAMINE OXIDASE INHIBITORS). It is used for the treatment of Parkinson's disease (*see* ANTIPARKINSONIAN DRUGS), either alone or in combination with *levodopa. It is available as tablets or a liquid on *prescription only.

Side effects: include low blood pressure on standing, nausea, dry mouth, confusion, and agitation.
Precautions: selegiline should not be taken by women who are pregnant or breastfeeding. The side effects of levodopa may be increased when a combination of selegiline and levodopa is used; the dose of levodopa may need to be reduced.
Interactions with other drugs:
Antidepressants: there is a risk of high blood pressure and overstimulation of the central nervous system if fluoxetine, fluvoxamine, paroxetine, sertraline, or venlafaxine are taken with selegiline; selegiline should be avoided for 1–5 weeks after stopping these drugs, which should not be started for 2 weeks after stopping selegiline; moclobemide should not be taken with selegiline.
Dopamine: there is a risk of a dangerous rise in blood pressure.
Pethidine: there is a risk of toxic effects on the central nervous system and this drug should not be used with selegiline.
Proprietary preparations: Eldepryl (tablets or liquid); Zelapar (freeze-dried tablets).

Selenase (Oxford Nutrition) *See* SELENIUM.

selenium A trace element that has important properties as an antioxidant, limiting damage to cells and tissues caused by toxic substances. Selenium deficiency usually results from inadequate diet or prolonged feeding by infusion of nutrients through a vein. A selenium supplement is available as an oral solution or an injection on *prescription only.
Proprietary preparation: Selenase.

selenium sulphide A drug with *antifungal properties that is applied to the scalp for the treatment of dandruff and seborrhoeic *eczema. It is available as a shampoo and can be obtained without a prescription, but only from pharmacies.
Precautions: selenium sulphide should not come into contact with the eyes or broken skin. It should not be used within 48 hours of using perming or hair-colouring lotions.
Proprietary preparation: Selsun.

Selexid (Leo Pharmaceuticals Limited) *See* PIVMECILLINAM HYDROCHLORIDE.

Selsun (Chattem UK) *See* SELENIUM SULPHIDE.

senna A *stimulant laxative, isolated from the fruit of the senna plant, used for the treatment of constipation; the active ingredients are chemicals called **sennosides**. It is available as tablets, granules, or a syrup and can be obtained without a prescription, but some preparations are available only from pharmacies.
Side effects and precautions: *see* STIMULANT LAXATIVES.
Proprietary preparations: Boots Natural Senna Tablets; Ex-Lax Senna (chocolate tablets); Senokot (tablets or syrup); *Boots Constipation Relief 1

Year Plus (combined with figs); *Califig California Syrup of Figs (combined with figs); *Manevac (combined with ispaghula husk); *Pripsen (combined with piperazine).

sennosides *See* SENNA.

Senokot (Forum Health Products) *See* SENNA.

Senselle (LRC Products) A proprietary non-hormonal water-based preparation used as a vaginal lubricant to relieve dryness of the vagina, which can occur at the menopause. Its effects last for up to 24 hours. Senselle is freely available *over the counter in the form of a liquid.

Sensodyne (GlaxoSmithKline) A proprietary combination of *triclosan (an antiseptic), *potassium chloride, and sodium *fluoride, used for the relief of pain from sensitive teeth and as an aid in preventing dental caries. It is freely available *over the counter as a toothpaste.

Septrin (GlaxoSmithKline) *See* CO-TRIMOXAZOLE.

Seractil (Genus Pharmaceuticals) *See* DEXIBUPROFEN.

Serc (Solvay Healthcare) *See* BETAHISTINE.

Serdolect (Lundbeck) *See* SERTINDOLE.

Serenace (IVAX) *See* HALOPERIDOL.

Seretide (Allen & Hanburys) A proprietary combination of *salmeterol (a bronchodilator) and *fluticasone propionate (a corticosteroid), used for the prevention of asthma and the treatment of chronic obstructive pulmonary disease. A *prescription only medicine, it is taken by inhalation (*see* INHALER) of a powder (**Seretide Accuhaler**) or an aerosol (**Seretide Evohaler**).
Side effects, precautions, and interactions with other drugs: *see* SALBUTAMOL; CORTICOSTEROIDS.

Serevent (Allen & Hanburys) *See* SALMETEROL.

S

Seroquel, Seroquel XL (AstraZeneca) *See* QUETIAPINE.

serotonin (**5-hydroxytryptamine**; **5HT**) A compound widely distributed in the tissues, particularly the brain and other parts of the nervous system, the blood platelets, and the intestinal wall. Serotonin is a transmitter of nerve impulses and also acts like a hormone. It causes contraction of smooth muscles (e.g. in the intestine) and constriction of blood vessels and may have a role in inflammation. Serotonin is thought to be involved in the development of a *migraine headache; drugs that act like serotonin (*see* $5HT_1$ AGONISTS) are used to treat migraine, while drugs that antagonize its effects (such as *pizotifen) are used to prevent migraine attacks. In the brain, concentrations of serotonin are believed to have important effects on mood. Drugs that act to prolong the effects of serotonin in the brain, such as the selective serotonin reuptake inhibitors (*see* SSRIs), are used in the treatment of depression.

Seroxat (GlaxoSmithKline) *See* PAROXETINE.

sertindole An atypical *antipsychotic drug used for the treatment of schizophrenia. Because it may cause serious abnormalities in heart rhythm (*arrhythmias), sertindole is now used only for treating patients who are taking part in clinical trials and who cannot be treated with other antipsychotic drugs. It is available as tablets on *prescription only.
Side effects: include arrhythmias, swelling of the ankles, weight gain, dizziness, low blood pressure on standing (which can cause fainting in some people), dry mouth, a running nose, nasal congestion, breathlessness, tingling in the fingers or toes, and (rarely) convulsions.
Precautions: sertindole should only be used for treating patients already taking it. It should not be taken by women who are pregnant or breastfeeding or by people with severe liver disease or arrhythmias. It should be used with caution in people with diabetes or mild or moderate liver disease. Heart activity should be monitored during treatment.
Interactions with other drugs:

Anaesthetics: their effect in lowering blood pressure is enhanced.
Anti-arrhythmic drugs: amiodarone and disopyramide should not be taken with sertindole as this combination increases the risk of arrhythmias.
Antibiotics: macrolides (such as erythromycin) and moxifloxacin increase the risk of arrhythmias and should not be taken with sertindole.
Antidepressants: tricyclic antidepressants increase the risk of arrhythmias; fluoxetine and paroxetine increase the effects of sertindole.
Antiepileptic drugs: their anticonvulsant effects are antagonized by sertindole; carbamazepine and phenytoin reduce the effects of sertindole.
Antifungal drugs: imidazoles and triazoles increase the risk of arrhythmias and should not be taken with sertindole.
Antipsychotic drugs: amisulpride and droperidol should not be taken with sertindole as this combination increases the risk of arrhythmias.
Antiviral drugs: fosamprenavir, indinavir, Kaletra, nelfinavir, ritonavir, and saquinavir increase the risk of arrhythmias and should not be taken with sertindole.
Atomoxetine: increases the risk of arrhythmias.
Cimetidine: increases the risk of arrhythmias and should not be taken with sertindole.
Diuretics: increase the risk of arrhythmias.
Ivabradine: increases the risk of arrhythmias.
Lithium: increases the risk of arrhythmias and should not be taken with sertindole.
Sedatives: the sedative effects of sertindole are increased if it is taken with anxiolytic or hypnotic drugs, or any other drug that causes sedation.
Sibutramine: increases the risk of adverse effects on the central nervous system.
Sotalol: increases the risk of arrhythmias.

Proprietary preparation: Serdolect.

sertraline An *antidepressant drug of the *SSRI group that is used for the treatment of depressive illness, obessive-compulsive disorder, and post-traumatic stress disorder. It is available as tablets on *prescription only.
Side effects and precautions: *see* SSRIs.
Interactions with other drugs:

Antipsychotic drugs: droperidol should not be taken with sertraline as this combination increases the risk of *arrhythmias; the plasma concentration of clozapine is increased.
Selegiline: there is an increased risk of hypertension and adverse effects on the central nervous system; selegiline should not be started until two weeks after stopping sertraline, which should not be started until two weeks after stopping selegiline.
Sumatriptan: there is an increased risk of adverse effects on the central nervous system and this drug should not be taken with sertraline.
See also SSRIs.

Proprietary preparation: Lustral.

sevelamer A *phosphate-binding agent used to reduce high levels of phosphate in the blood in people with kidney failure who are undergoing dialysis treatment. It is available as tablets on *prescription only.
Side effects: may include abdominal pain, constipation, diarrhoea, nausea, and vomiting.
Precautions: sevelamer should not be taken by people with an obstructed bowel and should be used with caution in people with bowel or stomach disorders and by women who are pregnant or breastfeeding.
Proprietary preparation: Renagel.

Sevikar (Daiichi Sankyo UK Limited) A proprietary combination of *olmesartan (an angiotensin II inhibitor) and *amlodipine (a calcium antagonist), used for the control of high blood pressure. It is available as tablets on *prescription only.
Side effects: *see* CALCIUM ANTAGONISTS; OLMESARTAN.
Precautions: *see* AMLODIPINE; OLMESARTAN.
Interactions with other drugs: *see* ACE INHIBITORS; CALCIUM ANTAGONISTS.

Sevredol (Napp Pharmaceuticals) *See* MORPHINE.

sibutramine A drug that acts on the central nervous system to suppress the appetite. It is used as an *adjunct for the treatment of obesity in people who have failed to respond to standard weight-reducing measures alone. Sibutramine is available as capsules on *prescription only.
Side effects: include a fast heart rate, palpitations, raised blood pressure, constipation, nausea, dry mouth, insomnia, light-headedness, and sweating.
Precautions: sibutramine should not be taken by people with a history of major eating disorders, coronary artery disease, congestive heart failure, a fast heart rate, peripheral artery disease, *arrhythmias, or stroke; by those with psychiatric illness, uncontrolled hypertension, underactivity of the thyroid

gland, severe liver or kidney disease, an enlarged prostate, or a history of drug or alcohol abuse; or by women who are pregnant or breastfeeding.
Interactions with other drugs:

Antidepressants and antipsychotics: increase the risk of toxic effects on the central nervous system.

Proprietary preparation: Reductil.

Siklos (Nordic) *See* HYDROXYCARBAMIDE.

sildenafil A drug that is taken by mouth in the treatment of impotence. It enhances the erectile response to sexual stimulation and is used for the treatment of men who have difficulty in obtaining or maintaining an erection. During sexual stimulation, it acts as a selective enzyme inhibitor, causing relaxation of smooth muscle and increasing blood flow to the erectile tissue of the penis. Sildenafil has been shown to be effective in a broad range of men, including the elderly and those with high blood pressure, diabetes, coronary artery disease, depression, spinal-cord injury, or prostate problems. Sildenafil has also been reported to increase the sensation of orgasm in women, but it is not licensed for use in women or in males under 18 years old. It is also used to treat high blood pressure in the vessels supplying the lungs. Sildenafil is available as tablets on *prescription only, and there are restrictions to its prescription for impotence on the NHS.
Side effects: include headache, flushing, dizziness, indigestion, nasal congestion, and visual disturbances (including effects on colour vision).
Precautions: sildenafil should not be used by people who are taking *nitrates (such as glyceryl trinitrate or isosorbide), or by those who have recently had a heart attack or a stroke, or who have cardiovascular conditions that make sexual activity inadvisable, severely impaired liver function, low blood pressure, or hereditary conditions that affect vision. It should be used with caution by men with abnormal anatomy of the penis, sickle-cell anaemia, multiple myeloma, leukaemia, and by men and women with active peptic ulcer, bleeding disorders, or impaired kidney function.
Interactions with other drugs:

Alpha blockers: their effect in lowering blood pressure is enhanced and they should not be started until four hours after stopping sildenafil.

Antibiotics: erythromycin, clarithromycin, and telithromycin increase the effect of sildenafil, whose dosage may therefore need to be reduced.

Antifungal drugs: ketoconazole and itraconazole increase the effect of sildenafil, whose dosage may therefore need to be reduced.

Antiviral drugs: atazanavir may increase the side effects of sildenafil; the plasma concentration of sildenafil is increased by indinavir and ritonavir (which should not be taken with it).

Cimetidine: increases the effect of sildenafil, whose dosage may therefore need to be reduced.

Nicorandil: sildenafil significantly enhances the effects of nicorandil in reducing blood pressure and should not be taken with this drug.

Nitrates: sildenafil significantly enhances the effects of these drugs in reducing blood pressure and it should not be taken with nitrates.
Proprietary preparations: Revatio; Viagra.

Silkis (Galderma (U.K) Ltd) *See* CALCITRIOL.

silver nitrate A *keratolytic used for the removal of warts and verrucas. It is available as a caustic pencil and can be obtained without a prescription, but only from pharmacies.
Side effects: silver nitrate stains skin and fabrics.
Precautions: silver nitrate should not be applied to facial or genital warts or to warts around the anus. Care should be taken to protect healthy skin and avoid broken skin during application.
Proprietary preparation: Avoca.

silver sulfadiazine <**silver sulphadiazine**> An *antibiotic that is active against a variety of bacteria; it has limited activity against viruses. It is used to prevent and treat infection in cases of severe burns and to disinfect skin graft sites, wounds, infected leg ulcers, and pressure sores. Silver sulfadiazine is available as a cream on *prescription only.
Side effects: discoloration of the skin has been reported; otherwise side effects are rare. However, if large areas of skin are treated enough sulfadiazine can be absorbed to cause the side effects of *sulphonamides.
Precautions: silver sulfadiazine should not be used during pregnancy or breastfeeding or on newborn babies. It should be used with caution by people with impaired kidney or liver function.
Interactions with other drugs: if large areas of skin are treated enough sulfadiazine can be absorbed to cause interactions (*see* SULPHONAMIDES).
Proprietary preparation: Flamazine.

simeticone *See* DIMETICONE.

Simulect (Novartis) *See* BASILIXIMAB.

Simvador (Discovery Pharmaceuticals) *See* SIMVASTATIN.

S

simvastatin A *statin used for the treatment of primary hypercholesterolaemia and mixed *hyperlipidaemia that has not responded to dietary intervention. It is also used to prevent the progression of *atherosclerosis in patients with coronary artery disease and to reduce the incidence of coronary events in susceptible individuals. It is available as tablets on *prescription only.
Side effects and precautions: *see* STATINS.
Interactions with other drugs:

Amiodarone: there is an increased risk of muscle damage if this drug is taken with simvastatin.
Antibiotics: there is an increased risk of muscle damage with clarithromycin, erythromycin, and telithromycin (which should not be taken with simvastatin) and fusidic acid.
Anticoagulants: the effects of warfarin and acenocoumarol are increased.

Antifungal drugs: the risk of muscle damage is increased if simvastatin is taken with itraconazole, ketoconazole, miconazole, and posaconazole (which should all be avoided).
Antiviral drugs: there is an increased risk of muscle damage with atazanavir, fosamprenavir, indinavir, Kaletra, nelfinavir, ritonavir, and saquinavir, and none of these drugs should be taken with simvastatin.
Danazol: increases the risk of muscle damage.
Verapamil: increases the risk of muscle damage.
See also STATINS.
Proprietary preparations: Simvador; Zocor; *Inegy (combined with ezetimibe).

Sinemet, Sinemet CR, Sinemet LS, Sinemet Plus (Bristol-Myers Squibb) *See* CO-CARELDOPA.

Sinepin (Marlborough) *See* DOXEPIN.

Singulair (Merck Sharp & Dohme) *See* MONTELUKAST.

Sinthrome (Alliance) *See* ACENOCOUMAROL.

Siopel (Centrapharm) A proprietary combination of *dimeticone (a water repellent) and *cetrimide (an antiseptic), used as a barrier cream (*see* BARRIER PREPARATIONS). It is freely available *over the counter.

sirolimus An *immunosuppressant that acts by inhibiting activation of T cells, a type of white blood cell involved in the immune response. It is used, initially in combination with *ciclosporin and a corticosteroid, to prevent rejection of kidney transplants. Sirolimus is available as tablets or an oral solution on *prescription only.
Side effects: include low blood cell and platelet counts, anaemia, fever, hypertension, urinary tract infection, raised blood lipids (*hyperlipidaemia), abdominal pain, joint pain, acne, diarrhoea, constipation, nausea, and headache.
Precautions: sirolimus should not be taken by women who are pregnant or breastfeeding and should be used with caution in people with liver disease.
Interactions with other drugs: drugs that strongly inhibit or induce an enzyme system in the liver that is involved in metabolizing sirolimus should be avoided, since they raise or lower plasma concentrations of sirolimus. These drugs include ketoconazole, voriconazole, itraconazole, telithromycin, and clarithromycin (inhibitors), and rifampicin and rifabutin (inducers).
Proprietary preparation: Rapamune.

sitagliptin An *oral hypoglycaemic drug used, in combination with other antidiabetic drugs, to control blood glucose levels in people with type 2 *diabetes mellitus. It works by increasing the secretion of *insulin and reducing the secretion of *glucagon. Sitagliptin is available as tablets on *prescription only.
Side effects: include nausea, vomiting, abdominal pain, and bowel upsets.
Precautions and interactions with other drugs: sitagliptin should not be

taken by people with kidney disease or by pregnant or breastfeeding women. There is a risk of *hypoglycaemia when sitagliptin is taken with other hypoglycaemic drugs.
Proprietary preparation: Januvia.

sitaxentan sodium A *vasodilator used to treat raised blood pressure within the blood vessels supplying the lungs; it has a similar action to *bosentan. Sitaxentan is used under specialist supervision; it is available as tablets on *prescription only.
Side effects: include headache, constipation, nasal congestion, dizziness, insomnia, flushing, and swollen ankles.
Precautions: sitaxentan should not be taken by people with liver disease or by breastfeeding women.
Interactions with other drugs:
Ciclosporin: its plasma concentration is increased and it should not be used with sitaxentan.
Warfarin: its anticoagulant effects are increased.
Proprietary preparation: Thelin.

Skelid (sanofi-aventis) *See* TILUDRONIC ACID.

Skinoren (Meda Pharmaceuticals) *See* AZELAIC ACID.

Slofenac SR (Merck Serono) *See* DICLOFENAC SODIUM.

Slo-Indo (Generics) *See* INDOMETACIN.

Slo-Phyllin (Merck Serono) *See* THEOPHYLLINE.

Slow-K (Alliance) *See* POTASSIUM CHLORIDE.

Slow Sodium (HK Pharma) *See* SODIUM CHLORIDE.

Slow-Trasicor (Amdipharm) *See* OXPRENOLOL HYDROCHLORIDE.

Slozem (Merck Serono) *See* DILTIAZEM HYDROCHLORIDE.

Sno Tears (Bausch & Lomb UK) *See* POLYVINYL ALCOHOL.

Sodiofolin (medac GmbH) *See* FOLINIC ACID.

sodium A mineral element that is an important constituent of the human body. Sodium ions (*see* ELECTROLYTE) control the volume of extracellular fluid in the body (i.e. the body fluids surrounding cells) and are also necessary for the functioning of nerves and muscles. The amount of sodium in the body is controlled by the kidneys. Sodium is contained in most foods, most commonly in the form of *sodium chloride (common salt). An excessive intake of sodium can lead to fluid retention (*see* OEDEMA) and may also be implicated in *hypertension (high blood pressure).

Sodium depletion is treated by means of oral or intravenous administration of sodium chloride or other sodium salts.

sodium acid phosphate A salt that is used as a *phosphate supplement. It

also acts as an *osmotic laxative, being administered rectally for the treatment of constipation and to clear the bowel before examination or surgery. It is available from pharmacies without a prescription in the form of tablets, enemas, or suppositories.
Side effects and precautions: *see* PHOSPHATE SUPPLEMENTS; PHOSPHATE LAXATIVES.
Proprietary preparations: *Carbalax (combined with sodium bicarbonate); *Fleet Ready-to-Use Enema (combined with sodium phosphate); *Phosphate-Sandoz (combined with sodium bicarbonate and potassium bicarbonate).

sodium alginate *See* ALGINIC ACID.

Sodium Amytal (Flynn Pharma) *See* AMOBARBITAL.

sodium aurothiomalate A salt of gold that is used for the treatment of active progressive rheumatoid arthritis and juvenile arthritis. Unlike *NSAIDs, sodium aurothiomalate does not have an immediate therapeutic effect and it may take 4–6 months to obtain a full response. It is available as a solution for intramuscular injection on *prescription only.
Side effects: gold salts can cause blood disorders and affect the kidneys; severe reactions occur in up to 5% of patients. The following symptoms should be reported to a doctor: rash or itching, a metallic taste, fever, sore throat or tongue, mouth ulcers, bleeding gums, bruising, heavy periods, and diarrhoea.
Precautions: blood counts and urine tests should be carried out regularly during treatment and treatment should be stopped if there are signs of blood disorders or protein in the urine. Gold should not be given to those with severe kidney or liver disease, blood disorders, exfoliative dermatitis, or pulmonary fibrosis. It should be used with caution in the elderly, in people with a history of urticaria, eczema, or colitis, and in women who are pregnant or breastfeeding.
Interactions with other drugs:
Penicillamine: increases the risk of adverse effects and should not be taken with aurothiomalate.
Proprietary preparation: Myocrisin.

sodium bicarbonate An *antacid used as an ingredient in many preparations for the relief of indigestion, heartburn, and the symptoms of ulcers; **sodium carbonate** has the same antacid action. Sodium bicarbonate is also used to treat metabolic acidosis (in which the acidity of the body fluids is abnormally high), such as occurs in kidney failure. For this it is given orally (as tablets or capsules) or, in severe cases, by intravenous injection or infusion. Solutions used to replace lost fluids or *electrolytes sometimes contain sodium bicarbonate. It is also taken orally to reduce the acidity of the urine in the treatment of mild infections of the urinary tract, such as cystitis. Sodium bicarbonate is also added to some preparations to make them effervescent, since it produces bubbles of carbon dioxide when dissolved in water. Oral preparations of sodium bicarbonate can be obtained without a prescription; infusions are available on *prescription only.

Side effects: antacid preparations cause belching. High doses of sodium bicarbonate may cause systemic alkalosis (in which the alkalinity of the body fluids is abnormally high).
Precautions: sodium bicarbonate should not be taken by people with kidney disease or by those who are on a low-sodium diet.
Interactions with other drugs: *see* ANTACIDS.
Proprietary preparations: Boots Gripe Mixture 1 Month Plus; Minijet Sodium Bicarbonate (injection); Peppermint Indigestion Tablets; *Bisodol Antacid Powder (combined with magnesium carbonate); *Bisodol Indigestion Relief Tablets (combined with calcium carbonate and magnesium carbonate); *Bisodol Extra Tablets (combined with calcium carbonate, magnesium carbonate, and simeticone); *Carbalax (combined with sodium acid phosphate); *Cymalon (combined with sodium citrate, sodium carbonate, and citric acid); *Electrolade (combined with sodium chloride, potassium chloride, and glucose); *Eno, Eno Lemon (combined with sodium carbonate and citric acid); *Gastrocote (combined with alginic acid, aluminium hydroxide, and magnesium trisilicate); *Gaviscon Double Action (combined with calcium carbonate and sodium alginate); *Gaviscon Liquid (combined with sodium alginate and calcium chloride); *Gaviscon Tablets (combined with alginic acid, aluminium hydroxide, and magnesium trisilicate); *Health Salt (combined with magnesium sulphate); *Jaap's Health Salts (combined with sodium potassium tartrate and tartaric acid); *Klean-Prep (combined with polyethylene glycol, sodium sulphate, sodium chloride, and potassium chloride); *Laxido Orange (combined with macrogol '3350', potassium chloride, and sodium chloride); *Molaxole (combined with macrogol '3350', sodium hydrogen carbonate, and potassium chloride); *Original Andrews Salts (combined with magnesium sulphate and citric acid); *Peptac (combined with alginic acid and calcium carbonate); *Phosphate-Sandoz (combined with sodium acid phosphate and potassium bicarbonate); *Resolve (combined with paracetamol, citric acid, potassium bicarbonate, and vitamin C); *Uriflex G (combined with citric acid, magnesium oxide, and disodium edetate); *Woodward's Gripe Water (combined with dill seed oil).

sodium calcium edetate **<sodium calciumedetate>** A drug used for the treatment of lead poisoning. Sodium calcium edetate is available as a form for intravenous infusion on *prescription only.
Side effects: include nausea and cramps; overdosage can cause kidney damage.
Precautions: sodium calcium edetate should be used with caution in people with kidney disease.
Proprietary preparation: Ledclair.

sodium carbonate *See* SODIUM BICARBONATE.

sodium chloride (**common salt**) A salt of *sodium that is present in all tissues and is important in maintaining the balance of *electrolytes in the body. Intravenous infusions of sodium chloride are the basis of fluid replacement therapy and treatment for conditions associated with sodium

depletion of electrolyte imbalance. Saline solutions of the correct concentration are similar to the body fluids and are therefore less disruptive to normal tissue structure and functioning than water. Sodium chloride in the form of a *nebulizer solution is used as a *mucolytic in people with cystic fibrosis. Sodium chloride can be combined with other ingredients (such as glucose, other sodium salts, and salts of potassium and calcium) in infusions. Sodium chloride can also be taken by mouth and is a basic ingredient of *oral rehydration therapy. Saline solutions are used widely to cleanse wounds and skin, irrigate the bladder, irrigate and lubricate the eyes (*see also* BALANCED SALT SOLUTION), flush out tubes and catheters, and as a mouthwash. They are also used for diluting drugs given by means of some *nebulizers. Sodium chloride is freely available *over the counter in the form of solutions, drops, or sprays; infusions are available on *prescription only.
Proprietary preparations: Irriclens; Irripod; Minims Saline (single-dose eye drops); Mucoclear 6% (solution for inhalation); Normasol; Saline Steri-Neb; Slow Sodium (tablets); Stericlens (spray); Steripod Sodium Chloride; Uriflex S; Uriflex SP; Uro-Tainer Sodium Chloride; *Boots Dual Action Diarrhoea Relief (sachets: combined with potassium chloride, sodium citrate, and citric acid); *Dioralyte Natural, Blackcurrent and Citrus GSL (combined with glucose, potassium chloride, and disodium hydrogen citrate); *Dioralyte Relief (combined with potassium chloride, sodium citrate, and precooked rice powder); *Electrolade (combined with potassium chloride, sodium bicarbonate, and glucose); *Laxido Orange (combined with macrogol '3350', sodium bicarbonate, and potassium chloride); *Minims Artificial Tears (combined with hydroxyethylcellulose); *Molaxole (combined with potassium chloride, sodium hydrogen carbonate, and macrogol '3350'); *Movicol (combined with polyethylene glycol, sodium sulphate, sodium bicarbonate, and potassium chloride).

sodium citrate A salt of sodium that is taken by mouth to make the urine alkaline in the treatment of cystitis and is instilled into the bladder to dissolve blood clots. It is also an *osmotic laxative used rectally to treat constipation. Sodium citrate is also an ingredient of electrolyte-replacement preparations used for the treatment of diarrhoea (*see* ORAL REHYDRATION THERAPY) and of *balanced salt solution for washing out the eyes. It can be obtained without a prescription in the form of granules to be dissolved in water or tablets (for cystitis) and as an enema.
Precautions: citrate tablets should be used with caution by elderly people, pregnant women, and by people with kidney or heart disease. Enemas should be used with caution in the elderly and should not be used by people with acute gastrointestinal conditions or inflammatory bowel disease.
Proprietary preparations: Boots Cystitis Relief (granules and tablets); Boots Dual Action Diarrhoea Relief (sachets: combined with sodium chloride, potassium chloride, and citric acid); *Cymalon (combined with citric acid, sodium bicarbonate, and sodium carbonate); *Dioralyte Relief (combined with sodium chloride, potassium chloride, and precooked rice powder); *Micolette Micro-enema (combined with sodium lauryl sulphoacetate);

*Micralax Micro-enema (combined with sodium alkylsulphoacetate); *Relaxit Micro-enema (combined with sodium lauryl sulphate).

sodium clodronate A *bisphosphonate used for the treatment of high blood concentrations of calcium and bone pain associated with primary or secondary bone cancers. It is available, on *prescription only, as tablets, capsules, or a solution for infusion.
Side effects: include nausea, diarrhoea, and (rarely) allergic skin reactions.
Precautions: sodium clodronate should not be taken by women who are pregnant or breastfeeding or by people with inflammatory conditions of the stomach or intestines. It should be used with caution in people with impaired kidney function.
Interactions with other drugs:
Aminoglycosides: in combination with sodium clodronate, they may cause abnormally low concentrations of calcium in the plasma.
Antacids: reduce the absorption of oral clodronate.
Calcium supplements: reduce the absorption of oral clodronate.
Estramustine: its plasma concentration is increased.
Iron supplements: oral supplements reduce the absorption of clodronate.
Proprietary preparations: Bonefos; Clasteon (capsules); Loron 520 (tablets).

sodium cromoglicate <sodium cromoglycate> A *chromone drug used to prevent attacks in the treatment of *asthma and a variety of other allergic conditions. It is available as aerosols for inhalation, sprays for the nose, and drops for the eyes. For food allergy sodium cromoglicate is given as capsules. It is available on *prescription and some preparations can be bought from pharmacies without a prescription.
Side effects: inhalation may cause local irritation of the throat, coughing, and transient wheezing and breathlessness. Taking capsules occasionally causes nausea, rashes, and joint pain. Local irritation may occur with preparations for the nose and eyes.
Proprietary preparations: Boots Hayfever Relief Eye Drops; Clariteyes (eye drops); Hay-Crom (eye drops); Intal CFC-free Inhaler; Nalcrom (capsules); Opticrom (eye drops); Optrex Allergy Eye Drops; Rynacrom (nasal spray); Vividrin (eye drops and nasal spray).

S

sodium dihydrogen phosphate dihydrate *See* PHOSPHATE LAXATIVES.

sodium feredetate <sodium ironedetate> An *iron supplement used for the treatment of iron-deficiency anaemia. It is available as an elixir without a prescription, but only from pharmacies.
Side effects, precautions, and interactions with other drugs: *see* IRON.
Proprietary preparation: Sytron.

sodium fluoride *See* FLUORIDE.

sodium fusidate *See* FUSIDIC ACID.

sodium hyaluronate A drug used for the treatment of dry eyes in people

with tear deficiency. It is freely available *over the counter in the form of eye drops.
Proprietary preparations: Clinitas; Hylo-Forte; Hylo-Tear; Ocusan; Oxyal; Vismed; Vismed Multi.

sodium lauryl sulphoacetate A detergent and wetting agent (*see* SURFACTANT). It is used as an ingredient of shampoos, skin cleansers, and in toothpastes. It is also included in some *osmotic laxative preparations.
Side effects: sodium lauryl sulphoacetate can be irritating when applied directly to the skin.
Proprietary preparations: *Micolette Micro-enema (combined with sodium citrate); *Relaxit Micro-enema (combined with sodium citrate).

sodium nitroprusside A cyanide-containing *vasodilator drug that is used in the emergency treatment of a sudden and severe rise in blood pressure (hypertensive crisis) and acute or chronic heart failure. It is also used by anaesthetists to control blood pressure during surgery. Nitroprusside does not have a *licence but is available from special order manufacturers as a solution for infusion on *prescription only.
Side effects: headache, dizziness, nausea, retching, abdominal pain, sweating, palpitations, and discomfort behind the breastbone are associated with rapid reduction of blood pressure induced by nitroprusside.
Precautions and interactions with other drugs: nitroprusside should not be used in people with severe vitamin B_{12} deficiency. It should be used with caution in women who are pregnant or breastfeeding, in people with an overactive thyroid gland, certain heart conditions, and liver or kidney disease, and in the elderly. The blood-pressure-lowering effect of nitroprusside is increased by a large number of drugs (including anaesthetics).

sodium oxybate A drug used for the treatment of narcolepsy with cataplexy (an extreme tendency to fall asleep combined with muscle weakness). It is used under specialist supervision and is available as an oral solution on *prescription only.
Side effects: include drowsiness, inattentiveness, depression, confusion, disorientation, nausea and vomiting, abdominal pain, diarrhoea, dizziness, and headache.
Precautions: sodium oxybate should not be taken by pregnant women. Activites that require mental alertness or motor coordination, such as driving, should be avoided for at least six hours after taking a dose of sodium oxybate.
Interactions with other drugs: barbiturates, benzodiazepines, and opioid analgesics increase the effects of sodium oxybate and should not be taken with it.
Proprietary preparation: Xyrem.

sodium phosphate *See* PHOSPHATE LAXATIVES.

sodium picosulfate **<sodium picosulphate>** A *stimulant laxative used for the treatment of constipation and for bowel evacuation before radiological examination, exploratory procedures, or surgery. It is available as an elixir or

capsules (for constipation) and as a *bowel-cleansing solution (with magnesium citrate) and can be obtained without a prescription, but only from pharmacies.
Side effects and precautions: *see* STIMULANT LAXATIVES.
Proprietary preparations: Dulcolax Liquid; Dulcolax Perles (capsules); *CitraFleet (combined with magnesium citrate) *Picolax (combined with magnesium citrate).

sodium polystyrene sulphonate A resin that exchanges potassium ions for sodium ions in the intestine when it is taken by mouth or by enema. It is used to reduce high concentrations of potassium in blood associated with failure of the kidneys to produce adequate quantities of urine or in patients on dialysis. It is available as a powder and can be obtained without a prescription, but only from pharmacies.
Side effects: include sodium retention, low plasma potassium and calcium concentrations, loss of appetite, nausea and vomiting, constipation, and diarrhoea. If constipation occurs, treatment should be stopped and magnesium-containing laxatives avoided.
Precautions: sodium polystyrene sulphonate should not be taken by people with obstructive bowel disease and should be used with caution in women who are pregnant or breastfeeding. Plasma electrolytes may need to be monitored.
Proprietary preparation: Resonium-A.

sodium potassium tartrate *See* TARTARIC ACID.

sodium pyrrolidone carboxylate A humectant (*see* EMOLLIENTS) used for the treatment of dry skin conditions. It is available as a cream and can be obtained without a prescription, but only from pharmacies. Some combined preparations are freely available *over the counter.
Proprietary preparation: *Hydromol Cream (combined with arachis oil, liquid paraffin, and sodium lactate).

S

sodium stibogluconate A drug containing antimony, used to treat leishmaniasis (a tropical infection affecting the skin and various internal organs). It is given by intravenous or intramuscular injection and is available on *prescription only.
Side effects: include nausea, vomiting, diarrhoea, abdominal pain, loss of appetite, muscle and joint pain, headache, lethargy, changes in heart rhythm, and cough.
Precautions: sodium stibogluconate should not be given to people with severe kidney disease. Allergic reactions may occur and facilities should be available for treatment. Sodium stibogluconate may cause *arrhythmias, therefore it should be used with caution in people with cardiovascular disease or ventricular arrhythmia. ECG monitoring should be performed during treatment. Sodium stibogluconate should be used with caution in pregnant and breastfeeding women.
Proprietary preparation: Pentostam.

sodium sulphate An *osmotic laxative that is combined with other laxatives in a *bowel-cleansing solution for rapid evacuation of the bowel before investigation or surgery. It is also used alone for the treatment of constipation. Sodium sulphate is available as a powder without a prescription, but only from pharmacies.
Precautions: sodium sulphate is not recommended for children.
Proprietary preparation: *Klean-Prep (combined with polyethylene glycol, sodium bicarbonate, sodium chloride, and potassium chloride).

sodium tetradecyl sulphate An irritant substance that is used in *sclerotherapy to treat varicose veins. It is available, on *prescription only, as a solution for slow injection into the vein.
Side effects and precautions: *see* ETHANOLAMINE OLEATE.
Proprietary preparation: Fibro-Vein.

sodium valproate An *anticonvulsant drug used in the treatment of all forms of epilepsy: it is a drug of choice in major, absence, and partial seizures. It is suitable for long-term use, does not cause sedation, and can be taken with oral contraceptives. Sodium valproate is available, on *prescription only, as tablets, crushable tablets, *modified-release tablets, granules, or capsules, a syrup, or a liquid for oral use and as an intravenous injection.
Side effects: include gastric irritation, nausea, unsteadiness, and weight gain. Transient hair loss, oedema, and blood disorders may occur; rare side effects are liver failure and bleeding disorders.
Precautions: patients who are planning on becoming pregnant, or who are already pregnant, should seek specialist advice. Liver function should be monitored before and during treatment.
Interactions with other drugs:
Anticonvulsants: taking two or more anticonvulsants together may increase their adverse effects. Valproate raises the plasma concentration of primidone and often raises (but may lower) the plasma concentration of phenytoin; phenytoin and primidone often lower the plasma concentration of valproate.
Antidepressants: reduce the anticonvulsant effect of sodium valproate; St John's wort should not be taken with valproate.
Antipsychotics: reduce the anticonvulsant effect of sodium valproate; olanzapine increases the risk of neutropenia (a blood disorder).
Aspirin: enhances the effect of sodium valproate.
Cimetidine: increases plasma concentration of sodium valproate.
Mefloquine: antagonizes the anticonvulsant effect of sodium valproate.
Proprietary preparations: Epilim; Epilim Intravenous; Episenta (modified-release capsules and granules); Orlept; *Epilim Chrono and Epilim Chronosphere (combined with valproic acid).

Sofradex (sanofi-aventis) A proprietary combination of *dexamethasone (a corticosteroid), *framycetin sulphate (an aminoglycoside antibiotic), and *gramicidin (an antibiotic), used for the treatment of inflammatory conditions of the eyes when infection is present or is likely to occur. It is also

used to treat infections of the outer ear. Sofradex is available, on *prescription only, as eye drops or ear drops.
Side effects: *see* TOPICAL STEROIDS; FRAMYCETIN SULPHATE.
Precautions: long-term use of Sofradex should be avoided in infants. *See also* TOPICAL STEROIDS.

Soft Corn Removal Pads (SSL International) *See* SALICYLIC ACID.

Solaraze (Almirall) *See* DICLOFENAC SODIUM.

Solian (sanofi-aventis) *See* AMISULPRIDE.

solifenacin succinate An *antimuscarinic drug used for the treatment of incontinence and increased frequency and urgency in passing urine. It is available as tablets on *prescription only.
Side effects: *see* ANTIMUSCARINIC DRUGS. There may also be acid reflux.
Precautions: *see* ANTIMUSCARINIC DRUGS. Solifenacin should not be taken by people with severe liver disease or by pregnant women.
Interactions with other drugs: *see* ANTIMUSCARINIC DRUGS.
Proprietary preparation: Vesicare.

Soliris (Alexion Pharma UK Ltd) *See* ECULIZUMAB.

Solpadeine Headache (GlaxoSmithKline) A proprietary combination of *paracetamol (an analgesic and antipyretic) and *caffeine (a stimulant), used for the relief of mild pain and feverish conditions. It is freely available *over the counter as tablets and soluble tablets.
Precautions: *see* PARACETAMOL; CAFFEINE.

Solpadeine Max (GlaxoSmithKline) A proprietary combination of *paracetamol (an analgesic) and *codeine (an opioid analgesic), used for the relief of moderate pain, including migraine, headache, toothache, period pains, backache, and arthritic pain. It is available as tablets and can be obtained without a prescription, but only from pharmacies.
Side effects: *see* CODEINE.
Precautions: *see* PARACETAMOL; OPIOIDS.
Interactions with other drugs: *see* OPIOIDS.

Solpadeine Migraine Ibuprofen & Codeine (GlaxoSmithKline) A proprietary combination of *ibuprofen (an NSAID) and *codeine (an opioid analgesic), used to relieve moderate pain, including rheumatic and muscular pain, backache, migraine, headache, toothache, and period pains. It is available as tablets and can be obtained without a prescription, but only from pharmacies.
Side effects and interactions with other drugs: *see* NSAIDs; CODEINE; OPIOIDS.
Precautions: this medicine is not recommended for children under 12 years old. *See also* NSAIDs; CODEINE; OPIOIDS.

Solpadeine Plus (GlaxoSmithKline) A proprietary combination of *paracetamol (an analgesic and antipyretic), *codeine (an opioid analgesic), and *caffeine (a stimulant), used for the relief of migraine, headache,

rheumatic pains, period pains, toothache, and the fever and pain associated with colds and influenza. It is available as capsules, tablets, or soluble tablets and can be obtained without a prescription, but only from pharmacies.
Side effects: *see* CODEINE.
Precautions: Solpadeine Plus is not recommended for children. *See also* PARACETAMOL; OPIOIDS; CAFFEINE.
Interactions with other drugs: *see* OPIOIDS.

Solpadol (sanofi-aventis) *See* CO-CODAMOL.

Soltamox (Rosemont Pharmaceuticals Limited) *See* TAMOXIFEN.

Solu-Cortef (Pharmacia) *See* HYDROCORTISONE.

Solu-Medrone (Pharmacia) *See* METHYLPREDNISOLONE.

Solvazinc (Galen Limited) *See* ZINC SULPHATE.

somatorelin *See* GROWTH HORMONE.

somatorelin acetate A synthetic form of *growth hormone releasing hormone (somatorelin), which stimulates the release of growth hormone from the pituitary gland. It is used in investigations of growth hormone deficiency, to distinguish whether this is due to disorders of the pituitary gland or the hypothalamus. An increase in the amount of growth hormone in the blood after intravenous injection of somatorelin acetate indicates a normally functioning pituitary gland. Somatorelin acetate is a *prescription only medicine.
Side effects: may include a feeling of warmth in the head, neck, and upper body, altered taste and smell, hot flushes, and raised or lowered blood pressure.
Precautions and interactions with other drugs: somatorelin acetate should not be given to women who are pregnant or breastfeeding. Drugs that affect the release of growth hormone should not be given with somatorelin acetate. These include atropine, clonidine, dopamine, glucagon, glucocorticoids, levodopa, propranolol, and somatostatin analogues.
Proprietary preparation: GHRH Ferring.

somatostatin *See* GROWTH HORMONE; LANREOTIDE; OCTREOTIDE.

somatropin A genetically engineered form of *growth hormone used for the treatment of children whose own secretion of growth hormone is insufficient to achieve normal stature. It is also used to treat underdevelopment of the ovaries or testes, Turner's syndrome (a genetic abnormality causing short stature and infertility in females), the poor growth seen in children with kidney insufficiency, and children who are considered small for their gestational age at birth. A *prescription only medicine, it is given by *subcutaneous injection; pens for self-injection are available.
Side effects: include headache, fluid retention, inhibition of the functioning of the thyroid gland (causing tiredness, lethargy, and weight gain), and reactions at the injection site.

Precautions: somatropin should not be taken by people who have had a kidney transplant or by those with cancer or by pregnant women; it should not be used to promote growth in children who have completed puberty. It should be used with caution in people with diabetes, poor thyroid function, or a history of malignant disease and by breastfeeding women.
Proprietary preparations: Genotropin; Humatrope; Norditropin; NutropinAq; Omnitrope; Saizen; Saizen Clickeasy; Zomacton.

Somatuline Autogel, Somatuline LA (Ipsen) *See* LANREOTIDE.

Somavert (Pfizer) *See* PEGVISOMANT.

Sominex (Actavis) *See* PROMETHAZINE HYDROCHLORIDE.

Somnite (Norgine) *See* NITRAZEPAM.

Sonata (Meda Pharmaceuticals) *See* ZALEPLON.

Soneryl (Flynn Pharma) *See* BUTOBARBITAL.

sorafenib A *tyrosine kinase inhibitor used for the treatment of kidney and liver cancers. It is taken as tablets under expert supervision and is available on *prescription only.
Side effects: *see* CYTOTOXIC DRUGS. There may also be diarrhoea, indigestion, rash, dry skin, hypertension, bleeding, and fatigue.
Precautions: *see* CYTOTOXIC DRUGS. Sorafenib should not be taken by women who are pregnant or breastfeeding. It should be used with caution in people with heart or liver disease.
Interactions with other drugs:

Clozapine: increases the risk of agranulocytosis (a blood disorder) and should not be used with sorafenib.

Warfarin: its anticoagulant effect may be increased by sorafenib.

Proprietary preparation: Nexavar.

Sotacor (Bristol-Myers Squibb) *See* SOTALOL HYDROCHLORIDE.

S

sotalol hydrochloride A non-cardioselective *beta blocker that is also a class III *anti-arrhythmic drug; it is used for the treatment and prevention of heart *arrhythmias. It is available as tablets or solution for injection on *prescription only.
Side effects and precautions: *see* BETA BLOCKERS.
Interactions with other drugs: the risk of ventricular arrhythmias is increased if sotalol is taken with certain drugs. Sotalol should therefore not be taken with the following drugs: amiodarone and disopyramide (anti-arrhythmic drugs), moxifloxacin, mizolastine, droperidol and zuclopenthixol (antipsychotic drugs), and atomoxetine. It should be used with caution with tricyclic antidepressants, diuretics, phenothiazines and certain other antipsychotics, tolterodine, and ivabradine. *See also* BETA BLOCKERS.
Proprietary preparations: Beta-Cardone; Sotacor.

soya oil An oil expressed from soya beans. It is used as an *emollient for the relief of dry skin conditions.
Proprietary preparations: Balneum (bath oil); *Balneum Plus Oil (combined with lauromacrogols).

spansule A capsule. The term is usually restricted to *modified-release capsules.

Spasmonal (Norgine) *See* ALVERINE CITRATE.

SpectraBan (Stiefel Laboratories) A proprietary *sunscreen preparation consisting of a lotion containing *aminobenzoic acid and padimate-O. It provides protection against UVB only (SPF 25). **SpectraBan Ultra Lotion** also contains oxybenzone and *titanium dioxide but no aminobenzoic acid. It protects against both UVA and UVB (SPF 28). Both lotions can be prescribed on the NHS or obtained without a prescription.

spermicidal contraceptives Preparations in which the active ingredient is a **spermicide** (an agent that kills sperm). These contraceptives are applied locally and should be used in conjunction with barrier forms of contraception (condoms or diaphragms) as an additional safeguard against pregnancy: they are not very effective as the sole means of contraception. However, some preparations may be used alone in the year following the final menstrual period, when protection is still advisable. Spermicidal contraceptives are available, without a prescription, in the form of creams, gels, foams, or pessaries (*see* NONOXINOL-9).
Side effects: there may be local sensitivity to the active ingredient or to the perfume in the preparation.

Spiriva (Boehringer Ingelheim Limited) *See* TIOTROPIUM.

spironolactone A *potassium-sparing diuretic that acts by inhibiting the activity of aldosterone, a hormone secreted by the adrenal gland that promotes potassium excretion and sodium retention by the kidneys. Spironolactone is used in the treatment of *oedema associated with cirrhosis of the liver, congestive *heart failure, kidney disorders, and primary hyperaldosteronism (a condition called Conn's syndrome, in which high concentrations of aldosterone occur as a result of increased activity of the adrenal gland). Its effects are slow and may only be seen after a few days' use. It may be given alone or in combination with *thiazide diuretics or *loop diuretics. Spironolactone is available as tablets or an oral suspension on *prescription only. *See also* CO-FLUMACTONE.
Side effects: nausea and vomiting are more common with spironolactone than with other potassium-sparing diuretics (affecting 10% of individuals). Potassium retention may occur, causing muscle weakness and numbness. Men may experience breast enlargement and reversible impotence. Less commonly menstrual irregularities, diarrhoea, headache, confusion, and rash can occur.
Precautions: spironolactone should not be taken by people with high plasma

concentrations of potassium or low concentrations of sodium or by those with severe kidney disease. *See also* POTASSIUM-SPARING DIURETICS.
Interactions with other drugs:
ACE inhibitors: *see* POTASSIUM-SPARING DIURETICS.
Digoxin: concentrations are increased, which may cause adverse effects. *See also* POTASSIUM-SPARING DIURETICS.
Proprietary preparations: Aldactone; Aldactide 25 and Aldactide 50 (*see* CO-FLUMACTONE); *Lasilactone (combined with furosemide).
See also DIURETICS.

Sporanox (Janssen-Cilag) *See* ITRACONAZOLE.

Sprilon (Ayrton Saunders) A proprietary combination of *dimeticone (a water repellent) and *zinc oxide (an astringent protective agent) in the form of a spray, used as a *barrier preparation to protect the skin around a *stoma after ileostomy or colostomy and for the treatment of eczema, leg ulcers, fissures (breaks in the skin), and pressure sores. It is freely available *over the counter.

Sprycel (Bristol-Myers Squibb) *See* DASATINIB.

squalane An oil that is included in some topical preparations to increase the absorption of the active ingredients. It is also a skin lubricant.

squill An extract from the bulb of a species of lily (*Urginea maritima*) that is used as an *expectorant in cough remedies. It is available as a liquid, syrup, medicated sweets, and throat lozenges that are freely available *over the counter.
Side effects: squill may cause nausea and vomiting.
Proprietary preparations: Buttercup Syrup Traditional; *Gee's Linctus (combined with opium tincture).

SSRIs (selective serotonin reuptake inhibitors) A class of *antidepressant drugs that act by inhibiting the reuptake of *serotonin (and possibly also of noradrenaline) and thus prolonging its action in the brain. They are less sedative than *tricyclic antidepressants (TCAs), with fewer *antimuscarinic side effects (dry mouth, blurred vision, constipation, and urinary retention), and fewer toxic effects on the heart. They do not cause weight gain. However, they have more gastrointestinal side effects (including nausea and vomiting) than the TCAs. The SSRIs are *citalopram, *escitalopram, *fluoxetine, *fluvoxamine maleate, *paroxetine, and *sertraline. *Duloxetine and *venlafaxine are related to the SSRIs.
Side effects: include dose-related gastrointestinal effects (diarrhoea, nausea and vomiting, dyspepsia, abdominal pain, constipation, and loss of appetite) and weight loss; headache, restlessness, nervousness, and anxiety may also occur. Other possible side effects are dry mouth, palpitation, tremor, confusion, dizziness, low blood pressure, mania, convulsions, interference with sexual function, sweating, and movement disorders. Allergic reactions (rash, itching, swelling of the face) should be reported to a doctor.

Precautions: SSRIs should be used with caution in people who have liver, kidney, or heart disease or epilepsy, in women who are pregnant or breastfeeding, and in patients who are undergoing electroconvulsive therapy. Dosage should be reduced gradually at the end of treatment.
Interactions with other drugs:
Anticoagulants: the effects of warfarin and acenocoumarol may be increased.
Antiepileptics: SSRIs increase the risk of convulsions recurring.
Lithium: can increase the toxic effects of SSRIs.
MAOIs: the effects of MAOIs are increased. SSRIs should not be started until two weeks after stopping MAOIs; MAOIs should not be started until at least a week after SSRIs have been stopped (at least five weeks for fluoxetine, two weeks for paroxetine and sertraline).
NSAIDs: the risk of bleeding is increased.
Pimozide: the risk of ventricular arrhythmias is increased; pimozide should not be taken with SSRIs.
Rasagiline: there is an increased risk of toxic effects on the nervous system.
Ritonavir: may increase plasma concentrations of SSRIs.
Sibutramine: there is an increased risk of toxic effects on the central nervous system.
Sumatriptan: there is an increased risk of toxic effects on the central nervous system.
Tramadol: the risk of toxic effects on the central nervous system is increased.
Other interactions are given in the entries for individual SSRIs.

Stalevo (Orion Pharma UK Limited) A proprietary combination of *co-careldopa and *entacapone (antiparkinsonian drugs), used for the treatment of Parkinson's disease and movement disorders not stabilized on co-careldopa alone. Entacapone enhances the effects of levodopa. Stalevo is available as tablets on *prescription only.
Side effects, precautions, and interactions with other drugs: *see* LEVODOPA; ENTACAPONE.

Staril (E.R. Squibb & Sons) *See* FOSINOPRIL.

Starlix (Novartis) *See* NATEGLINIDE.

statins A group of *lipid-lowering drugs that act by inhibiting the enzyme HMG Co-A (hydroxy-3-methylglutaryl coenzyme A, which is involved in the synthesis of *cholesterol. They lower total cholesterol (typically LDL-cholesterol is reduced by 40%) and, to a lesser extent, plasma *triglycerides, and also increase plasma HDL (*see* LIPOPROTEINS). They are more effective than *bile-acid sequestrants in lowering LDL-cholesterol, but less effective than *fibrates in reducing triglycerides and raising HDL-cholesterol. Statins are used to treat *hyperlipidaemias in which high cholesterol concentrations are the main feature and which have not responded to dietary measures. They are also used to prevent the progression of *atherosclerosis and to reduce the

incidence of untoward events in patients who have high cholesterol levels or known coronary artery disease. *See* ATORVASTATIN; FLUVASTATIN; PRAVASTATIN; ROSUVASTATIN; SIMVASTATIN.
Side effects: reversible muscle inflammation and rhabdomyolysis (a serious condition involving muscle breakdown) can occur, but this is rare. Other side effects include headache, abdominal pain, nausea, and vomiting.
Precautions and interactions with other drugs: rhabdomyolysis is more likely to occur in people who are also taking *ciclosporin, *colchicine, *nicotinic acid, or *fibrates. Any muscle pain, tenderness, or weakness should be reported to a doctor promptly. Statins should not be taken by people with active liver disease or by breastfeeding women and should be used with caution in those with a history of liver disease or alcoholism. Women should avoid pregnancy during and for one month after treatment.

status epilepticus *See* ANTICONVULSANT DRUGS.

stavudine An *antiviral drug that prevents retrovirus replication: it is a nucleoside analogue that inhibits the action of reverse transcriptase. Stavudine is used, in combination with other antiretroviral drugs, for the treatment of *HIV infection; it is available, on *prescription only, as capsules or an oral solution.
Side effects: include headache, fever, malaise, nausea, vomiting, diarrhoea, damage to peripheral nerves (causing weakness or numbness in the feet and hands), pancreatitis, chest pain, skin irritation and rash, and influenza-like symptoms.
Precautions: stavudine should be used with caution in people with a history of pancreatitis or disease of the peripheral nerves. It should not be taken by women who are breastfeeding.
Interactions with other drugs:
Antiviral drugs: ribavirin and zidovudine may inhibit the effect of stavudine; the side effects of stavudine may be increased by didanosine.
Hydroxycarbamide: increases the risk of adverse effects and should not be taken with stavudine.
Proprietary preparation: Zerit.

S

Stelara (Janssen-Cilag) *See* USTEKINUMAB.

Stelazine (Goldshield) *See* TRIFLUOPERAZINE.

Stemetil (sanofi-aventis) *See* PROCHLORPERAZINE.

sterculia A vegetable gum used as a *bulk-forming laxative for treating constipation and chronic diarrhoea caused by diverticular disease (a condition of the large intestine). It is freely available *over the counter in the form of granules.
Side effects and precautions: *see* ISPAGHULA HUSK.
Proprietary preparations: Normacol; *Normacol Plus (combined with frangula).

Stericlens (C D Medical) *See* SODIUM CHLORIDE.

Steripod Sodium Chloride (Medlock) *See* SODIUM CHLORIDE.

steroids A group of chemically related compounds that includes the *corticosteroids, the *androgens (male sex hormones) and *anabolic steroids, the *oestrogens and *progestogens (female sex hormones), and the bile acids. When used without qualification, the term 'steroid' usually refers to a corticosteroid.

Stesolid (Actavis) *See* DIAZEPAM.

Stiemycin (GlaxoSmithKline) *See* ERYTHROMYCIN.

stilboestrol *See* DIETHYLSTILBESTROL.

Stilnoct (sanofi-aventis) *See* ZOLPIDEM TARTRATE.

stimulant laxatives *Laxatives that stimulate motility of the intestines. They are used for the treatment of constipation and to clear the bowel before X-ray examination or surgery. Stimulant laxatives include *bisacodyl, *docusate sodium, *senna, and *sodium picosulfate. *See also* CASCARA; DANTRON; GLYCERIN.
Side effects and precautions: stimulant laxatives may cause colicky pains. They should not be taken by people with gastrointestinal obstruction and are best avoided in children. Long-term use can cause diarrhoea, low plasma *potassium concentrations, and colonic atony (a nonfunctioning large intestine), with black staining of the colon.

stimulants Drugs that promote the activity of a body system or function. The term usually refers to **central nervous system stimulants**, which increase activity in the brain and spinal cord, producing feelings of alertness. Central nervous system stimulants include *dexamfetamine sulphate, *methylphenidate hydrochloride, *atomoxetine, *modafinil, and *caffeine. **Respiratory stimulants** (also called **analeptic drugs**), mainly *doxapram hydrochloride, are occasionally used to stimulate breathing in comatose patients when mechanical ventilation cannot be used. They act on the central nervous system to stimulate the muscles involved in breathing, but since they also increase the activity of other muscles they may be harmful.

stiripentol An antiepileptic drug (*see* ANTICONVULSANT DRUGS) used in the treatment of severe myoclonic epilepsy in children (in which sudden muscle spasms occur between seizures). It is given as an *adjunct to *clobazam and *sodium valproate. Stiripentol is available, on *prescription only, as capsules or as a powder to produce an oral suspension.
Side effects: include loss of appetite, weight loss, insomnia, drowsiness, unsteady movements, and muscle disorders.
Precautions: stiripentol should not be taken by people with psychosis and delirium.
Interactions with other drugs: stiripentol affects several enzyme systems in the liver that are involved in metabolizing drugs; it therefore has the potential

to interact with many drugs. A doctor should be consulted before taking stiripentol with any other drug.
Proprietary preparation: Diacomit.

stoma The artificial opening created when part of the ileum or colon (small or large intestine, respectively) is brought to the surface of the body. The operation to create such an opening is an ileostomy or a colostomy. Various pouches and other appliances are designed to be used with stomas, and there is a variety of preparations, including *barrier preparations, for protecting the skin around a stoma.

Strattera (Eli Lilly & Co) *See* ATOMOXETINE.

Strefen (Reckitt Benckiser (UK) Ltd) *See* FLURBIPROFEN.

Strepsils (Reckitt Benckiser) A proprietary combination of the antiseptics *dichlorobenzyl alcohol and *amylmetacresol, used to relieve the symptoms of minor infections of the mouth and throat. It is freely available *over the counter in the form of lozenges (**Strepsils Original**, **Strepsils Cool**, **Strepsils Orange with Vitamin C**, and a variety of flavoured formulations).

Strepsils Extra (Reckitt Benckiser) *See* HEXYLRESORCINOL.

Streptase (CSL Behring) *See* STREPTOKINASE.

streptokinase A *fibrinolytic drug used for the treatment of deep-vein *thrombosis, pulmonary embolism, and an acute heart attack; treatment should be started rapidly (in the case of a heart attack, within 12 hours). It is available in a form for intravenous infusion on *prescription only. Because antibodies are formed against streptokinase, it is not usually used on more than one occasion.
Side effects: *see* FIBRINOLYTIC DRUGS. In addition, streptokinase may cause allergic reactions (such as rashes).
Precautions and interactions with other drugs: *see* FIBRINOLYTIC DRUGS.
Proprietary preparation: Streptase.

S

streptomycin An *aminoglycoside antibiotic used for the treatment of *tuberculosis that has failed to respond to standard therapy; it is given in combination with other antituberculosis drugs. Streptomycin is also used in conjunction with *doxycycline to treat brucellosis. It is available as a form for intramuscular injection on *prescription only; its use is restricted to specialists.
Side effects, precautions, and interactions with other drugs: *see* GENTAMICIN.

Striant SR (Ardana plc) *See* TESTOSTERONE.

Stronazon (Actavis) *See* TAMSULOSIN HYDROCHLORIDE.

Strong Co-danthramer (Napp Pharmaceuticals Limited) *See* CO-DANTHRAMER.

strontium ranelate A drug used for the treatment of postmenopausal

osteoporosis. It works by stimulating bone formation and decreasing the breakdown of bone. Strontium ranelate is taken orally between meals, to allow maximal absorption from the gut. It is available, on *prescription only, as granules to be dissolved in water.
Side effects: include nausea, diarrhoea, headache, dermatitis, and eczema.
Precautions: strontium ranelate increases the risk of venous thromboembolism (*see* THROMBOSIS), so should be used with caution in people at risk of this. There is also a risk of severe allergic reactions; if a rash develops, treatment should be stopped and a doctor consulted. Strontium ranelate should not be taken by people with severely impaired kidney function or by women who are pregnant or breastfeeding.
Proprietary preparation: Protelos.

Stugeron (McNeil Ltd) *See* CINNARIZINE.

styrax The balsam obtained from the bark of the liquidambar tree, which has mild *antiseptic properties. It is a component of *benzoin tincture compound.

subcutaneous injection The *injection of a drug under the skin, using a small volume of liquid (1–2 mL) and a narrow-gauge injection needle that is usually pushed through the skin at an angle of 45°. It is difficult and painful to inject larger volumes. A common site is the upper arm.

Subcuvia (Baxter) *See* IMMUNOGLOBULINS.

Subgam (BPL Bio Products Laboratory) *See* IMMUNOGLOBULINS.

Sublimaze (Janssen-Cilag) *See* FENTANYL.

sublingual Beneath the tongue: refers to a route of administration of tablets or capsules of certain drugs (such as nitrates) that are placed under the tongue and allowed to dissolve there.

Suboxone (Schering-Plough) A proprietary combination of *buprenorphine (an opioid analgesic) and *naloxone hydrochloride (an opioid antagonist), used for the treatment of people who are physically dependent on opioids (*see* DEPENDENCE). It is a *controlled drug, available as tablets.
Side effects and precautions: *see* BUPRENORPHINE; NALOXONE HYDROCHLORIDE.
Interactions with other drugs: *see* OPIOIDS.

Subutex (Schering-Plough) *See* BUPRENORPHINE.

sucralfate A substance that can coat and stick to mucous membranes. It has a *cytoprotectant action, forming a barrier between peptic ulcers and the stomach acid, which allows the ulcers to heal (*see* ACID-PEPTIC DISEASES). It is also used for the prevention of gastric bleeding due to stress ulceration in seriously ill patients, and can be used as mouthwash to coat sore patches or mouth ulcers, especially in people who have mouth problems due to radiotherapy or chemotherapy. Sucralfate is available, on *prescription only, as tablets or a suspension.

Side effects: include constipation, diarrhoea, nausea, indigestion, dry mouth, and rash.
Precautions: sucralfate should be used with caution in people with impaired kidney function and in women who are pregnant or breastfeeding.
Interactions with other drugs:
Digoxin: its absorption may be reduced by sucralfate.
Phenytoin: its absorption is reduced by sucralfate.
Tetracyclines: their absorption is reduced by sucralfate.
Theophylline: its absorption is reduced by sucralfate: an interval of two hours should be left between taking theophylline and sucralfate.
Warfarin: its absorption may be reduced by sucralfate.
Proprietary preparation: Antepsin.

Sudafed products *See* NON-DROWSY SUDAFED products.

Sudocrem (Forest Laboratories) A proprietary combination of *zinc oxide (an astringent protective agent) anhydrous *lanolin (an emollient), benzyl alcohol (an antiseptic), benzyl benzoate (which improves its spreading properties), and benzyl cinnamate (a preservative), used for the prevention and treatment of bed sores and napkin rash and for the relief of burns and *eczema. It is freely available *over the counter in the form of a cream.

Sulazine EC (Actavis) *See* SULFASALAZINE.

sulconazole An imidazole *antifungal drug that is active against a wide range of fungi. It is used for the treatment of fungal skin infections, especially tinea (ringworm), candidiasis (thrush), and pityriasis versicolor (a chronic fungal infection of the skin). Sulconazole is available as a cream on *prescription only.
Side effects: sulconazole may cause irritation, reddening, and blistering of the skin; if these are severe, treatment should be stopped.
Precautions: the cream should not come into contact with the eyes or mucous membranes.
Proprietary preparation: Exelderm.

sulfadiazine **<sulphadiazine>** A *sulphonamide antibiotic used to prevent the recurrence of rheumatic fever; it is also used for the treatment of toxoplasmosis (a protozoal infection that can cause blindness and mental retardation in a fetus), although it does not have a *licence in the UK for this. Sulfadiazine is available as tablets on *prescription only.
Side effects, precautions, and interactions with other drugs: *see* CO-TRIMOXAZOLE.

sulfadoxine A long-acting *sulphonamide antibiotic used in combination with *pyrimethamine for the treatment of malaria.
Side effects, precautions, and interactions with other drugs: *see* CO-TRIMOXAZOLE.
Proprietary preparation: *Fansidar (combined with pyrimethamine).

sulfamethoxazole **<sulphamethoxazole>** A *sulphonamide antibiotic

used in combination with the antibacterial drug trimethoprim (*see* CO-TRIMOXAZOLE) to treat serious infections.
Side effects, precautions, and interactions with other drugs: *see* CO-TRIMOXAZOLE.

sulfasalazine <**sulphasalazine**> A drug that is a combination of aminosalicylic acid and the sulphonamide sulfapyridine (*see* AMINOSALICYLATES). It is used for the treatment of the inflammatory bowel diseases ulcerative colitis and Crohn's disease. Sulfasalazine is also used for the treatment of active rheumatoid arthritis that has not responded to *NSAIDs alone; unlike NSAIDs, it does not have an immediate therapeutic effect and it may take 4–6 months to obtain a full response. Sulfasalazine is available, on *prescription only, as tablets, *enteric-coated tablets, a suspension, or suppositories.
Side effects: include nausea, diarrhoea, headache, rashes and more severe allergic reactions, fever, loss of appetite, blood disorders (see below), and damage to the kidneys and liver.
Precautions: blood counts and liver- and kidney-function tests should be carried out at the start of treatment and may be necessary during treatment. Sulfasalazine should not be taken by people who are allergic to aminosalicylates or sulphonamides and should be used with caution in those with a history of allergy or impaired liver or kidney function. Unexplained bleeding, bruising, sore throat, fever, or malaise should be reported to a doctor immediately as this may indicate a blood disorder. *See* AMINOSALICYLATES.
Proprietary preparations: Salazopyrin, Salazopyrin EN-Tabs; Sulazine EC.

sulfinpyrazone <**sulphinpyrazone**> A drug used for the long-term treatment of gout and recurrent gouty arthritis; it acts by increasing the amount of uric acid excreted in the urine. It is not used to control acute attacks, and may in fact exacerbate symptoms if started during an attack. Sulfinpyrazone may be used in conjunction with *allopurinol. It is available as tablets on *prescription only.
Side effects: include gastrointestinal disturbances and occasionally rashes and salt and water retention. Rarely, blood disorders and gastrointestinal ulcers and bleeding may occur.
Precautions: people taking sulfinpyrazone must maintain an adequate fluid intake (at least 2 litres a day) to prevent crystals of uric acid being passed in the urine (which can cause pain and bleeding). Sulfinpyrazone should not be taken by people with a history of blood disorders or who are allergic to *NSAIDs or by those with kidney stones or severe kidney disease.
Interactions with other drugs:
Anticoagulants: sulfinpyrazone enhances the anticoagulant effects of warfarin and acenocoumarol.
Aspirin: antagonizes the effect of sulfinpyrazone.
Ciclosporin: its plasma concentration is reduced.
Phenytoin: the plasma concentration of phenytoin is increased.

Sulphonylureas: their effects are enhanced by sulfinpyrazone.
Theophylline: the plasma concentration of theophylline is reduced.
Proprietary preparation: Anturan.

sulindac An *NSAID used for the treatment of pain and inflammation in rheumatoid arthritis and other disorders of the joints or muscles and to relieve the pain of acute gout. It is available as tablets on *prescription only.
Side effects: *see* NSAIDs. In addition, sulindac may occasionally cause discoloration of the urine.
Precautions: *see* NSAIDs. In addition, sulindac should be used with caution in people with a history of kidney stones, who should be advised to drink plenty of fluids.
Interactions with other drugs: *see* NSAIDs.

sulphadiazine *See* SULFADIAZINE.

sulphamethoxazole *See* SULFAMETHOXAZOLE.

sulphasalazine *See* SULFASALAZINE.

sulphinpyrazone *See* SULFINPYRAZONE.

sulphonamides A group of *antibiotics, derived from sulphanilamide (a red dye), that prevent the growth of bacteria (i.e. they are bacteriostatic). They act by inhibiting the production of an essential bacterial growth factor, folic acid. Most sulphonamides are taken orally and are short-acting, therefore they may need to be taken several times day. Topical sulphonamides are used in the treatment of infected burns.

A variety of side effects may occur with sulphonamide treatment, including nausea, vomiting, headache, and loss of appetite; more severe effects include blood disorders, skin rashes, and fever. Because of increasing bacterial resistance to sulphonamides and their adverse effects, and with the development of more effective less toxic antibiotics, the clinical use of these drugs has declined. Those still used include sulfamethoxazole (combined with trimethoprim as *co-trimoxazole), *sulfadiazine, *silver sulfadiazine, and sulfadoxine (combined with pyrimethamine as *Fansidar).

sulphonylureas A group of *oral hypoglycaemic drugs derived from sulphonamide. They act by stimulating *insulin secretion from functioning beta cells of the pancreas and are therefore used to treat people with type 2 (noninsulin-dependent) *diabetes mellitus, who are still producing some natural insulin. Sulphonylureas cause weight gain and should be used in conjunction with a carefully controlled diet; they should only be taken if strict dietary measures have failed to control blood-sugar levels. The main sulphonylureas are *glibenclamide, *gliclazide, *glimepiride, *glipizide, and *tolbutamide. They are available as tablets on *prescription only.
Side effects: these are usually mild and include stomach and bowel upsets (nausea, vomiting, diarrhoea, etc.) and headache. Allergic reactions (including transient rashes) may rarely occur.
Precautions: sulphonylureas should be used with caution in the elderly and

people with impaired liver or kidney function; they should not be taken by people with severe liver disease or by women who are pregnant or breastfeeding.

Interactions with other drugs:

Antibiotics: chloramphenicol enhances the effects of sulphonylureas; rifampicin and rifabutin accelerate the breakdown of sulphonylureas.

Anticoagulants: warfarin and acenocoumarol may enhance the effects of sulphonylureas.

Antifungal drugs: fluconazole and miconazole increase the plasma concentrations of sulphonylureas.

Corticosteroids: reduce the effects of sulphonylureas.

NSAIDs: enhance the effects of sulphonylureas.

Oral contraceptives: antagonize the effects of sulphonylureas.

Sulfinpyrazone: enhances the effects of sulphonylureas.

sulphur An element with *keratolytic and mild *antiseptic properties that also has some activity against fungi and kills parasites. It was formerly widely used in creams, lotions, and ointments to treat a variety of skin conditions, including acne, dandruff, psoriasis, scabies, and fungal infections. Sulphur has been replaced by more effective drugs for many purposes, although it is still used as an ingredient in some skin preparations.

Precautions: preparations containing sulphur should not be applied near the eyes or mouth.

Proprietary preparations: *Clearasil Treatment Cream Regular (combined with triclosan); *Cocois (combined with coal tar and salicylic acid); *Meted (combined with salicylic acid).

sulpiride An *antipsychotic drug used for the treatment of schizophrenia; it controls both the positive symptoms (e.g. delusions) and the negative symptoms (e.g. apathy) of the disease. Sulpiride is available as tablets or an oral solution on *prescription only.

Side effects: as for *chlorpromazine, but sulpiride is less sedating and does not cause jaundice or skin reactions.

Precautions: *see* CHLORPROMAZINE HYDROCHLORIDE.

Interactions with other drugs:

Anaesthetics: their effect in lowering blood pressure is enhanced.

Anti-arrhythmic drugs: there is an increased risk of *arrhythmias if sulpiride is taken with amiodarone or disopyramide.

Antidepressants: there is an increased risk of antimuscarinic effects and arrhythmias if sulpiride is taken with tricyclic antidepressants.

Antiepileptic drugs: their anticonvulsant effects are antagonized by sulpiride.

Antipsychotics: there is an increased risk of arrhythmias if sulpiride is taken with droperidol (which should be avoided), haloperidol, or pimozide.

Erythromycin: there is an increased risk of arrhythmias if this drug is given by injection with sulpiride.

Ritonavir: may increase the effects of sulpiride.

Sedatives: the sedative effects of sulpiride are increased if it is taken with anxiolytic or hypnotic drugs, or any other drug that causes sedation.
Sibutramine: there is an increased risk of adverse effects on the central nervous system if this drug is taken with sulpiride.
Sotalol: there is an increased risk of arrhythmias if sotalol is taken with sulpiride.

Proprietary preparations: Dolmatil (tablets); Sulpor (oral solution).

Sulpor (Rosemont Pharmaceuticals Limited) *See* SULPIRIDE.

sumatriptan A *5HT$_1$ agonist used for treating acute attacks of *migraine and cluster headaches. A single dose can relieve a migraine headache at any stage of the attack. Sumatriptan is available, on *prescription only, as tablets, a subcutaneous injection, or a nasal spray.
Side effects: include sensations of heaviness, pressure, heat, tingling, or tightness; if tightness in the chest or throat is severe, treatment should be stopped. Other side effects include flushing, fatigue, dizziness, and in increase in blood pressure (which does not last).
Precautions: sumatriptan should not be taken by people who have previously had a heart attack or stroke or who have uncontrolled high blood pressure. It should be used with caution in people with kidney or liver disease, heart conditions, or epilepsy, and in women who are pregnant or breastfeeding.
Interactions with other drugs:

Antidepressants: if MAOIs are taken with sumatriptan the risk of adverse effects on the central nervous system (CNS) is increased; sumatriptan should therefore not be started until two weeks after MAOIs have been stopped. SSRIs should not be taken with sumatriptan as this combination also has adverse effects on the CNS.
Ergotamine: the risk of spasm of the blood vessels, which can have serious consequences, is increased if ergotamine is taken with sumatriptan. Ergotamine should not be started for 6 hours after stopping sumatriptan, and sumatriptan should not be started for 24 hours after stopping ergotamine.

Proprietary preparations: Imigran; Imigran RADIS.

sunitinib A *tyrosine kinase inhibitor used for the treatment of gastrointestinal stromal tumours (a type of stomach cancer) that cannot be treated by surgery or *imatinib. It is available as capsules on *prescription only.
Side effects: *see* CYTOTOXIC DRUGS. Additional side effects include nausea, diarrhoea, vomiting, indigestion, insomnia, dizziness, peripheral neuropathy (causing numbness and tingling of the limbs), and hypertension.
Precautions: sunitinib should not be taken by breastfeeding women. If congestive heart failure develops, treatment should be stopped.
Interactions with other drugs:

Clozapine: should not be taken with sunitinib as this combination increases the risk of agranulocytosis (a blood disorder).

Proprietary preparation: Sutent.

sunscreen preparations Preparations that protect the skin against the harmful effects of the sun's ultraviolet (UV) radiation. The two ranges of solar UV wavelengths that cause skin damage are UVB (long wavelengths in the range 280–310 nanometres) and UVA (long wavelengths in the range 310–400 nm). UVB causes sunburn and contributes to the development of skin cancer but its strength varies during daylight depending on the extent to which it is filtered out by clouds and the atmosphere. UVA is not filtered by the atmosphere, does not cause sunburn, and penetrates more deeply into the skin, causing the wrinkles, yellowing, and blotching associated with ageing. It also causes some photosensitive reactions in patients taking such drugs as *amiodarone and *phenothiazines; it can also contribute to skin cancer.

Sunscreen preparations contain absorbent substances, such as *aminobenzoic acid, which absorb UVB only, or reflective substances, such as *zinc oxide and *titanium dioxide, which reflect both UVA and UVB radiation. The amount of protection to be expected from a sunscreen preparation effective against UVB is indicated by its sun protection factor (SPF). For example, a preparation with an SPF of 8 should enable a person to remain in the sun without burning eight times longer than an unprotected person. These preparations do not, however, protect against the long-term damage associated with UVA. Some manufacturers indicate the extent to which their product does offer UVA protection by means of an arbitrary star rating system. A four-star product can be expected to provide roughly equal UVA and UVB protection, while three, two, and one stars indicate greater protection against UVB than UVA roughly in proportion to the number of stars. Thus a three-star product will provide about 33% less protection to UVA than a four-star product.

The following proprietary preparations provide protection against both UVA and UVB: *Ambre Solaire, *Coppertone, *SpectraBan, and *Uvistat.

Sunya 20/75 (Stragen) A proprietary combination of *ethinylestradiol (20 mg) and *gestodene (75 mg), used as an *oral contraceptive. It is available as tablets on *prescription only.
Side effects, precautions, and interactions with other drugs: *see* ORAL CONTRACEPTIVES.

S

suppository A bullet-shaped plug containing a drug that is administered by insertion into the rectum. It is used when the drug needs to be delivered to the lining of the rectum or when an individual cannot take a drug by mouth, for example because he or she is unable to swallow or is vomiting. Since the lining of the rectum is well supplied with blood vessels, the absorption of a drug from a suppository is quite rapid. *Compare* PESSARY (vaginal suppository).

Supralip (Solvay Healthcare Limited) *See* FENOFIBRATE.

supraventricular tachycardia *See* ARRHYTHMIA.

Suprax (sanofi-aventis) *See* CEFIXIME.

Suprecur (sanofi-aventis) *See* BUSERELIN.

Suprefact (sanofi-aventis) *See* BUSERELIN.

surfactant A substance that is added to a cream or ointment to reduce its surface tension and thus increase its spreading or wetting properties. **Pulmonary** (or **lung**) **surfactant** is a complex mixture of proteins, fats, and carbohydrates that is made by cells in the lungs and prevents the lungs from collapsing by reducing surface tension. Premature babies often have difficulties in breathing because their lungs have not yet made enough surfactant. They are treated with synthetic pulmonary surfactants (*see* BERACTANT; PORACTANT ALFA).

Surgam (sanofi-aventis) *See* TIAPROFENIC ACID.

Surmontil (sanofi-aventis) *See* TRIMIPRAMINE.

Survanta (Abbott) *See* BERACTANT.

Suscard (Forest Laboratories) *See* GLYCERYL TRINITRATE.

sustained-release preparation *See* MODIFIED-RELEASE PREPARATION.

Sustanon 250 (Organon Laboratories) *See* TESTOSTERONE.

Sustiva (Bristol-Myers Squibb) *See* EFAVIRENZ.

Sutent (Pfizer) *See* SUNITINIB.

Symbicort (AstraZeneca) A proprietary combination of *budesonide (a corticosteroid) and *formoterol fumarate (a bronchodilator), used for the treatment of asthma. It is available as a powder in an *inhaler on *prescription only.
Side effects and precautions: *see* BUDESONIDE; FORMOTEROL FUMARATE.
Interactions with other drugs: *see* SALBUTAMOL.

Symmetrel (Alliance) *See* AMANTADINE HYDROCHLORIDE.

sympathetic nervous system A part of the nervous system that works in conjunction with another series of nerves (the parasympathetic system) to control the diameter of blood vessels and certain functions of the heart, lungs, intestines and pancreas, sweat glands, salivary glands, bladder, and genitalia. Both the sympathetic and parasympathetic nervous systems function automatically – we are not aware of their actions and have no voluntary control over them. The substances that relay information in the sympathetic nervous system are predominantly *noradrenaline and, to a lesser extent, *adrenaline. They act on very small specialized areas of the cells of the target tissues called *adrenoceptors. Many drugs act on the sympathetic nervous system, either by stimulating or by blocking these receptors or by increasing or preventing the release of noradrenaline from sympathetic nerve endings. *See* ALPHA BLOCKERS; BETA BLOCKERS; SYMPATHOMIMETIC DRUGS.

sympathomimetic drugs Drugs that mimic the effects of stimulating the *sympathetic nervous system. They act on the blood vessels, airways, and heart. There are two main types (although several drugs belong to both types).

The **alpha-adrenoceptor stimulants** (also called **alpha stimulants** or **alpha agonists**) stimulate the alpha *adrenoceptors; they are *vasoconstrictors and are used as nasal *decongestants (e.g. *ephedrine, *xylometazoline, *phenylephrine). Centrally acting alpha stimulants (e.g. *clonidine, *methyldopa) act on alpha receptors in the brain that control blood pressure, decreasing the sympathetic stimulation of arteries and thus causing them to relax. These drugs are used in treating *hypertension. **Beta-adrenoceptor stimulants** (also called **beta stimulants** or **beta agonists**) stimulate beta adrenoceptors. They are *bronchodilators (e.g. *salbutamol), used to treat asthma; heart stimulants (e.g. *dobutamine hydrochloride, *dopamine); or relaxants of uterine muscle (e.g. *ritodrine). Some drugs act by directly stimulating the release of noradrenaline. *See also* ADRENALINE; NORADRENALINE.

Synacthen, Synacthen Depot (Alliance) *See* TETRACOSACTIDE ACETATE.

Synagis (Abbott) *See* PALIVIZUMAB.

Synalar (GP Pharma) *See* FLUOCINOLONE ACETONIDE.

Synalar C (GP Pharma) A proprietary combination of *fluocinolone acetonide (a potent topical steroid) and *clioquinol (an antifungal agent), used for the treatment of infected conditions of the skin. It is available as a cream or an ointment on *prescription only.
Side effects and precautions: *see* TOPICAL STEROIDS; CLIOQUINOL.

Synalar N (GP Pharma) A proprietary combination of *fluocinolone acetonide (a potent topical steroid) and *neomycin sulphate (an antibiotic), used for the treatment of infected conditions of the skin. It is available as a cream or an ointment on *prescription only.
Side effects and precautions: *see* TOPICAL STEROIDS.

Synarel (Pfizer) *See* NAFARELIN.

Syndol (SSL International) A proprietary combination of *paracetamol and *codeine phosphate (analgesics), *doxylamine (an antihistamine), and *caffeine (a stimulant), used for the relief of headache, migraine, neuralgia, toothache, sore throat, period pains, and rheumatic aches and pains. It is available as tablets and can be obtained without a prescription, but only from pharmacies.
Side effects: *see* CODEINE; ANTIHISTAMINES; CAFFEINE.
Precautions: Syndol is not recommended for children. *See also* PARACETAMOL; ANTIHISTAMINES; CAFFEINE.
Interactions with other drugs: *see* ANTIHISTAMINES; OPIOIDS.

Synercid (Nordic) A proprietary combination of two antibiotics, quinupristin and dalfopristin, used for the treatment of severe infections, including meticillin-resistant *Staphylococcus aureus* (MRSA), that have not responded to other antibiotics. It is given by intravenous infusion and is available on *prescription only.

Side effects: may include reactions at the infusion site, nausea, vomiting, diarrhoea, headache, joint and muscle aches, rash, and itching.
Precautions: Synercid should not be given to people with high blood levels of bilirubin (a bile pigment) or severe liver disease or to breastfeeding women. It should be used with caution in pregnant women and in people with a history of *arrhythmias.
Interactions with other drugs:

Anti-arrhythmic drugs: Synercid increases the risk of arrhythmias if given with disopyramide or lidocaine.
Anxiolytic and hypnotic drugs: Synercid increases the plasma concentration (and therefore sedative effects) of midazolam and zopiclone.
Ergotamine tartrate: should not be given with Synercid.
Immunosuppresants: the plasma concentrations of ciclosporin and tacrolimus are increased.
Nifedipine: its plasma concentration is increased.

Syner-KINASE (Syner-Med (Pharmaceutical Products) Ltd) *See* UROKINASE.

Synflex (Roche Products) *See* NAPROXEN.

Synphase (Pfizer) A proprietary combination of *ethinylestradiol and *norethisterone, used as an *oral contraceptive of the triphasic type. These tablets are packaged in three phases, which differ in the amounts of the active ingredients they contain. Synphase is available on *prescription only.
Side effects, precautions, and interactions with other drugs: *see* ORAL CONTRACEPTIVES.

Syntaris (IVAX) *See* FLUNISOLIDE.

Syntocinon (Alliance) *See* OXYTOCIN.

Syntometrine (Alliance) A proprietary combination of *ergometrine maleate and *oxytocin, which causes contraction of the uterus and is used to stop the bleeding of an incomplete abortion or to assist delivery of the placenta in childbirth. It is available, on *prescription only, as a solution for intramuscular injection.
Side effects, precautions, and interactions with other drugs: *see* OXYTOCIN; ERGOMETRINE MALEATE.

Syprol (Rosemont Pharmaceuticals Limited) *See* PROPRANOLOL HYDROCHLORIDE.

systemic Throughout the body. A drug that is given systemically, e.g. by *injection or by mouth, is absorbed into the bloodstream and reaches most parts of the body; it therefore has effects on the body as a whole, rather than on individual tissues or organs. Drugs that are inhaled have systemic effects, as do those administered *transdermally or as *enemas, *suppositories, or *pessaries. Some drugs given by a *topical route of administration may have systemic effects.

Sytron (Archimedes Pharma UK Ltd) *See* SODIUM FEREDETATE.

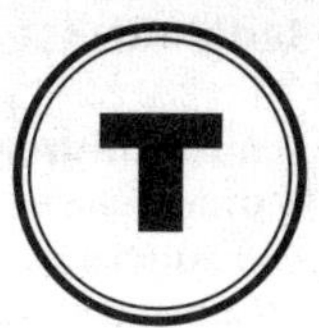

tablet A small disc or other shape containing one or more drugs, made by compressing a powdered form of the drug(s). It is usually taken by mouth but may be inserted into a body cavity (*see* PESSARY; SUPPOSITORY).

Tabphyn (ProStrakan) *See* TAMSULOSIN HYDROCHLORIDE.

tacalcitol An *analogue of *vitamin D that is used in the treatment of *psoriasis. It acts by slowing down the division of skin cells whose overgrowth causes the formation of scaly patches seen in this disease. Tacalcitol is available as an ointment or lotion on *prescription only.
Side effects: tacalcitol may irritate the skin, causing itching, reddening, or a burning sensation.
Precautions: tacalcitol should not be used by people with disorders of calcium metabolism. It should be used with caution by people with peeling psoriasis and by pregnant and breastfeeding women. Tacalcitol should not be used on the face, and excessive exposure to sunlight should be avoided after application.
Proprietary preparation: Curatoderm.

tacrolimus An *immunosuppressant, similar to *ciclosporin, used for the prevention of rejection in transplant patients. It is also used as a topical treatment for atopic *eczema. Tacrolimus is available as capsules, *modified-release capsules, or an ointment on *prescription only.
Side effects: the capsules may cause tremor, headache, tingling in the fingers and toes, kidney impairment, fatigue, gum swelling, gastrointestinal disturbances, and visual disturbances. There may be an increased susceptibility to infection. Application of the ointment may cause irritation, rash, and 'pins and needles'.
Precautions: tacrolimus should not be taken by women who are pregnant or breastfeeding. It may affect the performance of such skilled tasks as driving or operating machinery. Liver, kidney, and heart function should be monitored during treatment. People using the ointment should avoid alcohol (which may cause flushing and irritate the skin) and exposure to sunlight.
Interactions with other drugs (capsules): tacrolimus should be used with caution with NSAIDs, aminoglycosides, and amphotericin because these drugs increase the risk of kidney damage.

Antibiotics: the plasma concentration of tacrolimus is increased by chloramphenicol, clarithromycin, erythromycin, Synercid, and telithromycin and reduced by rifampicin.

Antifungal drugs: the plasma concentration of tacrolimus is increased by imidazoles and triazoles and reduced by caspofungin.

Antiviral drugs: the plasma concentration of tacrolimus may be increased by atazanavir, nelfinavir, ritonavir, and saquinavir and is altered by efavirenz.
Calcium antagonists: the plasma concentration of tacrolimus is increased by diltiazem and nifedipine.
Ciclosporin: should not be used in conjunction with tacrolimus because it increases the risk of kidney damage.
Droperidol: increases the risk of ventricular *arrhythmias and should not be taken with tacrolimus.
Hormonal contraceptives: tacrolimus may affect their contraceptive action; non-hormonal contraception should be used during treatment.
Phenobarbital: reduces the plasma concentration of tacrolimus.
Potassium-sparing diuretics and potassium supplements: the risk of high potassium plasma concentrations is increased.
St John's wort: reduces the plasma concentration of tacrolimus and should not be used with it.

Proprietary preparations: Advagraf (modified-release capsules); Prograf (capsules); Protopic (ointment).

tadalafil A drug with similar actions and effects to *sildenafil, used for the treatment of impotence. It is available as tablets on *prescription only.
Side effects: *see* SILDENAFIL. Additional side effects include heart failure, arrhythmias, and hypertension.
Precautions: *see* SILDENAFIL. In addition, tadalafil should not be taken by men with heart failure, hypertension, or arrhythmias and should be used with caution in men with impaired kidney function.
Interactions with other drugs:
Alpha blockers: tadalafil significantly enhances their effects in lowering blood pressure; doxazosin should not be taken with this drug.
See also SILDENAFIL.
Proprietary preparation: Cialis.

tafluprost A *prostaglandin analogue used to reduce pressure in the eye in the treatment of chronic (open-angle) *glaucoma and raised blood pressure in the eye. It is available as eye drops on *prescription only.
Side effects: tafluprost may increase the brown pigment of the iris, and people should be warned to notice any changes in eye colour. The eyes may become bloodshot, itchy, or painful, the eyelashes may become darker, longer, and thicker, and the skin around the eyes may become darker.
Precautions: tafluprost should not be used by pregnant women, and women capable of bearing children should use contraception during treatment.
Proprietary preparation: Saflutan.

Tagamet (Chemidax Pharma) *See* CIMETIDINE.

Tambocor, Tambocor XL (Meda Pharmaceuticals) *See* FLECAINIDE ACETATE.

Tamiflu (Roche Products) *See* OSELTAMIVIR.

tamoxifen An *oestrogen antagonist used to treat women with breast cancer, both before and after the menopause, in which oestrogen stimulates growth of the tumour. It is also used to prevent a recurrence of breast cancer, and for women at particularly high risk of developing the disease it may in some cases be a primary preventive treatment. Tamoxifen is also used, sometimes in conjunction with *human chorionic gonadotrophin, to treat infertility in women caused by failure of the ovaries to produce egg cells. As a side benefit, tamoxifen also reduces the risk of a heart attack. It is available as tablets on *prescription only.
Side effects: the most common are hot flushes, vaginal bleeding, and nausea or other stomach and bowel upsets; there may also be loss of periods, vaginal discharge or itching, light-headedness, loss of hair, rashes, and visual disturbances (in which case treatment should be stopped). Any abnormal vaginal bleeding or discharge or pelvic pain should be reported to a doctor promptly to exclude the possibility of cancer of the endometrium (womb lining).
Precautions: tamoxifen should not be used by women who are pregnant or breastfeeding. In women taking this drug there is a small increase in the risks of developing endometrial cancer and venous thrombosis (it should not be taken for infertility treatment by women at risk of thrombosis).
Interactions with other drugs:
Anticoagulants: tamoxifen increases the effects of warfarin and acenocoumarol.
Antidepressants: the effects of tamoxifen may be reduced by duloxetine, fluoxetine, and paroxetine, which should not be taken with it.
Bupropion: may reduce the effects of tamoxifen and should not be taken with it.
Droperidol: increases the risk of *arrhythmias and should not be taken with tamoxifen.
Proprietary preparations: Nolvadex Forte; Soltamox.

tamsulosin hydrochloride An *alpha blocker used to relieve urinary retention in men with an enlarged prostate gland. It is available as *modified-release tablets on *prescription only.
Side effects and interactions with other drugs: *see* ALPHA BLOCKERS.
Precautions: tamsulosin should not be taken by men with severe liver disease. *See also* ALPHA BLOCKERS.
Proprietary preparations: Flomaxtra; Stronazon; Tabphyn.

Tanatril (Chiesi) *See* IMIDAPRIL HYDROCHLORIDE.

tar A substance obtained from the distillation of the wood of various trees of the pine family. A *keratolytic that relieves itching, it is used in combination with other drugs in various preparations for the treatment or relief of a variety of skin disorders, including *eczema, *psoriasis, and dandruff.
Side effects and precautions: *see* COAL TAR.
Proprietary preparation: *Polytar (combined with cade oil, coal tar, arachis oil, and oleyl alcohol).

Tarceva (Roche Products) *See* ERLOTINIB.

Targinact (Napp Pharmaceuticals Limited) A proprietary combination of *oxycodone (an opioid analgesic) and *naloxone hydrochloride (an opioid antagonist), used for the treatment of severe pain. It is available as *modified-release tablets on *prescription only.
Side effects and precautions: *see* MORPHINE; NALOXONE HYDROCHLORIDE; OPIOIDS.
Interactions with other drugs: *see* OPIOIDS.

Targocid (sanofi-aventis) *See* TEICOPLANIN.

Targretin (Cephalon) *See* BEXAROTENE.

Tarivid (sanofi-aventis) *See* OFLOXACIN.

Tarka (Abbott) A proprietary combination of *verapamil hydrochloride (a calcium antagonist), in a modified-release form, and *trandolapril (an ACE inhibitor). It is used for the treatment of *hypertension in people who have been stabilized on the individual drugs at the same dosages and is available as capsules on *prescription only.
Side effects, precautions, and interactions with other drugs: *see* CALCIUM ANTAGONISTS; ACE INHIBITORS.

tartaric acid A weak acid with laxative properties used in the preparation of effervescent powders, granules, and tablets. Tartaric acid or its salt **sodium potassium tartrate** are ingredients of *antacid preparations used to relieve indigestion and heartburn and of mild *laxatives, which are freely available *over the counter.
Side effects: strong solutions are irritant and when swallowed can cause vomiting, diarrhoea, abdominal pains, and thirst.
Proprietary preparation: *Jaap's Health Salts (combined with sodium bicarbonate).

Tasigna (Novartis) *See* NILOTINIB.

Tasmar (Meda Pharmaceuticals) *See* TOLCAPONE.

tasonermin A genetically engineered form of tumour necrosis factor alpha, a protein produced by white blood cells that has a marked action against tumour cells. It is used, in combination with *melphalan, to treat soft-tissue tumours (*see* CANCER) of the limbs. It is given by intravenous infusion and is available on *prescription only.
Side effects: include infections, *arrhythmias, nausea, vomiting, fever, fatigue, chills, skin disorders, *oedema, limb pain, and nerve damage.
Precautions and interactions with other drugs: tasonermin should not be given to patients with cardiovascular or respiratory disease, peptic ulcers, severe ascites (*see* OEDEMA), severe blood disorders, liver or kidney disease, or raised blood-calcium levels, or to women who are pregnant or breastfeeding. Drugs that have adverse effects on the heart (e.g. anthracyclines) or cause lowering of blood pressure should not be used with tasonermin.

Proprietary preparation: Beromun.

Tavanic (sanofi-aventis) *See* LEVOFLOXACIN.

Tavegil (Novartis) *See* CLEMASTINE.

taxanes A group of drugs originally isolated from the bark of the Pacific yew (*Taxus brevifolia*). They are used for the treatment of advanced ovarian *cancer and advanced breast cancer, especially when standard treatment has failed. The common taxanes are *paclitaxel and *docetaxel.

Taxol (Bristol-Myers Squibb) *See* PACLITAXEL.

Taxotere (sanofi-aventis) *See* DOCETAXEL.

tazarotene A *retinoid used for the treatment of mild to moderate *psoriasis affecting up to 10% of the skin area. It is available as a gel on *prescription only.
Side effects: include local irritation, burning, redness, peeling of the skin, rash, dermatitis, and (rarely) skin pain.
Precautions: tazarotene should not be used by women who are pregnant or breastfeeding, and contraception must be used during treatment (*see* RETINOIDS). It should not be applied to skin folds, the face or scalp, normal or inflamed skin, or the eyes. Prolonged exposure to ultraviolet light (including sunlight) should be avoided.
Proprietary preparation: Zorac.

tazobactam An agent that inhibits the activity of of beta-lactamases, enzymes that are produced by bacteria and destroy *penicillins. It is given in combination with *piperacillin to prevent the destruction of this antibiotic (*see* TAZOCIN).

Tazocin (Pfizer) A proprietary combination of *piperacillin (a penicillin) and *tazobactam (a beta-lactamase inhibitor), used for the treatment of infections of the lower respiratory tract, urinary tract, and skin. It is available as an injection on *prescription only.
Side effects, precautions, and interactions with other drugs: *see* BENZYLPENICILLIN.

TCAs *See* TRICYCLIC ANTIDEPRESSANTS.

TCP Antiseptic Cream (Chefaro UK) A proprietary combination of *triclosan, *chloroxylenol, and *TCP Antiseptic Liquid, used for the treatment of minor cuts, grazes, scratches, insect bites, stings, spots, and blisters. It is freely available *over the counter.

TCP Antiseptic Liquid (Chefaro UK) A proprietary preparation of halogenated *phenols used an an *antiseptic for treating cuts, grazes, insect bites and stings, spots, mouth ulcers, and as a gargle for sore throats. It is freely available *over the counter.

TCP Sore Throat Lozenges (Chefaro UK) *See* HEXYLRESORCINOL.

Tears Naturale (Alcon Laboratories) A proprietary combination of *dextran and *hypromellose, used as a substitute for natural tears when the production of these is deficient. It is available as eye drops and can be obtained without a prescription, but only from pharmacies.
Precautions: the drops should not be used with soft contact lenses.

tegafur *See* UFTORAL.

Tegretol (Novartis) *See* CARBAMAZEPINE.

teicoplanin An *antibiotic, similar to *vancomycin, used for the treatment of serious infections, including those caused by meticillin-resistant *Staphylococcus aureus* (MRSA), endocarditis (infection of the heart membranes or valves), and peritonitis in dialysis patients, and to prevent infection after orthopaedic surgery. It is available, on *prescription only, as a solution for *intramuscular or *intravenous injection or infusion.
Side effects: include nausea, vomiting, diarrhoea, rash, fever, bronchospasm, anaphylactic reactions, dizziness, headache, blood disorders, and mild hearing loss.
Precautions: blood counts and liver and kidney function tests should be carried out during treatment; hearing tests are required for patients on long-term treatment. Teicoplanin should not be given to patients who are allergic to vancomycin, and it should be used with caution in people with kidney disease and in women who are pregnant or breastfeeding.
Proprietary preparation: Targocid.

Telfast (sanofi-aventis) *See* FEXOFENADINE HYDROCHLORIDE.

telithromycin An antibiotic derived from *erythromycin and having similar antibacterial activity to it (*see also* MACROLIDE ANTIBIOTICS). It is used to treat respiratory-tract infections and tonsillitis that are resistant to *first-line antibiotics. Telithromycin is available as tablets on *prescription only.
Side effects: include diarrhoea, dizziness, headache, nausea, vomiting, abdominal pain, and altered taste.
Precautions: telithromycin should not be taken by people with myasthenia gravis or *arrhythmias as it can exacerbate these conditions. It is not recommended for pregnant or breastfeeding women, and it should be used with caution in people with liver disease. Telithromycin may cause blurred vision, and people taking it should not drive or operate machinery if this occurs.
Interactions with other drugs: telithromycin should not be taken with a number of other drugs, including carbamazepine, phenytoin, eplerenone, ergot alkaloid derivatives (e.g. ergotamine), ivabradine, pimozide, sirolimus, and statins. A doctor should be consulted before taking it with any other drug.
Proprietary preparation: Ketek.

telmisartan An *angiotensin II inhibitor used for the treatment of *hypertension. It is available as tablets on *prescription only.

Side effects: *see* ANGIOTENSIN II INHIBITORS. There may also be headache and muscle and bone pain.
Precautions: telmisartan should not be taken by women who are pregnant or breastfeeding or by people with an obstructed bile duct or severe liver disease. It should be used with caution in people with kidney disease. *See also* ANTIHYPERTENSIVE DRUGS.
Interactions with other drugs: *see* ACE INHIBITORS; ANTIHYPERTENSIVE DRUGS.
Proprietary preparations: Micardis; *Micardis Plus (combined with hydrochlorothiazide).

Telzir (GlaxoSmithKline) *See* FOSAMPRENAVIR.

temazepam A short-acting *benzodiazepine used for the short-term treatment of insomnia and anxiety. It is also used to relax patients before operations. Temazepam is a *controlled drug, available as tablets or an oral solution.
Side effects and precautions: *see* BENZODIAZEPINES; DIAZEPAM.
Interactions with other drugs: *see* BENZODIAZEPINES.

Temgesic (Schering-Plough) *See* BUPRENORPHINE.

temocillin A penicillin that is resistant to beta-lactamase (*see* PENICILLINS). It is used for the treatment of infections due to penicillinase-producing bacteria, including septicaemia, urinary tract infections, and pneumonia. Temocillin is given by intravenous or intramuscular injection and is available on *prescription only.
Side effects: *see* BENZYLPENICILLIN.
Precautions: *see* BENZYLPENICILLIN. Temocillin should be used with caution in women who are pregnant or breastfeeding.
Proprietary preparation: Negaban.

Temodal (Schering-Plough) *See* TEMOZOLOMIDE.

temoporfin A drug used in the treatment of advanced head and neck *cancer that is resistant to or unsuitable for other treatments. It is injected into the bloodstream, accumulates in the cancer cells, and is then activated by laser light to destroy these cells. Temoporfin is a *prescription only medicine.
Side effects: *see* CYTOTOXIC DRUGS. There may also be constipation, difficulty in swallowing, giddiness, reddening or blistering of the skin, and pain at the injection site.
Precautions: *see* CYTOTOXIC DRUGS. This treatment makes the skin and eyes sensitive to light for up to several months, and patients should avoid exposure to direct sunlight or bright indoor light for at least 15 days after treatment. Temoporfin should not be given to pregnant or breastfeeding women or to people with porphyria.
Interactions with other drugs:
Fluorouracil: increases the sensitivity of the skin to light.
Proprietary preparation: Foscan.

temozolomide A *cytotoxic drug used for the treatment of glioblastoma

multiforme (a type of brain cancer). It is available as capsules on *prescription only.
Side effects and precautions: *see* CYTOTOXIC DRUGS. Temozolomide should not be taken by breastfeeding women.
Interactions with other drugs:

Clozapine: should not be taken with temozolomide as this combination increases the risk of agranulocytosis (a blood disorder).

Proprietary preparation: Temodal.

temsirolimus A derivative of *sirolimus used in the treatment of advanced kidney cancer. It is given by intravenous infusion and is available on *prescription only.
Side effects: *see* CYTOTOXIC DRUGS. There may also be rash, anaemia, abdominal pain, diarrhoea, loss of appetite, raised blood lipids, and allergic reactions, including flushing, chest pain, and breathlessness (which can be prevented by giving an antihistamine before treatment).
Precautions: temsirolimus should not be given to people with severe liver disease or to breastfeeding women.
Interactions with other drugs:

Clozapine: should not be given with temsirolimus as this combination increases the risk of agranulocytosis (a blood disorder).

Ketoconazole: increases the plasma concentration of temsirolimus and should not be used with it.

Rifampicin: reduces the plasma concentration of temsirolimus and should not be used with it.

Proprietary preparation: Torisel.

tenecteplase A *fibrinolytic drug used to dissolve blood clots in the coronary arteries (which supply the heart) in people who have had a heart attack; treatment should be started within 12 hours of the attack. Tenecteplase is given by intravenous injection or infusion and is available on *prescription only.
Side effects, precautions, and interactions with other drugs: *see* FIBRINOLYTIC DRUGS.
Proprietary preparation: Metalyse.

t

Tenif (AstraZeneca) A proprietary combination of *atenolol (a beta blocker) and *nifedipine (a calcium antagonist), used for the treatment of *angina or *hypertension, usually when a single drug has been inadequate. It is available as capsules on *prescription only.
Side effects, precautions, and interactions with other drugs: *see* BETA BLOCKERS; CALCIUM ANTAGONISTS.

See also ANTIHYPERTENSIVE DRUGS.

tenofovir disoproxil A nucleoside analogue reverse transcriptase inhibitor (*see* ANTIVIRAL DRUGS) used in the treatment of HIV infection (in combination with other antiretroviral drugs) and of chronic hepatitis B. It is available as tablets on *prescription only.

Side effects: include nausea, vomiting, abdominal pain, diarrhoea, liver damage, headache, insomnia, dizziness, fatigue, and blood disorders.
Precautions: tenofovir disoproxil should be used with caution in patients with chronic hepatitis B or C or impaired liver or kidney function and in pregnant women. It should not be given to breastfeeding women. Liver and kidney function should be monitored during treatment.
Interactions with other drugs:
Antiviral drugs: adefovir should not be taken with tenofovir. Tenofovir reduces the plasma concentration of atazanavir and its plasma concentration may be increased by atazanavir. Tenofovir increases the plasma concentration of didanosine and should not be taken with it. Kaletra increases the plasma concentration of tenofovir.
Proprietary preparations: Viread; *Atripla (combined with efavirenz and emtricitabine); *Truvada (combined with emtricitabine).

Tenoret 50 (AstraZeneca) *See* CO-TENIDONE.

Tenoretic (AstraZeneca) *See* CO-TENIDONE.

Tenormin (AstraZeneca) *See* ATENOLOL.

tenoxicam An *NSAID used for the treatment of pain and inflammation in rheumatoid arthritis and other disorders of the joints or muscles. It is available as tablets or an injection on *prescription only.
Side effects, precautions, and interactions with other drugs: *see* NSAIDs.
Proprietary preparation: Mobiflex.

Tensipine MR (Genus) *See* NIFEDIPINE.

Tensium (DDSA Pharmaceuticals) *See* DIAZEPAM.

Teoptic (Novartis) *See* CARTEOLOL HYDROCHLORIDE.

terazosin An *alpha blocker used to treat mild to moderate *hypertension and to relieve the obstruction of urine flow that can occur in men with an enlarged prostate gland. It is available as tablets on *prescription only.
Side effects, precautions, and interactions with other drugs: *see* ALPHA BLOCKERS.
Proprietary preparation: Hytrin.
See also ANTIHYPERTENSIVE DRUGS; VASODILATORS.

terbinafine An *antifungal drug used for the treatment of fungal infections of the skin, scalp, or nails. It is available as a cream, spray, gel, or tablets; the tablets are *prescription only medicines, but the other formulations can be obtained without a prescription.
Side effects: the tablets may cause stomach and bowel upsets, changes in taste, headache, and aches or pains in the muscles and joints. If any preparation causes a rash a doctor should be consulted, as treatment may need to be discontinued if the rash worsens.
Precautions: terbinafine should be used with caution by people with chronic

liver disease or impaired kidney function and by women who are pregnant or breastfeeding.
Interactions with other drugs:
Cimetidine: increases the plasma concentration of terbinafine.
Rifampicin: reduces the plasma concentration of terbinafine.
Proprietary preparations: Lamisil (tablets); Lamisil AT 1%; Lamisil Cream; Lamisil Once (single-application cream).

terbutaline sulphate A *sympathomimetic drug that stimulates beta *adrenoceptors in the airways. It is used mainly as a *bronchodilator to relieve constriction of the airways in attacks of *asthma and to alleviate wheezing and breathlessness in bronchitis and emphysema. It also relaxes the uterus and can be used in obstetrics to prevent or delay premature labour. Terbutaline is available, on *prescription only, as a metered-dose aerosol or as a powder for inhalation, as tablets, *modified-release tablets, or a syrup for oral use, as a solution for use in a *nebulizer or a ventilator, and as a solution for injection.
Side effects, precautions, and interactions with other drugs: *see* SALBUTAMOL.
Proprietary preparations: Bricanyl; Bricanyl Turbohaler (dry powder inhaler).

teriparatide A genetically engineered form of *parathyroid hormone, used for the treatment of osteoporosis in postmenopausal women and in men, and of people who are on long-term corticosteroid therapy and are at high risk of fractures. It is available as a form for subcutaneous injection on *prescription only.
Side effects: include palpitations, weakness, dizziness, headache, sciatica, vertigo, nausea, regurgitation of stomach acids, increased sweating, muscle cramps, and fatigue.
Precautions: teriparatide should not be given to people with severely impaired kidney function, metabolic bone disease (e.g. Paget's disease), high blood-calcium levels, or bone cancers or to pregnant or breastfeeding women.
Proprietary preparation: Forsteo.

terlipressin An analogue of *vasopressin that used for the treatment of bleeding varicose veins in the oesophagus. It is available in a form for injection on *prescription only.
Side effects: similar to those of *vasopressin, but milder.
Precautions and interactions with other drugs: *see* VASOPRESSIN.
Proprietary preparations: Glypressin; Variquel.

terpineol A constituent of various aromatic oils that has mild disinfectant properties. It is used in combination with other volatile agents in inhalations to relieve the congestion associated with colds and catarrh.
Proprietary preparation: *Karvol (combined with other aromatic substances and chlorobutanol).

Testim (Ferring Pharmaceuticals) *See* TESTOSTERONE.

Testogel (Bayer) *See* TESTOSTERONE.

testosterone The main *androgen (male sex hormone). It is available as a variety of esters (**testosterone enantate**, **propionate**, and **undecanoate**) for the treatment of underdevelopment of the testes or as replacement therapy in castrated men. It can also be used in postmenopausal women as an adjunct in *hormone replacement therapy and to treat women with low libido with surgically induced menopause. Testosterone is available, on *prescription only, as capsules, an intramuscular injection, a *depot implant, a topical gel, or *transdermal (skin) patches.
Side effects: include excessive frequency and duration of penile erections, sodium and fluid retention, increased bone growth, enlargement of the prostate, reduced production of sperm, headache, depression, anxiety, generalized tingling sensations, gastrointestinal bleeding, nausea, jaundice, changes in libido, abnormal hair growth in women, male pattern baldness, and acne.
Precautions: testosterone should not be taken by men with cancer of the breast or prostate or by women who are pregnant or breastfeeding. It should be used with caution in people who have heart, liver, or kidney disease, in elderly men and prepubertal boys, and in people who suffer from high blood pressure, epilepsy, or migraine.
Interactions with other drugs:
Anticoagulants: testosterone enhances the effects of warfarin, acenocoumarol, and phenindione.
Antidiabetic drugs: testosterone may increase their effects in lowering blood-sugar concentrations.
Proprietary preparations: Andropatch (transdermal patches); Intrinsa (skin patches); Nebido (injection); Restandol (capsules); Striant SR (modified-release *buccal tablets); Sustanon 250 (depot formulation); Testim (gel); Testogel (gel); Testosterone Enantate (injection); Testosterone Implant; Tostran (gel); Virormone (injection and patches).

Testosterone Enantate (Cambridge Laboratories) *See* TESTOSTERONE.

Testosterone Implant (Organon Laboratories Limited) *See* TESTOSTERONE.

tetrabenazine A drug that acts by reducing the amount of available *dopamine in the brain. It is used to control the jerky involuntary movements that occur in Huntington's disease and related disorders. Tetrabenazine is available as tablets on *prescription only.
Side effects: depression can develop (which may restrict the use of tetrabenazine); other side effects include drowsiness, nausea, vomiting, *extrapyramidal reactions, and low blood pressure.
Precautions: tetrabenazine should be used with caution in women who are pregnant and should not be taken by women who are breastfeeding. It may affect driving ability.
Interactions with other drugs:
MAOIs: stimulation of the central nervous system and increased blood pressure can occur if these antidepressants are taken with tetrabenazine.
Proprietary preparation: Xenazine 25.

tetracaine <**amethocaine**> A potent *local anaesthetic used in the form of a gel to anaesthetize the skin before intravenous injections or the insertion of a cannula. It is also used in eye drops to induce anaesthesia for minor eye operations and is an ingredient of a spray for treating mouth and throat conditions. Most preparations of tetracaine can be obtained without a prescription but eye drops are available on *prescription only.
Side effects: tetracaine may cause redness, itching, or irritation of the skin.
Precautions: tetracaine should not be applied to inflamed or damaged skin. It should not be used for prolonged periods or over extensive areas.
Proprietary preparations: Ametop (gel); Minims Tetracaine Hydrochloride (single-dose preservative-free eye drops); *Eludril Spray (combined with chlorhexidine); *Rapydan (combined with lidocaine).

tetracosactide acetate <**tetracosactrin acetate**> A drug that stimulates the adrenal glands to produce *corticosteroids; it is a synthetic form of the pituitary hormone corticotropin. Tetracosactide is used to test whether or not the adrenal glands are functioning normally to produce corticosteroids. It is available as an injection and a *depot injection on *prescription only.
Side effects: allergic reactions may occur. *See also* CORTICOSTEROIDS.
Precautions: tetracosactide should not be given to people who are allergic to it. *See also* CORTICOSTEROIDS.
Interactions with other drugs: *see* CORTICOSTEROIDS.
Proprietary preparations: Synacthen; Synacthen Depot.

tetracycline hydrochloride A broad-spectrum antibiotic that gave its name to the *tetracyclines. It is used for the treatment of chronic bronchitis, brucellosis, chlamydial infections, and infections due to mycoplasmas and rickettsias. It is also used to treat mouth ulcers and *acne. Tetracycline is available, on *prescription only, as tablets.
Side effects, precautions, and interactions with other drugs: *see* TETRACYCLINES.

tetracyclines A group of broad-spectrum antibiotics whose value has decreased since many infective organisms have developed resistance to them. However, they are still the treatment of choice against *Chlamydia* bacteria (which cause a variety of diseases, notably sexually transmitted infections, parrot disease, and eye infections), rickettsias (which cause Q fever and typhus), and mycoplasmas (bacteria that cause respiratory and genital infections). They are also used to treat brucellosis, Lyme disease, acne, gum disease, and exacerbations of chronic bronchitis. Tetracyclines act by inhibiting protein synthesis in sensitive organisms. *See* DEMECLOCYCLINE HYDROCHLORIDE; DOXYCYCLINE; LYMECYCLINE; MINOCYCLINE; OXYTETRACYCLINE; TETRACYCLINE HYDROCHLORIDE.
Side effects: include nausea and vomiting, diarrhoea, headache, and visual disturbances. If a rash occurs, treatment should be discontinued. A rash on exposure to sunlight may occur in rare cases.
Precautions: the tetracyclines are deposited in growing bones and teeth, causing discoloration. For this reason they should not be taken by children

under 12 years old or by women who are pregnant or breastfeeding. Absorption of most tetracyclines (except doxycycline and minocycline) from the stomach is reduced in the presence of milk and other dairy products. Most tetracyclines (except doxycycline and minocycline) can exacerbate kidney failure and should not be taken by people with kidney disease. They should also be avoided by people with porphyris.
Interactions with other drugs:
Antacids: reduce the absorption of tetracyclines.
Anticoagulants: the effects of warfarin, acenocoumarol, and phenindione may be enhanced by tetracyclines.
Calcium salts: reduce the absorption of tetracyclines.
Iron salts (oral): reduce the absorption of tetracyclines.
Oral contraceptives: there is a small risk that tetracyclines may reduce the effectiveness of oral contraceptives.
Retinoids: may increase pressure in the brain and should not be used with tetracyclines.
Zinc salts: reduce the absorption of tetracyclines.

tetrahydrofurfuryl salicylate *See* SALICYLATES.

Tetralysal 300 (Galderma) *See* LYMECYCLINE.

Teveten (Solvay Healthcare Limited) *See* EPROSARTAN.

T/Gel (Johnson & Johnson) *See* COAL TAR.

thalidomide A drug that modifies or regulates the immune system and has anti-inflammatory properties. It is used, in combination with *melphalan and *prednisone, for the treatment of multiple myeloma (cancer of antibody-forming cells in the bone marrow) in patients aged 65 years or more and in patients who cannot be given high-dose chemotherapy because of risk factors. It is available as capsules on *prescription only.
Side effects: include drowsiness, constipation, dry mouth, peripheral neuropathy (causing numbness and tingling of the limbs), tremor, dizziness, deep vein *thrombosis, breathlessness, and low white blood cell counts.
Precautions: because of the risk of deep vein thrombosis, patients should be given anticoagulants or antiplatelet drugs for at least the first five months of treatment. Signs of thrombosis (e.g. chest pain, limb swelling) should be reported to a doctor. Thalidomide can cause abnormalities in the fetus. Therefore women should use effective contraception for at least one month before, during, and for at least one month after treatment; men should use condoms during and for at least one week after treatment. Thalidomide should not be taken by women who are breastfeeding.
Proprietary preparation: Thalidomide Pharmion.

Thalidomide Pharmion (Celgene Ltd) *See* THALIDOMIDE.

Thelin (Encysive (UK) Limited) *See* SITAXENTAN SODIUM.

theophylline A *xanthine used for the treatment of *asthma and in some

cases of emphysema and chronic bronchitis (*see* BRONCHODILATORS). It is available as *modified-release tablets or capsules and can be obtained from pharmacies without a prescription.
Side effects: include nausea, headache, gastrointestinal disturbances, palpitation, and insomnia. *See also* XANTHINES.
Precautions: theophylline should be used with caution by people with some types of heart disease, liver disease, or peptic ulcer, and by women who are in late pregnancy or breastfeeding. There may be a need to monitor concentrations of plasma potassium.
Interactions with other drugs:

Antibiotics: the plasma concentration of theophylline is increased by ciprofloxacin, clarithromycin, and erythromycin; quinolones increase the risk of convulsions.
Antidepressants: the plasma concentration of theophylline is increased by fluvoxamine and reduced by St John's wort, and these drugs should not be taken with theophylline.
Antifungal drugs: fluconazole and ketoconazole may increase the plasma concentration of theophylline.
Calcium antagonists: may increase the plasma concentration of theophylline.
Cimetidine: increases the plasma concentration of theophylline.
Phenytoin: the plasma concentration of both drugs is reduced if phenytoin is taken with theophylline.
Ritonavir: reduces the plasma concentration of theophylline.

Proprietary preparations: Nuelin SA (modified-release tablets); Slo-Phyllin (modified-release capsules); Uniphyllin Continus (modified-release tablets); *Do-Do ChestEze (combined with ephedrine and caffeine).

thiamine (**vitamin B_1**) A vitamin of the B group (*see* VITAMIN B COMPLEX) that is taken orally (as **thiamine hydrochloride**) to treat vitamin B_1 deficiency. In combination with other B vitamins and vitamin C (ascorbic acid), it is given by injection to relieve severe deficiency states, such as those caused by alcoholism or occurring after acute infections, surgery, or in some psychiatric conditions; injections may also be needed by people undergoing kidney dialysis. Thiamine tablets are freely available *over the counter; the injection is a *prescription only medicine.
Side effects: rarely, an allergic reaction and anaphylactic shock (*see* ANAPHYLAXIS) can occur after injection.
Proprietary preparations: Benerva (tablets); *Pabrinex (combined with other B vitamins and ascorbic acid); *Yeast-Vite (combined with riboflavin, nicotinamide, and caffeine).

thiazide diuretics A class of *diuretics that bring about a moderate loss of fluid as urine. They are used for long-term treatment of such conditions as *hypertension or *oedema associated with congestive *heart failure. Thiazides and thiazide-like diuretics may be used for extended periods in the treatment of hypertension; in this situation their diuretic activity decreases but their *antihypertensive activity continues. *Potassium supplements may be required with the thiazide diuretics; alternatively, they may be used in combination with *potassium-sparing diuretics. Thiazide diuretics start to act within 1–2 hours of oral administration and have a duration of action of 12–24 hours. They are therefore usually given early during the day.

See BENDROFLUMETHIAZIDE; BENZTHIAZIDE; CHLORTALIDONE; CYCLOPENTHIAZIDE; HYDROCHLOROTHIAZIDE; HYDROFLUMETHIAZIDE; INDAPAMIDE; METOLAZONE; XIPAMIDE.

Side effects: if the loss of potassium, sodium, and water is too great, thiazide diuretics can cause weakness, lethargy, and cramps; dizziness may occur as a result of postural hypotension (low blood pressure on standing up from a sitting or lying posture); less commonly mild gastrointestinal upsets, rashes, photosensitivity (skin sensitivity to light), anorexia, reversible impotence, blood disorders, and pancreatitis may occur.

Precautions: thiazide diuretics should not be taken by people with certain liver or kidney disorders, and they can aggravate gout or diabetes. They should be used with caution by men with an enlarged prostate gland, women who are breastfeeding, and by elderly people. They should not be taken by women who are pregnant, as they can cause jaundice in the newborn baby and because they also cause a reduction in the total volume of the blood.

Interactions with other drugs:

Anti-arrhythmic drugs: if potassium loss occurs, amiodarone, disopyramide, flecainide, and sotalol are more likely to have adverse effects on the heart and the action of lidocaine is antagonized.

Antihypertensive drugs: their effects in lowering blood pressure are increased.

Antipsychotic drugs: if potassium loss occurs, amisulpride, pimozide, and sertindole are more likely to cause *arrhythmias.

Atomoxetine: the risk of arrhythmias is increased if potassium concentrations are low.

Corticosteroids: may further increase the loss of potassium when taken with thiazide diuretics.

Digitalis drugs: the adverse effects of these drugs may be increased if potassium concentrations are low.

Lithium: concentrations of lithium may be increased, leading to the risk of serious side effects.

NSAIDs: may reduce the diuretic effect of thiazides, requiring dosage modification, and the risk of kidney damage may be increased.

thioguanine *See* TIOGUANINE.

thiopental <thiopentone> *See* BARBITURATES.

thiotepa An *alkylating drug that is administered directly into the chest or abdomen to treat metastases in accumulations of fluid that are caused by certain *cancers. It is also instilled into the bladder to treat bladder cancer and is occasionally used to treat breast cancer. Thiotepa is available as an injection on *prescription only.

Side effects and precautions: *see* CYTOTOXIC DRUGS.
Interactions with other drugs:

Clozapine: increases the risk of agranulocytosis (a blood disorder) and should not be taken with thiotepa.

thromboembolism *See* THROMBOSIS.

thrombolytic drugs *See* FIBRINOLYTIC DRUGS.

thrombosis Blockage of a blood vessel by a blood clot (thrombus). Blood clots can form in arteries or veins. Thrombosis in an artery obstructs the blood flow to the tissue it supplies: obstruction of an artery to the brain is one of the causes of a stroke, and thrombosis in an artery supplying the heart (**coronary thrombosis**) results in a heart attack. Obstruction of a vein by a blood clot is most common in the deep veins of the calf of the leg (**deep-vein thrombosis**; **DVT**). A blood clot may form in one place, break off, and be carried in the blood to block another vessel some distance away; this is known as **thromboembolism**. For example, a blood clot that breaks off from a larger clot in a leg vein often lodges in the pulmonary artery, which brings blood to the lungs, resulting in **pulmonary embolism**.

Drugs used in the prevention and treatment of thrombosis and thromboembolism include *anticoagulants, *antiplatelet drugs, and *fibrinolytic drugs.

thrush *See* ANTIFUNGAL DRUGS.

Thwart (Alliance) *See* SALICYLIC ACID.

Thymoglobuline (Genzyme Therapeutics) *See* ANTI-HUMAN THYMOCYTE IMMUNOGLOBULIN.

thymol An aromatic liquid extracted from thyme oil. An antiseptic with antibacterial and antifungal activity, it is used in combination with *glycerin (**compound thymol glycerin**) as a mouthwash to relieve the pain of mouth ulcers and for general oral hygiene. It is also included, with other volatile substances, in inhalations for the relief of coughs, colds, and nasal congestion. Preparations containing thymol are freely available *over the counter.
Side effects: if swallowed, thymol may irritate the stomach.
Proprietary preparation: *Karvol (combined with other aromatic substances and chlorobutanol).

t

thymoxamine *See* MOXISYLYTE.

Thyrogen (Genzyme Therapeutics) *See* THYROTROPIN ALFA.

thyroid hormones Two iodine-containing hormones, **thyroxine** (**T_4**) and **triiodothyronine** (**T_3**), that are secreted by the thyroid gland. They are essential for normal metabolic processes and mental and physical development. Lack of these hormones, resulting from underactivity of the thyroid gland (**hypothyroidism**), causes mental and physical slowing, undue sensitivity to cold, slowing of the pulse, weight gain, and coarsening of the skin (**myxoedema**). Hypothyroidism may develop in those who have received treatment for an overactive thyroid gland. If present at birth, lack of thyroid hormones causes mental retardation and stunted growth (the condition of **cretinism**). Treatment of hypothyroidism is with *levothyroxine sodium or *liothyronine; affected babies must be treated promptly for normal development to occur.

Excessive amounts of thyroid hormones in the bloodstream causes **thyrotoxicosis**, producing a rapid heartbeat, sweating, tremor, anxiety, increased appetite, loss of weight, and intolerance of heat. Causes include simple overactivity of the thyroid gland (**hyperthyroidism**), a hormone-secreting tumour of the gland, and **Graves' disease**, in which there are additional symptoms, including swelling of the neck (**goitre**), due to enlargement of the gland, and protrusion of the eyes (**exophthalmos**). Treatment may be by the use of antithyroid drugs (*see* CARBIMAZOLE; PROPYLTHIOURACIL; IODINE), which interfere with the production of thyroid hormones. Alternatively, radioactive iodine is given by mouth to destroy some thyroid tissue, or part of the thyroid gland is surgically removed.

thyrotoxicosis *See* THYROID HORMONES.

thyrotropin alfa A genetically engineered form of thyroid-stimulating hormone used to detect remnants of thyroid tissue in patients with thyroid cancer who have had their thyroid gland removed by surgery. If remnants are present, thyrotropin alfa will stimulate them to produce thyroid hormones, which can be measured in the blood. Thyrotropin alfa is given by intramuscular injection and is available on *prescription only.
Side effects: may include nausea, vomiting, dizziness, and fatigue.
Precautions: thyrotropin alfa should not be given to women who are pregnant or breastfeeding.
Proprietary preparation: Thyrogen.

thyroxine sodium *See* LEVOTHYROXINE SODIUM.

tiagabine An *anticonvulsant drug used as an *adjunct in the treatment of partial epileptic seizures. It is available as tablets on *prescription only.
Side effects: include diarrhoea, dizziness, tiredness, difficulty in concentrating, tremor, mood changes, and impaired speech.
Precautions: tiagabine may impair driving ability and the performance of other skilled tasks. It should be used with caution in patients with liver disease.
Interactions with other drugs:
Antidepressants: antagonize the anticonvulsant effect of tiagabine.
Mefloquine: antagonizes the anticonvulsant effect of tiagabine.
Proprietary preparation: Gabitril.

tiaprofenic acid An *NSAID used for the treatment of pain and inflammation in rheumatoid arthritis and other disorders of the joints or muscles. It is available as tablets on *prescription only.
Side effects and precautions: *see* NSAIDs. Tiaprofenic acid may cause severe

cystitis and should not be taken by people with urinary disorders. If symptoms of cystitis develop (such as frequency or pain in passing urine or blood in the urine) treatment should be stopped and a doctor informed.
Interactions with other drugs: *see* NSAIDs.
Proprietary preparation: Surgam.

tibolone A synthetic steroid that mimics the effects of *oestrogens and *progestogens (it also has weak androgenic effects). It is used for the relief of hot flushes and other physical symptoms of the menopause and helps to relieve depression and decreased libido. It is also used to prevent osteoporosis in postmenopausal women. If natural periods have been absent for a year or more before taking tibolone, the lining of the uterus will not be stimulated and bleeding will not occur; otherwise there may be some irregular vaginal bleeding (*see* HORMONE REPLACEMENT THERAPY). Tibolone is available as tablets on *prescription only.
Side effects: include changes in body weight, dizziness, headache, migraine, visual disturbances, dermatitis, skin rashes and itching, vaginal bleeding, stomach upsets, and growth of facial hair.
Precautions: tibolone should not be taken during pregnancy or breastfeeding or by women with hormone-dependent tumours, undiagnosed vaginal bleeding, a history of cardiovascular disorders, or severe liver disorders. It should be taken with caution by women with epilepsy, migraine, or diabetes.
Interactions with other drugs:
Antiepileptic drugs: carbamazepine, phenobarbital, phenytoin, and primidone reduce the effect of tibolone.
Rifampicin: reduces the effect of tibolone.
Proprietary preparation: Livial.

ticarcillin A broad-spectrum *penicillin that is active against *Pseudomonas* and *Proteus* bacteria. It is used in combination with *clavulanic acid for the treatment of systemic (generalized) and local infections (such as infected wounds or burns) and respiratory and urinary-tract infections. Given by infusion, it is available on *prescription only. It is sometimes used in conjunction with an *aminoglycoside antibiotic.

Side effects, precautions, and interactions with other drugs: *see* BENZYLPENICILLIN.
Proprietary preparation: *Timentin (combined with clavulanic acid).

Tifaxin XL (Genus) *See* VENLAFAXINE.

tigecycline An antibiotic related to the *tetracyclines, used for the treatment of complicated skin, soft tissue, and abdominal infections that are resistant to other antibiotics, including meticilllin-resistant *Staphylococcus aureus* (MRSA). It is given by intravenous infusion and is available on *prescription only.
Side effects, precautions, and interactions with other drugs: *see* TETRACYCLINES.
Proprietary preparation: Tygacil.

Tiger Balm (SLL International) A proprietary combination of *camphor, *clove oil, *menthol, *peppermint oil, and *cajuput oil, used as a *rubefacient for the relief of minor muscular aches and pains. It is freely available *over the counter.
Side effects and precautions: *see* RUBEFACIENTS.

Tilade CFC-free Inhaler (sanofi-aventis) *See* NEDOCROMIL SODIUM.

Tildiem LA, Tildiem Retard (sanofi-aventis) *See* DILTIAZEM HYDROCHLORIDE.

Tiloryth (Tillomed Laboratories) *See* ERYTHROMYCIN.

tiludronic acid A *bisphosphonate used for the treatment of Paget's disease, in which the bones are deformed and fracture easily. It is available as tablets on *prescription only.
Side effects: include stomach pain, nausea, diarrhoea, and (rarely) weakness of the muscles, dizziness, headache, and rashes.
Precautions: tiludronic acid should not be taken by women who are pregnant or breastfeeding. It should be used with caution in people with kidney disease.
Interactions with other drugs:
Aminoglycosides: in combination with tiludronic acid, they may cause abnormally low concentrations of calcium in the plasma.
Antacids: reduce the absorption of tiludronic acid.
Calcium supplements: reduce the absorption of tiludronic acid.
Iron supplements (oral): reduce the absorption of tiludronic acid.
Proprietary preparation: Skelid.

Timentin (GlaxoSmithKline) A proprietary combination of *ticarcillin (a penicillin) and *clavulanic acid (a penicillinase inhibitor), used for the treatment of severe infections in hospitalized patients with suppressed or impaired immune systems (*see* TICARCILLIN). It is available, on *prescription only, in a form for injection or infusion.
Side effects, precautions, and interactions with other drugs: *see* BENZYLPENICILLIN.

Timodine (Forum Health Products Limited) A proprietary combination of *nystatin (an antifungal agent), *hydrocortisone (a corticosteroid), *benzalkonium chloride (an antiseptic), and *dimeticone (a water repellent), used for the treatment of a variety of skin conditions and napkin rash infected with *Candida*. It is available as a cream on *prescription only and should be stored in a refrigerator.
Side effects and precautions: *see* TOPICAL STEROIDS.

timolol maleate A *beta blocker used for the treatment of *hypertension, *angina, and after heart attacks to prevent recurrence. It is also used to prevent the occurrence of *migraine and as eye drops for the treatment of *glaucoma. Timodol is available, on *prescription only, as tablets or eye drops.

Side effects, precautions, and interactions with other drugs: *see* BETA BLOCKERS.
Proprietary preparations: Betim; Nyogel (eye drops); Timoptol (eye drops); Timoptol LA (long-acting eye drops); *Azarga (combined with brinzolamide); *Combigan (combined with brimonidine); *Cosopt (combined with dorzolamide); *DuoTrav (combined with travoprost); *Ganfort (combined with bimatoprot); *Prestim (combined with bendroflumethiazide); *Xalacom (combined with latanoprost).

See also ANTI-ARRHYTHMIC DRUGS.

Timoptol, Timoptol LA (Merck Sharp & Dohme) *See* TIMOLOL MALEATE.

tincture A medicinal preparation consisting of an extract of a drug derived from a plant in a solution of alcohol. Many plants contain active ingredients that are used as drugs and are extracted in this way.

tinea *See* ANTIVIRAL DRUGS.

tinidazole An *antibiotic that is active against protozoa (including amoebae) and some bacteria. It is similar to *metronidazole and has similar uses, including the treatment or prevention of intestinal amoebic infections (such as amoebic dysentery), giardiasis (a protozoal infection of the intestines), bacterial infections of the vagina or urethra, and ulceration of the gums and gingivitis. Tinidazole is longer acting than metronidazole and therefore needs to be taken only once daily. It is available as tablets on *prescription only.
Side effects: include nausea, vomiting, stomach upset, furred tongue, an unpleasant taste in the mouth, itching, swelling of the face, and darkening of the urine. Long-term therapy can decrease the numbers of white blood cells.
Precautions: the combination of alcohol and tinidazole may lead to vomiting, therefore alcohol should be avoided during treatment. Tinidazole should not be taken by women during the first three months of pregnancy and should be used with caution during the remainder of the pregnancy.
Proprietary preparation: Fasigyn.

t

tinzaparin sodium A *low molecular weight heparin used for the prevention and treatment of deep-vein *thrombosis and in the treatment of pulmonary embolism. It is also used in patients undergoing kidney dialysis, in order to prevent the formation of blood clots. Tinzaparin is available as a solution for subcutaneous injection on *prescription only.
Side effects, precautions, and interactions with other drugs: *see* HEPARIN.
Proprietary preparation: Innohep.

tioconazole An imidazole *antifungal drug that is active against a wide range of fungi. It is used for the treatment of fungal infections of the nail bed and is available, on *prescription only, as a solution for painting on the nails.
Side effects: there may be mild local irritation.
Precautions: tioconazole should not be used during pregnancy.
Proprietary preparation: Trosyl.

tioguanine <thioguanine> An *antimetabolite used for the treatment of acute myeloid and lymphocytic leukaemia (*see* CANCER), particularly in children. It is available as tablets on *prescription only.
Side effects and precautions: *see* MERCAPTOPURINE; CYTOTOXIC DRUGS.
Interactions with other drugs:
Clozapine: increases the risk of agranulocytosis (a blood disorder) and should not be taken with tioguanine.
Proprietary preparation: Lanvis.

tiotropium An *antimuscarinic drug used as a *bronchodilator for the treatment of chronic obstructive pulmonary disease. It is available as a powder or aerosol for inhalation on *prescription only.
Side effects and precautions: *see* IPRATROPIUM BROMIDE.
Proprietary preparation: Spiriva.

tipranavir A protease inhibitor (*see* ANTIVIRAL DRUGS) used, in combination with other antiretroviral drugs, for the treatment of HIV infection that has not responded to other protease inhibitors. It is available as capsules and an oral solution on *prescription only.
Side effects: include diarrhoea, nausea, vomiting, abdominal pain, indigestion, abdominal distension, liver damage, fatigue, itching, loss of appitite, peripheral neuropathy (causing tingling and numbness in the limbs), and dizziness.
Precautions: tipranavir should not be taken by people with impaired liver function or by women who are breastfeeding. It should be used during pregnancy only if the potential benefit justifies the potential risk to the fetus. Liver function tests should be carried out before and during treatment, which should be stopped if signs of liver damage (e.g. jaundice) occur.
Interactions with other drugs: tipranavir inhibits several enzymes systems in the liver that are involved in metabolizing drugs and also interacts with a number of other drugs. A doctor should therefore be consulted before tipranavir is taken with any other drug.
Proprietary preparation: Aptivus.

tirofiban An *antiplatelet drug used to prevent heart attacks in people with unstable *angina who have had recent chest pain (within the preceding 12 hours). Tirofiban is used only under specialist supervision. It is available as an intravenous infusion on *prescription only.
Side effects: include excessive bleeding.
Precautions: tirofiban should not be given to people who have had recent bleeding or a recent stroke (within the previous 30 days), or have any other risk factors for spontaneous bleeding. It should not be given to people with severely impaired liver function or to women who are breastfeeding. It should be used with caution in people who have had recent surgery or trauma, any condition that increases the risk of bleeding, severe heart failure, or anaemia. Platelet counts and haemoglobin concentrations should be monitored during treatment, which should be stopped if serious bleeding occurs.
Proprietary preparation: Aggrastat.

Tisept, Tisept Concentrate (Medlock Medical) Proprietary combinations of the antiseptics *chlorhexidine gluconate and *cetrimide, used for cleansing and disinfecting wounds and burns, changing dressings, and in obstetrical procedures. They are available as solutions without a prescription, but only from pharmacies.
Side effects: *see* CETRIMIDE.
Precautions: the solution should not come into contact with the eyes.

titanium dioxide A white compound that protects the skin and reflects sunlight. It is an ingredient of many *sunscreen preparations, since it protects the skin against the damaging effects of ultraviolet light (both UVA and UVB). It is also included in *barrier preparations for the prevention of napkin rash. Preparations containing titanium dioxide are freely available *over the counter.
Proprietary preparations: *Ambre Solaire (combined with UVB-absorbing agents); *Metanium (combined with a water-repellent emollient base); *SpectraBan (combined with UVB-absorbing agents); *Uvistat (combined with UVB-absorbing agents).

Tixylix Baby Syrup, Tixylix Toddler Syrup (Novartis) *See* GLYCERIN.

Tixylix Chesty Cough (Novartis) *See* GUAIFENESIN.

Tixylix Cough & Cold (Novartis) A proprietary combination of *chlorphenamine maleate (an antihistamine), *pholcodine (a cough suppressant), and *pseudoephedrine (a decongestant), used for the relief of dry irritating coughs and the running nose, congestion, and other symptoms associated with colds. It is available as a linctus without a prescription, but only from pharmacies.
Side effects and interactions with other drugs: *see* ANTIHISTAMINES; EPHEDRINE HYDROCHLORIDE; DECONGESTANTS; PHOLCODINE.
Precautions: this medicine is not recommended for children under one year old. *See also* ANTIHISTAMINES; EPHEDRINE HYDROCHLORIDE; DECONGESTANTS; OPIOIDS.

Tixylix Dry Cough (Novartis) *See* PHOLCODINE.

Tixylix Night Cough (Novartis) A proprietary combination of *pholcodine (a cough suppressant) and *promethazine hydrochloride (a sedative antihistamine), used to relieve the symptoms of coughs and colds, especially irritating dry coughs that interfere with sleep. It is available as a linctus without a prescription, but only from pharmacies. It cannot be prescribed on the NHS.
Side effects and interactions with other drugs: *see* PHOLCODINE; ANTIHISTAMINES.
Precautions: this medicine is not recommended for children under one year old. *See also* OPIOIDS; ANTIHISTAMINES.

tizanidine A *muscle relaxant that is used for the relief of spasticity

associated with multiple sclerosis or injury or disease of the spinal cord. It is available as tablets on *prescription only.
Side effects: include drowsiness, fatigue, dizziness, dry mouth, nausea, stomach upset, and low blood pressure.
Precautions: tizanidine should not be taken by people with severe liver disease, and should be used with caution in women who are pregnant or breastfeeding and in elderly people. Tizanidine enhances the sedative effects of alcohol.
Interactions with other drugs:
Antihypertensive drugs: tizanidine increases their effects in lowering blood pressure.
Anxiolytics and hypnotic drugs: tizanidine enhances their sedative effects.
Ciprofloxacin: increases the plasma concentration of tizanidine (and the risk of toxic effects) and should not be used with it.
Digoxin: heart rate may be slowed if digoxin is given with tizanidine.
Diuretics: tizanidine enhances their effects in lowering blood pressure.
Fluvoxamine: increases the plasma concentration of tizanidine (and the risk of toxic effects) and should not be used with it.
Proprietary preparation: Zanaflex.

Tobi (Novartis) *See* TOBRAMYCIN.

Tobradex (Alcon Laboratories (U.K) Limited) A proprietary combination of *dexamethasone (a corticosteroid) and *tobramycin (an aminoglycoside antibiotic), used to reduce inflammation and prevent infection during and following cataract operations. It is available as eye drops on *prescription only.
Side effects: include itching and swelling of the eyelid, reddening of the conjunctiva, and thinning of the cornea.
Precautions: Tobradex should not be used by people with viral, bacterial, or fungal infections of the eye.

tobramycin An *aminoglycoside antibiotic used for the treatment of serious infections that are resistant to *gentamicin. It is also used to treat eye infections. It is given as an *intramuscular or *intravenous injection, as a solution for use in a *nebulizer, or as eye drops and is available on *prescription only.
Side effects, precautions, and interactions with other drugs: *see* GENTAMICIN.
Proprietary preparations: Bramitob (nebulizer); Tobi (nebulizer); Tobravisc (eye drops); *Tobradex (combined with dexamethasone).

Tobravisc (Alcon Laboratories (U.K) Limited) *See* TOBRAMYCIN.

tocopherols *See* VITAMIN E.

Toctino (Basilea Pharmaceuticals Ltd) *See* ALITRETINOIN.

tolbutamide A *sulphonylurea used for the treatment of type II (noninsulin-dependent) *diabetes mellitus. It is available as tablets on *prescription only.

Side effects, precautions, and interactions with other drugs: *see* SULPHONYLUREAS.

tolcapone A *dopamine receptor agonist used as an *adjunct to *levodopa (with carbidopa or benserazide) for treating Parkinson's disease. It is used under specialist supervision and is available as tablets on *prescription only.
Side effects: include nausea, vomiting, abdominal pain, constipation, loss of appetite, liver damage (see Precautions below), somnolence, and involuntary muscle movements.
Precautions: among other conditions, tolcapone should not be given to people with liver disease or phaeochromocytoma (a tumour of the adrenal gland) or to breastfeeding women. There is a risk of liver damage, and liver function tests should be carried out every two weeks for the first year of treatment, then every four weeks for the next six months, and then every eight weeks. If symptoms of liver damage (e.g. itching, fatigue, dark-coloured urine) develop, a doctor should be consulted.
Proprietary preparation: Tasmar.

tolerance The reduction or loss of the normal response to a drug or other substance that usually provokes a reaction in the body. Tolerance may develop after taking a particular drug over a long period of time. In such cases the dosage of the drug may need to be increased in order to produce the desired effect. Examples of drugs that bring about tolerance are *ephedrine (used in nasal decongestants), *glyceryl trinitrate (for treating angina), and *opioids (used for pain relief). Tolerance does not imply *dependence, although some drugs that cause tolerance also cause dependence.

tolfenamic acid An *NSAID used to relieve the pain of *migraine attacks. It is available as tablets on *prescription only.
Side effects: *see* NSAIDs. Additional side effects may include difficulty or pain in passing urine (especially in men) and tremor.
Precautions and interactions with other drugs: *see* NSAIDs.
Proprietary preparation: Clotam Rapid.

tolnaftate An *antifungal drug that is active against a wide range of fungi, but not *Candida* (causing thrush). It is used for the treatment and prevention of various forms of tinea (ringworm) and pityriasis versicolor, a chronic fungal infection of the skin; it is not suitable for deep-seated infections of the nail bed. Tolnaftate is available, alone or in combination with other drugs, as a foot spray, ointment, powder, or cream; most preparations can be obtained without a prescription.
Proprietary preparations: Boots Dual Action Athlete's Foot Spray; Mycil Foot Spray; *Boots Dual Action Athlete's Foot Cream (combined with benzalkonium chloride); *Boots Dual Action Athlete's Foot Powder (combined with chlorhexidine hydrochloride).

tolterodine tartrate An *antimuscarinic drug used to treat urinary incontinence and abnormal frequency or urgency in passing urine. It is available as tablets or *modified-release capsules on *prescription only.

Side effects: include dry mouth, constipation, indigestion, nausea, abdominal discomfort, flatulence, vomiting, headache, dry skin, dry eyes, drowsiness, nervousness, tingling in the fingers, and (more rarely) blurred vision, chest pain, and difficulty in passing urine.
Precautions: tolterodine should not be taken by people with urinary retention, uncontrolled acute glaucoma, myasthenia gravis, or severe ulcerative colitis or by women who are pregnant or breastfeeding. It should be used with caution in people in whom the outlet of the bladder is obstructed (for example by an enlarged prostate) and in those with a hiatus hernia, disease of peripheral nerves, or impaired liver or kidney function.
Interactions with other drugs:
Anti-arrhythmic drugs: the risk of ventricular *arrhythmias is increased if amiodarone, disopyramide, or flecainide are taken with tolterodine.
Sotalol: increases the risk of ventricular arrhythmias if taken with tolterodine.
See also ANTIMUSCARINIC DRUGS.
Proprietary preparations: Detrusitol; Detrusitol XL (modified-release capsules).

tolvaptan A drug that blocks the action of *vasopressin (antidiuretic hormone), used to treat hyponatraemia (low levels of potassium in the blood) by promoting the excretion of water in the urine, Hyponatraemia is associated with congestive heart failure, cirrhosis, and syndrome of inappropriate antidiuretic hormone (SIADH; in which high plasma levels of vasopressin result in the retention of water). Tolvaptan is available as tablets on *presrcription only.
Side effects: include thirst, dry mouth, nausea, constipation, and decreased appetite.
Precautions: tolvaptan should not be taken by women who are pregnant or breastfeeding, and women capable of bearing children should use effective contraception during treatment.
Interactions with other drugs: tolvaptan is metabolized by an enzyme system in the liver that is inhibited by a number of other drugs, including ketoconazole, voriconazole, ritonavir, macrolide antibiotics, and diltiazam. These drugs therefore increase the plasma concentration of tolvaptan and should be used with caution.
Digoxin: its plasma concentration is increased by tolvaptan.
Proprietary name: Samsca.

Tomudex (Hospira) *See* RALTITREXED.

tonic A medicinal preparation purporting to increase vigour and liveliness and produce a feeling of wellbeing. Ingredients of tonics include bitters, which are supposed to increase the appetite; minerals, such as iron; and vitamins. Any beneficial effects of tonics, however, are likely to be due to their *placebo effect.

Topal (Pierre Fabre) A proprietary combination of *alginic acid, *aluminium

t

hydroxide, and *magnesium carbonate, used as an *antacid for the treatment of indigestion, heartburn and oesophagitis due to reflux, and gastritis (*see* ACID-PEPTIC DISEASES). It is freely available *over the counter in the form of tablets.
Side effects and interactions with other drugs: *see* ANTACIDS.
Precautions: Topal has a high sugar content and should therefore be used with caution by people with diabetes.

Topamax (Janssen-Cilag) *See* TOPIRAMATE.

topical Describing the route of administration of a drug that is applied directly to the surface of the body, where its effects are required. The term usually refers to application of a drug, in the form of a cream, ointment, or gel, to a region of skin, but is also used for application to the eyes, ears, nasal passages, and mouth cavity. Since a drug administered topically is intended to exert its effects only locally, any *systemic effects would be unwanted. Most drugs applied to the skin and other surfaces are not absorbed into the circulation and therefore do not reach other parts of the body. However, potent drugs (notably corticosteroids), for example in ointments and eye drops, can be absorbed and have systemic effects.

topical steroids *Corticosteroids formulated for use on the skin. They reduce inflammation and are effective for treating such conditions as *eczema, dermatitis, and *psoriasis. Steroids may also be used to reduce keloid scars and granulomas (growths of tissue that form over wounds or healing ulcers). Topical steroids may also be used in the nose, eyes, and ears; nasal preparations may be used for the treatment of hay fever. The side effects of topical steroids are less severe than those of systemic steroids, but care must still be taken; the number and degree of side effects will depend on the strength of the steroid, the duration of treatment, and the area of the body being treated. Topical steroids are classified in four groups: mild, moderately potent, potent, and very potent. More steroid is absorbed from the face, the genitals, and areas where skin surfaces rub together (as in the groin); there is little absorption from nose, ear, or eye preparations. Potent topical steroids are not usually used in children. Some compound preparations for topical use combine corticosteroids with antibiotics or antifungal agents; these must also be used with care, as the steroid will be absorbed.

See ALCLOMETASONE DIPROPIONATE; BECLOMETASONE DIPROPIONATE; BETAMETHASONE; CLOBETASOL PROPIONATE; CLOBETASONE BUTYRATE; DIFLUCORTOLONE VALERATE; FLUMETASONE PIVALATE; FLUOCINOLONE ACETONIDE; FLUOCINONIDE; FLUOCORTOLONE; FLUDROXYCORTIDE; HYDROCORTISONE; HYDROCORTISONE BUTYRATE; MOMETASONE FUROATE.
Side effects: there may be local irritation and allergic reactions at the site of application; disturbances in taste or smell may occur with nasal sprays. With long-term use of potent topical steroids, the most common side effect is atrophy (thinning) of the skin, with the development of stretch marks (striae) and possibly localized collections of fine blood vessels, which appear as red – sometimes spidery – spots. There may be increased growth of hair. Very potent

preparations may be absorbed through the skin and produce effects throughout the body (*see* CORTICOSTEROIDS).
Precautions: topical steroids should not be used to treat acne or rosacea (since they will exacerbate these conditions), dermatitis around the mouth, scabies, leg ulcers, ringworm, or viral skin diseases. They should not be used for bacterial or fungal infections unless antimicrobials are used as well. Topical steroids should not be used for ear or eye infections if viral, tuberculous, or purulent infections are present. Extensive use during pregnancy should be avoided. Use of steroids on the face and in children should be limited to five days unless a specialist has advised longer treatment; steroids should not be used for prolonged periods to treat nappy rash. Topical steroids should be withdrawn gradually after prolonged use.

topiramate A drug used alone or as an *adjunct in the treatment of tonic-clonic and partial seizures of epilepsy and (under specialist supervision) alone for the prevention of migraine attacks. It is available as tablets or capsules on *prescription only.
Side effects: include shaky movements, impaired concentration, confusion, dizziness, fatigue, tingling, agitation, and depression.
Precautions: topiramate should not be taken by women who are breastfeeding. Dosage should be reduced gradually at the end of treatment.
Interactions with other drugs:

Anticonvulsants: carbamazepine and phenytoin often lower the plasma concentration of topiramate; topiramate increases the plasma concentration of phenytoin.
Antidepressants: antagonize the anticoagulant effect of topiramate.
Mefloquine: antagonizes the anticoagulant effect of topiramate.
Oral contraceptives: the contraceptive effect of these drugs is reduced by topiramate.

Proprietary preparation: Topamax.

topoisomerase inhibitors A class of *cytotoxic drugs that block the action of topoisomerase, an enzyme that is required for DNA replication and hence cell division. Topoisomerase inhibitors are therefore used to treat *cancer, in which rapid cell division must be prevented. The drugs of this class are *irinotecan and *topotecan.

topotecan A *topoisomerase inhibitor used for the treatment of *cancer of the ovaries that has spread to other parts of the body and has not responded to other treatments. It may also be used to treat a certain form of lung cancer (small cell lung cancer) that has not responded to other therapy and (in combination with cisplatin) cervical cancer after radiotherapy. Topotecan is available as capsules and a form for intravenous infusion on *prescription only.
Side effects: include *bone marrow suppression, hair loss, nausea, abdominal pain, loss of appetite, sore mouth, fatigue, and weakness.
Precautions: topotecan should not be given to patients with severe liver or

kidney disease or bone marrow suppression, or to women who are pregnant or breastfeeding. *See also* CYTOTOXIC DRUGS.
Proprietary preparation: Hycamtin.

Toradol (Roche Products) *See* KETOROLAC TROMETAMOL.

torasemide A *loop diuretic used for the treatment of *oedema associated with liver or kidney disease and for pulmonary oedema (fluid in the spaces of the lungs causing breathing difficulties) associated with heart failure. It is also used to treat hypertension. It is available as tablets or an injection on *prescription only.
Side effects, precautions, and interactions with other drugs: *see* LOOP DIURETICS.
Proprietary preparation: Torem.
See also DIURETICS.

Torem (Meda Pharmaceuticals) *See* TORASEMIDE.

toremifene An *oestrogen antagonist used for the treatment of advanced breast cancer in postmenopausal women in which oestrogens stimulate growth of the tumour (*see* CANCER). It is available as tablets on *prescription only.
Side effects: include hot flushes, vaginal bleeding or discharge, sweating, nausea, vomiting, dizziness, fluid retention, and chest or back pain. Vaginal bleeding or discharge or pelvic pain should be reported to a doctor promptly to exclude the possibility of cancer of the endometrium (womb lining).
Precautions: toremifene should not be taken by women who are pregnant or breastfeeding or by those who have severe liver disease, hyperplasia (overgrowth) of the endometrium, or a history of arrhythmias. It should be used with caution in women with high concentrations of calcium in the blood or severe thromboembolic disease.
Interactions with other drugs:
Anticoagulants: toremifene increases the effects of warfarin and acenocoumarol.
Antiepileptic drugs: the effects of toremifene may be reduced by carbamazepine, phenobarbital, phenytoin, and primidone.
Thiazide diuretics: increase the risk of high concentrations of calcium in the blood, especially in women in whom the cancer has spread to the bones.
Proprietary preparation: Fareston.

Torisel (Pfizer) *See* TEMSIROLIMUS.

Tostran (ProStrakan) *See* TESTOSTERONE.

Toviaz (Pfizer) *See* FESOTERODINE.

trabectedin A *cytotoxic drug used for the treatment of advanced cancer of the soft tissues (including muscle). It is given by intravenous infusion, in

combination with *dexamethasone (which protects against nausea and liver damage), and is available on *prescription only.
Side effects: *see* CYTOTOXIC DRUGS. Other side effects may include abdominal pain, diarrhoea, constipation, indigestion, liver and gall bladder disorders, and 'pins and needles'.
Precautions: trabectedin should not be given to people with raised levels of bilirubin (a bile pigment) in the blood or kidney disease or to women who are pregnant or breastfeeding. Liver function and blood counts should be monitored and alcohol should be avoided during treatment.
Interactions with other drugs:
Clozapine: should not be given with trabectedin as this combination increases the risk of agranulocytosis (a blood disorder).
Proprietary preparation: Yondelis.

Tracleer (Actelion Pharmaceuticals UK) *See* BOSENTAN.

Tractocile (Ferring Pharmaceuticals) *See* ATOSIBAN.

Tradorec XL (Labopharm) *See* TRAMADOL HYDROCHLORIDE.

Tramacet (Janssen-Cilag) A proprietary combination of *paracetamol (a non-opioid analgesic) and *tramadol hydrochloride (an opioid analgesic), used for the relief of moderate to severe pain. It is available as tablets on *prescription only.
Side effects and precautions: *see* PARACETAMOL; TRAMADOL HYDROCHLORIDE.
Interactions with other drugs: *see* TRAMADOL HYDROCHLORIDE.

tramadol hydrochloride An *opioid analgesic used for the treatment of moderate to severe pain. It causes less depression of breathing and constipation than other opioids and is less likely to cause dependence. Tramadol is available, on *prescription only, as capsules, soluble tablets, dispersible tablets, *modified-release capsules and tablets, and an injection.
Side effects: include low blood pressure and (occasionally) high blood pressure, hallucinations, and confusion. *See also* MORPHINE.
Precautions: tramadol should not be given to people who have uncontrolled epilepsy and should be used with caution in women who are pregnant or breastfeeding. *See also* MORPHINE.
Interactions with other drugs:
Anticoagulants: the effects of warfarin and acenocoumarol are enhanced.
Antidepressants: the risk of convulsions may be increased if tramadol is taken with tricyclic antidepressants or SSRIs.
Carbamazepine: reduces the effects of tramadol.
See also OPIOIDS.
Proprietary preparations: Mabron (modified-release tablets); Tradorec XL (modified-release tablets); Tramake (capsules); Zamadol (capsules); Zamadol Melt (dispersible tablets); Zamadol SR, Zamadol 24hr (modified-release capsules); Zeridame SR (modified-release tablets); Zydol; Zydol SR, Zydol XL (modified-release tablets); *Tramacet (combined with paracetamol).

Tramake (Galen) *See* TRAMADOL HYDROCHLORIDE.

Trandate (UCB Pharma) *See* LABETALOL HYDROCHLORIDE.

trandolapril An *ACE inhibitor used after a heart attack to prevent deterioration of left ventricular function and to treat mild to moderate *hypertension. It is available as capsules on *prescription only.
Side effects, precautions, and interactions with other drugs: *see* ACE INHIBITORS.
Proprietary preparations: Gopten; *Tarka (combined with verapamil).
See also ANTIHYPERTENSIVE DRUGS.

tranexamic acid A drug that prevents the breakdown of blood clots in the circulation (fibrinolysis). It acts by preventing the activation of the enzyme that digests fibrin, the protein in blood clots, i.e. it is an antifibrinolytic drug (*see* HAEMOSTATIC DRUGS). Tranexamic acid is used to reduce excessive menstrual bleeding, especially when this is caused by an intrauterine contraceptive device (IUCD) and the woman does not wish to change to another form of contraception. It is also used to control excessive bleeding after surgery or tooth extraction. Tranexamic acid is available, on *prescription only, as tablets or a solution for intravenous injection or infusion.
Side effects: include nausea, vomiting, diarrhoea, and giddiness if the drug is injected rapidly.
Precautions: tranexamic acid should not be taken by people with thromboembolic disease (*see* THROMBOSIS) and should be used with caution in people with kidney disease or haematuria (blood in the urine).
Proprietary preparation: Cyklokapron.

Trangina XL (Actavis) *See* ISOSORBIDE MONONITRATE.

tranquillizers *See* ANTIPSYCHOTIC DRUGS; ANXIOLYTIC DRUGS.

transdermal Across the skin: describing a route of administration of drugs that enables them to be absorbed slowly and steadily into the circulation. Such drugs are usually incorporated into adhesive patches; examples are nicotine (for treating smoking dependence), female sex hormones for (*hormone replacement therapy), and nitrates (for angina).

Transiderm-Nitro (Novartis) *See* GLYCERYL TRINITRATE.

Transtec (Napp Pharmaceuticals Limited) *See* BUPRENORPHINE.

Transvasin Heat Rub (SSL International) A proprietary combination of *ethyl nicotinate, *hexyl nicotinate, and tetrahydrofurfuryl salicylate (*see* SALICYLATES), used as a *rubefacient for the relief of muscular aches and pains, sprains, and strains. It is freely available *over the counter in the form of a cream.
Side effects and precautions: *see* RUBEFACIENTS.

Transvasin Heat Spray (SSL International) A proprietary combination of

*2-hydroxyethyl salicylate, *diethylamine salicylate, and *methyl nicotinate, used as a *rubefacient for the relief of muscular aches and pains. It is freely available *over the counter.
Side effects and precautions: *see* RUBEFACIENTS.

tranylcypromine A *monoamine oxidase inhibitor used for the treatment of depressive illness. It is available as tablets on *prescription only.
Side effects and precautions: *see* MONOAMINE OXIDASE INHIBITORS. Tranylcypromine causes insomnia if taken in the evening; it should therefore not be taken later than 3 pm.
Interactions with other drugs: *see* MONOAMINE OXIDASE INHIBITORS.

Trasicor (Amdipharm) *See* OXPRENOLOL HYDROCHLORIDE.

Trasidrex (Goldshield) A proprietary combination of *oxprenolol hydrochloride (a beta blocker), and *cyclopenthiazide (a thiazide diuretic), used in the treatment of mild to moderate *hypertension. It is available as tablets on *prescription only.
Side effects, precautions, and interactions with other drugs: *see* BETA BLOCKERS; THIAZIDE DIURETICS.
See also ANTIHYPERTENSIVE DRUGS; DIURETICS.

trastuzumab A *monoclonal antibody used for the treatment of early and advanced breast cancer in which the tumour cells are covered with excess amounts of a protein, human epidermal growth factor 2 (HER2), that stimulates tumour growth. It works by binding to the HER2 receptors and thereby blocking their action. Trastuzumab is used alone or in combination with a *taxane or an *aromatase inhibitor. It is available as a form for intravenous infusion on *prescription only.
Side effects: include abdominal pain, weakness, chest pain, chills, fever, headache, muscle and joint pain, diarrhoea, nausea, vomiting, and rash.
Precautions and interactions with other drugs: there is a risk of allergic reactions during infusion and of heart damage, which may also occur if anthracyclines are given with trastuzumab. Therefore this medicine is not recommended for people with heart conditions, and heart function should be monitored during treatment. Trastuzumab should not be given to people with severe breathlessness or to breastfeeding women.
Proprietary preparation: Herceptin.

Travasept 100 (Baxter Healthcare) A proprietary combination of the antiseptics *chlorhexidine gluconate and *cetrimide, used for cleansing and disinfecting wounds and burns. It is available as a solution without a prescription, but only from pharmacies.
Side effects: *see* CETRIMIDE.
Precautions: the solution should not come into contact with the eyes.

Travatan (Alcon Laboratories (U.K) Limited) *See* TRAVOPROST.

travoprost A *prostaglandin analogue that is used to reduce the pressure inside the eye in the treatment of chronic (open-angle) *glaucoma and raised

blood pressure in the eye. It acts by increasing the outflow of aqueous fluid from the eye. Travoprost is available, on *prescription only, in the form of eye drops.
Side effects: travoprost may increase the brown pigment in the iris, and people should be warned to notice any changes in eye colour. The eye may become irritated, bloodshot, or itchy, and the eyelashes may become longer, darker, and thicker. There may also be headache.
Precautions: the drops may cause blurred vision and caution must be exercised when driving or operating heavy machinery. Travoprost should be used with caution in people with asthma and in women who are pregnant or breastfeeding.
Proprietary preparations: Travatan; *DuoTrav (combined with timolol).

Traxam, Traxam Pain Relief (Goldshield) *See* FELBINAC.

trazodone An *antidepressant drug, related to the *tricyclic antidepressants, used for the treatment of depressive illness, particularly when sedation is desirable, and anxiety. It is available, on *prescription only, as capsules, tablets, or a liquid.
Side effects: similar to those of *amitriptyline hydrochloride, but trazodone has fewer effects on the heart. Rarely, it can cause priapism (painful and persistent erection of the penis), in which case treatment should be stopped immediately.
Precautions and interactions with other drugs: *see* TRICYCLIC ANTIDEPRESSANTS.
Proprietary preparation: Molipaxin.

Tredaptive (Merck Sharp & Dohme Limited) A proprietary combination of *nicotinic acid (a lipid-lowering drug) and laropiprant (a *prostaglandin antagonist), used in the treatment of combined mixed dyslipidaemia and primary hypercholesterolaemia (*see* HYPERLIPIDAEMIA). It is available as *modified-release tablets on *prescription only.
Side effects, precautions, and interactions with other drugs: *see* NICOTINIC ACID.

Trental (sanofi-aventis) *See* PENTOXIFYLLINE.

treosulfan An *alkylating drug used for the treatment of ovarian *cancer. It is available, on *prescription only, as capsules or an injection.
Side effects: include pigmentation of the skin and (rarely) irritation and bleeding in the bladder. *See also* CYTOTOXIC DRUGS.
Precautions: *see* CYTOTOXIC DRUGS.

tretinoin A *retinoid used topically for the treatment of *acne and orally to treat certain types of leukaemia (*see* CANCER). A *prescription only medicine, it is available as a gel or as capsules.
Side effects: skin preparations may cause redness, local irritation, and peeling at the start of treatment, but this should not last; they may cause changes in skin pigmentation and make the skin more sensitive to light. Side effects

caused by the capsules include stomach upsets, irregular heart rhythms, flushing, headache, dry skin and mucous membranes, rash, visual impairment, hearing disturbances, confusion, dizziness, bone pain, and chest pain; the retinoic acid syndrome (including fever, breathlessness, and *oedema) requires immediate treatment.
Precautions: skin preparations should not be used on damaged or sunburnt skin, by people with eczema or a personal or family history of skin cancer, or by pregnant women. These preparations should not come into contact with the eyes, nostrils, or mouth, and exposure of treated skin to ultraviolet light (including excessive sunlight) should be avoided. Skin preparations should not be used with other topical agents (e.g. *keratolytics) that may cause irritation. Capsules should not be taken by women who are pregnant or breastfeeding, and contraception must be used for one month before and during treatment and for at least one month after stopping treatment (*see* RETINOIDS). They should be used with caution in people with liver or kidney disease. Blood tests to monitor concentrations of fats should be carried out during treatment; there is a risk of thrombosis during the first month of treatment.
Interactions with other drugs:
Keratolytics: see Precautions above.
Tetracyclines: may increase pressure in the brain and should not be used with tretinoin.
Proprietary preparations: Retin-A (gel); Vesanoid (capsules); *Aknemycin Plus (combined with erythromycin).

Triadene (Bayer) A proprietary combination of *ethinylestradiol and *gestodene used as an *oral contraceptive of the triphasic type. These tablets are packaged in three phases, which differ in the amounts of the active ingredients they contain. Triadene is available on *prescription only.
Side effects and interactions with other drugs: *see* ORAL CONTRACEPTIVES.
Precautions: Triadene should not be used by women who are at risk of developing thromboembolism, for example because they are very overweight or have varicose veins or a history of thrombosis. It should therefore only be taken by women who cannot tolerate other brands and who are prepared to accept the increased risk. *See also* ORAL CONTRACEPTIVES.

triamcinolone acetonide A potent glucocorticoid (*see* CORTICOSTEROIDS), similar to *prednisolone, used for the treatment of inflammatory disorders, including the swelling, pain, and stiffness associated with rheumatoid arthritis, osteoarthritis, bursitis, or tenosynovitis (inflammation of the tendon); and skin diseases, such as *eczema, *psoriasis, and dermatitis. It is also used for the prevention and treatment of allergic rhinitis (including hay fever). Triamcinolone is available, on *prescription only, as a solution for injection into joints or muscles, a skin cream or ointment, and a metered-dose nasal spray.
Side effects, precautions, and interactions with other drugs: *see* CORTICOSTEROIDS; TOPICAL STEROIDS.

Proprietary preparations: Adcortyl Intra-articular/Intradermal (injection); Kenalog Intra-articular/Intramuscular (injection); Nasacort (nasal spray); *Aureocort (combined with chlortetracycline).

Triam-Co (Norton Healthcare) A proprietary combination of *triamterene (a potassium-sparing diuretic) and *hydrochlorothiazide (a thiazide diuretic), used for the treatment of *hypertension and *oedema associated with heart failure, liver disease, or kidney disease. It is available as tablets on *prescription only.
Side effects, precautions, and interactions with other drugs: *see* THIAZIDE DIURETICS; POTASSIUM-SPARING DIURETICS.
See also ANTIHYPERTENSIVE DRUGS; DIURETICS.

triamterene A *potassium-sparing diuretic used for the treatment of *oedema associated with heart failure, liver disease, or kidney disease. It is often given with loop or thiazide diuretics. Triamterene is available as capsules on *prescription only.
Side effects, precautions, and interactions with other drugs: *see* POTASSIUM-SPARING DIURETICS.
Proprietary preparations: Dytac; *Dyazide (combined with hydrochlorothiazide); *Frusene (combined with furosemide); *Kalspare (combined with chlortalidone); *Triam-Co (combined with hydrochlorothiazide).
See also DIURETICS.

Triapin (Sanofi-aventis) A proprietary combination of *felodipine (a calcium antagonist) and *ramipril (an ACE inhibitor), used for the treatment of essential hypertension. It is available as tablets on *prescription only.
Side effects: *see* ACE INHIBITORS; CALCIUM ANTAGONISTS.
Precautions: *see* ACE INHIBITORS; ANTIHYPERTENSIVE DRUGS; CALCIUM ANTAGONISTS; FELODIPINE.
Interactions with other drugs: *see* ACE INHIBITORS; FELODIPINE.

tribavirin *See* RIBAVIRIN.

triclofos sodium A *hypnotic drug used for the short-term treatment of insomnia. It is taken by mouth and is available as a solution on *prescription only.

Side effects: similar to those of *chloral hydrate, but triclofos causes less stomach irritation and fewer other gastrointestinal side effects.
Precautions and interactions with other drugs: *see* CHLORAL HYDRATE.

triclosan An *antiseptic that is active against a wide range of bacteria and fungi. As a soap or liquid it is used as a preoperative hand wash for surgeons and for cleansing and disinfecting the skin of patients before surgery, injections, or taking blood samples. It is also included in various skin preparations to prevent infection of minor wounds and for treating such conditions as eczema and acne. Triclosan is freely available *over the counter.
Precautions: triclosan should not come into contact with the eyes.

Proprietary preparations: *Clearasil Treatment Cream Regular (combined with sulphur); *Dettol Antiseptic Cream (combined with chloroxylenol and edetic acid); *Oilatum Plus (combined with liquid paraffin and benzalkonium chloride; *Sensodyne (combined with sodium fluoride and potassium chloride); *TCP Antiseptic Cream (combined with chloroxylenol and TCP Antiseptic Liquid).

tricyclic antidepressants (TCAs) A class of *antidepressant drugs that block the reuptake of noradrenaline and serotonin into nerve endings, thus prolonging their action in the brain. TCAs can be divided roughly into two groups: those with sedative properties (*amitriptyline hydrochloride, *dosulepin hydrochloride, *doxepin, and *trimipramine), which tend to be of greater benefit to patients who are anxious and agitated; and those with only weakly sedative action (*clomipramine hydrochloride, *imipramine, *lofepramine, and *nortriptyline), which are more useful for treating lethargic and withdrawn patients. Related to the TCAs are the antidepressants *mianserin hydrochloride and *trazodone. Some TCAs are used to treat bedwetting in children and as an *adjunct for pain relief (*see also* MIGRAINE).
Side effects: all tricyclic antidepressants can have significant *antimuscarinic effects (dry mouth, blurred vision, drowsiness, constipation, and urinary retention), but *tolerance to these effects develops with continued use. Abnormal heart rhythms (*see* ARRHYTHMIA) and heart block can occasionally follow the use of TCAs, particularly amitriptyline. TCAs are sometimes associated with convulsions.
Precautions: TCAs and related antidepressants should not be taken by people who have recently suffered a heart attack, who have severe liver disease, or who are manic. They should be used with caution in people with heart disease, a history of epilepsy, thyroid disease, acute glaucoma, or a history of urinary retention, and in women who are pregnant or breastfeeding. Alcohol should be avoided, as it enhances the sedative effects of these drugs.
Interactions with other drugs:

Adrenaline and noradrenaline: the risk of ventricular arrhythmias is increased.

Anti-arrhythmics: TCAs increase the risk of recurrence of ventricular arrhythmias with amiodarone (which should be avoided), disopyramide, flecainide, and propafenone.

Anticoagulants: the effects of warfarin and acenocoumarol are reduced or enhanced.

Antiepileptics: TCAs increase the risk of convulsions recurring; plasma concentrations of some tricyclics are reduced.

Antiparkinsonian drugs: rasagiline and selegiline increase the risk of toxic effects on the central nervous system.

Antipsychotics: increase plasma concentrations of TCAs; droperidol and pimozide should be avoided.

Atomoxetine: increases the risk of ventricular arrhythmias.

Clonidine: TCAs antagonize its effect in lowering blood pressure.

MAOIs: cause restlessness and other signs of overactivity of the central

nervous system and should not be taken until at least a week after stopping a course of TCAs. TCAs should not be taken until two weeks after stopping an MAOI.
Moxifloxacin: increases the risk of ventricular arrhythmias and should not be taken with TCAs.
Pentamidine: increases the risk of ventricular arrhythmias and should not be taken with TCAs.
Ritonavir: increases the plasma concentrations of TCAs.
Sibutramine: increases the risk of toxic effects on the central nervous system and should not be taken with TCAs.
SSRIs: increase the plasma concentrations of some TCAs.
Sympathomimetics: cause raised blood pressure.
Tramadol: increases the risk of toxic effects on the central nervous system.

Tridestra (Orion Pharma) A proprietary preparation of *estradiol tablets and combined estradiol/*medroxyprogesterone tablets used as sequential combined *hormone replacement therapy for the relief of menopausal symptoms and prevention of osteoporosis in women who have not had a hysterectomy. The tablets, which are available on *prescription only, must be taken in the prescribed order.
Side effects, precautions, and interactions with other drugs: *see* HORMONE REPLACEMENT THERAPY.

trientine dihydrochloride A drug used to treat Wilson's disease (a condition in which copper accumulates in the body) in people who cannot tolerate treatment with *penicillamine. It is available as capsules on *prescription only.
Side effects: include nausea.
Precautions: trientine should be used with caution during pregnancy.
Interactions with other drugs:
Iron: the absorption of iron supplements given by mouth is reduced by trientine.
Zinc: the absorption of both drugs is reduced.

trifluoperazine An *antipsychotic drug used for the treatment of schizophrenia and other psychoses and for the short-term treatment of severe anxiety, agitation, and violent or dangerous behaviour. It is also used to treat severe nausea and vomiting. Trifluoperazine is available, on *prescription only, as tablets or a syrup.
Side effects: as for *chlorpromazine, but trifluoperazine is less sedating, has fewer antimuscarinic effects, and *extrapyramidal reactions are more frequent.
Precautions and interactions with other drugs: *see* CHLORPROMAZINE HYDROCHLORIDE.
Proprietary preparation: Stelazine.

triglycerides A class of important lipids consisting of glycerol combined with three fatty acids. Increased concentrations of triglycerides in the blood (**hypertriglyceridaemia**: *see* HYPERLIPIDAEMIA) are a risk factor for coronary heart disease, and very high levels can cause life-threatening pancreatitis (inflammation of the pancreas). Triglycerides are transported in the blood by *lipoproteins, and high circulating concentrations can be reduced by dietary modification, which is the usual first-line treatment. When triglyceride concentrations are particularly high, *lipid-lowering drugs may be used.

trihexyphenidyl hydrochloride <**benzhexol hydrochloride**> An *antimuscarinic drug used for the reversal of drug-induced *extrapyramidal reactions (*see* ANTIPARKINSONIAN DRUGS). It is available, on *prescription only, as tablets or a syrup.
Side effects: dry mouth, gastrointestinal disturbances, dizziness, and blurred vision are common; less common side effects are difficulty in urinating, slow heart rate, and nervousness. In high doses and in susceptible patients, mental confusion, excitement, and psychiatric disturbances can occur.
Precautions: trihexyphenidyl should not be taken by people with acute glaucoma, gastrointestinal obstruction, or enlargement of the prostate. It should be used with caution in those with heart, liver, or kidney disease.
Interactions with other drugs:
Antihistamines: increase the adverse effects of trihexyphenidyl.
Proprietary preparation: Broflex.

Triiodothyronine (Goldshield) *See* LIOTHYRONINE SODIUM.

Trileptal (Novartis) *See* OXCARBAZEPINE.

trilostane A drug that inhibits the production of both mineralocorticoids and glucocorticoids (*see* CORTICOSTEROIDS). It is therefore used to treat conditions that arise from overproduction of these hormones (such as Cushing's syndrome). It can also be used to treat postmenopausal breast cancer, in conjunction with corticosteroid replacement therapy. Trilostane is available as capsules on *prescription only.
Side effects: include flushing, nausea, a running nose, and diarrhoea.
Precautions: trilostane should not be taken by pregnant or breastfeeding women. It should be used with caution by people with impaired kidney or liver function. Nonhormonal contraception should be used (if appropriate) during treatment.
Interactions with other drugs:
Potassium-sparing diuretics: there is an increased risk of high concentrations of potassium in the blood.
Proprietary preparation: Modrenal.

trimeprazine tartrate (Withrop Pharmaceuticals Ltd) *See* ALIMEMAZINE TARTRATE.

trimethoprim An antibacterial drug whose action is similar to that of the *sulphonamides. It is used for the treatment of many bacterial infections, especially infections of the urinary and respiratory tracts. It is sometimes given as a combination with sulfamethoxazole (*see* CO-TRIMOXAZOLE);

however, it is currently recommended that trimethoprim alone is sufficient for the treatment of most infections and has fewer side effects. It is available, on *prescription only, as tablets or an oral suspension.
Side effects: gastrointestinal disturbances, including nausea and vomiting, may occur; other possible side effects are itching and rashes. Blood disorders may very rarely occur with long-term treatment – such symptoms as fever, sore throat, bruising, and rashes should be reported to a doctor immediately.
Precautions: trimethoprim should not be taken by patients with certain blood disorders and should be used with caution in people who have kidney disease, in women who are pregnant or breastfeeding, and in newborn babies. Blood counts are required for those on long-term therapy.
Interactions with other drugs: *see* CO-TRIMOXAZOLE.
Proprietary preparations: Trimopan; Bactrim (*see* CO-TRIMOXAZOLE); Septrin (*see* CO-TRIMOXAZOLE).

trimipramine A *tricyclic antidepressant drug used for the treatment of depressive illness, especially when sedation is required. It is available as tablets or capsules on *prescription only.
Side effects, precautions, and interactions with other drugs: *see* AMITRIPTYLINE HYDROCHLORIDE; TRICYCLIC ANTIDEPRESSANTS.
Proprietary preparation: Surmontil.

Trimopan (Teva) *See* TRIMETHOPRIM.

Trimovate (GlaxoSmithKline) A proprietary combination of *clobetasone butyrate (a moderately potent topical steroid), *nystatin (an antifungal agent), and *oxytetracycline (an antibiotic), used for the treatment of infected conditions of the skin in moist or covered areas. It is available as a cream on *prescription only.
Side effects and precautions: *see* TOPICAL STEROIDS.

TriNovum (Janssen-Cilag) A proprietary combination of *ethinylestradiol and *norethisterone used as an *oral contraceptive of the triphasic type. These tablets are packaged in three phases, which differ in the amounts of the active ingredients they contain. TriNovum is available on *prescription only.
Side effects, precautions, and interactions with other drugs: *see* ORAL CONTRACEPTIVES.

Trintek (Goldshield) *See* GLYCERYL TRINITRATE.

tripotassium dicitratobismuthate A bismuth-containing drug with *cytoprotectant action, used for the treatment of gastric and duodenal ulcers (*see* ACID-PEPTIC DISEASES). It is available as tablets and can be obtained without a prescription, but only from pharmacies.
Side effects: tripotassium dicitratobismuthate may cause blackening of the tongue and stools.
Precautions: this medicine should not be taken by people with kidney disease or by pregnant women.
Proprietary preparation: De-Noltab.

triprolidine hydrochloride One of the original (sedating) *antihistamines. It is available in combination with *pseudoephedrine for the treatment of hay fever and is also an ingredient in some cough medicines and decongestant preparations. Preparations containing triprolidine can be bought from pharmacies without a prescription.
Side effects, precautions, and interactions with other drugs: *see* ANTIHISTAMINES.
Proprietary preparations: *Multi-Action Actifed Chesty Coughs (combined with guaifenesin and pseudoephedrine); *Multi-Action Actifed Dry Coughs (combined with dextromethorphan and pseudoephedrine).

Triptafen (Goldshield) A proprietary combination of *amitriptyline hydrochloride (a *tricyclic antidepressant) and *perphenazine (an antipsychotic drug), used for the treatment of depression with anxiety. It is available as tablets on *prescription only. **Triptafen-M** is a similar preparation but contains a lower proportion of amitriptyline.
Side effects, precautions, and interactions with other drugs: *see* TRICYCLIC ANTIDEPRESSANTS; AMITRIPTYLINE HYDROCHLORIDE; PERPHENAZINE; CHLORPROMAZINE HYDROCHLORIDE.

triptans *See* $5HT_1$ AGONISTS.

triptorelin An analogue of *gonadorelin that is used for the treatment of *endometriosis, fibroids, and precocious puberty. It is also used to treat advanced prostate cancer, having an action similar to that of *leuprorelin. Triptorelin is given by *intramuscular or subcutaneous injection and is available on *prescription only.
Side effects: *see* GOSERELIN. Other side effects include dry mouth, excessive salivation, and difficulty in urinating.
Precautions: for women, *see* GOSERELIN. In cancer treatment, triptorelin should not be used by men in whom there is compression of the spinal cord or secondary tumours in the spinal cord.
Proprietary preparations: De-capeptyl SR; Gonapeptyl Depot.

Trisenox (Cephalon (UK) Limited) *See* ARSENIC TRIOXIDE.

Trisequens (Novo Nordisk) A proprietary preparation of combined *estradiol/*estriol tablets and combined estradiol/estriol/*norethisterone tablets used as sequential combined *hormone replacement therapy for the relief of menopausal symptoms in women who have not had a hysterectomy. The tablets, which are available on *prescription only, must be taken in the prescribed order.
Side effects, precautions, and interactions with other drugs: *see* HORMONE REPLACEMENT THERAPY.

Tritace (sanofi-aventis) *See* RAMIPRIL.

Trizivir (GlaxoSmithKline) A proprietary combination of the antiretroviral drugs *zidovudine, *abacavir, and *lamivudine, used in the treatment of *HIV infection. It is available as tablets on *prescription only.

Side effects, precautions, and interactions with other drugs: *see* ABACAVIR; LAMIVUDINE; ZIDOVUDINE.

tropicamide An *antimuscarinic drug that is applied to the eye to dilate the pupil before examination of the interior of the eye. It is shorter acting than *atropine sulphate and *cyclopentolate hydrochloride. Tropicamide is available as eye drops on *prescription only.
Side effects: tropicamide may cause transient stinging and an increase in pressure in the eye; with prolonged use local irritation and conjunctivitis can occur.
Precautions and interactions with other drugs: *see* ANTIMUSCARINIC DRUGS.
Proprietary preparations: Mydriacyl; Minims Tropicamide (single-dose eye drops).

Tropium (DDSA Pharmaceuticals) *See* CHLORDIAZEPOXIDE.

trospium chloride An *antimuscarinic drug used for the treatment of incontinence and frequency and urgency in passing urine. It is available as tablets or *modified-release capsules on *prescription only.
Side effects, precautions, and interactions with other drugs: *see* ANTIMUSCARINIC DRUGS.
Proprietary preparations: Regurin; Regurin XL (modified-release capsules).

Trosyl (Pfizer) *See* TIOCONAZOLE.

Trusopt (Merck Sharp & Dohme) *See* DORZOLAMIDE.

Truvada (Gilead Sciences Ltd) A proprietary combination of two antiretroviral drugs, *tenofovir disoproxil and *emtricitabine, used in the treatment of *HIV infection. It is available as tablets on *prescription only.
Side effects, precautions, and interactions with other drugs: *see* EMTRICITABINE; TENOFOVIR DISOPROXIL.

tryptophan An amino acid that appears to benefit some people with resistant depression (*see* ANTIDEPRESSANT DRUGS). It is available as tablets on *prescription only, and under hospital supervision, for those who are unsuited to alternative treatments. Patients and prescribers must be registered with the Optimax Information and Clinical Support Unit.
Side effects: include drowsiness, nausea, headache, and light-headedness. The risk of eosinophilia-myalgia syndrome (a blood disorder associated with muscle pain) has been reduced since nonprescription preparations containing tryptophan were withdrawn.
Precautions: dosage should be reduced gradually at the end of treatment to avoid withdrawal reactions.
Interactions with other drugs:

Other antidepressants: there is a risk of confusion, agitation, and nausea if MAOIs or SSRIs are taken with tryptophan.
Sibutramine: there is an increased risk of adverse effects on the central nervous system and this drug should not be used with tryptophan.

Proprietary preparation: Optimax.

tuberculosis An infectious disease caused by the bacillus *Mycobacterium tuberculosis* and characterized by the formation of nodular lesions (tubercles) in the tissues. In **pulmonary tuberculosis** the bacillus is inhaled into the lungs, where it sets up a primary tubercle and spreads to the nearest lymph nodes. Natural immune defences may heal it at this stage; alternatively the disease may smoulder for months or years and fluctuate with the patient's resistance. Many people become infected but show no symptoms. Others develop a chronic infection and can transmit the bacillus by coughing and sneezing. In some cases the bacilli spread from the lungs to the bloodstream, setting up millions of tiny tubercles throughout the body **miliary tuberculosis**, or migrate to the brain to cause **tuberculous meningitis**.

Tuberculosis is treated with a combination of antibiotics that should be continued for six months in order to prevent the development of drug-resistant strains of the bacillus. The recommended treatment is divided into two phases. In the first phase a combination of *isoniazid, *rifampicin, *pyrazinamide, and *ethambutol hydrochloride is taken for two months. This is followed by a combination of isoniazid and rifampicin, which is continued for four months. *See also* CAPREOMYCIN; CYCLOSERINE; RIFABUTIN; STREPTOMYCIN.

Tuinal (Flynn Pharma) A proprietary combination of the barbiturates *amobarbital and *secobarbital used for the short-term treatment of severe insomnia in patients who are already taking barbiturates. Tuinal is available as capsules; it is a *controlled drug.
Side effects, precautions, and interactions with other drugs: *see* BARBITURATES.

Tums (GlaxoSmithKline) *See* CALCIUM CARBONATE.

turpentine oil An aromatic oil that is an ingredient of *rubefacient liniments, embrocations, and creams for relief of aches, pains, and stiffness in muscles, tendons, and joints. It is also included in inhalant preparations to relieve the congestion caused by colds, catarrh, influenza, and hay fever. Preparations containing turpentine oil are freely available *over the counter.
Side effects and precautions: *see* RUBEFACIENTS.
Proprietary preparations: *Deep Heat Rub (combined with eucalyptus oil, menthol, and methyl salicylate); *Elliman's Universal Muscle Rub Lotion (combined with acetic acid); *Goddard's Muscle Lotion (combined with dilute ammonia solution and acetic acid); *Vicks Vaporub (combined with camphor, eucalyptus oil, and menthol).

Tygacil (Pfizer) *See* TIGECYCLINE.

Tylex (UCB Pharma Limited) *See* CO-CODAMOL.

tyrosine kinase inhibitors A group of drugs that interfere with cell growth in a variety of different ways to inhibit the action of tyrosine kinases, enzymes that have an important role in cell division and growth. Many tumour cells contain these enzymes, which can be targeted by tyrosine kinase inhibitors to prevent or reduce their growth and spread. Tyrosine kinase inhibitors are used to treat a range of advanced *cancers, including types of leukaemia (*dasatinib, *imatinib, *nilotinib), pancreatic cancer (*erlotinib), malignant gastrointestinal tumours (imatinib, *sunitinib), breast cancer (*lapatinib), kidney cancer (*sorafenib, sunitinib, *everolimus, *temsirolimus), and lung cancer (erlotinib, *gefitinib). Most of them can be taken by mouth and can easily be combined with other forms of chemotherapy.

tyrothricin An antibiotic that is too toxic to be taken systemically (into the body) but is used topically in low doses as an ingredient of lozenges for local treatment of infections of the skin and mouth.
Side effects: there may be blackening or soreness of the tongue.
Precautions: tyrothricin should not be used in the nose.
Proprietary preparations: *Boots Anaesthetic & Antibiotic Throat Lozenges (combined with benzocaine) *Tyrozets (combined with benzocaine).

Tyrozets (McNeil Ltd) A proprietary combination of *tyrothricin (an antibiotic) and *benzocaine (a local anaesthetic), used for the relief of sore throat and mild irritations of the mouth. It is available as lozenges and can be obtained without a prescription, but only from pharmacies.
Precautions: Tyrozets are not recommended for children under three years old.

Tysabri (Biogen Idec Ltd) *See* NATALIZUMAB.

Tyverb (GlaxoSmithKline) *See* LAPATINIB.

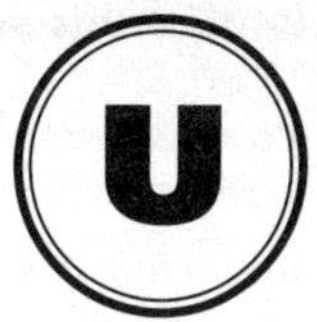

Ubretid (sanofi-aventis) *See* DISTIGMINE BROMIDE.

Ucerax (UCB Pharma) *See* HYDROXYZINE HYDROCHLORIDE.

Uftoral (Merck Serono) A proprietary combination of tegafur (a drug that is converted to *fluorouracil in the body) and uracil (which prevents the breakdown of fluorouracil), used – in combination with calcium folinate (*see* FOLINIC ACID) – for the *first-line treatment of advanced colorectal cancer. It is available as capsules on *prescription only.
Side effects: *see* CYTOTOXIC DRUGS; FLUOROURACIL.
Precautions: Uftoral should not be taken by women who are breastfeeding or by people with severe liver disease. *See also* CYTOTOXIC DRUGS.
Interactions with other drugs: *see* FLUOROURACIL.

ulipristal A drug that modifies *progesterone receptors. It is used for emergency contraception, being taken as a single dose within five days of unprotected sexual intercourse. Ulipristal is available as tablets on *prescription only.
Side effects: include nausea, vomiting, diarrhoea, abdominal pain, dizziness, headache, menstrual irregularities, and back pain.
Precautions: ulipristal should not be taken by women with severe liver disease and should be used with caution in those with severe asthma. Barrier contraception should be used until the next period.
Interactions with other drugs: ulipristal should not be used with the following drugs, which may reduce its contraceptive effects: antacids, ulcer-healing drugs, carbamazepine, phenobarbital, phenytoin, rifampicin, ritonavir, and St John's wort. Ulipristal may reduce the contraceptive effect of progestogens.
Proprietary preparation: EllaOne.

Ultiva (GlaxoSmithKline) *See* REMIFENTANIL.

Ultrabase (Meda Pharmaceuticals) A proprietary combination of *liquid paraffin and *white soft paraffin (both emollients) in the form of a cream, used for the treatment of dry skin conditions. It is freely available *over the counter.

Ultralanum Plain (Meadow) *See* FLUOCORTOLONE.

Ultraproct (Meadow) A proprietary combination of *fluocortolone (a corticosteroid) and *cinchocaine hydrochloride (a local anaesthetic), used to relieve the discomfort and pain of *haemorrhoids and itching of the anus. It is available as an ointment or suppositories on *prescription only.
Side effects: *see* CORTICOSTEROIDS.

Precautions: Ultraproct should not be used when viral or fungal infection is present; prolonged use should be avoided.

undecenoic acid An *antifungal drug. Undecenoic acid and its salts (mainly **zinc undecenoate**) are used to treat tinea (ringworm) infections of the skin, especially athlete's foot. Undecenoic acid and undecenoates are available in creams, dusting powders, sprays, paints, and shampoos, which can be obtained from pharmacies without a prescription.
Proprietary preparations: Mycota (cream, dusting powder, or spray); *Ceanel Concentrate (combined with cetrimide and phenylethyl alcohol).

Unguentum M (Almirall) A proprietary combination of *liquid paraffin, *white soft paraffin, and other *emollients and silicic acid (an anti-caking agent), used for the treatment of dry skin conditions and napkin rash. It is available without a prescription as a cream, but only from *pharmacies.

Uniphyllin Continus (Napp Pharmaceuticals) *See* THEOPHYLLINE.

Uniroid-HC (Chemidex Pharma) A proprietary combination of *hydrocortisone (a corticosteroid) and *cinchocaine hydrochloride (a local anaesthetic), used to relieve the discomfort and pain of *haemorrhoids and itching of the anus. It is available as an ointment or suppositories on *prescription only.
Side effects: *see* CORTICOSTEROIDS.
Precautions: Uniroid should not be used when viral or fungal infection is present and should be used for longer than seven days. It is not recommended for children under 12 years old.

Unisept (Medlock Medical) *See* CHLORHEXIDINE.

Univer (Cephalon) *See* VERAPAMIL HYDROCHLORIDE.

Urdox (Wockhardt UK) *See* URSODEOXYCHOLIC ACID.

urea A compound used alone or in combination with other drugs as a hydrating (moisturizing) agent in *emollient creams and lotions for treating dry skin conditions. It is also included in ear-drop preparations used for dissolving and washing out earwax (*see* UREA HYDROGEN PEROXIDE). Urea-containing preparations can be obtained without a prescription, but only from pharmacies.
Precautions: some people find the smell unpleasant. Urea may irritate sensitive skin.
Proprietary preparations: Aquadrate (cream); Eucerin (cream); Nutraplus (cream); *Alphaderm (combined with hydrocortisone); *Balneum Plus Cream (combined with lauromacrogols); *Boots Lip and Cold Sore Cream (combined with cimetidine, dimeticone, and chlorocresol); *Calmurid (combined with lactic acid); *Calmurid HC (combined with hydrocortisone and lactic acid); *E45 Itch Relief Cream (combined with lauromacrogol).

urea hydrogen peroxide A combination of *urea and *hydrogen peroxide in equal amounts, which releases hydrogen peroxide locally on application.

Its foaming action softens and facilitates the removal of earwax: it is therefore included in ear drops for this purpose. Urea hydrogen peroxide can be obtained without a prescription, but only from pharmacies.
Precautions: urea hydrogen peroxide may cause irritation; it should not be used on perforated eardrums.
Proprietary preparations: Otex; *Exterol (combined with glycerin).

Uriben (Rosemont Pharmaceuticals) *See* NALIDIXIC ACID.

Uriflex C (SSL International) *See* CHLORHEXIDINE.

Uriflex G (SSL International) A proprietary combination of *citric acid, *magnesium oxide, *sodium bicarbonate, and *disodium edetate in the form of a solution, used for flushing catheters. It is available from pharmacies without a prescription.

Uriflex R (SSL International) A proprietary combination of *citric acid, *magnesium carbonate, *gluconolactone, and *disodium edetate in the form of a solution, used for flushing catheters. It is available from pharmacies without a prescription.

Uriflex S, Uriflex SP (SSL International) *See* SODIUM CHLORIDE.

Urispas 200 (Recordati Pharmaceuticals Limited) *See* FLAVOXATE HYDROCHLORIDE.

urofollitropin <**urofollitrophin**> A preparation of follicle-stimulating hormone (a *gonadotrophin) used for the treatment of infertility in men and women that is due to underactivity of the pituitary gland (resulting in insufficient production of gonadotrophins). It is extracted from natural sources; a synthetic preparation (*see* FOLLITROPIN) is also available. Urofollitropin is also used to induce superovulation (production of a large number of eggs) in women undergoing fertility treatment, such as *in vitro* fertilization. It is available as an injection on *prescription only.
Side effects: include ovarian hyperstimulation (the uncontrolled production of large numbers of follicles in the ovaries) and multiple pregnancy; allergic reactions may occur in both sexes.
Precautions: urofollitropin should be used with caution in women with ovarian cysts and in people with thyroid or adrenal disorders or pituitary tumours.
Proprietary preparation: Fostimon.

urokinase A *fibrinolytic drug used for the treatment of deep vein *thrombosis and pulmonary embolism. It is also used to dissolve blood clots in the shunts used to connect patients to kidney dialysis equipment. Urokinase is available as a form for injection or infusion on *prescription only.
Side effects, precautions, and interactions with other drugs: *see* FIBRINOLYTIC DRUGS.
Proprietary preparation: Syner-KINASE.

Uromitexan (Baxter) *See* MESNA.

Uro-Tainer Chlorhexidine (B. Braun Medical)) *See* CHLORHEXIDINE.

Uro-Tainer Sodium Chloride (B. Braun (Medical)) *See* SODIUM CHLORIDE.

Uro-Tainer Suby G (B. Braun (Medical)) A proprietary combination of *citric acid, magnesium oxide, sodium bicarbonate, and *disodium edetate in the form of a solution, used for flushing catheters in the bladder to keep them unblocked. It is available from pharmacies without a prescription.

ursodeoxycholic acid A *bile acid used in the treatment of gallstones or to prevent recurrence after they have dissolved. Ursodeoxycholic acid is suitable for people with mild symptoms who cannot be treated by other means. It is also used, with limited effect, to treat primary biliary cirrhosis (a disease affecting the liver and bile ducts). It is available as tablets or capsules, or an oral suspension on *prescription only.
Side effects: diarrhoea may occur, but this is rare.
Precautions: ursodeoxycholic acid should not be taken by women who are pregnant or planning to become pregnant, or by people with inflammatory bowel or liver disease.
Interactions with other drugs:
Ciclosporin: its absorption is increased.
Proprietary preparations: Destolit; Urdox; Ursofalk; Ursogal.

Ursofalk (Dr. Falk Pharma) *See* URSODEOXYCHOLIC ACID.

Ursogal (Galen) *See* URSODEOXYCHOLIC ACID.

ustekinumab A *monoclonal antibody used for the treatment of severe *psoriasis that has not responded to other therapies (including anti-TNF drugs) or when other therapies cannot be used. It modifies the immune system by inhibiting the action of two *interleukins. Ustekinumab is given by subcutaneous injection and is available on *prescription only.
Side effects: include upper airways infections, dizziness, headache, diarrhoea, back or muscle pain, and itching.
Precautions: ustekinumab should not be given to people with active infection or to women who are pregnant or breastfeeding. It should be used with caution in people with tuberculosis, or who have previously received treatment for tuberculosis, or who are at high risk of this infection.
Interactions with other drugs:
Vaccines: should not be given to people who are receiving ustekinumab.
Proprietary preparation: Stelara.

Utinor (Merck Sharp & Dohme) *See* NORFLOXACIN.

Utovlan (Pfizer) *See* NORETHISTERONE.

Utrogestan (Ferring Pharmaceuticals) *See* PROGESTERONE.

Uvistat (LPC) A proprietary *sunscreen preparation that is available in a variety of forms. Uvistat cream, which contains ethylhexyl *p*-methoxycinnamate, avobenzone, and *titanium dioxide, offers protection against both UVA and UVB (SPF 22). Uvistat Ultrablock cream contains a higher proportion of *titanium dioxide and has an SPF of 30. A lotion, in which the cinnamate is replaced by methylbenzylidene camphor, has an SPF of 25. All these products can be prescribed on the NHS or obtained without a prescription.

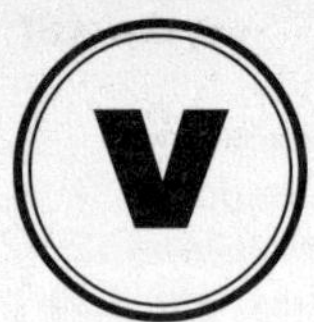

Vagifem (Novo Nordisk) *See* ESTRADIOL; HORMONE REPLACEMENT THERAPY.

Vaginyl (DDSA Pharmaceuticals) *See* METRONIDAZOLE.

Vagisil Medicated Creme (Combe International) *See* LIDOCAINE.

valaciclovir An *antiviral drug that is converted to *aciclovir in the body. It is used for the treatment of herpesvirus infections of the skin and mucous membranes, including shingles and genital herpes. Valaciclovir is available as tablets on *prescription only.
Side effects, precautions, and interactions with other drugs: *see* ACICLOVIR.
Proprietary preparation: Valtrex.

Valcyte (Roche Products) *See* VALGANCICLOVIR.

Valdoxan (Servier Laboratories Limited) *See* AGOMELATINE.

valganciclovir An *antiviral drug used for the treatment of cytomegalovirus eye infection in people with AIDS. It is rapidly metabolized to *ganciclovir in the body. Valganciclovir is available as tablets or an oral solution on *prescription only.
Side effects, precautions, and interactions with other drugs: *see* GANCICLOVIR.
Proprietary preparation: Valcyte.

Vallergan (Winthrop Pharmaceuticals UK Ltd) *See* ALIMEMAZINE TARTRATE.

Valni XL (Winthrop Pharmaceuticals UK Ltd) *See* NIFEDIPINE.

Valoid (Amdipharm) *See* CYCLIZINE.

valproic acid An *anticonvulsant drug used for the treatment of episodes of mania in people with bipolar disorder. Valproic acid is also used for the treatment of epilepsy. It is available as *enteric-coated capsules or tablets on *prescription only.
Side effects, precautions, and interactions with other drugs: *see* SODIUM VALPROATE.
Proprietary preparations: Convulex (capsules); Depakote (tablets); *Epilim Chrono (combined with sodium valproate).

valsartan An *angiotensin II inhibitor used mainly in the treatment of *hypertension. It is available as tablets on *prescription only.
Side effects and precautions: *see* ANGIOTENSIN II INHIBITORS.
Interactions with other drugs: *see* ACE INHIBITORS.

Proprietary preparations: Diovan; *Co-Diovan (combined with hydrochlorothiazide); *Exforge (combined with amlodipine).
See also ANTIHYPERTENSIVE DRUGS.

Valtrex (GlaxoSmithKline) *See* VALACICLOVIR.

Value Health Cold Relief (Boots) A proprietary combination of *paracetamol (an analgesic and antipyretic) and *vitamin C, used to relieve pain and reduce fever. It is available as an oral powder without a prescription, but only from Boots stores.
Side effects and precautions: *see* PARACETAMOL.

Vancocin (Flynn Pharma) *See* VANCOMYCIN.

vancomycin An *antibiotic used for the prevention and treatment of endocarditis (infection of the heart membranes and valves) and for the treatment of other serious infections, including staphylococcal infections resistant to other antibiotics. It is not absorbed after oral administration and must therefore be given intravenously for systemic infections. Vancomycin is also used for the treatment of pseudomembranous colitis, an inflammation of the large bowel associated with severe diarrhoea that is caused by broad-spectrum antibiotics. For this it can be given orally, as capsules (as it does not need to be absorbed). Vancomycin is available on *prescription only.
Side effects: high concentrations of vancomycin in the blood after injection can cause kidney damage and tinnitus (ringing in the ears; if this occurs treatment should be discontinued). Other side effects include blood disorders, nausea, chills, and fever; rashes and low blood pressure may occur if the drug is infused rapidly.
Precautions: rapid infusions should be avoided. Vancomycin should be used with caution in people who have impaired kidney function or who are deaf and in women who are pregnant or breastfeeding. Blood and urine tests are required to monitor kidney function.
Interactions with other drugs:
Antibiotics: aminoglycosides, capreomycin, and colistin increase the risk of ear and kidney damage.
Ciclosporin: increases the risk of kidney damage.
Loop diuretics: increase the risk of ear damage.
Proprietary preparation: Vancocin.

Vaniqa (Almirall) *See* EFLORNITHINE.

Vantas (Orion Pharma (UK) Limited) *See* HISTRELIN ACETATE.

vardenafil A drug with similar effects to *sildenafil but with a longer duration of action. It is available as tablets on *prescription only.
Side effects: *see* SILDENAFIL.
Precautions: *see* SILDENAFIL. In addition, vardenafil should not be taken by men with hereditary disorders of the retina or severely impaired liver function. It should be used with caution by men with bleeding peptic ulcers or bleeding disorders and by men who are susceptible to *arrhythmias.

Interactions with other drugs:

Alpha blockers: their effects are enhanced by vardenafil.

Antiviral drugs: the plasma concentration of vardenafil is increased by several antiviral drugs; indinavir and ritonavir should not be taken with it.

See also SILDENAFIL.

Proprietary preparation: Levitra.

varenicline A drug that is used to help smokers give up the habit. It works by acting as a partial *agonist at *nicotine receptors and is available as tablets on *prescription only.

Side effects: include increased appetite, abnormal dreams, insomnia, headache, somnolence, dizziness, altered taste, nausea, vomiting, constipation, diarrhoea, abdominal distension, stomach discomfort, indigestion, flatulence, dry mouth, and fatigue.

Precautions: varenicline should not be used during pregnancy. Treatment should be stopped if agitation, depression, or suicidal thoughts develop. Varenicline should be used with caution in people with a history of psychiatric illness or severely impaired kidney function.

Proprietary preparation: Champix.

Variquel (IS Pharmaceuticals Ltd) *See* TERLIPRESSIN.

Vascace (Roche Products) *See* CILAZAPRIL.

Vascalpha (Actavis) *See* FELODIPINE.

vascular endothelial growth factor (VEGF) A protein produced in the body that stimulates the formation of new blood vessels, in both normal and abnormal tissues (e.g. tumours). Several drugs inhibit the production of VEGF; they include *bevacizumab and some tyrosine kinase inhibitors (e.g. *everolimus), used for treating cancer, and *pegaptinib and *ranibizumab, used for treating age-related macular degeneration (ARMD). These drugs are known as **angiogenesis inhibitors** or **anti-VEGF drugs**.

vasoconstriction Narrowing of the blood vessels, especially arteries and arterioles (small arteries). Constricted blood vessels can cause insufficient blood supply to the tissues and can contribute to high blood pressure (*hypertension).

vasoconstrictor drugs (vasoconstrictors) Drugs that cause narrowing of blood vessels, reduction in blood flow, and an increase in blood pressure. They are used to increase blood pressure in disorders of the circulation, in cases of shock, or when blood pressure has fallen in lengthy surgical procedures. Some vasoconstrictors are *sympathomimetic drugs and are used to relieve nasal congestion.

vasodilatation An increase in the diameter of blood vessels, especially the arteries and arterioles (small arteries), brought about by relaxation of the muscle forming the vessel wall.

vasodilators Drugs that cause widening of blood vessels (mainly small

arteries) and therefore an increase in blood flow. Because blood pressure depends partly on the diameter of blood vessels, vasodilators are used to lower blood pressure in *hypertension. **Coronary vasodilators** increase the blood flow through the heart and are used to relieve or prevent *angina. **Peripheral vasodilators** affect the blood flow to the limbs and are used to treat conditions of poor circulation, such as acrocyanosis (purple-bluish discoloration of hands and feet due to slow circulation of blood in the skin), chilblains, and Raynaud's syndrome (poor circulation in hands and feet). Poor peripheral blood flow can also cause claudication (a cramp-like pain felt in the legs on walking or exercise). The main classes of vasodilator drugs are *alpha blockers, *nicotinic acid derivatives, *nitrates, class II *calcium antagonists, *potassium channel activators, and *ACE inhibitors. Potent vasodilators used in the treatment of severe hypertension include *ambrisentan, *bosentan, *diazoxide, *minoxidil, *sitaxentan sodium, and *hydralazine. The blood vessels are widened either by affecting the action of the muscles of the vessel walls (nitrates and calcium antagonists) or by interfering with nerve signals that govern the tone of the blood vessels (alpha blockers).
Side effects: flushing and headaches are common at the start of treatment. Dizziness and fainting can also occur as a result of lowered blood pressure. See also entries for individual classes of drugs.
Precautions: the major risk is that blood pressure may sometimes fall too low. See also entries for individual classes of drugs. *See also* ANTIHYPERTENSIVE DRUGS.

Vasogen Cream (Forest Laboratories) A proprietary combination of *zinc oxide (an astringent protective agent), *calamine (a mild astringent), and *dimeticone (a water repellent), used as a *barrier preparation for the prevention and treatment of bedsores and napkin rash and for the protection of the skin around a *stoma after an ileostomy or colostomy. It is freely available *over the counter.

vasopressin (**antidiuretic hormone**) A hormone, secreted by the pituitary gland, that decreases the excretion of water from the kidneys and also constricts blood vessels. A lack of vasopressin results in **diabetes insipidus**, a condition in which the patient passes large amounts of urine and is always thirsty. Synthetic vasopressin (**argipressin**) is used to treat diabetes insipidus and to stop the bleeding from varicose veins in the oesophagus, which can in serious cases be life-threatening. It is given by subcutaneous or intramuscular injection or by intravenous infusion and is available on *prescription only.

Synthetic analogues of vasopressin include *terlipressin and *desmopressin.
Side effects: include pallor, nausea, belching, abdominal cramps, an urge to defecate, and headache; allergic reactions (such as rash) may rarely occur, and vasopressin may cause constriction of coronary vessels, resulting in angina.
Precautions: vasopressin should not be given to people with vascular disease or chronic kidney disease; it should be used with caution in those with

asthma, heart failure, hypertension, epilepsy, migraine, or poor kidney function and in pregnant women.
Proprietary preparation: Pitressin.

Vectavir (Novartis) *See* PENCICLOVIR.

Vectibix (Amgen) *See* PANITUMUMAB.

Veganin (Chefaro UK) A proprietary combination of *aspirin and *paracetamol (analgesics and antipyretics) and *codeine (an opioid analgesic), used to treat the symptoms of influenza and to relieve mild to moderate pain, such as headache, period pains, rheumatic pains, and toothache. It is available as tablets and can be obtained without a prescription.
Side effects and precautions: *see* ASPIRIN; PARACETAMOL; CODEINE.
Interactions with other drugs: *see* ASPIRIN; OPIOIDS.

VEGF *See* VASCULAR ENDOTHELIAL GROWTH FACTOR.

vehicle Any substance that acts as the medium in which a drug is administered. Examples are sterile water, isotonic sodium chloride, and dextrose solutions.

Velbe (Genus) *See* VINBLASTINE SULPHATE.

Velcade (Janssen-Cilag) *See* BORTEZOMIB.

Velosef (E.R. Squibb & Sons) *See* CEFRADINE.

Venaxx XL (Goldshield) *See* VENLAFAXINE.

venlafaxine An *antidepressant drug that is related to the *SSRI group; it inhibits the reuptake of *serotonin and *noradrenaline. It is used for the treatment of depressive illness (and may be more effective for treating resistant depression than the SSRIs) and of generalized anxiety disorder. Venlafaxine is available as tablets or *modified-release capsules or tablets on *prescription only.
Side effects: include nausea, constipation, headache, insomnia, drowsiness, dizziness, weakness, sweating, itching, and nervousness. At the end of treatment, dosage should be reduced gradually.
Precautions: venlafaxine should not be taken by people with arrhythmias or uncontrolled hypertension, by those with severely impaired liver or kidney function, or by women who are pregnant. It should be used with caution in people with heart disease and in women who are breastfeeding. Driving ability may be impaired.

Interactions with other drugs:

Clozapine: its plasma concentration is increased.

MAOIs: venlafaxine should not be taken with MAOIs and should not be started until two weeks after stopping MAOIs; MAOIs should not be started until at least a week after stopping venlafaxine.

Moclobemide: should not be started until one week after stopping venlafaxine.
NSAIDs: increase the risk of bleeding.
Selegiline: increases the risk of hypertension and excitation of the central nervous system; it should not be started until one week after stopping venlafaxine, which should not be started until two weeks after stopping selegiline.
Sibutramine: increases the risk of adverse effects on the central nervous system and should not be used with venlafaxine.
Warfarin: its anticoagulant effect may be enhanced.

Proprietary preparations: Efexor XL (capsules); Foraven XL (capsules); Politid XL (capsules); Tifaxin XL (capsules); Venaxx XL (capsules); Venlalic XL (modified-release tablets); ViePax (tablets); ViePax XL (capsules); Winfex XL (capsules).

Venlalic XL (Dallas Burston Ashbourne) *See* VENLAFAXINE.

Venofer (Syner-Med) *See* FERRIC HYDROXIDE SUCROSE.

Ventavis (Bayer) *See* ILOPROST.

ventilator A piece of equipment that is mechanically operated to maintain a flow of air into and out of the lungs of a patient who is unable to breathe normally.

Ventmax SR (Chiesi) *See* SALBUTAMOL.

Ventolin, Ventolin Accuhaler, Ventolin Evohaler, Ventolin Nebules (Allen & Hanburys) *See* SALBUTAMOL.

ventricular tachycardia *See* ARRHYTHMIA.

Vepesid (Bristol-Myers Squibb) *See* ETOPOSIDE.

Veracur (Typharm) *See* FORMALDEHYDE.

verapamil hydrochloride A class I *calcium antagonist used for the treatment of mild to moderate *hypertension, *angina, and supraventricular tachycardia (*see* ARRHYTHMIA). It is available, on *prescription only, as short-acting and *modified-release tablets or capsules, as an oral solution, and as an injection.

Side effects: constipation is the most common side effect. *See also* CALCIUM ANTAGONISTS.

Precautions: verapamil should not be taken by people with low blood pressure, a slow heart rate, a history of heart failure, or certain other heart conditions. *See also* CALCIUM ANTAGONISTS; ANTIHYPERTENSIVE DRUGS.

Interactions with other drugs:
Anaesthetics: verapamil increases the effect of general anaesthetics in lowering blood pressure.
Anti-arrhythmic drugs: verapamil increases the risk of amiodarone slowing the heart rate and having other adverse effects on the heart; the risk of the

heart ceasing to beat is increased if verapamil is taken with disopyramide or flecainide.
Antibiotics: the adverse effects of verapamil may be increased by clarithromycin and erythromycin; rifampicin reduces the effects of verapamil.
Antiepileptic drugs: verapamil enhances the effects of carbamazepine; the effects of verapamil are reduced by phenytoin, primidone, and phenobarbital.
Beta blockers: verapamil should not be taken with beta blockers as this combination increases the risk of a severe fall in blood pressure, leading to heart failure.
Ciclosporin: its plasma concentration is increased by verapamil.
Digoxin: its plasma concentration is increased by verapamil; bradycardia (slowing of heart rate) is increased.
Ivabradine: its plasma concentration is increased and it should not be given with verapamil.
Simvastatin: the risk of muscle damage is increased.
Sirolimus: the plasma concentrations of both drugs are increased.
Theophylline: its effects are enhanced by verapamil.
See also CALCIUM ANTAGONISTS.

Proprietary preparations: Cordilox; Half Securon SR (modified-release tablets); Securon; Securon SR (modified-release tablets); Univer (modified-release capsules); Verapress MR (modified-release tablets); Vertab SR (modified-release tablets); Zolvera (oral solution); *Tarka (combined with trandolapril).

Verapress MR (Dexcel Pharma) *See* VERAPAMIL HYDROCHLORIDE.

Vermox (Janssen-Cilag) *See* MEBENDAZOLE.

Verruca Removal System (SSL International) *See* SALICYLIC ACID.

Verrugon (Ransom) *See* SALICYLIC ACID.

Versatis (Grunenthal Ltd) *See* LIDOCAINE.

Vertab SR (Chiesi manu) *See* VERAPAMIL HYDROCHLORIDE.

verteporfin A light-sensitive drug used in the treatment of wet age-related macular degeneration, an eye disorder in which abnormal new blood vessels grow under the retina and leak blood and fluid into it, disrupting the visual function of the macula (the most sensitive part of the retina). Verteporfin is given by intravenous infusion and passes to the abnormal vessels, where it is activated by laser light and seals these vessels, preventing further damage to the macula. It is available on *prescription only.
Side effects: include blurred vision, decreased vision, flashes of light, back pain, nausea, and itching.
Precautions: verteporfin should not be given to people with porphyria or severe liver disease or to breastfeeding women. The skin and eyes should be protected from bright light during and for two days after treatment.
Proprietary preparation: Visudyne.

Vesanoid (Roche Products) *See* TRETINOIN.

Vesicare (Astellas Pharma Ltd) *See* SOLIFENACIN SUCCINATE.

Vexol (Alcon Laboratories (U.K) Limited) *See* RIMEXOLONE.

Vfend (Pfizer) *See* VORICONAZOLE.

Viagra (Pfizer) *See* SILDENAFIL.

Viazem XL (Genus) *See* DILTIAZEM HYDROCHLORIDE.

Vibramycin-D (Pfizer) *See* DOXYCYCLINE.

Vicks Cold & Flu Care Medinite Complete (Procter & Gamble) A proprietary combination of *dextromethorphan (a cough suppressant), *pseudoephedrine (a decongestant), *doxylamine (an antihistamine), and *paracetamol (an analgesic and antipyretic), used to relieve the symptoms of colds and influenza, including nasal congestion, irritating coughs, headache, fever, and aches and pains. It is available as a syrup and can be obtained without a prescription, but only from pharmacies.
Side effects: *see* DEXTROMETHORPHAN; EPHEDRINE HYDROCHLORIDE; DECONGESTANTS; ANTIHISTAMINES.
Precautions: this syrup should not be taken by children under 10 years old. *See also* OPIOIDS; DECONGESTANTS; ANTIHISTAMINES; PARACETAMOL.
Interactions with other drugs: *see* OPIOIDS; EPHEDRINE HYDROCHLORIDE; ANTIHISTAMINES.

Vicks Cough Lozenges with Honey (Procter & Gamble) *See* DEXTROMETHORPHAN.

Vicks Cough Syrup for Chesty Coughs (Procter & Gamble) *See* GUAIFENESIN.

Vicks Cough Syrup with Honey for Dry and Irritating Coughs (Procter & Gamble) *See* MENTHOL.

Vicks Inhaler (Procter & Gamble) A proprietary combination of *menthol and *camphor, used to relieve nasal congestion. It is freely available *over the counter in the form of a stick; this is inserted into the nostril, and the vapour is inhaled.

Vicks Sinex (Procter & Gamble) *See* OXYMETAZOLINE.

Vicks Vaporub (Procter & Gamble) A proprietary combination of *menthol, *camphor, *eucalyptus oil, and *turpentine oil, used to relieve nasal and catarrhal congestion associated with colds. It can be rubbed on the chest or back or added to hot water and used as an inhalation. Vicks Vaporub is freely available *over the counter.
Side effects and precautions: *see* RUBEFACIENTS.

Victanyl (Actavis) *See* FENTANYL.

Victoza (Novo Nordisk Limited) *See* LIRAGLUTIDE.

Vidaza (Celgene Ltd) *See* AZACITIDINE.

Videne (Ecolab) *See* POVIDONE–IODINE.

Videx (Bristol-Myers Squibb) *See* DIDANOSINE.

ViePax, ViePax XL (Dexcel Pharma Ltd) *See* VENLAFAXINE.

vigabatrin An *anticonvulsant drug used, under specialist supervision, as an *adjunct for the treatment of partial epilepsy that has not been controlled by other anticonvulsants and alone for the treatment of infantile spasms. It is available, on *prescription only, for oral use as tablets or a powder to be made into a solution.
Side effects: include drowsiness, fatigue, dizziness, nervousness, irritability, agitation, depression, headache, and impaired concentration. Less commonly, confusion, aggression, memory disturbance, and disturbances of vision (including loss of visual field) may occur.
Precautions: vigabatrin should be used with caution in people who have kidney disease. Visual-field tests should be performed before and during treatment, and patients should report any new visual symptoms to a doctor. Women who are planning to become pregnant, or who are already pregnant, should seek specialist advice. Vigabritin is not recommended for women who are breastfeeding. Dosage should be reduced gradually at the end of treatment.
Interactions with other drugs:
Anticonvulsants: taking two or more anticonvulsants together may increase their adverse effects; vigabatrin often lowers the plasma concentration of phenytoin.
Antidepressants: may increase the risk of convulsions; St John's wort should not be taken with vigabatrin.
Mefloquine: antagonizes the anticonvulsant effect of vigabatrin.
Proprietary preparation: Sabril.

Vigam (BPL) *See* IMMUNOGLOBULINS.

Vigranon B (Wallace) A proprietary combination of *nicotinamide (a B vitamin), *riboflavin (vitamin B_2), *pyridoxine hydrochloride (vitamin B_6), *thiamine hydrochloride (vitamin B_1), and pantothenol (a B vitamin), used to prevent vitamin B deficiency (*see* VITAMIN B COMPLEX). It is available as tablets and can be bought without a prescription, but only from pharmacies.

vildagliptin An *oral hypoglycaemic drug used, in combination with other antidiabetic drugs, to control blood glucose levels in people with type 2 *diabetes mellitus. It works by increasing the secretion of *insulin and reducing the secretion of *glucagon. Vildagliptin is available as tablets on *prescription only.
Side effects: include dizziness, nausea, headache, and tremor.
Precautions and interactions with other drugs: vildagliptin is not recommended for people with liver or kidney disease or moderate to severe heart failure or for pregnant or breastfeeding women. Liver function tests

should be carried out before and during treatment. There is a risk of *hypoglycaemia when vildagliptin is taken with other hypoglycaemic drugs.
Proprietary preparations: Galvus; *Eucreas (combined with metformin).

Vimpat (UCB Pharma Limited) *See* LACOSAMIDE.

vinblastine sulphate A *vinca alkaloid used for the treatment of acute leukaemias, lymphomas, and some solid tumours (*see* CANCER). It is available as a form for intravenous injection on *prescription only.
Side effects and precautions: *see* VINCA ALKALOIDS; CYTOTOXIC DRUGS.
Interactions with other drugs:

Clozapine: there is an increased risk of agranulocytosis (a blood disorder) and this drug should not be used with vinblastine.

Erythromycin: increases the adverse effects of vinblastine and should not be used with it.

Posaconazole: the risk of neurological side effects is increased.

Proprietary preparation: Velbe.

vinca alkaloids A class of *cytotoxic drugs originally extracted from the periwinkle plant (*Catharanthus roseus*; formerly called *Vinca rosea*). They are used to treat acute lymphomas, acute leukaemias, and some solid tumours, such as breast and lung cancer (*see* CANCER). The commonly used vinca alkaloids are *vinblastine sulphate, *vincristine sulphate, *vindesine sulphate, and *vinorelbine. They are usually given by intravenous injection or infusion and are available on *prescription only. *See also* ETOPOSIDE.
Side effects: vinca alkaloids commonly cause reversible peripheral neurological side effects, which include tingling of the fingers or toes, abdominal pain, constipation, and muscle weakness. Other side effects include *bone marrow suppression and reversible hair loss. There may also be pain and irritation at the injection site. *See also* CYTOTOXIC DRUGS.
Precautions: vinca alkaloids should not be given to women who are pregnant or breastfeeding. The dosage may need to be reduced for people with liver disease. Any signs of fever, sore throat, or infection should be reported to a doctor. *See also* CYTOTOXIC DRUGS.

vincristine sulphate A *vinca alkaloid used for the treatment of acute leukaemias, lymphomas, and some solid tumours (*see* CANCER). It is available as a solution for intravenous injection on *prescription only.
Side effects and precautions: *see* VINCA ALKALOIDS; CYTOTOXIC DRUGS.
Interactions with other drugs:

Antifungal drugs: itraconazole and posaconazole may increase the risk of neurological side effects of vincristine.

Clozapine: there is an increased risk of agranulocytosis (a blood disorder) and this drug should not be given with vincristine.

Proprietary preparation: Oncovin.

vindesine sulphate A *vinca alkaloid used for the treatment of acute leukaemias, lymphomas, and some solid tumours (*see* CANCER). It is available as a form for intravenous injection on *prescription only.

Side effects and precautions: *see* VINCA ALKALOIDS; CYTOTOXIC DRUGS.
Proprietary preparation: Eldisine.

vinorelbine A semisynthetic *vinca alkaloid used for the treatment of some forms of lung cancer and also for advanced breast cancer when treatment with anthracyclines (*cytotoxic antibiotics) has failed. It is available as capsules or a concentrate for intravenous infusion or injection on *prescription only.
Side effects: *see* VINCA ALKALOIDS; CYTOTOXIC DRUGS.
Precautions: the capsules should not be taken by patients who have had major surgery of the stomach or bowel. *See also* VINCA ALKALOIDS; CYTOTOXIC DRUGS.
Interactions with other drugs:
Clozapine: the risk of agranulocytosis (a blood disorder) is increased and this drug should not be given with vinorelbine.
Proprietary preparation: Navelbine.

Viracept (Roche Products) *See* NELFINAVIR.

Viramune (Boehringer Ingelheim) *See* NEVIRAPINE.

Virazole (Meda Pharmaceuticals) *See* RIBAVIRIN.

Viread (Gilead Sciences Ltd) *See* TENOFOVIR DISOPROXIL.

Virgan (Chauvin) *See* GANCICLOVIR.

Viridal (UCB Pharma Limited) *See* ALPROSTADIL.

Virormone (Nordic Pharma Limited) *See* TESTOSTERONE.

Virovir (Opus) *See* ACICLOVIR.

Visclair (Ranbaxy) *See* METHYLCYSTEINE HYDROCHLORIDE.

Viscotears (Novartis) *See* CARBOMER.

Viskaldix (Amdipharm) A proprietary combination of *pindolol (a non-cardioselective beta blocker) and clopamide (a *thiazide diuretic), used in the treatment of mild to moderate *hypertension. It is available as tablets on *prescription only.
Side effects, precautions, and interactions with other drugs: *see* BETA BLOCKERS; THIAZIDE DIURETICS.

See also ANTIHYPERTENSIVE DRUGS; DIURETICS.

Visken (Amdipharm) *See* PINDOLOL.

Vismed (TRB Chemedica) *See* SODIUM HYALURONATE.

Vistabel (Allergan) *See* BOTULINUM TOXIN TYPE A.

Vistamethasone (Martindale Pharmaceuticals) *See* BETAMETHASONE.

Vistide (Gilead Sciences Ltd) *See* CIDOFOVIR.

Visudyne (Novartis) *See* VERTEPORFIN.

vitamin Any of a group of substances that are required, in very small amounts, for healthy growth and development: they cannot be synthesized by the body and are therefore essential constituents of the diet. Vitamins are divided into two groups, according to whether they are soluble in water or fat. The water-soluble group includes the vitamin B complex and vitamin C; the fat-soluble vitamins are vitamins A, D, E, and K. Lack of sufficient quantities of any of the vitamins in the diet results in specific vitamin deficiency diseases.

Vitamin supplements are readily available for treating and preventing vitamin deficiencies.

vitamin A (**retinol**) A fat-soluble vitamin that is necessary for healthy vision, particularly vision in dim light. It is also essential for growth and the integrity of mucous tissue (in the mouth, eyes, nose, and genitals). Vitamin A deficiency causes stunted growth, night blindness, and drying and thickening of the cornea, which can progress eventually to blindness. The vitamin occurs in foods of animal origin, especially milk products, egg yolk, and liver, and it can be formed in the body from beta-carotene, a pigment found in vegetables, especially carrots, cabbage, and lettuce. Deficiency is rare in the UK.

Supplements of vitamin A are given usually in combination with *vitamin D as tablets or capsules of fish oils (*see* HALIBUT-LIVER OIL) for adults and children; these are freely available *over the counter.

Side effects: none reported in low doses, but vitamin A is one of the few vitamins that can be toxic in overdose, causing rough dry skin, dry hair, and an enlarged liver.

Precautions: there is evidence suggesting that vitamin A may cause birth defects, therefore women who are pregnant or planning to become pregnant should not take vitamin A supplements (unless advised to by a doctor) or eat large amounts of liver products, such as paté.

Interactions with other drugs:

Retinoids: the risk of vitamin A poisoning is increased.

Proprietary preparation: *Vivioptal (combined with vitamin C, vitamin D, vitamin E, B-complex vitamins, and various minerals and trace elements).

See also HEALTHY START CHILDREN'S VITAMIN DROPS.

vitamin B_1 *See* THIAMINE; VITAMIN B COMPLEX.

vitamin B_2 *See* RIBOFLAVIN; VITAMIN B COMPLEX.

vitamin B_6 *See* PYRIDOXINE; VITAMIN B COMPLEX.

vitamin B_{12} *See* VITAMIN B COMPLEX.

vitamin B complex A group of water-soluble vitamins that, although not chemically related, are often found together in the same kinds of food (including milk, liver, and cereals).

Vitamin B_1 (*see* THIAMINE) is required for carbohydrate metabolism; a deficiency leads to beriberi. **Vitamin B_2** (*see* RIBOFLAVIN) is important for oxygen exchange in the tissues. **Vitamin B_6** (*see* PYRIDOXINE) is involved in protein metabolism. **Vitamin B_{12}** (*see* CYANOCOBALAMIN; HYDROXOCOBALAMIN) is necessary for the synthesis of nucleic acids (DNA and RNA), the maintenance of myelin (an important component of certain nerve cells), and the proper functioning of *folic acid. B_{12} can be absorbed only in the presence of **intrinsic factor**, a protein secreted in the stomach. A deficiency of vitamin B_{12} affects nearly all the body tissues, particularly those containing rapidly dividing cells. The most serious effects of a deficiency are pernicious *anaemia (due to deficiency of intrinsic factor) and degeneration of the nervous system. Vitamin B_{12} is contained only in foods of animal origin. Other members of the B complex include *nicotinamide, *aminobenzoic acid, **pantothenic acid**, **panthenol**, **inositol**, and **biotin**.

B group vitamins are used to treat specific diseases due to deficiencies of these vitamins and also to prevent deficiency in people considered to be at risk (e.g. pregnant women). They are available as specific vitamin supplements and are also included in numerous multivitamin preparations; many *iron supplements also contain B group vitamins.
Proprietary preparations: *Vigranon B; *Abidec Multivitamin Drops (combined with vitamins A, C, and D); *Dalivit (combined with vitamins A, C, and D); *Pabrinex (combined with vitamin C); *Vivioptal (combined with vitamin A, vitamin C, vitamin D, vitamin E, and various minerals and trace elements); *Yeast-Vite (combined with caffeine).

vitamin C (**ascorbic acid**) A water-soluble vitamin that is essential for maintaining healthy connective tissues and the integrity of cell membranes: it is necessary for the synthesis of collagen, which is required to produce connective tissue. Vitamin C has antioxidant properties, i.e. it neutralizes oxygen free radicals, which are produced by various disease processes and toxic substances and have damaging effects on the body. Vitamin C occurs in fruits and vegetables, especially citrus fruits. Elderly people may suffer mild vitamin C deficiency, which leads to an increased susceptibility to infection. Severe vitamin C deficiency causes scurvy. There have been claims that large doses of vitamin C help to prevent colds and influenza, and consequently vitamin C is often included in cold preparations, but these claims are unproven. Vitamin C is freely available *over the counter as tablets or effervescent tablets; these cannot be prescribed on the NHS. It is included as an ingredient in numerous multivitamin preparations. Vitamin C is also available as an injection.

Proprietary preparations: Redoxon; *Pabrinex (combined with B group vitamins); *Vivioptal (combined with vitamin A, vitamin D, vitamin E, B-complex vitamins, and various minerals and trace elements); plus many other proprietory preparations.

See also HEALTHY START CHILDREN'S VITAMIN DROPS.

vitamin D A fat-soluble *vitamin that promotes the absorption of *calcium and phosphorus from the intestine and their deposition in bone. It occurs in the form of a group of closely related steroid-based compounds, including

vitamin D_2 (*ergocalciferol), manufactured from ergosterol by plants when exposed to ultraviolet light, and **vitamin D_3** (*colecalciferol), which is formed from a derivative of cholesterol by the action of sunlight on the skin. Deficiency of vitamin D interferes with the absorption of calcium from the intestine, causing rickets in children and osteomalacia (softening of the bones) in adults. Vitamin D supplements may be required by people who do not get enough sunlight (for example, the housebound elderly and members of certain ethnic groups or cultures who always keep their skin covered) and menopausal women. People who have kidney disease, especially those on dialysis, may also need vitamin D therapy to avoid bone disease.

Simple vitamin D deficiency is treated with oral supplements of ergocalciferol or colecalciferol. Deficiency caused by poor absorption of calcium from the intestines or chronic liver disease is treated with *calciferol tablets. People with kidney disease or poorly functioning parathyroid glands (which produce *parathyroid hormone) are treated with *alfacalcidol, *calcitriol, *dihydrotachysterol, or *paricalcitol. Since vitamin D promotes absorption of calcium from food, care must be taken to ensure that not too much calcium is absorbed, which may cause adverse effects (see below); blood tests may be necessary. *See also* CALCIPOTRIOL.

Side effects: these are most commonly related to increased concentrations of calcium in the blood, caused by overdosage of vitamin D. Symptoms of overdosage include loss of appetite, tiredness, nausea, vomiting, stomach pains, thirst, headache, dizziness, and excessive urination.

Precautions: vitamin D preparations should not be taken by people with high plasma concentrations of calcium or calcification due to malignant disease. Plasma calcium may need to be monitored during treatment. Vitamin D should be used with caution during pregnancy and breastfeeding.

Interactions with other drugs:

Antiepileptic drugs: carbamazepine, phenobarbital, phenytoin, and primidone reduce the effects of vitamin D: increased dosage of vitamin D may be required.

Thiazide diuretics: increase the risk of absorbing too much calcium.

Proprietary preparations: *Abidec Multivitamin Drops (combined with vitamins A, B, and C); *Dalivit (combined with vitamins A, B, and C); *Vivioptal (combined with vitamin D, vitamin E, B-complex vitamins, and various minerals and trace elements).

See also HEALTHY START CHILDREN'S VITAMIN DROPS.

vitamin E (**tocopherols**) A group of fat-soluble vitamins that stabilize cell membranes by protecting them from the damaging effects of oxygen free radicals, which are produced by various disease processes and toxic substances, i.e. they have antioxidant effects. The most important member of the vitamin E group is **alpha-tocopherol**, which is found in vegetable oils, eggs, butter, and wholemeal cereals. There is evidence to suggest that it may reduce the risk of a heart attack in susceptible individuals. It is available, as **alpha tocopheryl acetate**, in the form of a suspension or tablets that can be obtained without a prescription, but only from pharmacies.

Side effects: there may be diarrhoea and abdominal pain with higher dosages.
Proprietary preparations: *Forceval (combined with other vitamins); *Ketovite (combined with other vitamins); *Vivioptal (combined with vitamin D, vitamin E, B-complex vitamins, and various minerals and trace elements).

vitamin K A fat-soluble vitamin that is necessary for the production of factors (including prothrombin) that are essential for blood clotting. Because vitamin K dissolves in fat, people who do not absorb fat properly also do not absorb vitamin K and become deficient in the vitamin. In such people vitamin K can be replaced orally by a soluble synthetic form, *menadiol sodium phosphate. An injectable form of the vitamin, *phytomenadione, is given to premature newborn babies to protect against haemorrhage and to people taking anticoagulant therapy to counteract the effects of an overdosage of *warfarin sodium.

Vivaglobin (CSL Behring) *See* IMMUNOGLOBULINS.

Vividrin (Pharma-Global) *See* SODIUM CROMOGLICATE.

Vivioptal (Iris Healthcare Ltd) A proprietary combination of *vitamin A, *vitamin C, *vitamin D, *vitamin E, the B complex vitamins biotin, inositol, pantothenic acid (*see* VITAMIN B COMPLEX), *folic acid, *nicotinic acid, *pyridoxine, *riboflavin, and *thiamine, and various minerals, including *calcium, iron, magnesium, *potassium, and *zinc, used to treat vitamin and mineral deficiency. It is freely available *over the counter as tablets.

Volibris (GlaxoSmithKline) *See* AMBRISENTAN.

Volsaid Retard (Novartis) *See* DICLOFENAC SODIUM.

Voltarol (Novartis) *See* DICLOFENAC SODIUM.

von Willebrand factor A protein that acts as a blood-clotting factor and is required for normal platelet function. Deficiencies of the factor result in several diseases characterized by excessive and uncontrolled bleeding. A concentrated form of this factor is used to treat these diseases.
Proprietary preparations: *Haemate P (combined with Factor VIII); *Optivate (combined with Factor VIII).

voriconazole A triazole *antifungal drug used for the treatment of generalized aspergillosis and candidiasis. It is available, on *prescription only, as tablets, an oral suspension, and a form for intravenous infusion.

Side effects: include nausea, vomiting, abdominal pain, diarrhoea, chest pain, headache, dizziness, blood disorders, blurred vision, sensitivity to light, and itching.
Precautions: voriconazole should not be given to people with porphyria or to breastfeeding women. It should be used with caution in people with a history of *arrhythmias or liver or kidney disease and in pregnant women. People being treated should avoid exposure to sunlight and undergo liver and kidney function tests.
Interactions with other drugs: voriconazole inhibits an enzyme system in the

liver that is involved in metabolizing a number of drugs, whose plasma concentrations (and therefore adverse effects) are therefore increased. These drugs include pimozide, sertindole, phenytoin, ciclosporin, lapatinib and nilotinib, ergotamine, atorvastatin and simvastatin, sirolimus, tacrolimus, and omeprazole. Pimozide, sertindole, and ergotamine should not be taken with voriconazole. In addition, the plasma concentrations of voriconazole are reduced by some drugs, including St John's wort, ranolazine, carbamazepine and primidone, ritonavir, and phenobarbital (none of which should be taken with voriconazole), phenytoin, efavirenz, and the sulphonylureas.
Proprietary preparation: Vfend.

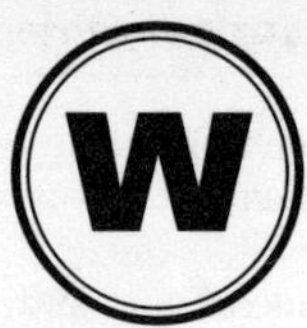

warfarin sodium An oral *anticoagulant used for the prevention and treatment of deep-vein *thrombosis and pulmonary embolism and for the prevention of embolism in people with atrial fibrillation (*see* ARRHYTHMIA) and in those who have an artificial heart valve or a cardiac aneurysm (a weakness in the wall of a coronary artery). Warfarin is available as tablets on *prescription only.

Side effects: excessive bleeding is the most serious side effect (*see* ANTICOAGULANTS); if this occurs, immediate medical advice should be sought and *phytomenadione may need to be given. Other side effects include allergic reactions and rashes.

Precautions: patients are required to have regular blood tests to ensure that they are on a suitable dose of warfarin. Warfarin should not be used during the first three months or the last three months of pregnancy or by women who are trying to become pregnant, unless the patient's condition makes this unavoidable. It should also be avoided in people with peptic ulcer and severe hypertension and used with caution in people with kidney or liver disease and in women who are breastfeeding. Excessive consumption of alcohol increases the anticoagulant effects of warfarin, and radical changes in diet can affect the anticoagulant effect of warfarin; cranberry juice should not be consumed by people taking warfarin as it may increase its anticoagulant effect.

Interactions with other drugs: warfarin interacts with many other drugs, the most important of which are listed below. If warfarin and the interacting drug are both taken regularly, the dosage of warfarin will need to be adjusted to take this into account. Short courses of interacting drugs may also affect the dose of warfarin needed.

Acitretin: may reduce the anticoagulant effect of warfarin.

Anabolic steroids: enhance the anticoagulant effect of warfarin.

Analgesics: NSAIDs and tramadol may enhance the anticoagulant effect of warfarin; azapropazone, intravenous diclofenac, and ketorolac should not be taken with warfarin.

Anti-arrhythmic drugs: amiodarone and propafenone enhance the anticoagulant effect of warfarin.

Antibiotics: the anticoagulant effect of warfarin is enhanced by chloramphenicol, metronidazole, tetracyclines, cephalosporins, sulphonamides, macrolides, quinolones, and possibly by certain other antibiotics. Rifampicin reduces the anticoagulant effect of warfarin.

Antidepressants: SSRIs and venlafaxine may enhance the anticoagulant effect of warfarin; St John's wort reduces the anticoagulant effect of warfarin and should not be taken with it.

Antiepileptic drugs: carbamazepine, phenobarbital, and primidone reduce

the anticoagulant effect of warfarin; valproate enhances its anticoagulant effect; phenytoin may either reduce or enhance the anticoagulant effect of warfarin.
Antifungal drugs: griseofulvin reduces the anticoagulant effect of warfarin; fluconazole, itraconazole, ketoconazole, miconazole, and voriconazole enhance its anticoagulant effect.
Antiplatelet drugs: clopidogrel and dipyridamole enhance the anticoagulant effect of warfarin.
Antiviral drugs: nevirapine and ritonavir enhance or reduce the anticoagulant effect of warfarin.
Aspirin: increases the risk of excessive bleeding.
Azathioprine: may reduce the anticoagulant effect of warfarin.
Colestyramine: may enhance or reduce the anticoagulant effect of warfarin.
Corticosteroids: may alter the anticoagulant effect of warfarin.
Cytotoxic drugs: etoposide, ifosfamide, fluorouracil, and sorafenib may enhance the anticoagulant effect of warfarin; mercaptopurine and mitotane may reduce the anticoagulant effect of warfarin; erlotinib increases the risk of bleeding.
Danazol: increases the anticoagulant effect of warfarin.
Disulfiram: enhances the anticoagulant effect of warfarin.
Entacapone: enhances the anticoagulant effect of warfarin.
Flutamide: increases the anticoagulant effect of warfarin.
Glucosamine: enhances the anticoagulant effect of warfarin and should not be taken with it.
Levamisole: may enhance the anticoagulant effect of warfarin.
Lipid-lowering drugs: fibrates, fluvastatin, and simvastatin enhance the anticoagulant effect of warfarin.
Methylphenidate: may enhance the anticoagulant effect of warfarin.
Oral contraceptives: may reduce or enhance the anticoagulant effect of warfarin.
Sitaxentan: enhances the anticoagulant effect of warfarin.
Sulfinpyrazone: enhances the anticoagulant effect of warfarin.
Tamoxifen: increases the anticoagulant effect of warfarin.
Testosterone: enhances the anticoagulant effect of warfarin.
Thyroid hormones: enhance the anticoagulant effect of warfarin.
Toremifene: may enhance the anticoagulant effect of warfarin.
Ulcer-healing drugs: cimetidine, esomeprazole, and omeprazole enhance the anticoagulant effect of warfarin; sucralfate reduces the anticoagulant effect of warfarin.
Vitamin K: reduces the anticoagulant effect of warfarin.

Proprietary preparation: Marevan.

Warticon (Stiefel Laboratories) *See* PODOPHYLLOTOXIN.

Wasp-Eze Ointment (SSL International) *See* ANTAZOLINE.

Wasp-Eze Spray (SSL International) A proprietary combination of

*mepyramine maleate (an antihistamine) and *benzocaine (a local anaesthetic), used for the relief of insect stings. It is available from pharmacies without a prescription.
Side effects: the spray may occasionally cause allergic reactions.
Precautions: the spray should not be applied to the eyes, mouth, or other mucous membranes or to broken skin.

Waxsol (Norgine) *See* DOCUSATE SODIUM.

Welldorm (Alphashow) *See* CLORAL BETAINE.

Welldorm Elixir (Alphashow) *See* CHLORAL HYDRATE.

Wellvone (GlaxoSmithKline) *See* ATOVAQUONE.

white soft paraffin (**white petroleum jelly**) A purified mixture of hydrocarbons obtained from petroleum. A bleached version of *yellow soft paraffin, it is used as an *emollient and as a base for ointments. It is odourless when rubbed into the skin and not readily absorbed.
Side effects: very rarely it may cause allergic reactions or acne.
Proprietary preparations: *Cetraben Emollient Cream (combined with liquid paraffin); *Diprobase (combined with liquid paraffin); *E45 Cream (combined with lanolin and liquid paraffin); *Emollin (combined with liquid paraffin); *50:50 Ointment (combined with liquid paraffin); *Hewletts Cream (combined with zinc oxide); *Lacri-Lube (combined with liquid paraffin and wool fat); *Lipobase (combined with liquid paraffin); *Lubri-Tears (combined with liquid paraffin and wool fat); *Ultrabase (combined with liquid paraffin and stearyl alcohol); *Unguentum M (combined with silicic acid, liquid paraffin, and other emollients).

Wilzin (Orphan Europe) *See* ZINC ACETATE.

Wind-eze (GlaxoSmithKline) *See* DIMETICONE.

Winfex XL (Winthrop Pharmaceuticals) *See* VENLAFAXINE.

witch hazel *See* HAMAMELIS.

withdrawal symptoms *See* DEPENDENCE.

Woodward's Gripe Water (SSL International) A proprietary combination of *sodium bicarbonate and *dill seed oil, used for the relief of wind pain in babies and children over one month old. It is freely available *over the counter.

wool fat *See* LANOLIN.

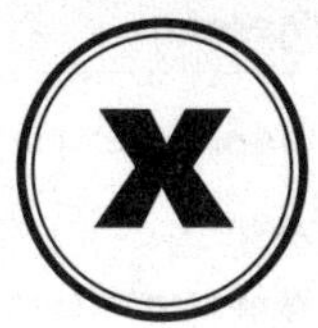

Xagrid (Shire Pharmaceuticals) *See* ANAGRELIDE.

Xalacom (Pharmacia) A proprietary combination of *latanoprost (a prostaglandin analogue) and *timolol maleate (a beta blocker), used to reduce the pressure inside the eye in people with *glaucoma and to treat high blood pressure in the eye. It is used when beta blockers alone have failed to reduce the pressure and is available as eye drops on *prescription only.
Side effects and precautions: *see* BETA BLOCKERS; LATANOPROST.
Interactions with other drugs: *see* BETA BLOCKERS.

Xalatan (Pharmacia) *See* LATANOPROST.

Xamiol (Leo Pharmaceuticals Limited) A proprietary combination of *calcipotriol (an analogue of vitamin D) and *betamethasone (a corticosteroid), used for the treatment of psoriasis of the scalp. It is available as a scalp gel on *prescription only.
Side effects and precautions: *see* CALCIPOTRIOL; TOPICAL STEROIDS.
Interactions with other drugs: *see* TOPICAL STEROIDS.

Xanax (Pharmacia) *See* ALPRAZOLAM.

xanthines A group of nitrogen-containing compounds found widely in nature. Natural xanthines include *caffeine and theobromine, which are consumed in tea and coffee. Xanthine drugs relax smooth muscle, especially in the airways (*see* BRONCHODILATORS), and are therefore used primarily in the treatment of *asthma (*see also* PHOSPHODIESTERASE INHIBITORS). *Modified-release formulations are particularly useful for the prevention of nocturnal asthma attacks. *See* AMINOPHYLLINE; THEOPHYLLINE; PENTOXIFYLLINE.
Side effects: up to one-third of children experience gastrointestinal disturbances, sleep disruption, and/or psychological changes. Adults experience gastrointestinal upset, nausea, headaches, vertigo, and flushes.
Precautions: smoking and alcohol shorten the duration of action of xanthines and higher doses may be necessary in smokers. The duration of action is increased in heart failure, cirrhosis of the liver, and viral infections, in the elderly, and by certain drugs.

Xarelto (Bayer) *See* RIVAROXABAN.

Xatral, Xatral XL (sanofi-aventis) *See* ALFUZOSIN HYDROCHLORIDE.

Xeloda (Roche Products) *See* CAPECITABINE.

Xenazine 25 (Cambridge Laboratories) *See* TETRABENAZINE.

Xenical (Roche Products) *See* ORLISTAT.

Xeomin (Merz Pharma UK Ltd) *See* BOTULINUM TOXIN TYPE A.

Xepin (CHS) *See* DOXEPIN.

Xerotin (SpePharm) A proprietary combination of sorbitol (a sugar), carboxymethylcellulose (a protective agent; *see* CARMELLOSE), and salts of potassium, sodium, magnesium, and calcium, used as an artificial saliva to relieve the symptoms of dry mouth. It is freely available *over the counter as an oral spray.

Xigris (Lilly) *See* DROTRECOGIN ALFA.

xipamide A thiazide-like diuretic (*see* THIAZIDE DIURETICS) used for the treatment of *hypertension and *oedema associated with heart failure, liver disease, or kidney disease. More potent than many of the thiazide diuretics, it is available as tablets on *prescription only.
Side effects, precautions, and interactions with other drugs: *see* THIAZIDE DIURETICS.
Proprietary preparation: Diurexan.
See also DIURETICS.

Xismox 60 XL (Genus Pharmaceuticals) *See* ISOSORBIDE MONONITRATE.

Xolair (Novartis) *See* OMALIZUMAB.

Xomolix (ProStrakan) *See* DROPERIDOL.

xylitol A sugar, obtained from birch and other trees, that increases the production of saliva and inhibits bacterial growth. It is used as a bulk sweetener in foods and a toothpaste and as a component of artificial salivas.
Proprietary preparations: *Oralbalance (combined with oxidase enzymes); *Saliva Orthana (combined with mucin).

Xylocaine (AstraZeneca) *See* LIDOCAINE.

xylometazoline A *sympathomimetic drug that stimulates alpha *adrenoceptors. It is used for the treatment of nasal congestion (*see* DECONGESTANTS) and is also used in combination with other drugs to treat allergic conjunctivitis. It is available from pharmacies without a *prescription in the form of a nasal spray or drops and eye drops.
Side effects: include nasal irritation, headache, and increased heart rate. Prolonged use may cause rebound congestion.
Precautions: prolonged use should be avoided.
Interactions with other drugs: *see* DECONGESTANTS.
Proprietary preparations: Non-Drowsy Sudafed Decongestant Nasal Spray; Otrivine (adult nasal drops, children's nasal drops, and adult nasal spray); *Otrivine-Antistin (combined with antazoline sulphate).

Xyloproct (AstraZeneca) A proprietary combination of *zinc oxide and aluminium acetate (astringents), *lidocaine (a local anaesthetic), and *hydrocortisone acetate (a corticosteroid), used to relieve the discomfort of

*haemorrhoids, itching of the anus or vulva, and the pain of anal fissures. It is available as an ointment on *prescription only.
Side effects: Xyloproct may cause dermatitis. *See also* CORTICOSTEROIDS.
Precautions: Xyloproct should not be used when viral or fungal infection is present; prolonged use should be avoided.

Xyrem (UCB Pharma Limited) *See* SODIUM OXYBATE.

Xyzal (UCB Pharma Limited) *See* LEVOCETIRIZINE.

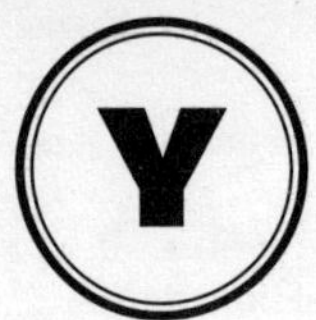

8Y (BPL) *See* FACTOR VIII.

Yasmin (Bayer) A proprietary combination of *ethinylestradiol and drospirenone (a synthetic *progestogen), used as an *oral contraceptive. It is available as tablets on *prescription only.
Side effects, precautions, and interactions with other drugs: *see* ORAL CONTRACEPTIVES.

Yeast-Vite (Actavis) A proprietary combination of *thiamine, *riboflavin, and *nicotinamide (all B vitamins) and *caffeine (a stimulant), used to prevent vitamin B deficiency (*see* VITAMIN B COMPLEX) and to relieve fatigue and drowsiness. It is available as tablets and can be obtained without a prescription but only from *pharmacies.

yellow soft paraffin (**yellow petroleum jelly**) A purified mixture of hydrocarbons obtained from petroleum. Semisolid, pale yellow to amber, and translucent, it is used as an *emollient and as a base for ointments. It is odourless when rubbed into the skin and not readily absorbed.
Side effects: very rarely it may cause allergic reactions or acne.
Proprietary preparation: *Epaderm (combined with liquid paraffin and wax).

Yentreve (Eli Lilly & Co) *See* DULOXETINE.

Yondelis (Pharma Mar, S.A.) *See* TRABECTEDIN.

Yutopar (Durbin) *See* RITODRINE.

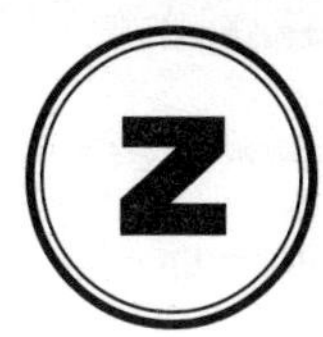

Zacin (Cephalon) *See* CAPSAICIN.

Zaditen (Novartis) *See* KETOTIFEN.

zafirlukast A *leukotriene receptor antagonist used for the treatment of mild to moderate asthma that is not adequately controlled by the usual combination of an inhaled *corticosteroid and a beta stimulant (such as *salbutamol). It should not be used to treat acute attacks. Zafirlukast is available as tablets on *prescription only.
Side effects: include abdominal pain, headache, insomnia, and (rarely) allergic reactions (including rashes) and severe asthma.
Precautions: zafirlukast should not be taken by people with liver disease or by women who are breastfeeding. It should be used with caution in the elderly, in people with kidney disease, and in pregnant women.
Interactions with other drugs:
Aspirin: increases the plasma concentration of zafirlukast.
Erythromycin: reduces the plasma concentration of zafirlukast.
Theophylline: reduces the plasma concentration of zafirlukast; the plasma concentration of theophylline may be increased by zafirlukast.
Warfarin: its anticoagulant effect is increased by zafirlukast.
Proprietary preparation: Accolate.

zaleplon A very short-acting drug used for the short-term treatment of insomnia (*see* HYPNOTIC DRUGS). It acts in the same way as benzodiazepines but takes a shorter time to react and has little or no hangover effect. Zaleplon is available as capsules on *prescription only.
Side effects: include amnesia, 'pins and needles', drowsiness, nausea, and vomiting. *Dependence may rarely occur with prolonged use.
Precautions: zaleplon should not be taken by people with severe liver disease, sleep apnoea syndrome (in which airflow to the lungs is obstructed during sleep), depressed breathing, or myasthenia gravis or by children under 18 years of age. It should be used with caution in people with a history of drug abuse or depression.
Interactions with other drugs: the sedative effects of zaleplon may be increased by a number of drugs, including general anaesthetics, opioid analgesics, some antidepressants, antihistamines, and the antiviral drug ritonavir.
Proprietary preparation: Sonata.

Zamadol (Meda Pharmaceuticals) *See* TRAMADOL HYDROCHLORIDE.

Zanaflex (Cephalon) *See* TIZANIDINE.

zanamivir An *antiviral drug used for the treatment and prevention of influenza. It is most effective when taken within two days of the symptoms first appearing (for treatment) and within 36 hours of exposure to influenza (for prevention). Zanamivir acts by reducing replication of the virus. It is available, on *prescription only, as a powder for inhalation.
Precautions: zanamivir should not be taken by people with severe asthma and should be used with caution in people with chronic obstructive pulmonary disease and in women who are pregnant or breastfeeding.
Proprietary preparation: Relenza.

Zanidip (Recordati Pharmaceuticals Limited) *See* LERCANIDIPINE.

Zantac (GlaxoSmithKline) *See* RANITIDINE.

Zaponex *See* CLOZAPINE.

Zarontin (Pfizer) *See* ETHOSUXIMIDE.

Zarzio (Sandoz) *See* FILGRASTIM.

Zavedos (Pharmacia) *See* IDARUBICIN.

Zavesca (Actelion) *See* MIGLUSTAT.

ZeaSORB (Stiefel Laboratories) A proprietary combination of aldioxa (aluminium dihydroxyallantoinate; an astringent), *chloroxylenol (an antiseptic), and powdered maize core. It is used as an antiperspirant dusting powder to prevent excessive sweating of the feet, hands, and armpits. ZeaSORB can be obtained without a prescription, but only from pharmacies.

Zeffix (GlaxoSmithKline) *See* LAMIVUDINE.

Zelapar (Cephalon) *See* SELEGILINE.

Zemon XL (Neolab) *See* ISOSORBIDE MONONITRATE.

Zemplar (Abbott) *See* PARICALCITOL.

Zemtard (Galen) *See* DILTIAZEM HYDROCHLORIDE.

Zeridame SR (Actavis) *See* TRAMADOL HYDROCHLORIDE.

Zerit (Bristol-Myers Squibb) *See* STAVUDINE.

Zestoretic (AstraZeneca) A proprietary combination of *lisinopril (an ACE inhibitor) and *hydrochlorothiazide (a thiazide diuretic), used in the treatment of mild to moderate *hypertension. A *prescription only medicine, it is available as tablets of two strengths: **Zestoretic 10** and **Zestoretic 20**.
Side effects, precautions, and interactions with other drugs: *see* ACE INHIBITORS; THIAZIDE DIURETICS.

Zestril (AstraZeneca) *See* LISINOPRIL.

Zevalin (Bayer) *See* IBRITUMONAB TIUXETAN.

Ziagen (GlaxoSmithKline) *See* ABACAVIR.

Zibor (Archimedes Pharma UK Ltd) *See* BEMIPARIN SODIUM.

ziconotide acetate An analgesic used for the treatment of severe chronic pain; it functions as a *calcium antagonist. Ziconotide is given, under expert supervision, by infusion into the membranes surrounding the spinal cord. It is available on *prescription only.
Side effects: include dizziness, nausea, nystagmus, confusion, abnormal gait, memory impairment, blurred vision, headache, vomiting, and somnolence.
Precautions: ziconotide should be used with caution in people with impaired liver or kidney function and in pregnant or breastfeeding women. As it may cause somnolence, people treated with ziconotide should not drive or operate machinery.
Proprietary preparation: Prialt.

Zidoval (Meda Pharmaceuticals) *See* METRONIDAZOLE.

zidovudine (**azidothymidine**; **AZT**) An *antiviral drug that prevents retrovirus replication: it is a nucleoside analogue that inhibits reverse transcriptase. One of the oldest antiviral drugs, zidovudine is used, in combination with other antiretrovirals, for the treatment of *HIV infection and to prevent transmission of HIV from mother to fetus. Zidovudine is available, on *prescription only, as tablets, capsules, a syrup, or a solution for infusion.
Side effects: include anaemia, nausea and vomiting, loss of appetite, abdominal pain, indigestion, headache, rash, fever, aching muscles, pigmentation of the skin, nails, and mouth, and reduced production of white blood cells.
Precautions: zidovudine should not be given to people with severe anaemia or a very low white-blood-cell count; blood tests are required during the first three months of treatment. It should be used with caution in those with kidney or liver disease and in pregnant women; breastfeeding is not recommended during treatment.
Interactions with other drugs:
Analgesics: methadone increases the plasma concentration (and therefore side effects) of zidovudine; NSAIDs increase the risk of blood disorders.
Antiviral drugs: ganciclovir greatly reduces production of blood cells in the bone marrow; ribavirin increases the risk of anaemia and should not be used with zidovudine; stavudine may inhibit the effects of zidovudine; tipranavir reduces the plasma concentration of zidovudine.
Clarithromycin: reduces the absorption of zidovudine.
Fluconazole: increases the plasma concentration (and risk of adverse effects) of zidovudine.
Phenytoin: the plasma concentration of phenytoin is altered.
Probenecid: increases the plasma concentration of zidovudine.
Proprietary preparations: Retrovir; *Combivir (combined with lamivudine); *Trizivir (combined with abacavir and lamivudine).

Zimbacol XL (Archimedes Pharma UK Ltd) *See* BEZAFIBRATE.

Zimovane (sanofi-aventis) *See* ZOPICLONE.

Zinacef (GlaxoSmithKline) *See* CEFUROXIME.

zinc A metallic element required in minute amounts for the normal functioning of many enzymes in the body. Deficiency is rare with a balanced diet but it may occur in people with some forms of kidney disease or conditions in which absorption of food substances from the intestine is reduced or it may result from burns or trauma. Zinc deficiency can affect the skin, oesophagus (gullet), or eyes. It is treated with supplementary *zinc sulphate.

zinc acetate A drug that blocks the absorption of copper from the diet, used in treating Wilson's disease, in which copper cannot be metabolized and accumulates in the liver and brain. It is available as capsules on *prescription only; treatment is started under the supervision of a specialist.
Side effects: include irritation of the stomach.
Precautions: zinc acetate should not be taken by women who are breastfeeding.
Proprietary preparation: Wilzin.

zinc oxide A soothing and protective agent that is mildly *astringent and used in the form of a cream, ointment, or dusting power to treat napkin rash, urine rashes, *eczema, *haemorrhoids, and mild skin abrasions. Creams and ointments often also contain *emollients, such as castor oil, arachis oil, and wool fat. Zinc oxide is also used as a paste in medicated bandages to treat leg ulcers. Combined with *coal tar or *ichthammol, it is used as a paste to treat *psoriasis or eczema. Zinc oxide reflects sunlight and is therefore included in some *sunscreen preparations. Zinc oxide can be obtained without a prescription but some compound preparations are *prescription only medicines.
Proprietary preparations: Zincaband (medicated bandage); *Anugesic-HC (combined with pramocaine hydrochloride, hydrocortisone acetate, benzyl benzoate, Peru balsam, and bismuth oxide); *Anugesic-HC Suppositories (combined with pramocaine hydrochloride, hydrocortisone acetate, benzyl benzoate, bismuth oxide, and bismuth subgallate); *Anusol (combined with bismuth oxide, bismuth subgallate, and Peru balsam); *Anusol-HC (combined with bismuth oxide, bismuth subgallate, Peru balsam, benzyl benzoate, and hydrocortisone acetate); *Benadryl Skin Allergy Relief Cream (combined with diphenhydranine and camphor); *E45 Wash Cream (combined with light liquid paraffin); *Germolene Antiseptic Ointment (combined with methyl salicylate, octafonium chloride, and phenol); *Germoloids (combined with lidocaine); *Haemorrhoid Relief Ointment (combined with lidocaine); *Hewletts Cream (combined with white soft paraffin); *Icthopaste (combined with ichthamol); *Morhulin (combined with cod liver oil); *Sudocrem (combined with anhydrous lanolin, benzyl benzoate, benzyl cinnamate, and benzyl alcohol); *Vasogen Cream (combined with calamine and dimeticone); *Xyloproct (combined with lidocaine, aluminium acetate, and hydrocortisone).
See also LASSAR'S PASTE.

zinc sulphate A salt of zinc used as a supplement for treating *zinc deficiency. It is also used as an *astringent for the treatment of excessive tear production or watery eyes. Zinc sulphate is available as effervescent tablets without a prescription, but only from pharmacies; an injection is available on *prescription only.
Side effects: oral preparations may cause abdominal pain and indigestion.
Precautions: oral zinc sulphate should be used with caution by people with kidney disease.
Interactions with other drugs:
Iron supplements: reduce the absorption of zinc and their own absorption is reduced by zinc.
Penicillamine: reduces the absorption of zinc and its own absorption is reduced by zinc.
Quinolone antibiotics: the absorption of ciprofloxacin, levofloxacin, moxifloxacin, norfloxacin, and ofloxacin is reduced.
Tetracyclines: reduce the absorption of zinc and their own absorption is reduced by zinc.
Proprietary preparation: Solvazinc (tablets).

zinc undecenoate *See* UNDECENOIC ACID.

Zindaclin (Crawford) *See* CLINDAMYCIN.

Zineryt (Astellas Pharma) A proprietary combination of *erythromycin (a macrolide antibiotic) and zinc acetate (an *astringent), used for the treatment of *acne. It is available as a solution for topical application on *prescription only.
Side effects: local irritation may occur.
Precautions: when applying the solution, care should be taken to avoid the eyes and mucous membranes.
Interactions with other drugs: *see* ERYTHROMYCIN.

Zinnat (GlaxoSmithKline) *See* CEFUROXIME.

Zirtek (UCB Pharma Limited) *See* CETIRIZINE HYDROCHLORIDE.

Zispin SolTab (Organon Laboratories) *See* MIRTAZAPINE.

Zithromax (Pfizer) *See* AZITHROMYCIN.

Zocor (Merck Sharp & Dohme) *See* SIMVASTATIN.

Zofran (GlaxoSmithKline) *See* ONDANSETRON.

Zoladex (AstraZeneca) *See* GOSERELIN.

zoledronic acid A *bisphosphonate used mainly for the treatment of osteoporosis in postmenopausal women and in men and osteoporosis associated with long-term treatment with glucocorticoids. It is also used to reduce bone damage and pain in advanced bone cancer. Zoledronic acid is available as a solution for infusion on *prescription only.
Side effects: include headache, anaemia, dizziness, fever, flu-like symptoms,

chills, fatigue, weakness, pain, malaise, nausea, vomiting, diarrhoea, muscle, bone, and back pain, low concentrations of phosphate in the blood, and arrhythmias.
Precautions: zoledronic acid should not be given to people with low plasma-calcium concentrations or to women who are pregnant or breastfeeding. It is not recommended for people with severely impaired kidney function.
Proprietary preparations: Aclasta; Zometa.

Zoleptil (Healthcare Logistics) *See* ZOTEPINE.

Zollinger-Ellison syndrome *See* ACID-PEPTIC DISEASES.

zolmitriptan A *5HT$_1$ agonist used for treating acute attacks of *migraine. A single dose can relieve a migraine headache at any stage of the attack. Zolmitriptan is available as tablets, dispersible tablets, or a nasal spray on *prescription only.
Side effects: include sensations of heat, heaviness, pressure, tingling or tightness; if tightness in the chest or throat is severe, treatment should be stopped. Other side effects may include drowsiness, an increase in blood pressure (which does not last), and (rarely) dry mouth and muscle weakness.
Precautions: zolmitriptan should not be taken for 12 hours before or after taking other 5HT$_1$ agonists. It should not be taken by people who have previously had a heart attack or who have uncontrolled high blood pressure or certain heart conditions. Zolmitriptan should be used with caution in people with liver disease and in women who are pregnant or breastfeeding.
Interactions with other drugs:

Ergotamine: the risk of spasm of the blood vessels, which can have serious consequences, is increased if ergotamine is taken with zolmitriptan. Ergotamine should not be started for six hours after stopping zolmitriptan, and zolmitriptan should not be started for 24 hours after stopping ergotamine.

Fluvoxamine: this antidepressant may enhance the effects of zolmitriptan, whose dosage should therefore be reduced.

MAOIs: increase the risk of adverse effects on the central nervous system; the dosage of zolmitriptan should be reduced if it is taken with moclobemide.

Proprietary preparations: Zomig; Zomig Nasal Spray; Zomig Rapimelt (dispersible tablets).

zolpidem tartrate A short-acting drug that is used for the short-term treatment (up to four weeks) of insomnia (*see* HYPNOTIC DRUGS). It acts in the same way as *benzodiazepines, but takes a shorter time to act and has little or no hangover effect. Zolpidem is available as tablets on *prescription only.
Side effects: include diarrhoea, nausea, vomiting, vertigo, dizziness, headache, daytime drowsiness, memory disturbances, and nightmares. *Dependence can occur with prolonged use.
Precautions: zolpidem should not be taken by people with obstructive sleep apnoea (in which airflow from the nose to the lungs is obstructed during sleep), myasthenia gravis, severe liver or lung disease, or psychosis, by women

who are pregnant or breastfeeding, or by children aged under 18. It should be used with caution by people with a history of drug abuse or depression. *See also* HYPNOTIC DRUGS.
Interactions with other drugs: the sedative effects of zolpidem are increased by a number of drugs, including general anaesthetics, opioid analgesics, some antidepressants, antihistamines, antipsychotics, and most importantly by ritonavir, which increases the plasma concentration of zolpidem, causing profound sedation; these two drugs should therefore not be taken together.
Proprietary preparation: Stilnoct.

Zolvera (Rosemont Pharmaceuticals Limited) *See* VERAPAMIL HYDROCHLORIDE.

Zomacton (Ferring Pharmaceuticals) *See* SOMATROPIN.

Zometa (Novartis) *See* ZOLEDRONIC ACID.

Zomig (AstraZeneca) *See* ZOLMITRIPTAN.

Zomorph (Archimedes Pharma UK) *See* MORPHINE.

Zonegran (Eisai) *See* ZONISAMIDE.

zonisamide A sulphonamide *anticonvulsant drug used as an *adjunct in the treatment of partial epileptic seizures, tonic-clonic seizures, and infantile spasms. It is available as capsules on *prescription only.
Side effects: include drowsiness, loss of appetite, dizziness, headache, nausea, and agitation.
Precautions: zonisamide should not be taken by women who are breastfeeding or by people with severe liver disease.
Interactions with other drugs:
Antidepressants: increase the risk of convulsions; St John's wort should not be taken with zonisamide.
Antimalarial drugs: chloroquine, hydroxychloroquine, and mefloquine increase the risk of convulsions.
Proprietary preparation: Zonegran.

zopiclone A short-acting drug that is used for the short-term treatment (up to four weeks) of insomnia (*see* HYPNOTIC DRUGS). It acts in the same way as *benzodiazepines, but takes a shorter time to act and has little or no hangover effect. Zopiclone is available as tablets on *prescription only.
Side effects: include a bitter or metallic taste, diarrhoea, nausea, vomiting, vertigo, dizziness, headache, irritability, confusion, daytime drowsiness, memory disturbances, and nightmares. *Dependence can occur with prolonged use.
Precautions: zopiclone should not be taken by people with depressed breathing, severe obstructive sleep apnoea (in which the airflow from mouth to lungs is obstructed during sleep), myasthenia gravis, or severe liver disease, by women who are pregnant or breastfeeding, or by children aged under 18. It

should be used with caution by people with a history of drug abuse or depression. *See also* HYPNOTIC DRUGS.
Interactions with other drugs: the sedative effects of zopiclone are enhanced by a number of other drugs, including erythromycin, ritonavir, anaesthetics, opioid analgesics, some antidepressants, antihistamines, and antipsychotic drugs.
Proprietary preparation: Zimovane.

Zorac (Allergan) *See* TAZAROTENE.

zotepine An atypical *antipsychotic drug used for the treatment of schizophrenia. It is available as tablets on *prescription only.
Side effects: include weight gain, dizziness, low blood pressure on standing (which can cause fainting in some people), constipation, indigestion, dry mouth, a fast heart rate, headache, insomnia, drowsiness, and fever. Zotepine may also prolong a certain phase of the heartbeat (the QT interval) and cause blood disorders.
Precautions: zotepine should not be given to those suffering from acute gout, to people who have had kidney stones, or to women who are breastfeeding. It should be used with caution in people with cardiovascular disease, a history of epilepsy or Parkinson's disease, liver or kidney disease, an enlarged prostate gland, or acute glaucoma, and in pregnant women. It should also be used with care in people taking other drugs that prolong the QT interval (since this may give rise to *arrhythmias; see below) or that cause loss of potassium (such as some diuretics).
Interactions with other drugs:

Anaesthetics: their effect in lowering blood pressure is increased.
Anti-arrhythmic drugs: there is an increased risk of arrhythmias if these drugs are taken with zotepine.
Antidepressant drugs: there is an increased risk of arrhythmias if zotepine is taken with tricyclic antidepressants; fluoxetine increases the plasma concentration of zotepine.
Antiepileptic drugs: zotepine antagonizes the effects of these drugs in controlling seizures.
Atomoxetine: there is an increased risk of arrhythmias if zotepine is taken with this drug.
Methadone: there is an increased risk of arrhythmias if this drug is taken with zotepine.
Ritonavir: may increase the effects of zotepine.
Sedatives: the sedative effects of zotepine are increased if it is taken with anxiolytic or hypnotic drugs; diazepam increases the plasma concentration of zotepine.
Sibutramine: increases the risk of adverse effects on the central nervous system and should not be taken with zotepine.

Proprietary preparation: Zoleptil.

Zoton FasTab (Pfizer) *See* LANSOPRAZOLE.

Zovirax (GlaxoSmithKline) *See* ACICLOVIR.

zuclopenthixol A thioxanthene *antipsychotic drug. **Zuclopenthixol dihydrochloride** is used for the treatment of schizophrenia and other psychoses, especially in patients who are agitated, hostile, or aggressive (it should not be given to patients who are apathetic or withdrawn); **zuclopenthixol decanoate** is given by *depot injection for the maintenance treatment of such patients. **Zuclopenthixol acetate** is given by injection for the short-term treatment of acute psychosis, mania, or exacerbations of chronic psychosis; it is used to stabilize patients and treatment should not last longer than two weeks. Zuclopenthixol is available, on prescription only, as tablets or injections.
Side effects and precautions: *see* CHLORPROMAZINE HYDROCHLORIDE.
Interactions with other drugs:
Anaesthetics: their effect in lowering blood pressure is enhanced.
Anti-arrhythmic drugs: there is an increased risk of arrhythmias if zuclopenthixol is taken with amiodarone, disopyramide, or sotalol, which should therefore be avoided.
Antibiotics: there is an increased risk of arrhythmias if zuclopenthixol is taken with erythromycin or moxifloxacin, which should therefore be avoided.
Antidepressants: there is an increased risk of antimuscarinic effects and arrhythmias if zuclopenthixol is taken with tricyclic antidepressants.
Antiepileptic drugs: their anticonvulsant effects are antagonized by zuclopenthixol.
Ritonavir: may increase the effects of zuclopenthixol.
Sedatives: the sedative effects of zuclopenthixol are increased if it is taken with anxiolytic or hypnotic drugs, or any other sedating drug.
Sibutramine: there is an increased risk of adverse effects on the central nervous system and this drug should not be taken with zuclopenthixol.
Proprietary preparations: Clopixol (tablets or depot injection); Clopixol Acuphase (injection); Clopixol Conc. (depot injection).

Zumenon (Solvay Healthcare) *See* ESTRADIOL; HORMONE REPLACEMENT THERAPY.

Zyban (GlaxoSmithKline) *See* BUPROPION HYDROCHLORIDE.

Zydol, Zydol SR, Zydol XL (Grünenthal) *See* TRAMADOL HYDROCHLORIDE.

Zyloric (GlaxoSmithKline) *See* ALLOPURINOL.

Zyomet (Goldshield) *See* METRONIDAZOLE.

ZypAdhera (Eli Lilly & Co) *See* OLANZAPINE.

Zyprexa (Eli Lilly & Co) *See* OLANZAPINE.

Zyvox (Pharmacia) *See* LINEZOLID.

Appendices

1. Some proprietary preparations containing aspirin and/or paracetamol

Preparation	Active Ingredients	Form
Alka-Seltzer	aspirin	effervescent tablets
Alka-Seltzer XS	aspirin, caffeine, paracetamol	effervescent tablets
Alvedon	paracetamol	suppositories
Anadin	aspirin, caffeine	tablets
Anadin Extra, Anadin Extra Soluble	aspirin, caffeine, paracetamol	tablets, soluble tablets
Anadin Paracetamol	paracetamol	tablets
Angettes 75	aspirin	tablets (75 mg antiplatelet)
Bayer Aspirin	aspirin	tablets
Beechams All-in-One	paracetamol, guaifenesin, phenylephrine	liquid
Beechams Flu-Plus Hot Lemon, Beechams Flu-Plus Hot Berry Fruits	paracetamol, phenylephrine	powders
Beechams Flu-Plus Caplets	paracetamol, caffeine, phenylephrine	tablets
Beechams Powders	aspirin, caffeine	powders
Beechams Powders Capsules	paracetamol, caffeine, phenylephrine	capsules
Benylin Day & Night Tablets	paracetamol, diphenhydramine, pseudoephedrine	tablets
Benylin Four Flu	paracetamol, diphenhydramine, pseudoephedrine	tablets, liquid
Boots Children's Pain Relief Syrup	paracetamol	liquid
Boots Cold Relief Hot Blackcurrent, Boots Cold Relief Hot Lemon	paracetamol	powders

Preparation	Active Ingredients	Form
Boots Infant Pain Relief	paracetamol	oral suspension
Boots Max Strength Cold & Flu Capsules	paracetamol, caffeine, phenylephrine	capsules
Boots Night Cold Comfort	paracetamol, diphenhydramine pholcodine, pseudoephedrine	tablets
Calcold	paracetamol, diphenhydramine	tablets
Calpol 6 Plus, Calpol Paediatric	paracetamol	oral suspension
Caprin	aspirin	enteric-coated tablets (75 mg antiplatelet; 300 mg standard)
*Codipar	paracetamol, codeine [co-codamol]	tablets
Codis 500	aspirin, codeine	dispersible tablets
Coldrex Tablets	paracetamol, caffeine, phenylephrine	tablets
Day and Night Nurse	paracetamol, dextromethorphan, pholcodine, promethazine, pseudoephedrine	capsules
Day Nurse	paracetamol, pholcodine, pseudoephedrine	capsules, liquid
Disprin, Disprin Direct	aspirin	dispersible tablets
Disprin Extra	aspirin, paracetamol	soluble tablets
Disprol Paediatric Suspension	paracetamol	sugar-free suspension for children
Disprol Soluble Paracetamol Tablets	paracetamol	dispersible tablets for children
Feminax Period Pain Capsules	paracetamol, codeine	capsules
Fennings Children's Cooling Powders	paracetamol	powders
Flamasacard	aspirin	modified-release capsules (162.5 mg antiplatelet)
Hedex Caplets, Hedex Tablets	paracetamol	tablets
Hedex Extra	paracetamol, caffeine	tablets

Preparation	Active Ingredients	Form
*Kapake	paracetamol, codeine [co-codamol]	tablets, capsules
Lemsip Cold & Flu Capsules	paracetamol, caffeine, phenylephrine	capsules
Lemsip Cold & Flu Lemon	paracetamol, phenylephrine, vitamin C	powders
Lemsip Max Flu Lemon	paracetamol, pseudoephedrine	powders
Medinol Over 6	paracetamol	oral suspension for children
Medinol Paediatric	paracetamol	sugar-free suspension for children
Medised	paracetamol, promethazine	liquid (standard or sugar-free)
Micropirin	aspirin	tablets (75 mg antiplatelet)
Migraine Relief	paracetamol, codeine	capsules
Migraleve	paracetamol, codeine, buclizine	tablets (pink)
	paracetamol, codeine	tablets (yellow)
Night Nurse	paracetamol, dextromethorphan, promethazine	capsules, liquid
Non-Drowsy Sinutab	paracetamol, pseudoephedrine	tablets
Non-Drowsy Sudafed Congestion and Headache Capsules	paracetamol, caffeine, phenylephrine	capsules
Non-Drowsy Sudafed Congestion, Cold and Flu Tablets	paracetamol, pseudoephedrine	tablets
Nu-Seals Aspirin	aspirin	enteric-coated tablets (75 mg antiplatelet; 300 mg standard)
Paldesic	paracetamol	suspension for children
Panadol, Panadol Soluble	paracetamol	capsules, tablets, soluble tablets, sugar-free suspension

Preparation	Active Ingredients	Form
Panadol Extra	paracetamol, caffeine	tablets, soluble tablets
Panadol Night	paracetamol, diphenhydramine	tablets
Panadol Ultra	paracetamol, codeine	tablets
*Paracodol	paracetamol, codeine [co-codamol]	capsules
Paradote	paracetamol, methionine [co-methiamol]	tablets
Paramol	paracetamol, dihydrocodeine	tablets
Resolve	paracetamol, citric acid, sodium and potassium salts, vitamin C	effervescent granules
Solpadeine Headache	paracetamol, caffeine	soluble tablets
Solpadeine Max	paracetamol, codeine	tablets
Solpadeine Plus	paracetamol, caffeine, codeine	tablets, soluble tablets, capsules
*Solpadol	paracetamol, codeine [co-codamol]	tablets, effervescent tablets
Syndol	paracetamol, caffeine, codeine	tablets
*Tylex	paracetamol, codeine [co-codamol]	capsules, effervescent tablets
Veganin	aspirin, paracetamol, codeine	tablets
Vick's Cold & Flu Care Medinite Complete	paracetamol, dextromethorphan, doxylamine, pseudoephedrine	syrup

* prescription only medicine

† controlled drug

2. Abbreviations

ACE	angiotensin-converting enzyme
ADHD	attention deficit hyperactivity disorder
AIDS	acquired immune deficiency syndrome
AZT	azidothymidine (= zidovudine); azathioprine; azithromycin
BAN	British Approved Name
BNF	British National Formulary
CD	controlled drug
CNS	central nervous system
CR	continuous release (= modified release)
D3	vitamin D_3
DMARD	disease-modifying antirheumatic drug
EC	enteric-coated
ECG	electrocardiogram
EEG	electro-encephalogram
FSH	follicle-stimulating hormone
5FU	fluorouracil
G-CSF	granulocyte-colony stimulating factor
GnRH	gonadotrophin-releasing hormone
G6PD	glucose 6-phosphate dehydrogenase
GSL	general sales list
H	histamine
HC	hydrocortisone
HDL	high-density lipoproteins
HIV	human immunodeficiency virus
HRT	hormone replacement therapy
5HT	5-hydroxytryptamine (= serotonin)
IM, i.m.	intramuscular
INR	International Normalized Ratio
IV, i.v.	intravenous
IZS	insulin zinc suspension
LA	= modified release
LDL	low-density lipoproteins
LH-RH	luteinizing hormone-releasing hormone
MAOI	monoamine oxidase inhibitor

mcg	micrograms
mg	milligrams
MHRA	Medicines and Healthcare products Regulatory Agency
MR	modified release
NICE	National Institute for Health and Clinical Excellence
NSAID	non-steroidal anti-inflammatory drug
ORT	oral rehydration therapy
OTC	over the counter
P	pharmacy medicine
POM	prescription only medicine
PZI	protamine zinc insulin
rINN	Recommended International Non-proprietary Name
RSV	respiratory syncytial virus
SC, s.c.	subcutaneous
SR	sustained release (= modified release)
SSRI	selective serotonin reuptake inhibitor
TCA	tricyclic antidepressant
TNF	tumour necrosis factor
TTS	= skin patch
TNF	tumour necrosis factor
VEGF	vascular endothelial growth factor
XL	= modified release

Abbreviations used in prescriptions

a. c.	ante cibum (before food)
b. d.	bis die (twice daily)
o. d.	omni die (every day)
o. m.	omni mane (every morning)
o. n.	omni nocte (every night)
p. c.	post cibum (after food)
p. r. n.	pro re nata (when required)
q. d. s.	quater die sumendum (to be taken four times daily)
q. q. h.	quarta quaque hora (every four hours)
stat	immediately
t. d. s.	ter die sumendum (to be taken three times daily)
t. i. d.	ter in die (three times daily)

3. New British Approved Names of medicines

Former BAN	New BAN
amethocaine	tetracaine
aminacrine	aminoacridine
amoxycillin	amoxicillin
amphetamine	amfetamine
amylobarbitone	amobarbital
amylobarbitone sodium	amobarbital sodium
beclomethasone	beclometasone
bendrofluazide	bendroflumethiazide
benorylate	benorilate
benzhexol	trihexyphenidyl
benztropine	benzatropine
busulphan	busulfan
butobarbitone	butobarbital
carticaine	articaine
cephalexin	cefalexin
cephradine	cefradine
chloral betaine	cloral betaine
chlorbutol	chlorobutanol
chlormethiazole	clomethiazole
chlorpheniramine	chlorphenamine
chlorthalidone	chlortalidone
cholecalciferol	colecalciferol
cholestyramine	colestyramine
clomiphene	clomifene
colistin sulphomethate sodium	colistimethate sodium

Former BAN	New BAN
corticotrophin	corticotropin
cyclosporin	ciclosporin
cysteamine	mercaptamine
danthron	dantron
desoxymethasone	desoximetasone
dexamphetamine	dexamfetamine
dibromopropamidine	dibrompropamidine
dicyclomine	dicycloverine
dienoestrol	dienestrol
dimethicone(s)	dimeticone
dimethyl sulphoxide	dimethyl sulfoxide
dothiepin	dosulepin
doxycycline hydrochloride (hemihydrate hemiethanolate)	doxycycline hyclate
eformoterol	formoterol
ethamsylate	etamsylate
ethinyloestradiol	ethinylestradiol
ethynodiol	etynodiol
flumethasone	flumetasone
flupenthixol	flupentixol
flurandrenolone	fludroxycortide
frusemide	furosemide
gestronol	gestonorone
guaiphenesin	guaifenesin
hexachlorophane	hexachlorophene
hexamine hippurate	methenamine hippurate
hydroxyurea	hydroxycarbamide
indomethacin	indometacin
lignocaine	lidocaine

Former BAN	New BAN
lysuride	lisuride
methotrimeprazine	levomepromazine
methyl cysteine	mecysteine
methylene blue	methylthioninium chloride
mitozantrone	mitoxantrone
mustine	chlormethine
nicoumalone	acenocoumarol
oestradiol	estradiol
oestriol	estriol
oestrone	estrone
oxpentifylline	pentoxifylline
phenobarbitone	phenobarbital
pipothiazine	pipotiazine
polyhexanide	polihexanide
potassium clorazepate	dipotassium clorazepate
pramoxine	pramocaine
procaine penicillin	procaine benzylpenicillin
prothionamide	protionamide
quinalbarbitone	secobarbital
riboflavine	riboflavin
salcatonin	calcitonin (salmon)
sodium calciumedetate	sodium calcium edetate
sodium cromoglycate	sodium cromoglicate
sodium ironedetate	sodium feredetate
sodium picosulphate	sodium picosulfate
sorbitan monostearate	sorbitan stearate
stibocaptate	sodium stibocaptate
stilboestrol	diethylstilbestrol
sulphacetamide	sulfacetamide
sulphadiazine	sulfadiazine

Former BAN	New BAN
sulphamethoxazole	sulfamethoxazole
sulphapyridine	sulfapyridine
sulphasalazine	sulfasalazine
sulphathiazole	sulfathiazole
sulphinpyrazone	sulfinpyrazone
tetracosactrin	tetracosactide
thiabendazole	tiabendazole
thioguanine	tioguanine
thiopentone	thiopental
thymoxamine	moxisylyte
thyroxine sodium	levothyroxine sodium
tribavirin	ribavirin
trimeprazine	alimemazine
urofollitrophin	urofollitropin

4. SI units

TABLE 4.1 Base and supplementary SI units

Physical quantity	Name of unit	Symbol for unit
length	metre	m
mass	kilogram	kg
time	second	s
electric current	ampere	A
thermodynamic temperature	kelvin	K
luminous intensity	candela	cd
amount of substance	mole	mol
*plane angle	radian	rad
*solid angle	steradian	sr

*supplementary units

TABLE 4.2 Derived SI units with special names

Physical quantity	Name of unit	Symbol for unit
frequency	hertz	Hz
energy	joule	J
force	newton	N
power	watt	W
pressure	pascal	Pa
electric charge	coulomb	C
electric potential difference	volt	V
electric resistance	ohm	W
electric conductance	siemens	S
electric capacitance	farad	F
magnetic flux	weber	Wb
inductance	henry	H
magnetic flux density (magnetic induction)	tesla	T
luminous flux	lumen	lm
illuminance (illumination)	lux	lx
absorbed dose	gray	Gy
activity	becquerel	Bq
dose equivalent	sievert	Sv

TABLE 4.3 Decimal multiples and submultiples to be used with SI units

Submultiple	Prefix	Symbol	Multiple	Prefix	Symbol
10^{-1}	deci	d	10^{1}	deca	da
10^{-2}	centi	c	10^{2}	hecto	h
10^{-3}	milli	m	10^{3}	kilo	k
10^{-6}	micro	μ	10^{6}	mega	M
10^{-9}	nano	n	10^{9}	giga	G
10^{-12}	pico	p	10^{12}	tera	T
10^{-15}	femto	f	10^{15}	peta	P
10^{-16}	atto	a	10^{16}	exa	E
10^{-21}	zepto	z	10^{21}	zetta	Z
10^{-24}	yocto	y	10^{24}	yotta	Y

TABLE 4.4 Conversion of units to and from SI units

From	To	Multiply by
in	m	0.0254
ft	m	0.3048
sq in	m^2	0.00064516
sq ft	m^2	0.092903
cu in	m^3	0.0000164
cu ft	m^3	0.0283168
l(itre)	m^3	0.001
gal(lon)	m^3	0.0045609
gal(lon)	litres	4.5609
lb	kg	0.453592
$g\ cm^{-3}$	$kg\ m^{-3}$	1000
lb/in^3	$kg\ m^{-3}$	27679.9
mmHg	Pa	133.322
cal	J	4.1868
m	in	39.3701
cm	in	0.393701
cm^2	sq in	0.155
m^2	sq in	1550
m^2	sq ft	10.7639
m^3	cu in	61023.6

TABLE 4.4 (cont.)

From	To	Multiply by
m^2	sq ft	10.7639
m^3	cu in	61023.6
m^3	cu ft	35.3146
m^3	l(itre)	1000
m^3	gal(lon)	219.969
kg	lb	2.20462
$kg\ m^{-3}$	$g\ cm^{-3}$	0.001
$kg\ m^{-3}$	lb/in^3	0.0000363
Pa	mmHg	0.0075006
J	cal	0.238846

Temperature conversion

°C (Celsius) = 5/9(°F – 32)

°F (Fahrenheit) = (9/5 × °C) + 32

5. Online resources

SEE WEB LINKS

The following is a selection of authoritative, quality-controlled, freely accessible sites that provide key information on medicines licensed for use in the UK. These range from specialist databases designed for the use of health-care professionals to more general sites providing advice for patients and their families. To access any of these websites, go to the dictionary's web page at www.oup.com/uk/reference/resources/medicinaldrugs, click on the **Web links** in the Resources section, go to **Appendix web links**, and then click through to the relevant site.

- Bandolier: evidence-based information on medicines and other interventions for both professionals and consumers.
- BestTreatments: latest research evidence about the effectiveness of thousands of drugs and other treatments. Developed by the British Medical Journal in partnership with NHS Direct.
- British National Formulary: up-to-date, authoritative information for health-care professionals regarding the selection, prescribing, and administration of medicines. The BNF is a joint publication of the British Medical Association and the Royal Pharmaceutical Society of Great Britain
- ClinicalTrials: an online registry of research trials organized by the US National Institutes of Health. Many health-care journals now demand that trials of medicines and other interventions are registered at ClinicalTrials as a prerequisite for publication.
- Cochrane Collaboration: systematic evidence-based reviews of medicines and other interventions; mainly for professionals, but with plain-language summaries for laypeople.
- Dictionary of Medicines and Devices (dm+d): a database hosted by the Prescription Pricing Division of the NHS Business Services Authority.
- Electronic Medicines Compendium (eMC): up-to-date information on medicines licensed for use in the UK. Content is supplied by pharmaceutical companies and checked by the UK Medicines and Healthcare products Regulatory Agency (MHRA) or the European Medicines Agency.

- Medicine Guides: up-to-date information on most medicines currently available in the UK: developed by the Medicines Information Project in partnership with NHS Direct.pp
- NetDoctor Medicines Database: an A-Z listing of some 3000 branded and generic medicines.
- NHS Direct Online: an A–Z guide to common medical conditions including information on the generic drugs typically prescribed for their treatment.
- X-PIL: an online compendium of the Patient Information Leaflets included with UK medicines. These are also made available in formats designed for the blind or visually impaired.

Oxford Paperback Reference

Concise Medical Dictionary

Over 12,000 clear entries covering all the major medical and surgical specialities make this one of our best-selling dictionaries.

'"No home should be without one" certainly applies to this splendid medical dictionary'

Journal of the Institute of Health Education

'An extraordinary bargain'

New Scientist

'Excellent layout and jargon-free style'

Nursing Times

A Dictionary of Nursing

Comprehensive coverage of the ever-expanding vocabulary of the nursing professions. Features over 10,000 entries written by medical and nursing specialists.

An A–Z of Medicinal Drugs

Over 4,000 entries cover the full range of over-the-counter and prescription medicines available today. An ideal reference source for both the patient and the medical professional.